Estrogen/Antiestrogen Action and Breast Cancer Therapy

ESTROGEN/ ANTIESTROGEN ACTION AND BREAST CANCER THERAPY

Edited by V. Craig Jordan

The University of Wisconsin Press

Published 1986

The University of Wisconsin Press
114 North Murray Street
Madison, Wisconsin 53715

The University of Wisconsin Press, Ltd.
1 Gower Street
London WC1E 6HA, England

First printing

Printed in the United States of America

For LC CIP information see the colophon

ISBN 0-299-10480-X

By studying the old, one can discover the new.
—Confucius

The Editor

V. Craig Jordan, Ph.D., D.Sc., is Professor of Human Oncology and Pharmacology at the University of Wisconsin–Madison and leader of the pharmacology program at the Wisconsin Clinical Cancer Center.

Dr. Jordan graduated with a first-class honors degree (1969) and a Ph.D. (1972) from the Department of Pharmacology, Leeds University Medical School. From 1972 to 1974, he was a visiting scientist at the Worcester Foundation for Experimental Biology in Shrewsbury, Massachusetts, and then he returned to the University of Leeds as Lecturer in Pharmacology. In 1979, he accepted a one-year appointment as Head of the Endocrinology Unit at the Ludwig Institute for Cancer Research in Berne, Switzerland, before joining the faculty at the University of Wisconsin in 1980.

Dr. Jordan is a Fellow of the Royal Society of Chemistry and the American Institute of Chemists. In 1984 he was awarded a University of Wisconsin H. I. Romnes Faculty Fellowship and in 1985 a Doctor of Science degree by the University of Leeds. Dr. Jordan is currently a member of the Therapeutics and Cancer Prevention Study Section of the American Cancer Society and a core member of the Breast Cancer Task Force of the European School of Oncology.

Contents

Contributors   xi
Preface   xvii
Acknowledgments   xxiii

I. Chemistry and Biochemistry

1. Estrogen Receptors—Highlights of Their History,
   Properties, and Actions   3
   Gerald C. Mueller

2. Structure-Activity Relationships of Nonsteroidal Estrogens
   and Antiestrogens   19
   V. Craig Jordan, Rick Koch, and Mara E. Lieberman

3. Nuclear Localization of Unoccupied Estrogen Receptors   43
   Mara E. Lieberman, Wade V. Welshons, and Jack Gorski

4. Multiple Binding Sites for Estrogen in Target Tissues   55
   Barry M. Markaverich, James H. Clark, R. R. Roberts,
   and M. A. Alejandro

5. Radiolabeled Antiestrogens and Other Probes for the
   Estrogen Receptor   73
   John A. Katzenellenbogen

II. Antiestrogen Binding Sites

6. Properties of High Affinity Intracellular Binding Sites for
   Antiestrogens   93
   Colin K. W. Watts, Leigh C. Murphy, and
   Robert L. Sutherland

7. Antiestrogen Action and Antiestrogen Binding Sites 115
James H. Clark, Barry M. Markaverich, S. C. Guthrie,
and R. C. Winneker

8. Antiestrogen Binding to Estrogen Receptors and Additional
Antiestrogen Binding Sites in Human Breast Cancer Cells 127
Margaret Ann Miller, Yhun Yhong Sheen, Alaka Mullick,
and Benita S. Katzenellenbogen

III. *Pharmacology*

9. The Progesterone Receptor as a Marker for Estrogen and
Antiestrogen Activity *in Vivo* and *in Vitro* 151
Carolyn A. Campen, V. Craig Jordan, and Jack Gorski

10. Antiestrogen Action in the Chicken 171
C. B. Lazier and P. R. Murphy

11. Metabolism of Nonsteroidal Antiestrogens 191
Stewart D. Lyman and V. Craig Jordan

12. Inhibitors of the Aromatase Enzyme System: Basic and
Clinical Studies with 4-Hydroxyandrostenedione 221
A. M. H. Brodie, L. Y. Wing, M. Dowsett, P. Goss,
and R. C. Coombes

IV. *Laboratory Models to Study Hormone-Dependent
Breast Cancer*

13. Estrogens Regulate Production of Specific Growth Factors
in Hormone-Dependent Human Breast Cancer 237
Marc E. Lippman, Karen K. Huff, Raimund Jakesz,
Toby Hecht, Attan Kasid, Susan Bates, and
Robert B. Dickson

14. Different Efficacy of Antiestrogens on Estrogen-Regulated
Proteins in Human Breast Cancer Cell Lines 249
H. Rochefort, F. Vignon, S. Bardon, F. May, and
B. Westley

15. Effects of Antiestrogens on Cell Cycle Progression 265
    Robert L. Sutherland, Roger R. Reddel,
    Leigh C. Murphy, and Ian W. Taylor

16. Animal Models to Study the Therapy of Hormone-
    Dependent Breast Cancer 283
    Marco M. Gottardis and V. Craig Jordan

V. *Hormone Receptors: Clinical Applications*

17. Estrogen Receptor Studies: Laboratory Investigations and
    Clinical Applications 303
    Eugene R. DeSombre, William J. King, Geoffrey L.
    Greene, Susan M. Thorpe, Carsten Rose, and
    Elwood V. Jensen

18. Estrogen Receptor Determinations: Studies in Relation to
    Rapidly Progressive Carcinoma of the Breast 325
    K. Griffiths, R. I. Nicholson, R. W. Blamey, and
    C. W. Elston

19. Progesterone Receptor Determinations: A Refinement of
    Predictive Tests for Hormone Dependency of Breast Cancer 341
    C. F. LeMaistre and W. L. McGuire

VI. *Antibodies to Steroid Hormone Receptors*

20. Antibodies to Estrogen Receptor: New Probes for the
    Analysis of Receptor Structure and Function 357
    Geoffrey L. Greene, William J. King, Michael F. Press,
    and Elwood V. Jensen

21. The Generation of Antibodies Against Partially Purified
    Estradiol Receptor from Human Myometrium 375
    R. J. B. King and A. I. Coffer

22. Monoclonal Antibodies Raised Against Chick Oviduct
    Progesterone Receptor: Cross Reaction with Human Antigen 395
    Dean P. Edwards, Nancy L. Weigel, William T. Schrader,
    Sarah Peleg, Bert W. O'Malley, and W. L. McGuire

VII. *Advanced and Adjuvant Breast Cancer Therapy*

23. Endocrine Treatment of Advanced Breast Cancer   417
    Baha'Uddin M. Arafah and Olof H. Pearson

24. Combined Chemohormonotherapy Approaches for Breast
    Cancer   431
    D. C. Tormey

25. Antihormone Therapy as an Adjuvant to Mastectomy   451
    Nolvadex Adjuvant Trial Organization—
    Paper Presented by Diana Brinkley

26. The Ludwig Breast Cancer Studies: Adjuvant Therapy for
    Early Breast Cancer   459
    Franco Cavalli, Aron Goldhirsch, and Richard Gelber,
    for the Ludwig Breast Cancer Study Group

27. Adjuvant Tamoxifen and Chemotherapy in Stage II Breast
    Cancer: Interim Findings from NSABP Protocol B–09   471
    Norman Wolmark and Bernard Fisher

28. Breast Cancer 1984: Role of Tamoxifen   483
    Paul P. Carbone

VIII. *Summary*

29. Laboratory and Clinical Research on the Hormone
    Dependence of Breast Cancer: Current Studies and Future
    Prospects   501
    V. Craig Jordan, N. F. Fritz, Marco M. Gottardis,
    D. M. Mirecki, P. M. Ravdin, and Wade V. Welshons

Index   523

Contributors

M. A. Alejandro
Department of Cell Biology, Baylor College of Medicine, Houston, Texas 77030

Baha'Uddin M. Arafah
Department of Medicine, University Hospitals, Case Western Reserve University School of Medicine, Cleveland, Ohio 44106

S. Bardon
Unité d'Endocrinologie Cellulaire et Moléculaire, 60 rue de Navacelles, 34100 Montpellier, France

Susan Bates
Medical Breast Cancer Section, Medicine Branch, National Cancer Institute, Bethesda, Maryland 20205

R. W. Blamey
Department of Surgery, City Hospital, Nottingham, Great Britain

Diana Brinkley
Consultant Radiotherapist, King's College Hospital, Denmark Hill, London SE5 9RS, Great Britain

A. M. H. Brodie
Department of Pharmacology and Experimental Therapeutics, University of Maryland School of Medicine, Baltimore, Maryland 21201

Carolyn A. Campen
The Salk Institute, San Diego, California 92138

Paul P. Carbone
Department of Human Oncology, University of Wisconsin Medical School, University of Wisconsin Clinical Cancer Center, Madison, Wisconsin 53792

Franco Cavalli
Servizio Oncologico, Ospedale San Giovanni, Bellinzona, Switzerland

James H. Clark
Department of Cell Biology, Baylor College of Medicine, Houston, Texas 77030

xi

A. I. Coffer

Hormone Biochemistry Department, Imperial Cancer Research Fund, Lincoln's Inn Fields, London WC2A 3PX, Great Britain

R. C. Coombes

Ludwig Institute for Cancer Research Laboratories, St George's Hospital Medical School, Tooting, London SW 18, Great Britain

Eugene R. DeSombre

The Ben May Laboratory for Cancer Research, The University of Chicago, Chicago, Illinois 60637

Robert B. Dickson

Medical Breast Cancer Section, Medicine Branch, National Cancer Institute, Bethesda, Maryland 20205

M. Dowsett

Chelsea Hospital for Women, London, Great Britain

Dean P. Edwards

Department of Pathology, University of Colorado Health Sciences Center, Denver, Colorado 80262

C. W. Elston

Department of Pathology, City Hospital, Nottingham, Great Britain

Bernard Fisher

Department of Surgery, University of Pittsburgh School of Medicine, Pittsburgh, Pennsylvania 15261

N. F. Fritz

Department of Human Oncology, University of Wisconsin Medical School, University of Wisconsin Clinical Cancer Center, Madison, Wisconsin 53792

Richard Gelber

Division of Biostatistics and Epidemiology, Dana-Farber Cancer Institute and Harvard School of Public Health, Boston, Massachusetts 02115

Aron Goldhirsch

Ludwig Institute for Cancer Research, Bern Branch, Inselspital, CH-3010 Bern, Switzerland

Jack Gorski

Department of Biochemistry and Department of Meat and Animal Science, University of Wisconsin-Madison, Madison, Wisconsin 53706

P. Goss

Department of Medicine, Princess Margaret Hospital, Toronto, Canada

Marco M. Gottardis

Department of Human Oncology, University of Wisconsin Medical School, University of Wisconsin Clinical Cancer Center, Madison, Wisconsin 53792

Geoffrey L. Greene

The Ben May Laboratory for Cancer Research, The University of Chicago, Chicago, Illinois 60637

K. Griffiths

Tenovus Institute for Cancer Research, University of Wales College of Medicine, Heath Park, Cardiff CF4 4XX, Wales, Great Britain

S. C. Guthrie

Department of Cell Biology, Baylor College of Medicine, Houston, Texas 77030

Toby Hecht

Medical Breast Cancer Section, Medicine Branch, National Cancer Institute, Bethesda, Maryland 20205

Karen K. Huff

Medical Breast Cancer Section, Medicine Branch, National Cancer Institute, Bethesda, Maryland 20205

Raimund Jakesz

Medical Breast Cancer Section, Medicine Branch, National Cancer Institute, Bethesda, Maryland 20205

Elwood V. Jensen

Research Director, Ludwig Institute for Cancer Research, Zurich, Switzerland

V. Craig Jordan

Department of Human Oncology, University of Wisconsin Medical School, University of Wisconsin Clinical Cancer Center, Madison, Wisconsin 53792

Attan Kasid

Medical Breast Cancer Section, Medicine Branch, National Cancer Institute, Bethesda, Maryland 20205

Benita S. Katzenellenbogen

Department of Physiology and Biophysics, University of Illinois and University of Illinois College of Medicine, Urbana, Illinois 61801

John A. Katzenellenbogen

School of Chemical Sciences, University of Illinois, Urbana, Illinois 61801

R. J. B. King

Hormone Biochemistry Department, Imperial Cancer Research Fund, Lincoln's Inn Fields, London WC2A 3PX, Great Britain

William J. King

Abbott Laboratories, North Chicago, Illinois 60064

Rick Koch

Department of Human Oncology, University of Wisconsin Medical School, University of Wisconsin Clinical Cancer Center, Madison, Wisconsin 53792

C. B. Lazier

Department of Biochemistry, Dalhousie University, Halifax, Nova Scotia B3H 4H7, Canada

C. F. LeMaistre

Department of Medicine, University of Texas Health Science Center at San Antonio, San Antonio, Texas 78284

Mara E. Lieberman

Department of Human Oncology, University of Wisconsin Medical School, University of Wisconsin Clinical Cancer Center, Madison, Wisconsin 53792

Marc E. Lippman

Medical Breast Cancer Section, Medicine Branch, National Cancer Institute, Bethesda, Maryland 20205

Stewart D. Lyman

Department of Human Oncology, University of Wisconsin Medical School, University of Wisconsin Clinical Cancer Center, Madison, Wisconsin 53792

W. L. McGuire

Department of Medicine, University of Texas Health Science Center at San Antonio, San Antonio, Texas 78284

Barry M. Markaverich

Department of Cell Biology, Baylor College of Medicine, Houston, Texas 77030

F. May

Unité d'Endocrinologie Cellulaire et Moléculaire, 60 rue de Navacelles, 34100 Montpellier, France

Margaret Ann Miller

Department of Physiology and Biophysics, University of Illinois and University of Illinois College of Medicine, Urbana, Illinois 61801

D. M. Mirecki

Department of Human Oncology, University of Wisconsin Medical School, University of Wisconsin Clinical Cancer Center, Madison, Wisconsin 53792

Gerald C. Mueller

McArdle Laboratory for Cancer Research, University of Wisconsin-Madison, Madison, Wisconsin 53706

Alaka Mullick

Department of Physiology and Biophysics, University of Illinois and University of Illinois College of Medicine, Urbana, Illinois 61801

Leigh C. Murphy

Department of Physiology, University of Manitoba, Winnipeg R3E OW3, Canada

P. R. Murphy

Department of Biochemistry, Dalhousie University, Halifax, Nova Scotia B3H 4H7, Canada

R. I. Nicholson

Tenovus Institute for Cancer Research, University of Wales College of Medicine, Heath Park, Cardiff CF4 4XX, Wales, Great Britain

Bert W. O'Malley

Department of Cell Biology, Baylor College of Medicine, Houston, Texas 77030

Olof H. Pearson

Department of Medicine, University Hospitals, Case Western Reserve University School of Medicine, Cleveland, Ohio 44106

Sarah Peleg

Department of Cell Biology, Baylor College of Medicine, Houston, Texas 77030

Michael F. Press

Department of Pathology, The University of Chicago, Chicago, Illinois 60637

P. M. Ravdin

Department of Human Oncology, University of Wisconsin Medical School, University of Wisconsin Clinical Cancer Center, Madison, Wisconsin 53792

Roger R. Reddel

Laboratory of Human Carcinogenesis, National Institutes of Health, Bethesda, Maryland 20205

R. R. Roberts

Department of Cell Biology, Baylor College of Medicine, Houston, Texas 77030

H. Rochefort

Unité d'Endocrinologie Cellulaire et Moléculaire, 60 rue de Navacelles, 34100 Montpellier, France

Carsten Rose

Finsen Institute, Copenhagen, Denmark

William T. Schrader

Department of Cell Biology, Baylor College of Medicine, Houston, Texas 77030

Yhun Yhong Sheen

Department of Physiology and Biophysics, University of Illinois and University of Illinois College of Medicine, Urbana, Illinois 61801

Robert L. Sutherland

Garvan Institute of Medical Research, St. Vincent's Hospital, Darlinghurst, Sydney, N.S.W. 2010, Australia

Ian W. Taylor

Queensland Institute of Medical Research, Bramston Terrace, Herston, Brisbane, Australia

Susan M. Thorpe

Finsen Institute, Copenhagen, Denmark

D. C. Tormey

Department of Human Oncology, University of Wisconsin Medical School, University of Wisconsin Clinical Cancer Center, Madison, Wisconsin 53792

F. Vignon

Unité d'Endocrinologie Cellulaire et Moléculaire, 60 rue de Navacelles, 34100 Montpellier, France

Colin K. W. Watts

Garvan Institute of Medical Research, St. Vincent's Hospital, Darlinghurst, Sydney, N.S.W. 2010, Australia

Nancy L. Weigel

Department of Cell Biology, Baylor College of Medicine, Houston, Texas 77030

Wade V. Welshons

Department of Human Oncology, University of Wisconsin Medical School, University of Wisconsin Clinical Cancer Center, Madison, Wisconsin 53792

B. Westley

Unité d'Endocrinologie Cellulaire et Moléculaire, 60 rue de Navacelles, 34100 Montpellier, France

L. Y. Wing

Department of Physiology, National Cheng Kung University, Medical College, Tainan, Taiwan 200, Republic of China

R. C. Winneker

Endocrinology Division, Sterling-Winthrop Research Institute, Rensselaer, New York 12144

Norman Wolmark

Department of Surgery, University of Pittsburgh School of Medicine, Pittsburgh, Pennsylvania 15261

Preface

I N June 1984, the Wisconsin Clinical Cancer Center in Madison hosted a satellite symposium entitled "Estrogen and Antiestrogen Action: Basic and Clinical Aspects" as part of the events surrounding the Seventh International Congress of Endocrinology in Montreal, Canada. The three-day symposium was opened by the Honorable Fred A. Risser, President, Wisconsin Senate (Madison) and Dr. Robert M. Bock, Dean of the University of Wisconsin–Madison Graduate School, at a reception held in the Wisconsin Capitol Rotunda for the 25 invited speakers and more than 100 other registrants.

An international meeting at this time was particularly important. The models to describe the early events in estrogen action were being reviewed to propose that the estrogen receptor is a nuclear protein. In addition, new technologies to detect steroid hormone receptors using monoclonal antibodies were just entering clinical evaluation. Furthermore, the results of adjuvant clinical trials for breast cancer were showing advantages for tamoxifen-treated patients, and laboratory and pilot clinical experiences suggested that prolonged or indefinite treatment with adjuvant tamoxifen therapy may be the best treatment strategy. It was, therefore, important to bring together many of the leading laboratory scientists in the area of estrogen and antiestrogen action to share their experience with leaders in the clinical research of breast cancer therapy. The aim was to review the evolution of our ideas about the hormonal control of breast cancer and to establish new friendships among colleagues from around the world in the relaxed and informal atmosphere of the University of Wisconsin at Madison.

This book marks one of the achievements of the conference. It is not intended to be a meeting proceedings but is a historical review of the development of this field of endeavor during the past 30 years. The chapters have been written by many of the leading experts in the field who were asked to recount the development of a particular area or laboratory idea in which they had been personally involved. The book is intended to provide both scientists and clinicians with a single-volume overview of both the basic principles of hormonal control of breast cancer and the recent clinical results from cooperative groups around the world.

The University of Wisconsin has a long history of commitment to hormone action and cancer therapy. Many faculty members have been involved over the years and each has played an important role in the development of our understanding of hormone-dependent breast cancer growth. Dr. Harold Rusch, the founder and first director of the McArdle Laboratory for Cancer Research, later became the director of the Wisconsin Clinical Cancer Center. His drive and enthusiasm developed the science of cancer research at the University of Wisconsin. Dr. Paul Carbone, the present director of the Wisconsin Clinical Cancer Center, has been instrumental in developing the clinical program at the University of Wisconsin and as chairman of the Eastern Cooperative Oncology Group has developed a nationwide mechanism to test new therapeutic strategies in the clinic. Dr. Gerald Mueller was recruited to the McArdle Laboratory in the 1940s by Harold Rusch and his distinguished career has focused upon estrogen action and growth regulation. His laboratory has been fertile ground for scientific training. Dr. Jack Gorski completed postdoctoral research with Gerald Mueller before moving to the University of Illinois. He returned to Wisconsin in the early 1970s and is currently Professor of Biochemistry. After taking his medical degree at the University of Wisconsin, Dr. Douglass Tormey trained with Gerald Mueller to obtain a Ph.D. in oncology from the McArdle Laboratory. Dr. Tormey later joined the National Cancer Institute in Bethesda, where, as Head of the Breast Service, he worked closely with Paul Carbone, who was Chief of the Medicine Branch. In the mid-1970s, Dr. Tormey returned to Madison to work with Dr. Carbone and accepted an appointment in the Department of Human Oncology. Dr. Tormey is currently Professor of Human Oncology and Medicine and is leader of the breast program at the Wisconsin Clinical Cancer Center.

These colleagues have provided a critical resource for the University of Wisconsin and they have acted as the catalyst to develop many of the ideas expressed in this volume.

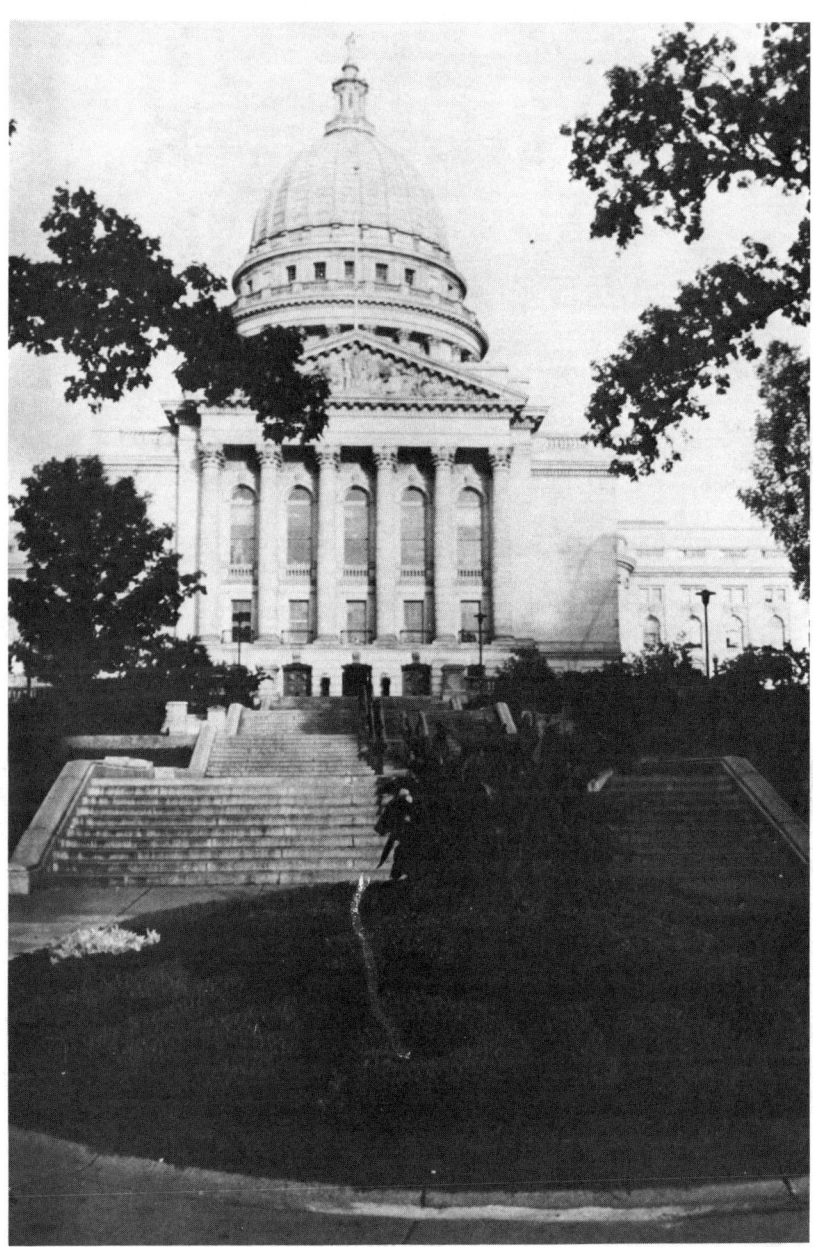

The Wisconsin State Capitol in the center of Madison. The ground was broken in 1907 for a building project which took 10 years to complete. The welcoming reception for the Breast Cancer Conference was held in the Capitol Rotunda.

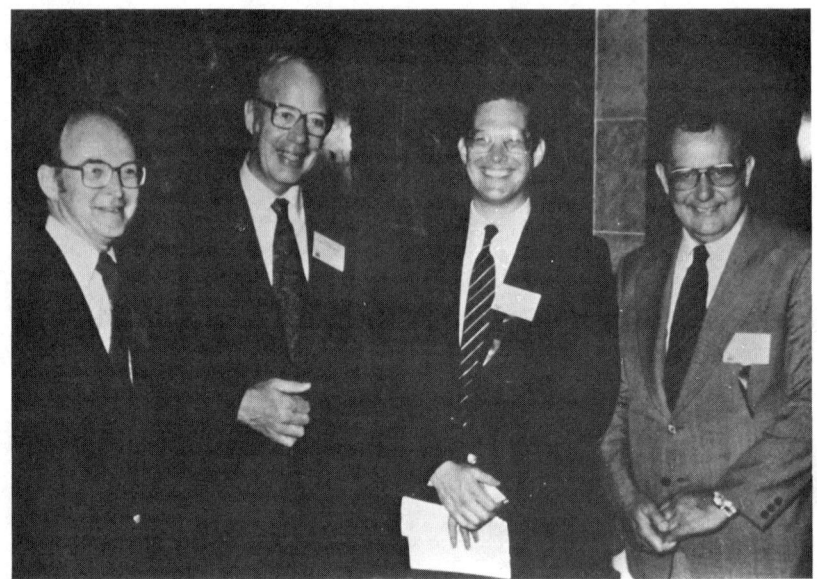

Speakers involved in the opening ceremony for the conference at the Wisconsin State Capitol. *Left to right:* Dean Robert M. Bock, Senator Fred A. Risser, Dr. V. Craig Jordan, and Dr. Paul P. Carbone.

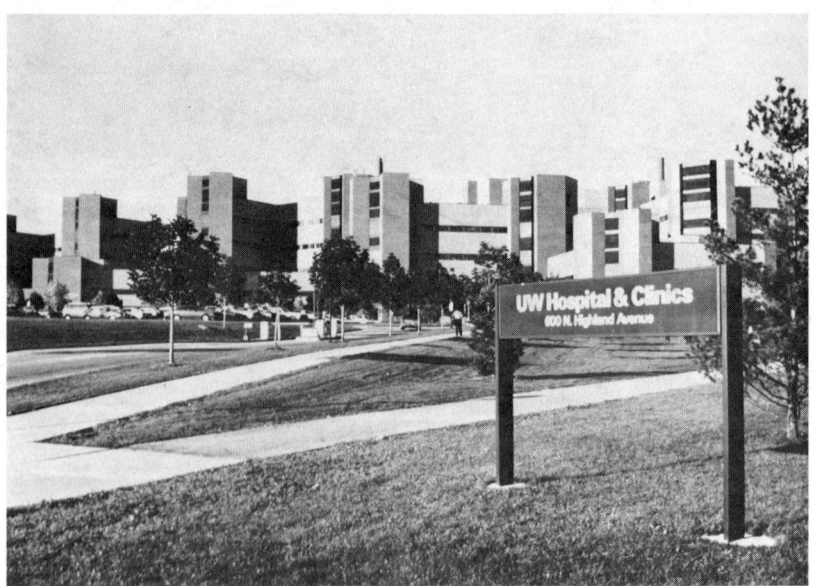

The University of Wisconsin Hospital and Clinics situated at the west end of the University campus. The buildings were opened in the late 1970s.

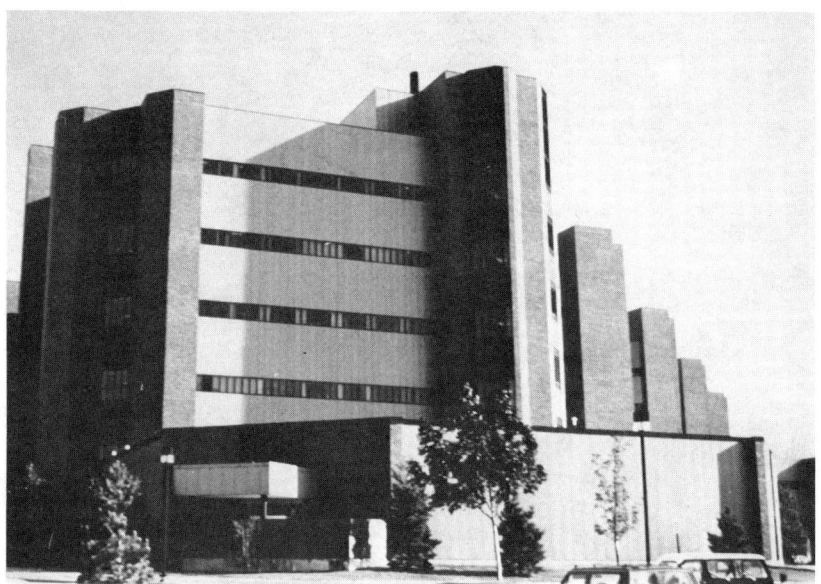

The University of Wisconsin Clinical Cancer Center. The animal facility adjoining the Cancer Center is in the foreground.

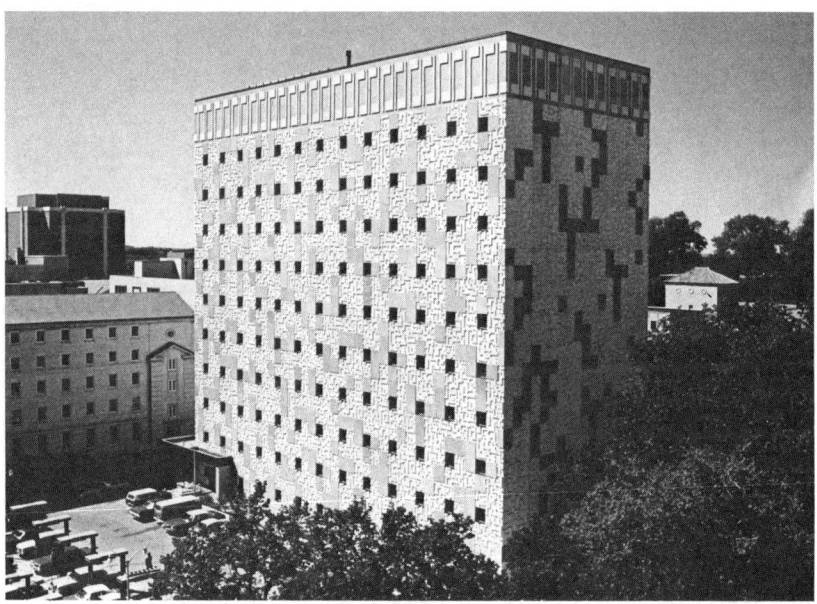

The McArdle Laboratory for Cancer Research on the University of Wisconsin–Madison campus.

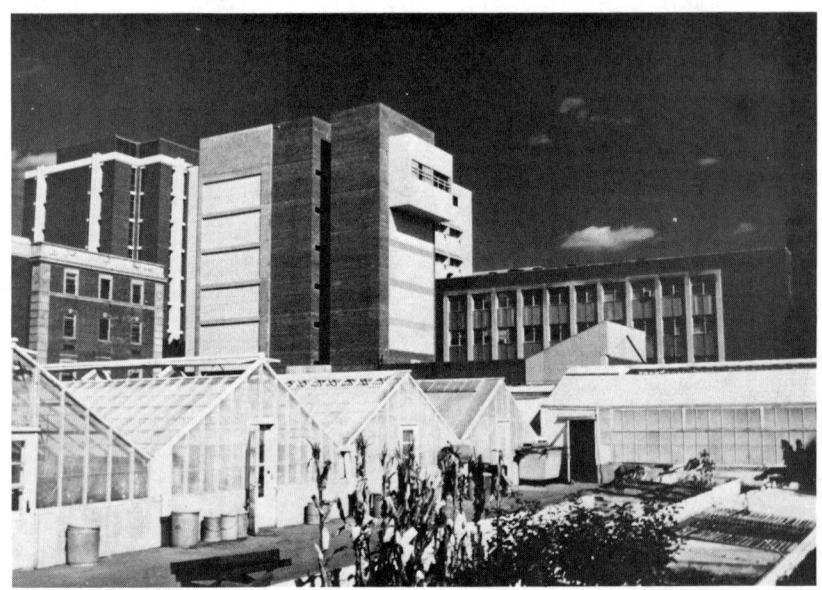

The new Biochemistry Department buildings on the University of Wisconsin–Madison campus.

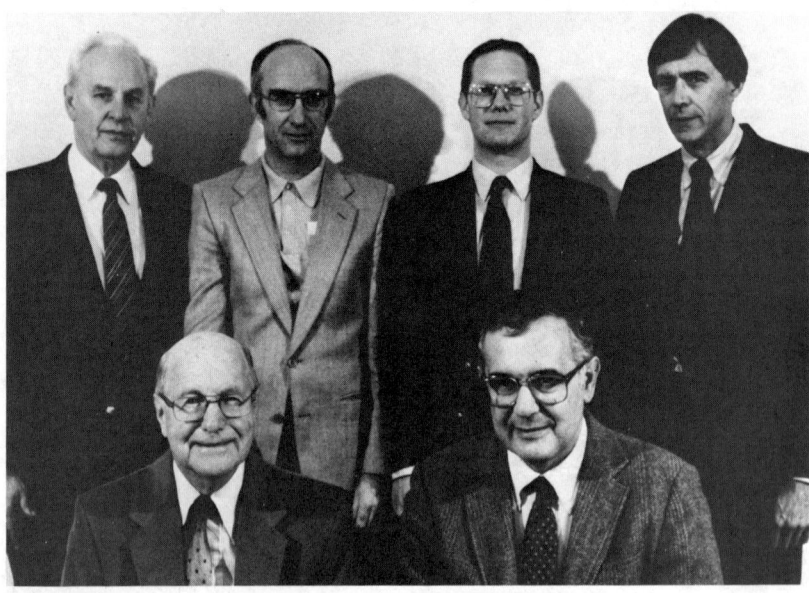

University of Wisconsin Cancer Center faculty involved in hormone action and breast cancer therapy. *Back row, left to right:* Dr. Gerald C. Mueller, Dr. Jack Gorski, Dr. V. Craig Jordan, and Dr. Douglass C. Tormey; *seated, left to right:* Dr. Harold Rusch and Dr. Paul P. Carbone.

Acknowledgments

THE symposium and this book would not have been possible without the major contributions provided by

   Imperial Chemical Industries, Cheshire, England
   Stuart Pharmaceuticals, Wilmington, Delaware
   Abbott Laboratories, North Chicago, Illinois

Additional sponsorship was provided by Amersham, New England Nuclear (Du Pont), Eli Lilly, Sorval (Du Pont), CIBA-Geigy, Bristol Myers, Smith Kline Beckman, Mead Johnson, and Merrell-Dow.

Local support for the symposium was provided by

   Bessimer America, Inc., Belmont, Wisconsin
   Coca Cola Bottling Company, Madison, Wisconsin
   Curran Cheese Corporation, Browntown, Wisconsin
   Heileman Brewery, La Crosse, Wisconsin
   Kendall/Hunt Publishers, Dubuque, Iowa
   S and R Cheese Corporation, Plymouth, Wisconsin
   Swiss Colony, Monroe, Wisconsin

Special thanks are due to Sandy Schwartz, whose tireless efforts helped to make the symposium in Madison such a success. Mary Carbone, Marion Jordan, and Pat Tormey provided outstanding support during the symposium to make the social program so memorable for all our guests.

Last, but by no means least, I would like to acknowledge gratefully the efforts of Elizabeth Steinberg, Chief Editor, University of Wisconsin Press, and Jane Behrend, Editorial Assistant, University of Wisconsin Press, during the development of this book. The photograph of McArdle Laboratory was taken by Norman Lenburg of the Office of Information Services, University of Wisconsin–Madison; the other photographs of the University of Wisconsin and Madison were provided by Rick Koch.

I

Chemistry and Biochemistry

1

Estrogen Receptors— Highlights of Their History, Properties, and Actions

GERALD C. MUELLER

I. HISTORICAL PERSPECTIVES CONCERNING ESTROGEN RECEPTORS   4
II. A SUMMARY OF ESTROGEN RECEPTOR PROPERTIES   6
III. ESTROGEN RECEPTORS AS DYNAMIC MOLECULES   8
IV. CONCLUDING COMMENTS—RECEPTORS AS TRANSDUCERS   13
    REFERENCES   15

3

I. Historical Perspectives
Concerning Estrogen Receptors

IN 1950, when the author first became interested in the problem of steroid hormone action, the endocrinological literature abounded with new findings on the synthesis and metabolism of steroid hormones—however, there were few, if any, insights into the basic cellular and molecular mechanisms by which these entities brought about their remarkable biological responses. Among the different steroid hormones, the estrogens looked most promising for an investigation of hormone action because they were clearly active in a target tissue within the hour and were effective at vanishingly low concentrations. Studies were also well in progress by such pioneers as E. B. Astwood (1938), Clara Szego and Sidney Roberts (1953), M. A. Telfer (1953), and Claude Villee (1956) which established that the uterus of an estrogen-treated animal, a remarkably sensitive target tissue, rapidly imbibed fluid containing nutrients and electrolytes and then mobilized the intermediate metabolism of these components for a growth response. The initial phase of the response was characterized by an acceleration of RNA and protein synthesis (Mueller 1953; Mueller and Herranen 1956; Jervell et al. 1958)—and was accompanied, as well, by an accumulation of structural phospholipids. This hypertrophy of uterine cells was followed in turn by a wave of DNA synthesis and mitotic activity after an interval of 18–34 hours—the hyperplasia of estrogenic action (Mueller 1953).

Although in the light of present-day knowledge the acceleration of RNA and protein synthesis is clearly the product of hormone influences on gene expression mechanisms, it was not so evident in the early days. Insights into the synthesis and interactions of messenger RNA with ribosomes, transfer RNA, and activated amino acids were just beginning to emerge. The observations that blocking protein synthesis with puromycin (Mueller et al. 1961) or limiting RNA synthesis with actinomycin (Ui and Mueller 1963) prevented the majority of estrogen effects came somewhat later. Even so, it was evident at that time that there had to be a mechanism for communicating between the hormone on the cell periphery and the genes of the cell nucleus and the expression mechanism in the cytoplasm.

In 1952 Dr. Ilse Riegel and I, anticipating this need, had initiated a deliberate search for such a communication pathway. We reasoned that the high activity of estradiol and the unique responsiveness of target tissues was evidence for either a steroid-concentrating mechanism or a unique metabolism of this steroid in the rat uterus. At that time only ^{14}C-labeled estradiol was available; unfortunately, it had too low a specific activity for the inquiry that we mounted. At the time, we calculated that there would have to be some mechanism for concentrating more than 25,000 molecules of estradiol per cell before we would be above background levels at the concentrations of steroids used. It is of interest now to note how closely this figure approximates the average number of receptors in sensitive cells. Restricted by this dilemma, we were forced to settle for studies of estradiol metabolism in liver and kidney (Riegel and Mueller 1954).

It remained for Dr. Elwood Jensen and Dr. Herbert Jacobson, who were able to synthesize [3H]estradiol of high specific activity from the newly available tritium, to make the dramatic announcement in 1959 that target tissues did indeed concentrate and selectively retain this steroid (Jensen and Jacobson 1960). Figure 1.1 illustrates the momentous data which activated the search for and characterization of receptors of all types

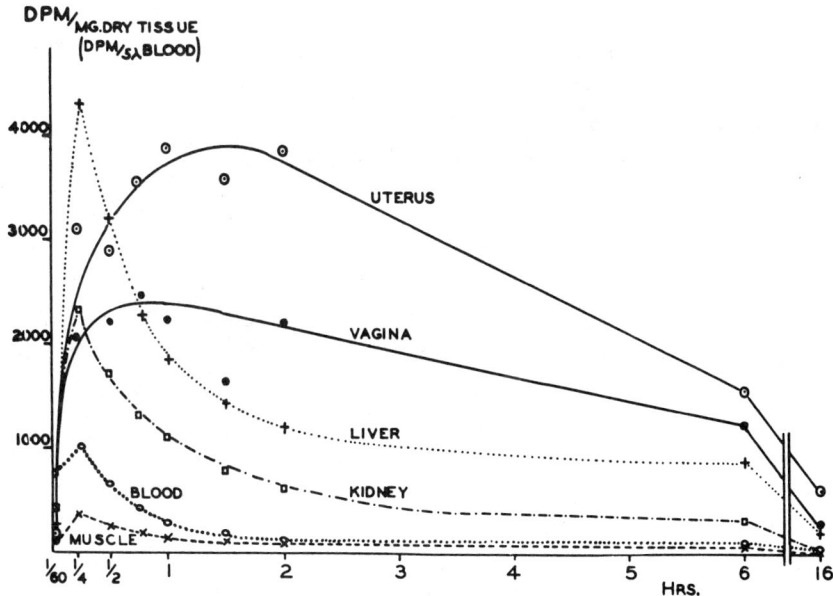

Figure 1.1. The selective concentration of [3H]estradiol by target tissues (Jensen and Jacobson 1960).

in practically all areas of cell biology. Although the quest extended rapidly
to androgens, progesterone, and glucocorticoids—and then to vitamins,
insect hormones, peptide hormones, and growth factors—the initial progress was most rapid in the estrogen receptor field. Homogenization of uteri
from estradiol-treated rats revealed that the majority of the hormone was
in the nucleus with only 20–30% residing in the cytosol (Noteboom and
Gorski 1965; King and Gordon 1966; Stumpf 1968). In each location the
hormone was retained by a noncovalent association with protein. Toft and
Gorski (1966) provided the first real physical evidence on the properties
of the receptor. They showed that the receptor-estradiol complex sedimented as a 9.5S component in low salt sucrose density gradients—and
that the complex was reversibly dissociable into 4S units in the presence
of 0.4 M KCl.

At the onset of these studies, I remember receiving a telephone call
from Jack Gorski, who asked me what I thought of Elwood Jensen's findings. I remarked that they were extremely interesting—and that they ac-
corded very well with our early expectations. I also stated that since some
of the receptor was present in a soluble form, the task of isolating the pure
receptor should be quite feasible. Indeed, Elwood was clearly engaged in
this research and so why not let him finish the job. Some 20-plus years
later, it is abundantly clear that Jack Gorski made a wise decision in not
accepting this advice, since the problem of isolating and characterizing
estrogen receptors turned out to be much more difficult than I anticipated.
Instead, he and his associates went on to make many basic contributions
to the estrogen receptor and estrogen action field.

II. A Summary of Estrogen Receptor Properties

In the interval following their discovery (i.e., some 25 years) we have
come to know the estrogen receptors by their properties as set forth in
Table 1.1. Many investigators have contributed to our present insight. One
of the most striking observations was that receptors in combination with
estradiol at 37°C undergo "activation." In this process they expose groups
which enable them to form tight complexes with both acidic and basic
macromolecules—with DNA, certain acidic polysaccharides, histones,
and certain other basic proteins. Most important, the transformation process is correlated with the development of a high affinity of the receptors
for the cell nucleus, whether the activation occurred *in vivo* or is carried

out in the test tube. Activation also correlates with a shift in the sedimentation character in high salt sucrose gradients from 4S to 5S forms. Recent studies have proven convincingly that this shift results from a dimerization of the receptor subunits (Scholl and Lippman 1984). As will be explored more exhaustively in the following chapters, it was also found that estradiol receptors competitively form high affinity complexes with estrogen antagonists such as nafoxidine, CI 628 (Parke-Davis), and tamoxifen metabolites (Lunan and Green 1974; Jordan and Dowse 1976). In fact, the demonstration of these competitive interactions has provided some of the best evidence that estrogen receptors do mediate the hormonal responses. These interactions have been studied extensively by the following scientists and their associates: Jordan, Notides, Sutherland, McGuire, Horwitz, Katzenellenbogen, and Lippman. The majority of their conclusions stem from binding kinetics, receptor localization of ^{3}H-labeled hormone or analogues, and the sedimentation properties of receptor-ligand complexes. While these results implicate the estrogen receptors in the responses, they do not really tell us how receptors work.

Table 1.1. Important events in estrogen receptor characterization

First demonstration of an estrogen-concentration mechanism in target tissues	Jensen and Jacobson 1960
Preliminary evidence for estrogen receptors in both nuclei and cytosol	Talwar et al. 1964; Noteboom and Gorski 1965; King and Gordon 1966
Salt dissociation and analysis of cytosolic estrogen receptors by sedimentation in sucrose gradients	Toft and Gorski 1966
Early evidence for activation of estrogen receptors	Puca and Bresciani 1968; Jensen et al. 1968; DeSombre et al. 1972; Notides and Nielson 1974
Early evidence that estrogen antagonists combine with estrogen receptors	Korenman 1970; Skidmore et al. 1972; Clark et al. 1973; Lunan and Green 1974; Jordan and Dowse 1976
Demonstration that activated receptors have affinity for DNA	Yamamoto and Alberts 1975; Rochefort et al. 1980; Evans et al. 1982
Development of antibodies to estrogen receptors	Greene et al. 1977; Greene et al. 1980; Moncharmont et al. 1982
Physical evidence that the turnover of estrogen receptors is rapid in cells	Eckert et al. 1982; Scholl and Lippman 1984
Injection of estrogen receptors into *Xenopus* liver nuclei activates gene expression	Knowland et al. 1984

III. *Estrogen Receptors as Dynamic Molecules*

The remainder of this overview will be devoted to a description of some less-appreciated properties of estrogen receptors which I feel are fundamental in understanding their function. The first property is the ability of estrogen receptors to recognize other molecules in their environment besides estrogens and antiestrogens. The fact that estrogen receptors form such high affinity complexes with their ligands ($K_d = \sim 10^{-9}$ M), in my opinion, has lulled investigators into viewing them like the Rock of Gibraltar. To the contrary, estrogen receptors should be viewed as highly adaptive and conformationally active molecules—exhibiting an ability to interact with other molecules in their milieu in a manner which alters in turn their binding of the hormone. For example, *p*-secondary amyl phenol (*p*SAP), a flexible analog of the A and B rings of estradiol, interacts with receptors both to prevent the binding of estradiol and to displace estradiol which has already been bound (Mueller and Kim 1978). The finding that tightly bound estradiol is rapidly displaced by *p*SAP at 0°C (Fig. 1.2) without itself forming a high affinity complex with the receptor suggests two things: (1) the phenol binding site on the receptor is open to an approach by *p*SAP even though the receptor is otherwise occupied by estradiol; (2) the approach of *p*SAP to this region of the receptor induces structural changes in the receptor which extend to the region of the receptor responsible for the high affinity binding of the resident estradiol molecule.

In a series of other studies it was observed that 2-tetrahydronaphthol, a rigid analog of the A and B rings of estradiol, could prevent the binding of estradiol without itself forming a stable complex with the receptor. This compound, in contrast to *p*SAP, was nevertheless ineffective as a displacer of prebound estradiol. Together, these results with simple phenols (i.e., pseudoligands) argue for induced conformational changes in receptors already occupied by estradiol—and suggest that binding and release of the estradiol molecule involves an ordered sequence of ligand-induced conformational changes. In brief, the path of the steroid entering the receptor differs from its path of exit.

A second interesting property of receptors is their ability to interact with nonsteroids in a manner that alters their affinity for estradiol. By testing a wide series of compounds it was found that tetracaine and related local anesthetic agents were remarkable in their ability to lower the temperature required for estradiol exchange on occupied receptors (Fig. 1.3) (Kim et al. 1982). In addition, it was found that heparin and other sulfated

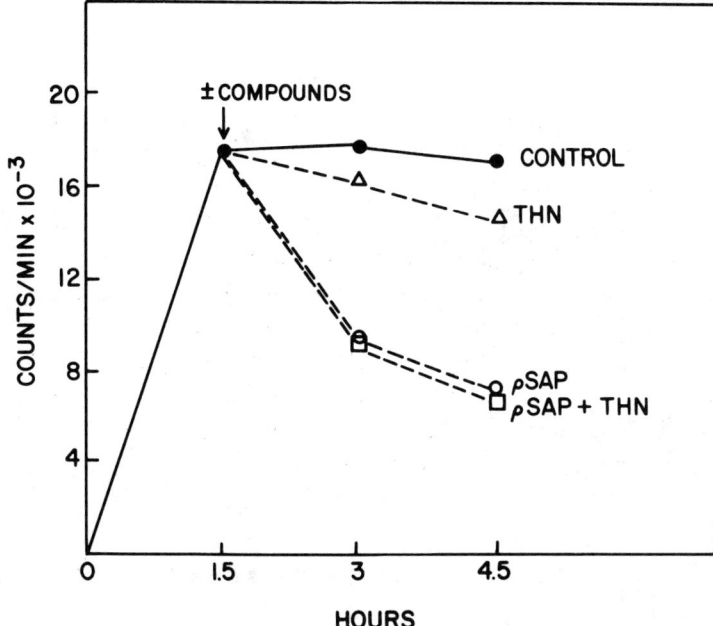

Figure 1.2. Displacement of [³H]estradiol from estrogen receptors by tetrahydronaphthol (THN) and *p*-secondary amyl phenol (*p*SAP) at 0°C. A cytosol preparation from mature rabbit uteri was pretreated with [³H]estradiol (1×10^{-3} µg/ml) for 1.5 hours to label the estrogen receptors. This preparation was then treated with 50 µg/ml THN, *p*SAP, or the combination of THN plus *p*SAP, and the incubation was continued at 0°C. At the indicated times, 0.1 ml aliquots of the cytosol were assayed by the hydroxyapatite assay for the amount of receptor-bound [³H]estradiol. Data are expressed as counts per minute/0.1 ml cytosol (Mueller and Kim 1978).

polysaccharides clearly synergize with tetracaine to produce this effect; the combination of both agents can even cause release of prebound estradiol at 0°C (Fig. 1.4) (Van Oosbree et al. 1984a). The existence of a recognition site in the receptors for the sulfated polysaccharide is further indicated by the dependence of the release on the structure of this class of macromolecules.

This synergism between a charged hydrophilic macromolecule and a charged hydrophobic small molecule in relaxing the receptor structure suggests that the receptor contains two classes of charged domains—one hydrophilic and another hydrophobic. Both domains seem to influence the structure of the receptor but appear to be distinct from the actual binding site for the steroid. Clearly these domains provide potential sites for estro-

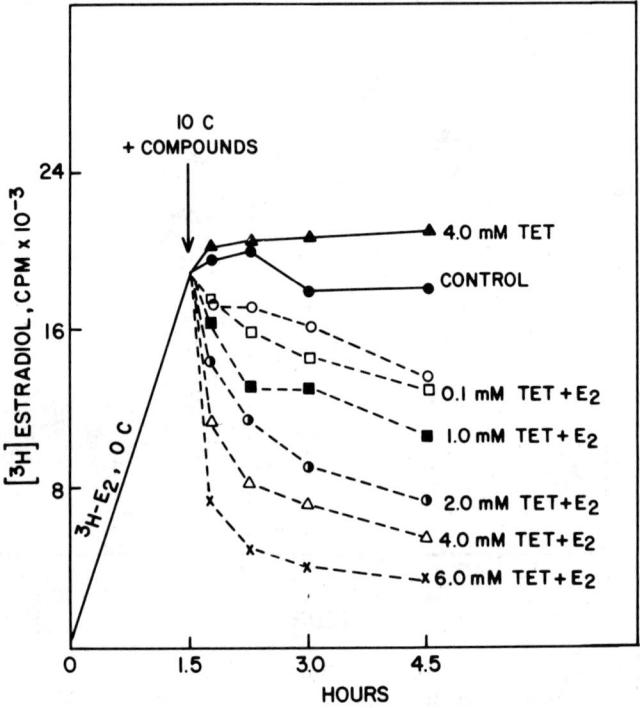

Figure 1.3. Effect of tetracaine (TET) concentration on the exchange of receptor-bound [³H]estradiol. Rabbit uterine cytosol was pretreated at 0°C with [³H]estradiol. After this interval the indicated levels of tetracaine were added ± a diluting pool of unlabeled estradiol and the temperature of the system was elevated to 10°C. At the indicated times, aliquots were assayed by the hydroxyapatite method for receptor-bound [³H]estradiol. The data are expressed as cpm × 10⁻³ of receptor-bound [³H]estradiol (Kim et al. 1982).

gen receptor interaction with other cellular molecules—possibly the molecules involved in the regulation of gene expression.

To gain more insight into this realm, our laboratory devised a simple one-step adsorption-elution procedure using diethylstilbestrol-agarose for the preparation of estrogen receptors in high purity (Van Oosbree et al. 1984b). An electropherogram of these isolated receptor proteins is shown in Figure 1.5. Two proteins appear to account for the estrogen binding in the preparations of rat and rabbit uterine cytosols—a 65 K and a 50 K protein. Limited proteolysis experiments with V-8 protease, trypsin, and N-chlorosuccinimide have revealed that the proteins are structurally related (Olsen et al. 1986). It is not yet known, however, whether one or the other arises as a product of posttranscriptional modification, or has its

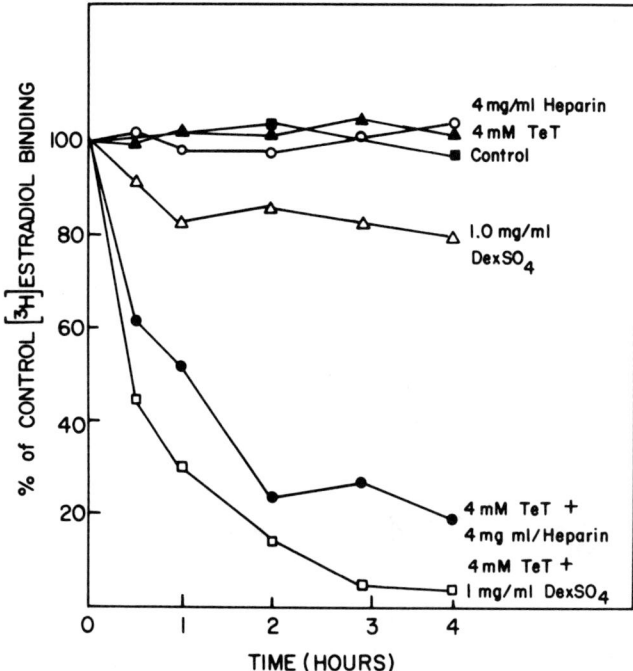

Figure 1.4. Displacement of [³H]estradiol from estrogen receptors by the combination of tetracaine and sulfated polysaccharides. Rabbit uterine cytosol was pretreated with [³H]estradiol to label the estrogen receptors. The preparation was then treated with 4 mM tetracaine (TeT), 4 mg/ml heparin, 1 mg/ml dextran sulfate (DexSO₄), 4 mM tetracaine plus 4 mg/ml heparin, or 4 mM tetracaine plus 1 mg/ml dextran sulfate at 0°C. The amount of receptor-bound [³H]estradiol remaining in each preparation was measured over the next 4 hours by using the hydroxyapatite assay (Van Oosbree et al. 1984a).

origin in the transcription process itself (i.e., different structural genes or an altered transcription of the same gene).

Even though the characterization of the primary structure of these proteins is being pursued in the interest of determining their exact amino acid sequence, and ultimately for the purpose of using this information to isolate the estrogen receptor gene(s), the isolated receptors have already proven useful for studies of their interaction with both DNA and histones. As presented in Figure 1.6, histones interact with the purified receptors to stabilize the estradiol receptor complexes. A comparison of the individual calf-thymus histones has also revealed that histones H2A and H2B are most effective in this action. In contrast, histones H3, H4, and H1 exhibit a destabilizing effect when added to the receptor preparation (K. Bhatta-

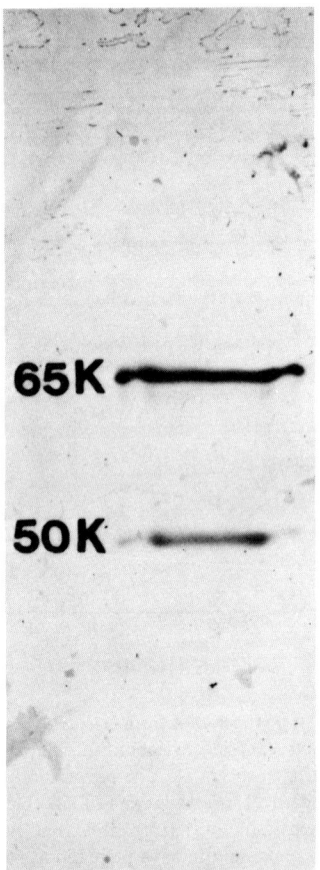

Figure 1.5. Estrogen-binding proteins purified from rabbit uterine cytosol by affinity chromatography on diethylstilbestrol-agarose (Van Oosbree et al. 1984b).

charyya and G. C. Mueller, unpublished observations). Although these actions are not yet understood, it is clear that the histones require the presence of estradiol for their responses—unoccupied receptors do not appear to be targets.

In a separate study the receptors were tested for their ability to bind DNA (T. R. Van Oosbree and G. C. Mueller, unpublished observations). [3H]Thymidine-labeled DNA from HeLa cells was added to rabbit uterine cytosol in the presence and absence of a receptor-titrating level of estradiol. The mixtures were then passed over diethylstilbestrol-agarose to adsorb unoccupied estrogen receptors and any DNA which might be combined to them. A significant level of radioactive DNA was retained on the

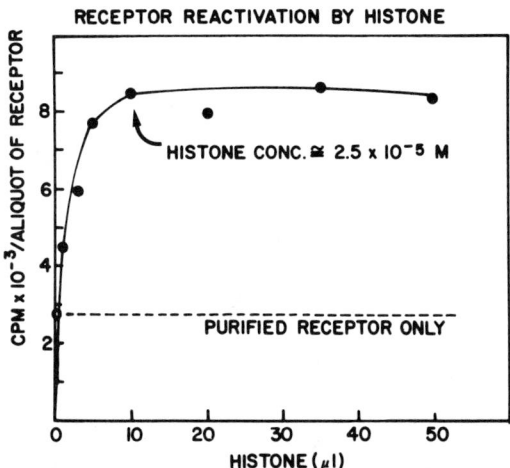

Figure 1.6. Effect of histones on estrogen binding by purified receptors. Receptor proteins were isolated by affinity chromatography over diethylstilbestrol-agarose (Van Oosbree et al. 1984b) and tested for their ability to bind [³H]estradiol in the presence of added levels of histones (histone concentration = 0.37 μg/μl; Sigma H2B). Estradiol binding was measured by the hydroxyapatite assay (K. Bhattacharyya and G. C. Mueller, unpublished observations).

affinity resin; however, when the cytosol preparation was pretreated with estradiol to block the adsorption of the receptors, the DNA was not retained. DNA adsorption was thus a function of the selective retention of the receptors.

This study has been extended using restriction fragments of lambda phage DNA containing the cloned 5' region of the prolactin gene. In this case the prolactin-DNA segment was retained selectively, suggesting a specificity of the interaction of the receptor with this DNA sequence. Although these results are preliminary, the observations that estrogen receptors can recognize both DNA segments and histone types provide a molecular-mechanical basis for perturbing the structure of chromatin which might contain genes of interest to hormonal responses (T. R. Van Oosbree, T. J. Schuh, and G. C. Mueller, unpublished observations).

IV. Concluding Comments—Receptors as Transducers

More than 25 years have elapsed since Jensen and Jacobson (1960) first clearly demonstrated the presence of estrogen receptors in target tissues.

DOMAINS

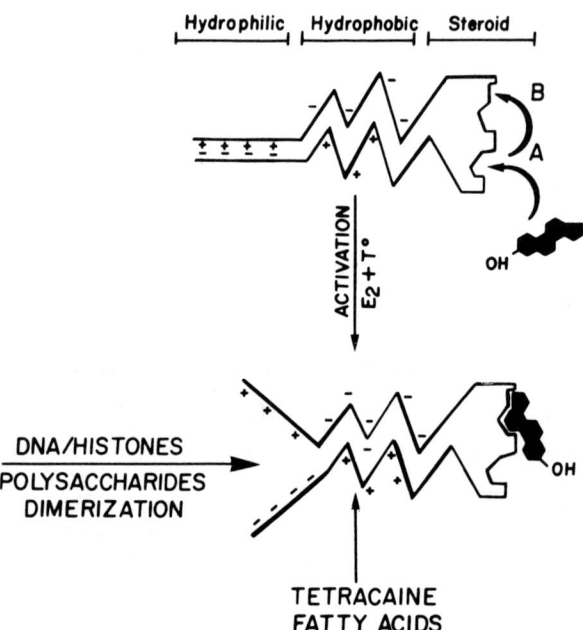

Figure 1.7. Hypothetical structure of the estrogen receptor. Studies with compounds that modulate estradiol binding suggest that the receptor protein contains three separate but interactive domains. The steroid-binding domain recognizes sequentially the A-ring of the hormone (site A) with the high affinity binding occurring at site B. A second domain, noncompeting with estradiol, recognizes nonpolar, hydrophobic compounds such as tetracaine and long chain fatty acids such as arachidonic acid. On activation with estradiol and 37°C heating, a third, hydrophilic domain becomes exposed for interaction selectively with certain DNA sequences, histones, and sulfated polysaccharides. The hydrophilic domain appears also to be involved in the dimerization of activated receptors. It is proposed that the receptor protein is highly active conformationally—responding adaptively to the simultaneous interaction of ligands at each of the three domains. In this manner, the receptor can function as a molecular transducer among components determining the structure and activity of chromosomal complexes.

Summarizing the progress in this interval, we have come to know the receptors, mainly from sedimentation and binding studies, as proteins with an unusually high affinity for estradiol and competing antiestrogens. Easily extracted in the cytosolic fractions from estrogen-deficient cells, they sediment as ~ 9.5S molecular aggregates in low salt sucrose gradients but readily dissociate to ~ 4S units in the presence of 0.4 M KCl. In this state, they have a relatively low affinity for DNA or nucleochromatin. Treatment of the cells or the isolated receptors with estradiol at 37°C, however, activates the receptors for dimerization and exposes groups which facilitate their binding to DNA and other hydrophilic-charged polymers—both acidic and basic. In the activation process, the affinity for estradiol is not grossly altered. This situation suggests that the exposed DNA binding sites in a hydrophilic domain and the estradiol binding site are separated significantly in the native estrogen receptors.

The findings that tetracaine and similar local anesthetic agents, as well as fatty acids like arachidonic acid, strikingly decrease the affinity of the receptors for estradiol argues for the presence of a separate charged hydrophobic domain; this region of the receptor is proximate to, but not identical with, the estrogen binding site. In addition, it would appear that both the hydrophilic and hydrophobic domains can synergize to modulate the affinity of the estrogens.

A hypothetical view of the estrogen receptor molecule, illustrating the interaction of these domains in receptor function, is depicted in Figure 1.7. Most important, this diagram attempts to show estrogen receptors as highly dynamic structures, sensing simultaneously quite separate classes of molecules in their environment and responding to each entity by conformational changes which alter in turn their affinity for the different ligands—estrogens, antiestrogens, DNA, histones, and charged lipidlike molecules. Impressed by this capacity to complex with and respond conformationally to such a diversity of compounds, we propose that receptors function as molecular transducers, combining the signals of the incoming estrogen, antiestrogen, and other small molecules to perturb or stabilize those macromolecular associations of DNA and protein which regulate the catalyzed expression of specific genes.

Acknowledgments

The author wishes to acknowledge the many contributions of past and present associates; with respect to the work currently in progress, I am particularly grateful to Dr. Thomas Van Oosbree, Mrs. Uh Hee Kim, Mr. Mark Olsen, and Dr. Kalyan Bhattacharyya. I also thank Mary A. LeMahieu for her expert assistance in the preparation of the manuscript. This work was supported by grants CA-07175 and CA-23076 from the National Cancer Institute, USPHS, and NIH Training Grants CA-09020 and CA-09230. G.C.M. is the recipient of a Research Career Award, CA-00685, from the National Cancer Institute.

References

Astwood, E. B. 1938. A six-hour assay for the quantitative determination of estrogen. *Endocrinology* 23:25–31.
Clark, J. H., J. Anderson, and E. J. Peck. 1973. Estrogen receptor antiestrogen complex:

a typical binding by uterine nuclei and effect on uterine growth. *Steroids* 22:707–718.

DeSombre, E. R., S. Mohla, and E. V. Jensen. 1972. Estrogen-independent activation of the receptor protein of calf uterine cytosol. *Biochemical and Biophysical Research Communications* 48:1601–1608.

Eckert, R. L., E. A. Rorke, and B. S. Katzenellenbogen. 1982. Determination of the rates of synthesis and turnover of the estrogen receptor in MCF-7 breast cancer cells using a density shift technique. *Sixty-fourth Annual Meeting of the Endocrine Society,* San Francisco, Calif., p. 87.

Evans, E., P. P. Baskevitch, and H. Rochefort. 1982. Estrogen-receptor-DNA-interaction. *European Journal of Biochemistry* 128:185–191.

Greene, G. L., L. E. Closs, H. Fleming, E. R. DeSombre, and E. V. Jensen. 1977. Antibodies to estrogen receptor: immunochemical similarity of estrophilin from various mammalian species. *Proceedings of the National Academy of Sciences* 74:3681–3685.

Greene, G. L., C. Nolan, J. P. Engler, and E. V. Jensen. 1980. Monoclonal antibodies to human estrogen receptor. *Proceedings of the National Academy of Sciences* 77:5115–5119.

Jensen, E. V., and H. I. Jacobson. 1960. Fate of steroid estrogens in target tissues. In *Biological activities of steroids in relation to cancer,* ed. G. Pincus and E. P. Vollmer, 161–178. New York: Academic Press.

Jensen, E. V., T. Suzuki, T. Kawashima, W. E. Stumpf, P. W. Jungblut, and E. R. DeSombre, 1968. A two-step mechanism for the interaction of estradiol with rat uterus. *Proceedings of the National Academy of Sciences* 59:632–638.

Jervell, K. F., C. R. Diniz, and G. C. Mueller. 1958. The determination of uridine and thymine in small samples of nucleic acid-protein residue. *Archives of Biochemistry and Biophysics* 78:157–164.

Jordan, V. C., and L. J. Dowse. 1976. Tamoxifen as an antitumour agent: effect on oestrogen binding. *Journal of Endocrinology* 68:297–303.

Kim, U. H., T. R. Van Oosbree, and G. C. Mueller, 1982. Influence of tetracaine on the structure and function of estrogen receptors. *Endocrinology* 111:260–268.

King, R. J. B., and J. Gordon. 1966. The localization of $[6,7-^3H]$oestradiol-17β in rat uterus. *Journal of Endocrinology* 34:431–437.

Knowland, J., I. Theulaz, C. V. E. Wright, and W. Wahli. 1984. Injection of partially purified estrogen receptor protein from *Xenopus* liver nuclei into oocytes activates the silent vitellogenin locus. *Proceedings of the National Academy of Sciences* 81:5777–5781.

Korenman, S. G. 1970. Relation between estrogen inhibiting activity and binding to cytosol of rabbit and human uterus. *Endocrinology* 87:1119–1123.

Lunan, C. B., and B. Green. 1974. $[^3H]$Oestradiol uptake in vivo by human uterine endometrium: effect of tamoxifen (ICI 46,474). *Clinical Endocrinology* 3:465–480.

Moncharmont, B., J.-L. Su, and I. Parikh. 1982. Monoclonal antibodies against estrogen receptor: interaction with different molecular forms and functions of the receptor. *Biochemistry* 21:6916–6921.

Mueller, G. C. 1953. Incorporation of glycine-2-C^{14} into protein by surviving uteri from α-estradiol-treated rats. *Journal of Biological Chemistry* 204:77–90.

Mueller, G. C., and A. Herranen. 1956. Metabolism of 1-carbon fragments by surviving uteri from estradiol-treated rats. *Journal of Biological Chemistry* 219:585–594.

Mueller, G. C., and U. H. Kim. 1978. Displacement of estradiol from estrogen receptors by simple alkyl phenols. *Endocrinology* 102:1429–1435.

Mueller, G. C., J. Gorski, and Y. Aizawa. 1961. The role of protein synthesis in early estrogen. *Proceedings of the National Academy of Sciences* 47:164–169.

Noteboom, W. D., and J. Gorski. 1965. Stereospecific binding of estrogens in the rat uterus. *Archives of Biochemistry and Biophysics* 111:559–568.

Notides, A. C., and S. Nielson. 1974. The molecular mechanism of the in vitro 4S to 5S transformation of the uterine estrogen receptor. *Journal of Biological Chemistry* 249:1866–1873.

Olsen, M. R., T. R. Van Oosbree, and G. C. Mueller. 1986. Characterization of rabbit uterine estrogen receptor proteins by radioiodination and partial peptide mapping. Submitted for publication.

Puca, G. A., and F. Bresciani. 1968. Receptor molecule for oestrogens from rat uterus. *Nature* (London) 218:967–969.

Riegel, I. L., and G. C. Mueller. 1954. Formation of a protein-bound metabolite of estradiol-16-C^{14} by rat liver homogenates. *Journal of Biological Chemistry* 210:249–257.

Rochefort, H., J. Andre, P. P. Basekvitch, J. Kallos, F. Vignon, and B. Westley. 1980. Nuclear translocation and interactions of the estrogen receptor in uterus and mammary tumors. *Journal of Steroid Biochemistry* 12:135–142.

Scholl, S., and M. E. Lippman. 1984. The estrogen receptor in MCF-7 cells: evidence from dense amino acid labeling for rapid turnover and a dimeric model of activated nuclear receptor. *Endocrinology* 115:1295–1301.

Skidmore, J. R., A. L. Walpole, and J. Woodburn. 1972. Effect of some triphenylethylenes on oestradiol binding in vitro to macromolecules from uterus and anterior pituitary. *Journal of Endocrinology* 52:289–298.

Stumpf, W. E. 1968. Subcellular distribution of ^{3}H-estradiol in rat uterus by quantitative autoradiography: a comparison between ^{3}H-estradiol and ^{3}H-norethynodrel. *Endocrinology* 83:777–782.

Szego, C. M., and S. Roberts. 1953. Steroid action and interaction in uterine metabolism. *Recent Progress in Hormone Research* 8:419–469.

Talwar, G. P., S. J. Segal, A. Evans, and O. W. Davidson. 1964. The binding of oestradiol in the uterus: a mechanism for depression of RNA synthesis. *Proceedings of the National Academy of Sciences* 52:1059–1066.

Telfer, M. A. 1953. Influence of estradiol on nucleic acids, respiratory enzymes, and the distribution of nitrogen in the rat uterus. *Archives of Biochemistry and Biophysics* 44:111–119.

Toft, D., and J. Gorski. 1966. A receptor molecule for estrogens: isolation from the rat uterus and preliminary characterization. *Proceedings of the National Academy of Sciences* 55:1574–1581.

Ui, H., and G. C. Mueller. 1963. The role of RNA synthesis in early estrogen action. *Proceedings of the National Academy of Sciences* 50:256–260.

Van Oosbree, T. R., U. H. Kim, and G. C. Mueller. 1984a. Release of receptor-bound estradiol by heparin or dextran sulfate in combination with tetracaine. *Journal of Receptor Research* 3:727–743.

Van Oosbree, T. R., U. H. Kim, and G. C. Mueller. 1984b. Affinity chromatography of estrogen receptors on diethylstilbestrol-agarose. *Analytical Biochemistry* 136:321–327.

Villee, C. A., and E. E. Gordon. 1956. The stimulation by estrogens of a DPN-linked isocritic dehydrogenase from human placenta. *Bulletin of the Society of Chemistry of Belgium* 65:186–201

Yamamoto, K., and B. M. Alberts. 1975. The interaction of estradiol-receptor protein with the genome: an argument for the existence of undetected specific sites. *Cell* 4:301–310.

2

Structure-Activity Relationships of Nonsteroidal Estrogens and Antiestrogens

V. Craig Jordan, Rick Koch, and Mara E. Lieberman

I.	Introduction	20
II.	Historical Perspective	20
III.	Phytoestrogens	23
IV.	Pesticides	27
V.	Nonsteroidal Antiestrogens	28
VI.	Regulation of Prolactin Synthesis *In Vitro*—An Assay to	
	Study Structure-Activity Relationships	30
VII.	Structure-Activity Relationships	32
VIII.	Conclusions	36
	References	37

I. Introduction

Fᴏʀ more than half a century, there has been a growing interest in the structure-activity relationships of estrogenic compounds. This chapter reviews the evolution of structure-activity relationship studies and suggests estrogen receptor models to predict biological activity. A brief survey of the structure-activity relationships of phytoestrogens, pesticides, and antiestrogens will be used to demonstrate the recurrent molecular features necessary for a compound (1) to bind to the estrogen receptor and (2) to produce conformational changes in the estrogen receptor complex which result in agonistic or antagonistic actions.

II. Historical Perspective

The pioneering studies by Sir Charles Dodds laid the foundation for all the subsequent research on the structure-activity relationships of nonsteroidal estrogens. The 1930s saw a remarkable expansion of knowledge that culminated in the description of the optimal structural requirement in a simple molecule to produce estrogen action. The first compound of known structure (1-keto-1,2,3,4 tetrahydrophenanthrene) (Fig. 2.1, Compound 2) to be found to have estrogenic activity was tested because of its structural similarity to the presumed structure of ketohydroxy estrin (Fig. 2.1, Compound 1) (Cook et al. 1933). As it turned out, the presumed structure of the natural steroid (estrone) was incorrect, but this did not matter because the fact that nonsteroidal compounds can exhibit estrogenic properties was established. However, by reference to the steroid nucleus, it was believed that a phenanthrene nucleus might be necessary for estrogenic activity. This hypothesis was found to be incorrect because simple bisphenolic compounds are active estrogens (Fig. 2.1, Compounds 3–6) (Dodds and Lawson 1936); as will be seen, this is a recurrent feature of many nonsteroidal estrogens. The finding that hydroxystilbenes (Fig. 2.1, Compounds 7–9) possess potent estrogenic activity provided a valuable clue that stimulated a systematic investigation to find the ideal substitution for optimal estrogenic activity. At this time, an interesting side issue occurred that deserves comment because it illustrates how parallel endeav-

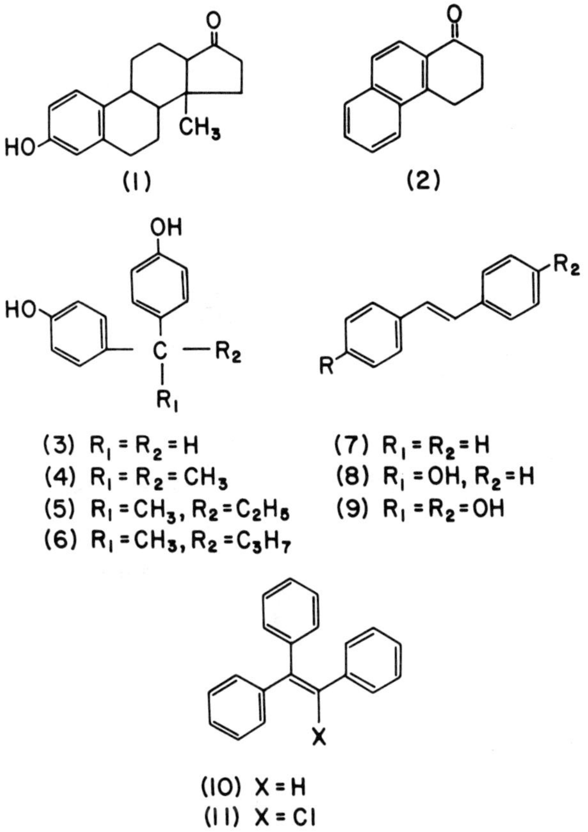

Figure 2.1. The formulae of compounds found in the 1930s to have estrogenic activity *in vivo*. Compound 1 was believed to be the molecular structure of ketohydroxyestrin (estrone). This is now known to be incorrect.

ors can eventually resolve a research problem and reach the same conclusion. Anol, a simple phenol derived from anethole (Fig. 2.2), was reported to possess extremely potent estrogenic activity with 1 μg inducing estrus in all rats (Dodds and Lawson 1937a). These results were not confirmed by other investigations using different preparations of anol (Dodds and Lawson 1937b; Zondek and Bergman 1938), but it was found that dimerization of anol to dianol (Fig. 2.2) can occur and this impurity, which was known to have potent estrogenic properties (Campbell et al. 1938a), was the compound responsible for the controversy (Campbell et al. 1938b). At this time, Dodds reported that diethyl substitution at the ethylenic bond of stilbestrol (Fig. 2.2) produces an extremely potent estro-

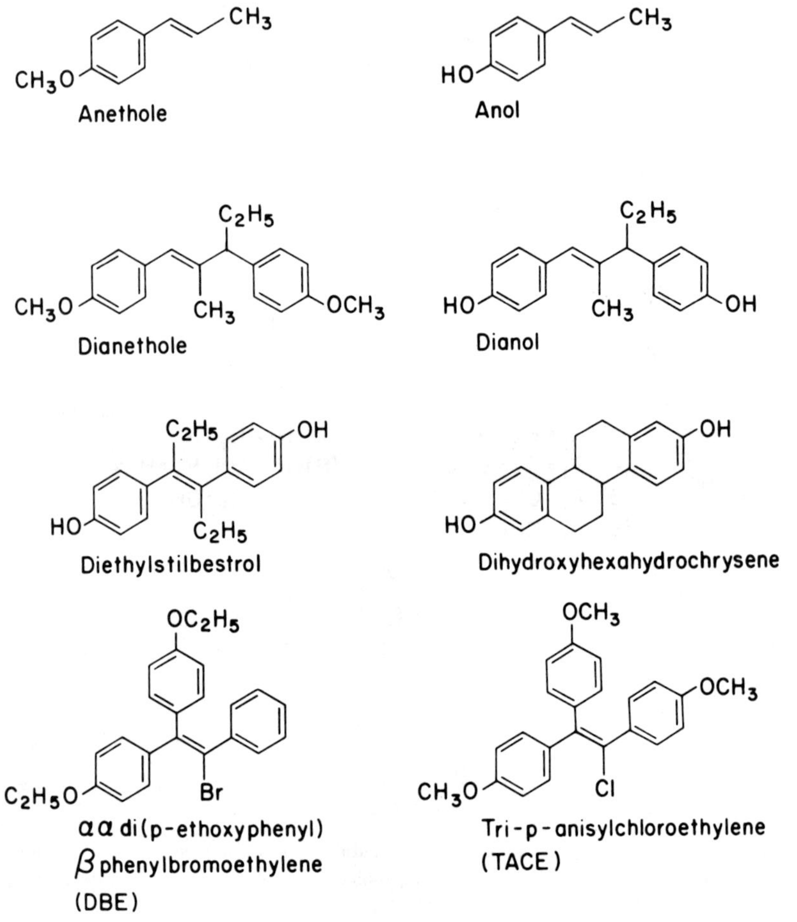

Figure 2.2. The formulae of nonsteroidal compounds with estrogenic (or suspected) activity *in vivo*.

gen (Dodds et al. 1938a,d); other substitutions produce less active compounds (Dodds et al 1938b). The structural similarity between diethylstilbestrol and estradiol (the formula was established by 1938) was noted (Dodds et al. 1938a), but an attempt to mimic the rigid steroid structure by the synthesis of dihydroxyhexahydrochrysene (Fig. 2.2) demonstrated a drop in estrogenic potency. Dihydroxyhexahydrochrysene is approximately 1/2000 as potent as diethylstilbestrol.

There has been considerable interest in the development of a long-acting synthetic estrogen because of the potential for clinical application.

The duration of action of diethylstilbestrol can be increased by esterification of the phenolic groups (Dodds et al. 1938c). Ten μg of diethystilbestrol diproprionate can produce estrus for more than 50 days whereas the phenol, at the same dose, is active for only 5 days.

The simple hydrocarbon triphenylethylene is a weakly active estrogen (Robson and Schonberg 1937), but 10 mg can produce vaginal cornification in mice for up to 9 weeks. Replacement of the free ethylenic hydrogen with chlorine (Fig. 2.1) increases the potency and duration of action by subcutaneous administration (Robson et al. 1938), but when administered orally, triphenylchloroethylene has a duration of action similar to diethylstilbestrol or estradiol benzoate. In the search for orally active agents, Robson and Schonberg (1942) showed that α,α-di-(p-ethoxyphenyl)βphenylbromoethylene (DBE) (Fig. 2.2) was a very effective estrogen. The long duration of action is related to depot formation in body fat (Robson and Ansari 1943), but DBE did not reach clinical trial. The related compound, trianisylchloroethylene (TACE) is, however, available clinically as a long-acting estrogen (Fig. 2.2). TACE, like DBE, is stored in body fat for prolonged periods (Thompson and Werner 1951; Greenblatt and Brown 1952; Thompson and Werner 1953).

The issue of oral activity for estrogens has been resolved by the identification of estrone and estriol as the primary metabolites of estradiol (Fig. 2.3). The recognition that estradiol is oxidized to estrone led to the introduction of 17α ethinyl estradiol and mestranol (Fig. 2.3) as the orally active estrogenic components of oral contraceptives. It is believed that mestranol is demethylated (metabolically activated) to ethinyl estradiol (Hahn et al. 1971; Eisenfeld 1974). However, although mestranol has a low binding affinity for the estrogen receptor, the steroid can initiate prolactin synthesis by primary cultures of dispersed rat pituitary cells (Fig. 2.4). It is unlikely that mestranol is metabolically activated in the pituitary cell prolactin assay system. The concept of metabolic activation is a recurrent feature of the pharmacology of phytoestrogens, selected estrogenic pesticides, and the nonsteroidal antiestrogens.

III. *Phytoestrogens*

Plants contain estrogens that are suspected of contributing to infertility problems in farm animals (Farnsworth et al. 1975). Aside from the potentially harmful effects of estrogens, they are apparently important to im-

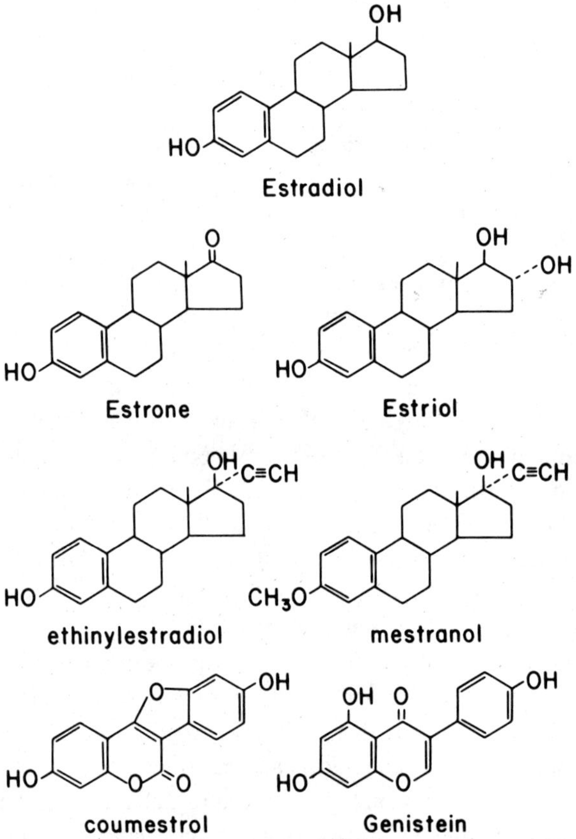

Figure 2.3. The formulae of some steroidal estrogens and the phytoestrogens coumestrol and genistein.

prove the quality of meat. Grazing animals in areas that are rich in phytoestrogens could provide economic advantages. It is also possible that phytoestrogens in the diet can contribute to the growth of hormone-dependent breast tumors in postmenopausal patients (Martin et al. 1978).

There are three major chemical types of phytoestrogens in plants: coumestans, flavones, and isoflavones. Coumesterol (Fig. 2.3) is the most potent of the estrogens in forage crops (Bickoff et al. 1957) and, consistent with this observation, has a higher binding affinity for the estrogen receptor than genistein (Shemesh et al. 1972; Shutt and Cox 1972). In contrast, the flavones are very weak estrogens. The methoxyflavone tricin is a constituent of alfalfa (Bickoff et al. 1964) but is very weakly estrogenic in the

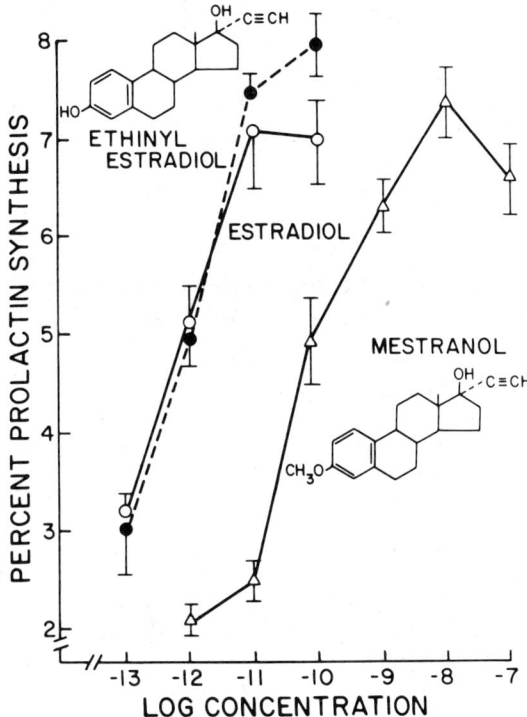

Figure 2.4. The ability of estradiol, ethinyl estradiol, and mestranol to stimulate prolactin synthesis in primary cultures of dispersed immature rat pituitary gland cells.

mouse. The isoflavone derivatives have attracted much attention as estrogenic compounds in clover. The early studies of the structure-activity relationships have been reviewed by Bradbury and White (1955). Genistein (Fig. 2.3) is the most active estrogen in this group and has the highest binding affinity (RBA 0.9) for the estrogen receptor (Shutt and Cox 1972). The methoxy derivative, Biochanin A, does not bind to the estrogen receptor but is estrogenic *in vivo* (Cheng et al. 1954; Shutt and Cox 1972). Similarly, diadzein (Fig. 2.5) has a higher binding affinity for the estrogen receptor than the methoxy derivative, formononetin (Fig. 2.5). Both compounds are weak estrogens *in vivo* (Cheng et al. 1954; Shutt and Cox 1972) but are directly estrogenic *in vitro* using the prolactin synthesis assay in primary cultures of rat pituitary cells. The estrogenic activities of diadzein and formononetin are compared with coumestrol and genistein in Figure 2.6.

The metabolism of formononetin and Biochanin A by microorganisms

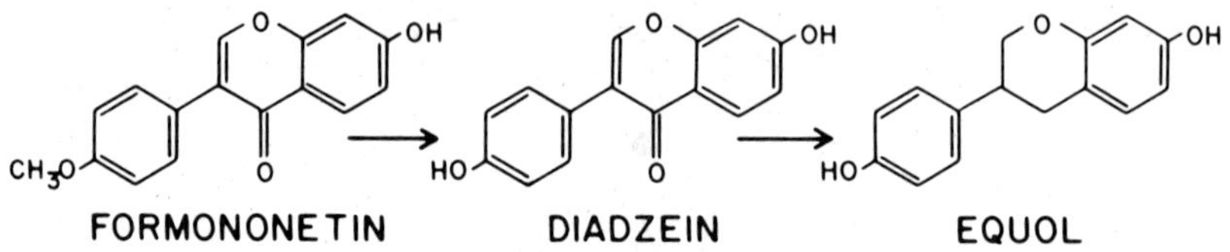

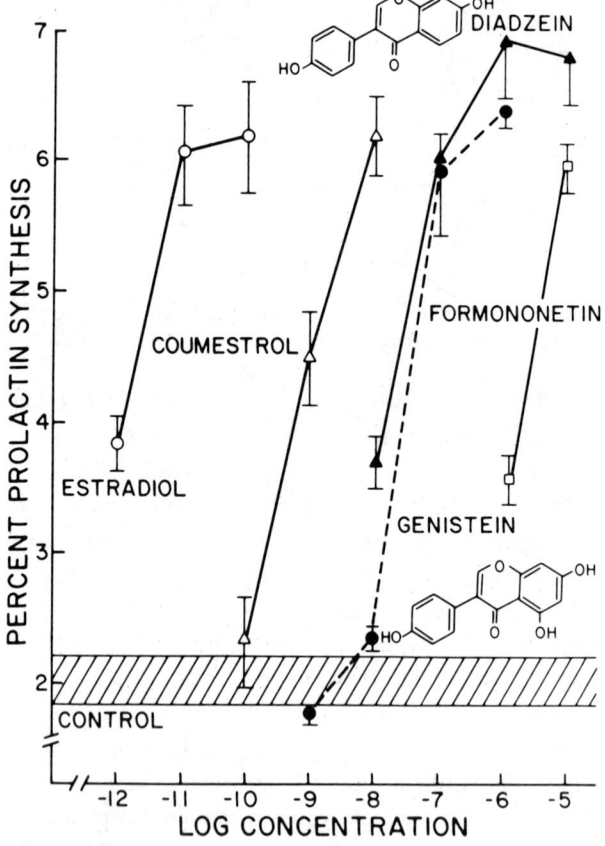

FORMONONETIN   DIADZEIN   EQUOL

Figure 2.5. The metabolic activation of the phytoestrogen formononetin to diadzein and equol.

in the sheep rumen has been described (Shutt 1976); however, diadzein is further reduced to equol (Fig. 2.5). Currently there is much interest in the detection of phytoestrogens in human urine because of the possibility that changes in diet might cause the activation of hormone-dependent breast

Figure 2.6. The ability of estradiol and different phytoestrogens to stimulate prolactin synthesis in primary cultures of dispersed immature rat pituitary gland cells.

cancer. Several studies have reported phytoestrogens in the urine (Adler-creutz et al. 1982; Bannwart et al. 1984); however, a recent report by Setchell and coworkers (1984) is particularly interesting because it documents that certain individuals have the ability to produce equol from soya products. Clearly this will be a significant area of research in the future.

IV. Pesticides

Various investigators showed that the chlorinated pesticides alter the reproductive capacity of animals by an interaction with estrogen target tissues (Kupfer 1975; Nelson et al. 1978; Bulger and Kupfer 1983). The o,p' isomer of DDT (Ireland et al. 1980), methoxychlor (Bulger et al. 1978), and kepone (Hammond et al. 1979) all have estrogenic activity in rat uterine weight assays. p,p'DDT (Fig. 2.7) has extremely low affinity for the estrogen receptor, but the o,p' isomer of DDT is active and will inhibit the binding of [³H]estradiol to estrogen receptors *in vivo* (Nelson 1974) and *in vitro* (Kupfer and Bulger 1976; Ireland et al. 1980). The related compound, methoxychlor (Fig. 2.7), is estrogenic in the rat; however, its mono- and didemethylated metabolites, as would be expected

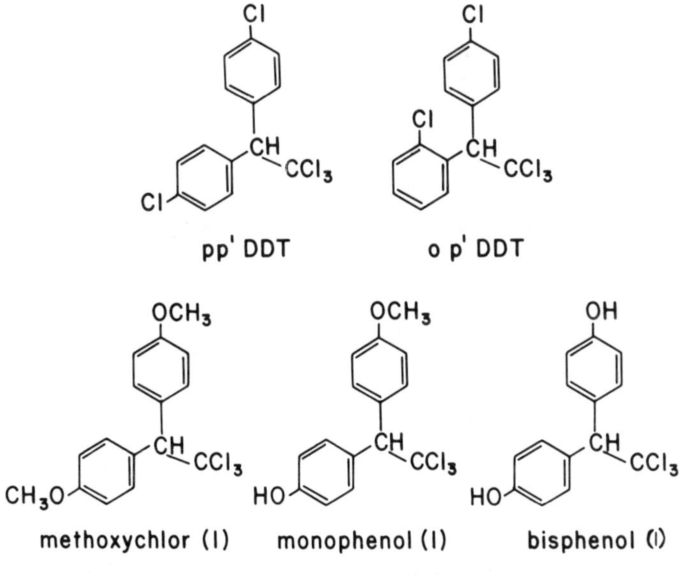

Figure 2.7. The formulae of some polychlorinated pesticides and the hydroxy metabolites of methoxychlor.

from the structure (cf. the early work of Dodds, Fig. 2.1), are capable of inhibiting the binding of [^{3}H]estradiol to its receptor *in vivo* (Ousterhout et al. 1981) and *in vitro* (Bulger et al. 1978; Kupfer and Bulger 1979). However, the recent report by Bulger and coworkers (1985) underlines the necessity for using ultrapure materials when examining the estrogenic actions of methoxychlor. Fifteen compounds which constitute, with methoxychlor, 99.5% of total technical-grade methoxychlor were examined *in vivo* and *in vitro*. Two compounds were estrogenic *per se:* 1,1-dichloro-2-(4-hydroxyphenyl)-2-(4-methoxyphenyl)ethylene and 1,1,1-trichloro-2(4-hydroxyphenyl)-2-(4-methoxyphenyl)ethane; and two compounds required metabolic transformation: 1,1-dichloro-2,2-bis(4-methoxyphenyl)ethene and methoxychlor.

V. *Nonsteroidal Antiestrogens*

In 1958, Lerner and coworkers described the pharmacological properties of the first nonsteroidal antiestrogen, MER 25. The compound is antiestrogenic in all species tested and also has antifertility properties in laboratory animals (Lerner et al. 1958; Segal and Nelson 1958; Chang 1959). Clinical trials with MER 25 confirmed its antiestrogenic activity in patients; however, the low potency and the occurrence of central nervous system side effects (Kistner and Smith 1961) caused a search for other agents. Clomiphene (MRL 41) is more potent than MER 25 but has some estrogenic properties in laboratory animals (Holtkamp et al. 1960). Clomiphene has antifertility properties in animals, but the drug induces ovulation in subfertile women (Greenblatt et al. 1962). The commercial preparation, Clomid, is routinely used for the induction of ovulation in subfertile women (Huppert 1979).

Many structural derivatives of triphenylethylene have been tested for antifertility and antiestrogenic activity in laboratory animals. Nafoxidine (Duncan et al. 1963; Lednicer et al. 1967) and CI 628 (Callantine et al. 1966) (Fig. 2.8) are both effective agents and can be classified as partial agonists based on immature rat uterine weight tests. These compounds have been used routinely as research tools for studies of estrogen and antiestrogen action.

The pharmacology of the antiestrogens is extremely complex and often paradoxical. The triphenylethylene derivative, tamoxifen (ICI 46,474) (Fig. 2.8) (Harper and Walpole 1966), is a complete estrogen antagonist

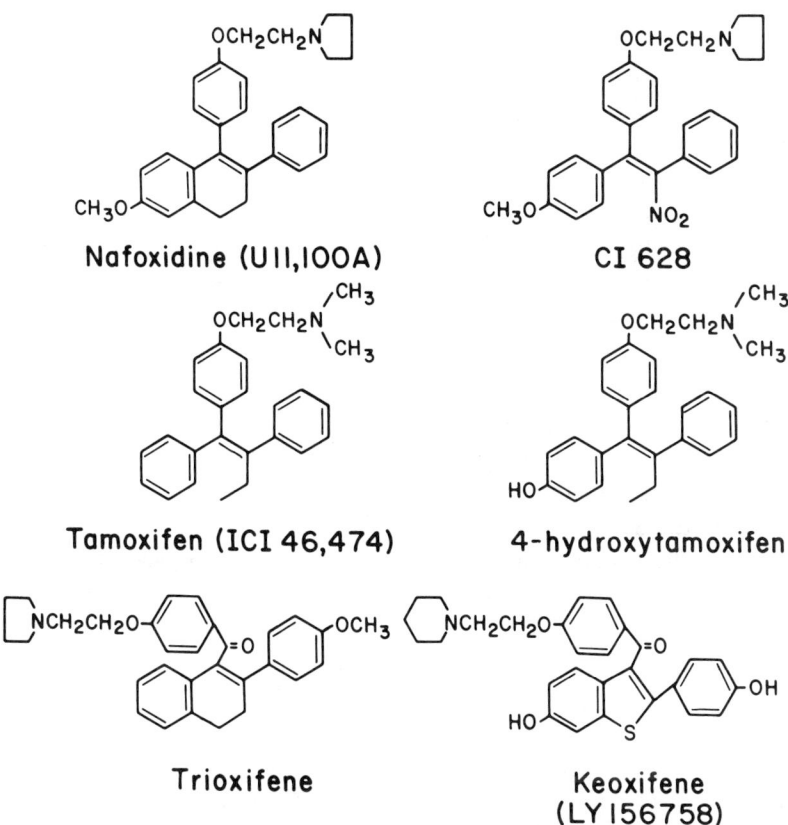

Figure 2.8. Nonsteroidal antiestrogens.

in the chick oviduct (Sutherland et al. 1977), a partial agonist with antiestrogenic activity in the immature (Harper and Walpole 1967) and ovariectomized rat (Jordan and Koerner 1976), and a full estrogen in the immature (Terenius 1971) and ovariectomized mouse uterus (Jordan et al. 1978). However, the biological actions of tamoxifen within rodent species are even more complex. Tamoxifen is fully estrogenic in the Allen-Doisy vaginal assay using ovariectomized mice (Harper and Walpole 1966), but large doses of tamoxifen produce a prolonged vaginal refractoriness to estrogen after an initial short period of estrogenic stimulation (Emmens 1971; Jordan 1975). In contrast, antiestrogens produce a mixture of estrogenic and antiestrogenic actions in the rat. Although antiestrogens can inhibit estradiol-stimulated increases in uterine wet weight (Harper and Walpole 1967), there is a simultaneous stimulation of luminal epithelial cell hypertrophy (Kang et al. 1975) and progesterone receptor synthesis (Dix and Jordan 1980; Jordan and Gosden 1982).

Several antiestrogens have been tested clinically as agents for breast cancer therapy. In the 1960s, clomiphene (Herbst et al. 1964), nafoxidine (EORTC 1972), and tamoxifen (Cole et al. 1971) were tested in phase I and phase II trials but only tamoxifen is available for general use.

Recently, the compound trioxifene (Fig. 2.8), which has antiestrogenic (Jones et al. 1979; Jordan and Gosden 1982) and antitumor actions (Rose et al. 1981) in laboratory animals, was tested in phase I and phase II trials (Manni et al. 1981) but is not available for therapy.

Current interest in the antiestrogens focuses upon the development of compounds with a high affinity for the estrogen receptor and, as a result, increased potency. Tamoxifen has a low binding affinity for the estrogen receptor; however, hydroxylation to produce 4-hydroxytamoxifen dramatically increases the affinity of the compound for the receptor and improves the antiestrogenic activity (Jordan et al. 1977). Similarly, polyhydroxylated antiestrogens like LY 117018 and LY 156758 (keoxifene) (Fig. 2.8) have high affinity for the estrogen receptor and an increased potency *in vitro*. One of the interesting biological properties of the new generation of antiestrogens (LY 117018 and LY 156758) is a decreased estrogenic activity in the rat and mouse uterus (Black and Goode 1980; Black et al. 1983; Jordan and Gosden 1983a), but these advantages may be offset by a decrease in the biological half-life of the polyhydroxylated antiestrogens (Jordan and Gosden 1983b). The multiple hydroxyl groups increase the solubility of the compounds and increase the probability of conjugation and excretion.

VI. *Regulation of Prolactin Synthesis* in Vitro— *An Assay to Study Structure-Activity Relationships*

Primary cultures of rat pituitary cells respond to physiological concentrations of estradiol by a specific increase in prolactin synthesis (Lieberman et al. 1978). This model system for estrogen action has been validated for the study of structure-activity relationship within groups of nonsteroidal estrogens and antiestrogens. The antiestrogens, tamoxifen and 4-hydroxytamoxifen, competitively and reversibly inhibit estradiol-stimulated prolactin synthesis (Lieberman et al. 1983a). Their potencies are consistent with their relative binding affinities for the estrogen receptor; 4-hydroxytamoxifen is 30 times more potent than tamoxifen. To avoid the possibility that tamoxifen is metabolically activated to 4-hydroxytamoxifen *in vitro,* several *para*-substituted derivatives to tamoxifen (4-methyl, chloro, and fluoro) that are unlikely to be metabolized to 4-hydroxytamoxifen (Allen et al. 1980; Lieberman et al. 1983a) have been tested. The substitution does not affect the binding of the compounds to the estrogen receptor (Allen et al. 1980; Lieberman et al. 1983a) and the derivatives of tamoxifen inhibit estradiol-stimulated prolactin synthesis consistent with their relative binding affinities for the receptor. Although it is an advantage for tamoxifen to be metabolized to 4-hydroxytamoxifen, it is clearly not a requirement for antiestrogenic activity.

The effects of estradiol and 4-hydroxytamoxifen, in the prolactin synthesis assay have been used to develop drug receptor models. In their simplest form, the current theories of drug interaction with receptors are based upon the fundamental studies by Clark (1926) and Gaddum (1926), who suggest that the response to a drug is proportional to the number of receptors occupied. However, the occupancy theory was modified by Stephenson (1956) and Ariens and Simonis (1964) into two steps: receptor binding (dependent upon the affinity of the drug for the receptor) followed by the production of a response (dependent upon the efficacy or intrinsic activity of the drug receptor complex). Thus, within a series of nonsteroidal estrogens (i.e., the intrinsic activity $\alpha = 1$), which have progressively lower affinities for the estrogen receptor than estradiol, their log dose-response curves in an assay system will be progressively shifted to the right of estradiol's curve. However, for a group of compounds with intrinsic activities progressively less than 1.0, the maximal responses in their log dose-response curves will be progressively lower. These are partial agonists. However, the ideal antagonist would have a high affinity for the estrogen receptor but would have an intrinsic activity of zero. This ideal has been achieved with antiestrogens in the pituitary prolactin synthesis assay *in vitro.* The receptor interaction of estradiol and 4-hydroxytamoxifen can be represented by the hypothetical scheme illustrated in Figure 2.9. Estradiol first interacts via the C-3 phenolic group with a phenolic site on the receptor, which then directs the steroid to the correct position at the binding site on the protein. The initial binding step is followed by a change in the tertiary structure of the protein that locks the steroid into the receptor; this change develops the intrinsic activity of the receptor complex. The antiestrogen, 4-hydroxytamoxifen, binds with high

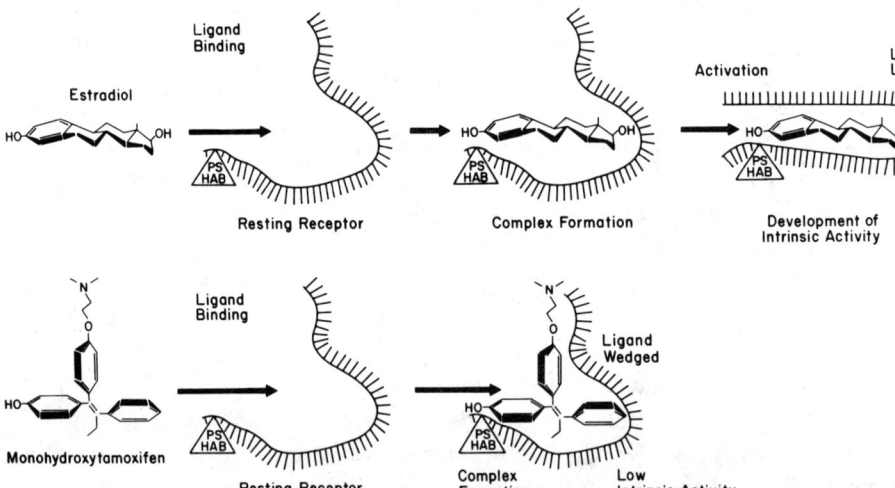

Figure 2.9. Hypothetical models to describe the binding of estradiol or 4-hydroxy-tamoxifen with the ligand binding site on the estrogen receptor. Estrogen can induce a conformational change in the receptor to lock the ligand into the receptor, whereas the antiestrogen prevents these changes from occurring. (From Jordan 1984.)

affinity via the interaction of the phenolic group with the phenolic site on the receptor. However, the tertiary changes in the receptor necessary to develop intrinsic activity in the complex is prevented by the alkyl-aminoethoxy side chain.

This hypothetical model has served as a basis for all our subsequent structure-activity relationship studies.

VII. *Structure-Activity Relationships*

A hypothetical model of the ligand interaction with the estrogen receptor binding site has been developed to describe the structural features necessary to initiate or to inhibit prolactin synthesis *in vitro*. Among the tri-phenylethylenes, compounds that have *cis* and *trans* geometric isomers are extremely important for the development of a ligand receptor model because the isomeric molecules encompass estrogenic and antiestrogenic actions (Harper and Walpole 1966; Jordan et al. 1981). The *trans* isomers, i.e., tamoxifen and enclomiphene (Fig. 2.10), are antiestrogens with zero intrinsic activity, whereas the *cis* isomers ICI 47,699 and zuclomiphene (Fig. 2.10), are estrogens with an intrinsic activity of 1.

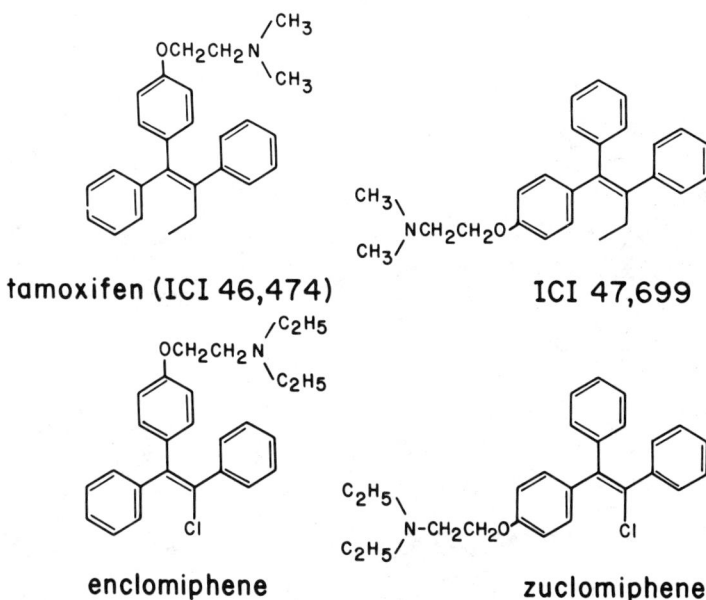

tamoxifen (ICI 46,474)   ICI 47,699

enclomiphene   zuclomiphene

Figure 2.10. The geometric isomers of substituted triphenylethylenes.

To describe the interaction of the geometric isomers with the estrogen receptor, the *trans* stilbenelike structure of tamoxifen and enclomiphene could sit loosely at the binding site with a low affinity interaction so that the phenyl ring substituted with the p-alkylaminoethoxy side chain is projected away from the binding site (Fig. 2.11). The estrogenic ligands, zuclomiphene and ICI 47,699, with their low affinity for the estrogen receptor, can create a *trans* stilbenelike structure with the *para*-substituted phenyl ring. In this binding state, the aminoethoxy side chain would lie next to the phenolic site on the receptor with a weak interaction through the ether oxygen (Fig. 2.11). There would be no interaction of the side chain with a hypothetical antiestrogen region of the receptor and, as a result, no inhibition of estrogen action. The tertiary changes that are necessary to develop a high intrinsic activity for the complex can occur unimpeded (Lieberman et al. 1983b).

Clearly, a correctly placed alkylaminoethoxy side chain is important to prevent the initiation of prolactin synthesis via the estrogen receptor. We have focused upon this area of interaction at the ligand binding site and found that the compounds related to bisphenol (4-hydroxytamoxifen without the alkylaminoethyl side chain) are particularly interesting, as they are all partial agonists *in vitro* (Jordan and Lieberman 1984; Jordan et al.

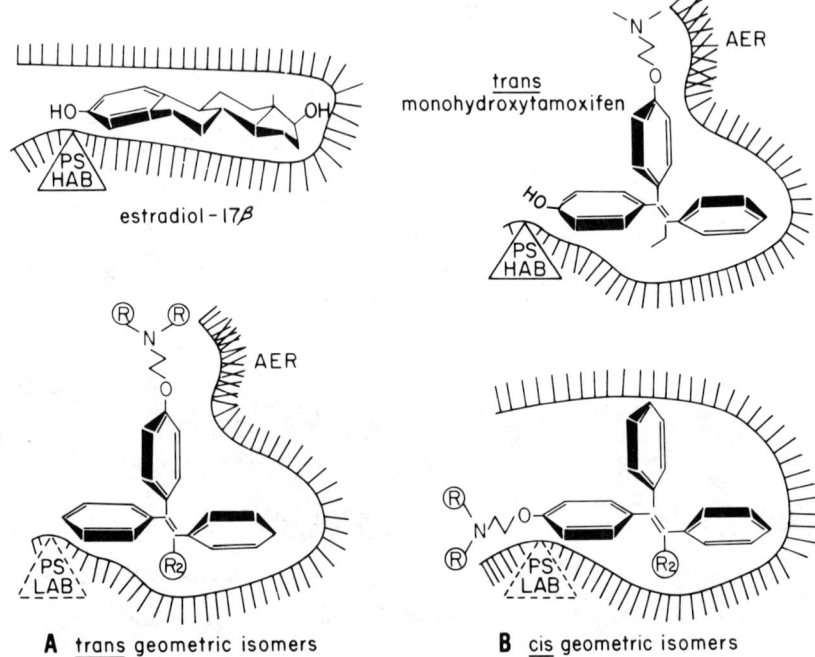

A <u>trans</u> geometric isomers   **B** <u>cis</u> geometric isomers

Figure 2.11. Hypothetical models for estrogenic and antiestrogenic ligands binding to the estrogen receptor. 17β-Estradiol is anchored at a phenolic site (PS) with high affinity binding (HAB). *trans*-Monohydroxytamoxifen has the same high affinity binding but this antiestrogenic ligand binds to the receptor site so that the alkylaminoethoxy side chain can interact with a hypothetical antiestrogen region (AER) on the protein. Compounds without a phenolic hydroxyl have low affinity binding (LAB). The *trans* and *cis* geometric isomers refer to (A) tamoxifen (R = CH_3, R_2 = C_2H_5) and enclomiphene (R = C_2H_5, R = C1); (B) ICI 47,699 (R = CH_3, R = C_2H_5) and zuclomiphene (R = C_2H_5, R_2 = C1).

1984). Belleau's macromolecular perturbation theory (Belleau 1964), which was originally proposed to explain agonistic, partial agonistic, and antagonistic activity of drugs at the muscarinic cholinergic receptor, may be used to explain partial agonists in terms of the estrogen receptor model. According to Belleau's hypothesis, antagonists bind to the receptor and produce a nonspecific conformational perturbation (NSCP) and the complex has zero intrinsic activity. An agonist, on the other hand, binds to the receptor and induces a specific conformational perturbation (SCP). Between these extremes, a partial agonist binds to the receptor and produces an equilibrium mix of agonistic and antagonistic receptor complexes. Applying these definitions to the estrogen receptor (Fig. 2.12), estradiol binds with high affinity to the resting receptor and induces a SCP, which

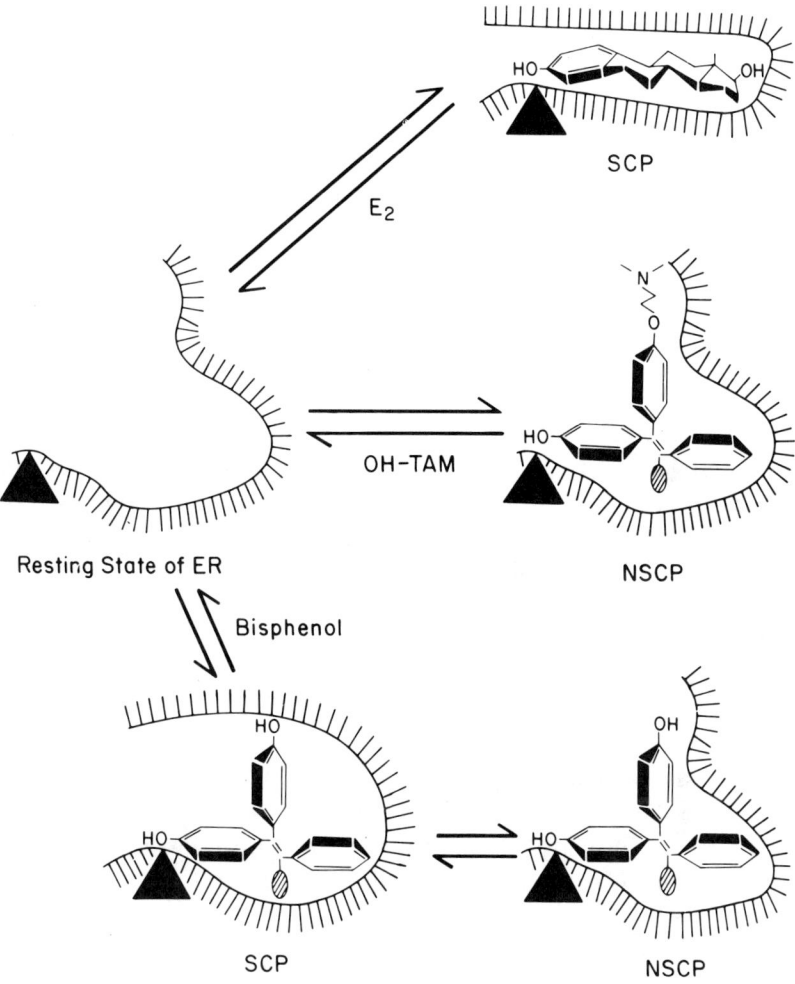

Figure 2.12. Adaptation of Belleau's macromolecular perturbation theory to describe the interaction of agonists, antagonists, and partial agonists with the estrogen receptor (ER). The phenol group on the ligand interacts with the phenolic site on the ER (▲) and produces a high affinity interaction if the geometry of the ligand is correct. Estradiol (E_2), an agonist, induces a specific conformational perturbation (SCP), whereas 4-hydroxytamoxifen (OH-TAM), an antagonist, only induces a nonspecific conformational perturbation (NSCP). Bisphenol (partial agonist) produces a mixture of SCP and NSCP in the ER. (From Jordan 1984.)

results in the ligand being locked into the binding site. 4-Hydroxytamoxifen (antagonist) wedges into the resting receptor and only produces an NSCP. Bisphenol (partial agonist) interacts at the ligand binding site, and although some of the receptors can be induced to lock the ligand into the protein, other ligand interactions are only able to induce an NSCP in the complex.

Thus, nonsteroidal compounds can now be classified experimentally into agonists and antagonists and partial agonists based upon their structures. An adequate assay system is established and validated to dissect the structural constraints in a ligand to modulate estrogen-dependent events via the estrogen receptor.

VIII. *Conclusions*

In order to understand the control of estrogen-dependent events, it is important to be able to evaluate the role of metabolic alterations and structure-activity relationships upon the subsequent pharmacology of a ligand in an isolated system. This is now possible using primary cultures of rat pituitary gland cells to assay the modulation of estrogen-stimulated prolactin synthesis. As a result, a simplified ligand model (Fig. 2.13) has been developed to describe the pharmacology of test compounds *in vitro*.

As with other drugs, the substituents that determine potency are different from those that determine pharmacological activity. A phenolic hydroxyl, equivalent to the C-3 phenol of estradiol, is extremely important for high affinity binding to the estrogen receptor. This structural feature is necessary to anchor the drug to the receptor binding site, which ultimately permits a variety of "spacing groups" to be present in the drug. These groups provide a rigid skeleton to permit the correct hinging of protein receptor to produce the occupancy of the binding site. Conversion of the

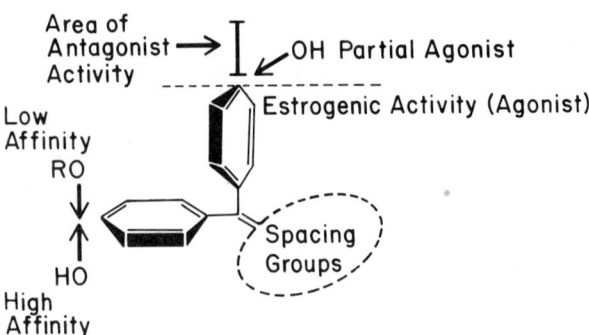

Figure 2.13. A general ligand model to describe the structural requirements to control biological activity *in vitro*. (From Jordan 1984.)

phenols to ether reduces the binding affinity for the receptor *in vitro;* however, these compounds are active longer *in vivo.* Substitution of the phenyl ring extending away from the binding site governs pharmacological activity. (1) A *bis para* hydroxyl predicts estrogenic activity *in vivo* but partial agonistic activity *in vitro.* (2) Extension of a side chain predicts partial agonistic and antagonistic activity *in vivo* but complete antagonistic activity *in vitro.*

The simple receptor binding site map provides a useful insight into the regulation of an estrogen-stimulated gene product. Future studies in similar isolated systems will undoubtedly provide an understanding of each facet of the mechanisms of hormone-dependent events. These facets can be integrated to develop a clear understanding of the growth mechanisms of breast cancer, which can be countered by new therapeutic strategies.

Acknowledgments

Supported by NIH grant R01-CA-32713.

References

Adlercreutz, H., T. Fotsis, R. Heikkinen, J. T. Dwyer, M. Woods, B. R. Goldin, and S. L. Gorbach. 1982. Excretion of the lignans, enterolactone and enterodiol and of equol in omnivorous and vegetarian postmenopausal women and in women with breast cancer. *Lancet* 11:1295–1299.

Allen, K. E., E. R. Clark, and V. C. Jordan. 1980. Evidence for the metabolic activation of non-steroidal antioestrogens: a study of structure-activity relationships. *British Journal of Pharmacology* 71:83–91.

Ariens, E. J., and A. M. Simonis. 1964. A molecular basis for drug action. *Journal of Pharmacy and Pharmacology* 16:137–157.

Bannwart, C., T. Fotsis, R. Heikkinen, and H. Adlercreutz. 1984. Identification of the isoflavonic phytoestrogen daidzein in human urine. *Clinica Chimica Acta* 136:165–172.

Belleau, B. 1964. A molecular theory of drug action based on induced conformational perturbations of receptors. *Journal of Medicinal Chemistry* 7:776–784.

Bickoff, E. M., A. N. Booth, R. L. Lyman, A. L. Livingston, C. R. Thompson, and F. DeEds. 1957. Coumestrol, a new estrogen isolated from forage crops. *Science* 126:969–970.

Bickoff, E. M., A. L. Livingston, and A. N. Booth. 1964. Tricin from alfalfa—isolation and physiological activity. *Journal of Pharmaceutical Sciences* 53:1411–1412.

Black, L. J., and R. L. Goode. 1980. Uterine bioassay of tamoxifen, trioxifene and a new estrogen antagonist (LY 117018) in rats and mice. *Life Sciences* 26:1453–1458.

Black, L. J., C. D. Jones, and J. F. Falcone. 1983. Antagonism of estrogen action with a new benzothiophene-derived antiestrogen. *Life Sciences* 32:1031–1036.

Bradbury, R. B., and D. E. White. 1955. Estrogens and related substances in plants. *Vitamins and Hormones* 12:207–233.

Bulger, W. H., and D. Kupfer. 1983. Estrogenic action of DDT analogs. *American Journal of Industrial Medicine* 4:163–173.

Bulger, W. H., R. M. Muccitelli, and D. Kupfer. 1978. Studies on the *in vivo* and *in vitro* estrogenic activities of methoxychlor and its metabolites. Role of hepatic monooxygenase in methoxychlor activation. *Biochemical Pharmacology* 27:2417–2423.

Bulger, W. H., V. J. Feil, and D. Kupfer. 1985. Role of hepatic monooxygenases in generating estrogenic metabolites from methoxychlor and from its identified contaminants. *Molecular Pharmacology* 27:115–124.

Callantine, M. R., R. R. Humphrey, S. L. Lee, B. L. Windsor, N. H. Schottin, and O. P. O'Brien. 1966. Action of an estrogen antagonist on reproductive mechanisms in the rat. *Endocrinology* 79:153–169.

Campbell, N. R., E. C. Dodds, and W. Lawson. 1938a. Oestrogenic activity of dianol, a dimeride of p-propenyl-phenol. *Nature* (London) 141:78.

Campbell, N. R., E. C. Dodds, and W. Lawson, 1938b. Oestrogenic activity of anol: a highly active phenol isolated from the byproducts. *Nature* (London) 142:1121.

Chang, M. C. 1959. Degeneration of ova in the rat and rabbit following oral administration of 1-(p-2-diethylaminoethoxyphenyl)-1-phenyl-2-p-anisyl-ethanol. *Endocrinology* 65:339–342.

Cheng, E., L. Yoder, C. D. Story, and W. Burrough. 1954. Estrogenic activity of some isoflavone derivatives. *Science* 120:575–577.

Clark, A. J. 1926. The reaction between acetyl choline and muscle cells. *Journal of Physiology* 61:530–546.

Cole, M. P., C. T. A. Jones, and I. D. H. Todd. 1971. A new anti-oestrogenic agent in late breast cancer. *British Journal of Cancer* 25:270–275.

Cook, J. W., E. C. Dodds, and C. L. Hewett. 1933. A synthetic oestrus-exciting compound. *Nature* (London) 131:56.

Dix, C. J., and V. C. Jordan. 1980. Modulation of rat uterine hormone receptors by estrogen and antiestrogen. *Endocrinology* 107:2011–2020.

Dodds, E. C., and W. Lawson, 1936. Synthetic oestrogenic agents without the phenanthrene nucleus. *Nature* (London) 137:996.

Dodds, E. C., and W. Lawson. 1937a. A simple aromatic oestrogenic agent with an activity of the same order as oestrone. *Nature* (London) 139:627.

Dodds, E. C., and W. Lawson. 1937b. Oestrogenic activity of p-hydroxypropenyl-benzene (anol). *Nature* (London) 139:1068.

Dodds, E. C., L. Golberg, W. Lawson, and R. Robinson, 1938a. Oestrogenic activity of certain synthetic compounds. *Nature* (London) 141:247–248.

Dodds, E. C., L. Golberg, W. Lawson, and R. Robinson. 1938b. Oestrogenic activity of alkylated stilbestrols. *Nature* (London) 142:34.

Dodds, E. C., L. Golberg, W. Lawson, and R. Robinson. 1938c. Oestrogenic activity of esters of diethylstilbestrol. *Nature* (London) 142:211–212.

Dodds, E. C., W. Lawson, and R. L. Noble. 1938d. Biological effects of the synthetic oestrogenic substance 4:4′-dihydroxy-α:β-diethylstilbene. *Lancet* 1:1389–1391.

Duncan, G. W., S. C. Lyster, J. J. Clark, and D. Lednicer. 1963. Antifertility activities of two diphenyl-dihydronaphthalene derivatives. *Proceedings of the Society for Experimental Biology and Medicine* 112:439–442.

Eisenfeld, A. 1974. Oral contraceptives: ethinyl estradiol binds with higher affinity than mestranol to macromolecules from the sites of antifertility action. *Endocrinology* 94:803–807.

Emmens, C. W. 1971. Compounds exhibiting prolonged antioestrogenic and antifertility activity in mice and rats. *Journal of Reproduction and Fertility* 26:175–182.

European Organisation for Research on Treatment of Cancer (EORTC). 1972. Breast Cancer Group. Clinical trial of nafoxidine, an oestrogen antagonist in advanced breast cancer. *European Journal of Cancer* 8:387–389.

Farnsworth, N. R., A. S. Bingell, G. A. Cordell, F. A. Crone, and H. H. S. Fong. 1975. Potential value of plants as sources of new antifertility agents. II. *Journal of Pharmaceutical Sciences* 64:717–754.

Gaddum, J. H. 1926. The action of adrenalin and ergotamine on the uterus of the rabbit. *Journal of Physiology* 61:141–150.

Greenblatt, R. B., and N. H. Brown. 1952. The storage of estrogen in human fat after estrogen administration. *American Journal of Obstetrics and Gynecology* 63:1361–1363.

Greenblatt, R. B., S. Roy, V. B. Mahesh, W. E. Barfield, and E. C. Jungck. 1962. Induction of ovulation. *American Journal of Obstetrics and Gynecology* 84:900–912.

Hahn, D. W., J. L. McGuire, F. C. Greenslade, and G. D. Turner. 1971. Molecular parameters involved in the estrogenicity of mestranol and ethinyl estradiol. *Proceedings of the Society for Experimental Biology and Medicine* 137:1180–1185.

Hammond, B., B. S. Katzenellenbogen, N. Krauthammer, and J. McConnell. 1979. Estrogenic activity of the insecticide chlordecane (kepone) and interaction with uterine estrogen receptors. *Proceedings of the National Academy of Sciences* 76:6641–6645.

Harper, M. J. K., and A. L. Walpole. 1966. Contrasting endocrine activities of *cis* and *trans* isomers in a series of substituted triphenylethylenes. *Nature* (London) 212:87.

Harper, M. J. K., and A. L. Walpole. 1967. A new derivative of triphenylethylene: effect on implantation and mode of action in rats. *Journal of Reproduction and Fertility* 13:101–119.

Herbst, A. L., C. T. Griffiths, and R. W. Kistner. 1964. Clomiphene citrate (NSC-35770) in disseminated mammary carcinoma. *Cancer Chemotherapy Reports* 43:39–41.

Holtkamp, D. E., S. C. Greslin, C. A. Root, and L. J. Lerner. 1960. Gonadotropin inhibiting and antifercundity effects of chloramiphene. *Proceedings of the Society for Experimental Biology and Medicine* 105:197–201.

Huppert, L. C. 1979. Induction of ovulation with clomiphene citrate. *Fertility and Sterility* 31:1–8.

Ireland, J. S., V. R. Mukku, A. K. Robinsin, and G. M. Stancel. 1980. Stimulation of uterine deoxyribonucleic acid synthesis by 1,1,1-trichloro-2-(p-chlorophenyl)-2-(O-chlorophenyl)ethane(o,p'-DDT). *Biochemical Pharmacology* 24:1469–1474.

Jones, C. D., T. Suarez, E. H. Massey, L. J. Black, and F. C. Tinsley, 1979. Synthesis and antiestrogenic activity of [3,4-dihydro-2-(4-methoxyphenyl)-1-naphthenyl] [4-(2-(1-pyrrolidinyl)ethoxy)-phenyl]ethanone methanesulfane acid salt. *Journal of Medicinal Chemistry* 22:962–966.

Jordan, V. C. 1975. Prolonged antioestrogenic activity of ICI 46,474 in the ovariectomized mouse. *Journal of Reproduction and Fertility* 52:251–258.

Jordan, V. C. 1984. Biochemical pharmacology of antiestrogen action. *Pharmacological Reviews* 36:245–276.

Jordan, V. C., and B. Gosden. 1982. Importance of the alkylaminoethoxy side chain for the estrogenic and antiestrogenic actions of tamoxifen and trioxifene in the immature rat uterus. *Molecular and Cellular Endocrinology* 27:291–306.

Jordan, V. C., and B. Gosden. 1983a. Differential antiestrogen action in the immature rat uterus: a comparison of hydroxylated antiestrogens with high affinity for the estrogen receptor. *Journal of Steroid Biochemistry* 19:1249–1258.

Jordan, V. C., and B. Gosden. 1983b. Inhibition of the uterotropic activity of estrogens and antiestrogens by the short acting antiestrogen, LY 117018. *Endocrinology* 113:463–468.

Jordan, V. C., and S. Koerner. 1976. Tamoxifen as an antitumor agent: role of oestradiol and prolactin. *Journal of Endocrinology* 68:305–310.

Jordan, V. C., and M. E. Lieberman. 1984. Estrogen-stimulated prolactin synthesis *in vitro*. *Molecular Pharmacology* 26:279–285.

Jordan, V. C., M. M. Collins, L. Rowsby, and G. Prestwich. 1977. A monohydroxylated metabolite of tamoxifen with potent antioestrogenic activity. *Journal of Endocrinology* 75:305–316.

Jordan, V. C., L. Rowsby, C. J. Dix, and G. Prestwich. 1978. Dose-related effects of nonsteroidal antioestrogens and oestrogens on the measurement of cytoplasmic oestrogen receptors in the rat and mouse uterus. *Journal of Endocrinology* 78:71–81.

Jordan, V. C., B. Haldeman, and K. E. Allen. 1981. Geometric isomers of substituted triphenylethylenes and antiestrogen action. *Endocrinology* 108:1353–1361.

Jordan, V. C., M. E. Lieberman, E. Cormier, R. Koch, J. R. Bagley, and P. C. Ruenitz. 1984. Structural requirements for the pharmacological activity of nonsteroidal antiestrogens *in vitro*. *Molecular Pharmacology* 26:272–278.

Kang, Y. H., W. A. Anderson, and E. R. DeSombre. 1975. Modulation of uterine morphology and growth by estradiol-17β and estrogen antagonist. *Journal of Cell Biology* 64:682–691.

Kistner, R. W., and O. W. Smith. 1961. Observations on the use of a nonsteroidal estrogen antagonist, MER25. *Fertility and Sterility* 12:121–141.

Kupfer, D. 1975. Effects of pesticides and related compounds on steroid metabolism and function. *CRC Critical Reviews in Toxicology* 4:83–124.

Kupfer, D., and W. H. Bulger. 1976. Studies on the mechanism of estrogenic actions of o,p'DDT: Interactions with the estrogen receptor. *Pesticide Biochemistry and Physiology* 6:561–570.

Kupfer, D., and W. H. Bulger. 1979. A novel *in vitro* method for demonstrating proestrogens metabolism of methoxychlor and o,p'DDT by liver microsomes in the presence of uteri and effects on intracellular distribution of estrogen receptors. *Life Sciences* 25:975–984.

Lednicer, D., S. C. Lyster, and G. W. Duncan. 1967. Mammalian antifertility agents. IV. Basic 3,4–dihydronaphthalenes and 1,2,3,4-tetrahydro-1-naphthols. *Journal of Medicinal Chemistry* 10:78–86.

Lerner, L. J., J. F. Holthaus, and C. R. Thompson. 1958. A non-steroidal estrogen antagonist 1-(p-2-diethylaminoethoxyphenyl)-1-phenyl-2-p-methoxyphenylethanol. *Endocrinology* 63:295–318.

Lieberman, M. E., R. A. Maurer, and J. Gorski. 1978. Estrogen control of prolactin synthesis *in vitro*. *Proceedings of the National Academy of Sciences* 75:5946–5949.

Lieberman, M. E., J. Gorski, and V. C. Jordan. 1983a. An estrogen receptor model to describe the regulation of prolactin synthesis by antiestrogens *in vitro*. *Journal of Biological Chemistry* 258:4741–4745.

Lieberman, M. E., V. C. Jordan, M. Fritsch, M. A. Santos, and J. Gorski. 1983b. Direct and reversible inhibition of estradiol-stimulated prolactin synthesis by antiestrogens *in vitro*. *Journal of Biological Chemistry* 258:4734–4740.

Manni, A., B. Arafah, and O. H. Pearson. 1981. Changes in endocrine status following antioestrogen administration to premenopausal and postmenopausal women. In *Nonsteroidal antioestrogens: molecular pharmacology and antitumour activity,* ed. R. L. Sutherland and V. C. Jordan, 435–452. Sydney: Academic Press.

Martin, P. M., K. B. Horwitz, D. S. Ryan, and W. L. McGuire. 1978. Phytoestrogen interaction with estrogen receptors in human breast cancer cells. *Endocrinology* 103:1860–1867.

Nelson, J. A. 1974. Effects of dichlorodiphenyl trichloroethane (DDT) analogs and polychlorinated biphenyl (PCB) mixtures on 17β-[^{3}H] estradiol binding to rat uterine receptor. *Biochemical Pharmacology* 23:447–451.

Nelson, J. A., R. F. Struck, and R. James. 1978. Estrogenic activities of chlorinated hydrocarbons. *Journal of Toxicology and Environmental Health* 4:325–339.

Ousterhout, J., R. F. Struck, and J. A. Nelson. 1981. Estrogenic activities of methoxychlor metabolites. *Biochemical Pharmacology* 30:2869–2871.

Robson, J. M., and M. Y. Ansari. 1943. The fate of D.B.E. (α,α-di-(p-ethoxyphenyl)β-phenyl bromo-ethylene) in the body. *Journal of Pharmacology and Experimental Therapeutics* 79:340–345.

Robson, J. M., and A. Schonberg. 1937. Oestrous reactions including mating produced by triphenylethylene. *Nature* (London) 140:196.

Robson, J. M., and A. Schonberg. 1942. A new synthetic oestrogen with prolonged action when given orally. *Nature* (London) 150:22–23.

Robson, J. M., A. Schonberg, and H. A. Fahim. 1938. Duration of action of natural and synthetic oestrogens. *Nature* (London) 142:292–293.

Rose, D. P., A. H. Fischer, and V. C. Jordan. 1981. Activity of the antioestrogen trioxifene against N-nitrosomethylurea-induced rat mammary carcinomas. *European Journal of Cancer and Clinical Oncology* 17:893–898.

Segal, J. S., and W. O. Nelson. 1958. An orally active component with antifertility effects in rats. *Proceedings of the Society for Experimental Biology and Medicine* 98:431–436.

Setchell, K. D. R., S. P. Borriello, P. Hulme, D. N. Kirk, and M. Axelson. 1984. Nonsteroidal estrogens of dietary origin: possible roles in hormone-dependent disease. *American Journal of Clinical Nutrition* 40:569–578.

Shemesh, M., H. R. Lindner, and N. Ayalon. 1972. Affinity of rat uterine oestradiol receptor for phyto-oestrogens and its use in a competitive protein-binding radioassay for plasma coumestrol. *Journal of Reproduction and Fertility* 29:1–9.

Shutt, D. A. 1976. The effects of plant oestrogens on animal reproduction. *Endeavor* 35:110–113.

Shutt, D. A., and R. I. Cox. 1972. Steroid and phyto-oestrogen binding to sheep uterine receptors *in vitro*. *Journal of Endocrinology* 52:299–310.

Stephenson, R. P. 1956. A modification of receptor theory. *British Journal of Pharmacology* 11:379–392.

Sutherland, R. L., J. Mester, and E. E. Baulieu. 1977. Tamoxifen is a potent "pure" antioestrogen in the chick oviduct. *Nature* (London) 267:434–435.

Terenius, L. 1971. Structure-activity relationships of antioestrogens with regard to interaction with 17β oestradiol in the mouse uterus and vagina. *Acta Endocrinologica* Suppl. 66:431–447.

Thompson, C. R., and H. W. Werner. 1951. Studies of estrogen tri-p-anisylchloroethylene. *Proceedings of the Society for Experimental Biology and Medicine* 77:494–497.

Thompson, C. R., and H. W. Werner. 1953. Fat storage of an estrogen in women following orally administered tri-p-anisylchloroethylene. *Proceedings of the Society for Experimental Biology and Medicine* 84:491–492.

Zondek, B., and C. Bergman. 1938. Phenol methyl ethers as oestrogenic agents. *Biochemical Journal* 32:641–645.

3

Nuclear Localization of Unoccupied Estrogen Receptors

Mara E. Lieberman, Wade V. Welshons, and Jack Gorski

I. Introduction   44
II. Intracellular Distribution of the Estrogen Receptor in
GH₃ Cells   45
  A. Preparation of Cytoplasts and Nucleoplasts   45
  B. Receptor Studies in Whole Cells, Cytoplasts, and Cells +
      Nucleoplasts   48
  References   53

I. Introduction

Steroid hormones, which can enter all cells by passive diffusion from the blood stream, are retained in responsive cells by high affinity binding to specific receptor proteins, thought to be cytoplasmic. Binding of the ligand to its receptor is thought to induce a conformational change (transformation) enabling the hormone-receptor complex to move into the nucleus, resulting in an alteration in the pattern of gene expression.

This hypothetical scheme of steroid hormone receptor action, known as the translocation or two-step model, was first proposed for the estrogen receptor (Gorski et al. 1968; Jensen et al. 1968) on the basis of the observations detailed below. Following the detection of the estrogen receptor in the rat uterus (Toft and Gorski 1966), it was observed that when tissues from immature or ovariectomized animals were fractionated, most of the unoccupied receptor was found in the cytosol (Toft et al. 1967), whereas after administration of estrogen, the ligand-bound receptor was recovered in the nuclear fraction, concomitant with a loss of receptor from the cytosol (Gorski et al. 1968; Jensen et al. 1968). Autoradiographic studies were interpreted as supporting the biochemical evidence for the apparent movement of the receptor from the cytoplasm into the nucleus (Jensen et al. 1968; Stumpf 1968). Subsequently, studies were extended to numerous other steroid hormone receptor systems with similar conclusions, leading to the universal acceptance of the two-step theory of steroid hormone receptor action (Liao and Fang 1969; O'Malley et al. 1970; Wilson and Gloyna 1970).

Over the years, a number of reports have appeared in the literature which could not be easily reconciled with the two-step model. Siiteri et al. (1973) and Linkie and Siiteri (1978) presented evidence indicating that transformation of the receptor from the 4S (i.e., cytosolic) to the 5S (nuclear) form, an essential feature of the two-step hypothesis, might be taking place in the nucleus. McCormack and Glasser (1980) reported that in dispersed uterine cells, the distribution of unfilled receptor in nuclear fractions was much higher than expected. Sheridan et al. (1979) were able to localize a large proportion of estrogen receptors in the nucleus by autoradiography under nontranslocating conditions, leading them to propose an equilibrium model with unoccupied receptors in both cytoplasmic and nuclear compartments. Furthermore, Martin and Sheridan (1982) presented evidence that the predominance of cytosolic receptor may be due to dilution of homogenates during their preparation. Pietras and Szego (1979) reported that hypotonic buffers, which are usually employed in tissue homogenization, yielded receptors in the cytosol, whereas in 0.25 M sucrose, receptors partitioned predominantly with the nuclear fraction. Cell lines have been described in which unfilled estrogen receptors are nuclear in homogenized cells (Zava and McGuire 1977) until nuclei are washed and extracted more rigorously (Edwards et al. 1980).

In the absence of their ligands, receptors for thyroid hormones (Samuels and Tsai 1973; Oppenheimer et al. 1976), ecdysteroid (Yund et al. 1978), and vitamin D_3 (Walters et al. 1980) have been reported to be predominantly nuclear. It is relevant, however, that in the latter study, the salt concentration in the extraction buffer had a pronounced effect on the cytoplasmic partitioning of the vitamin D_3 receptor.

The above-cited findings lead one to conclude that "cytosolic" and "nuclear" receptors ought to be viewed as operational terms related to the techniques of cell fractionation and extraction, and that the distribution and dynamics of receptor movement in the living cell remain an unresolved issue. Recently, two different experimental methods have been employed which do not involve cell breakage with its attendant artifacts. In this report, we describe studies carried out in our laboratory in which we examined the intracellular distribution of the estrogen receptor using cytochalasin B–induced enucleation as the experimental approach. The second new approach, the immunocytochemical localization of the estrogen receptor using monoclonal antibodies to "estrophilin," is described elsewhere in this volume.

II. *Intracellular Distribution of the Estrogen Receptor in GH₃ Cells*

A. PREPARATION OF CYTOPLASTS AND NUCLEOPLASTS

Cytochalasin B-induced enucleation in several cell lines has been described in detail (Poste 1973; Bossart et al. 1975). Because of its effect on microfilament structure, cytochalasin B causes nuclei to bud out of the cytoplasm, and the separation achieved by shearing during centrifugation yields enucleated cells (cytoplasts) and a portion of cells containing the nucleus surrounded by a thin rim of cytoplasm (nucleoplasts). Both cytoplasts and nucleoplasts are bounded by an intact plasma membrane and can be fused to reform a viable cell (Veomett et al. 1974). This method was used to demonstrate that DNA polymerase α, an enzyme essential in DNA replication that is found to a variable extent in the cytosol of fractionated cells, is in fact a nuclear protein (Herrick et al. 1976).

Although many cell lines have been successfully enucleated, freshly dispersed uterine or pituitary cells, or primary cultures prepared from such cells, do not enucleate satisfactorily (Lieberman, Welshons, and Gorski, unpublished observations). We, therefore, used GH_3 cells, a clonal line derived from an estrogen-induced rat pituitary tumor (Tashjian et al. 1970). GH_3 cells contain estrogen receptor that is found in the cytosol by the usual cell disruption method (Haug et al. 1978; Noteboom et al. 1982). The specific strain used in these experiments was shown to respond to estrogen by increased prolactin synthesis (Tate et al. 1984).

For the preparation of cytoplasts and nucleoplasts, we followed the scheme shown in Figure 3.1. (For a detailed experimental protocol, see Welshons et al. 1984.) Before enucleation, a narrow density range of cells

PREPARATION OF CYTOPLASTS

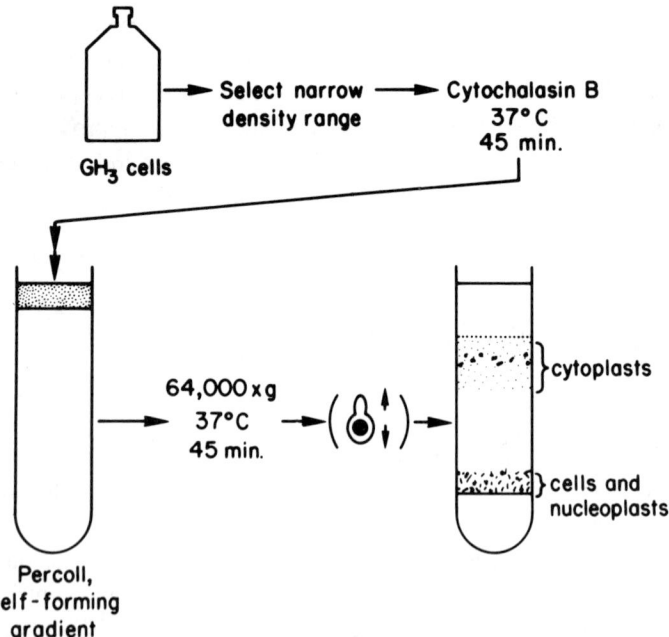

Figure 3.1. Enucleation procedure for GH_3 cells. (From Shull et al. 1985.)

was selected by centrifugation on a step gradient of Percoll. A Feulgen-stained preparation of these cells is shown in Figure 3.2A. After incubation of cells in cytochalasin-containing medium and centrifugation on a self-forming Percoll gradient, approximately 85% of the cells became enucleated, forming cytoplasts that were on average one-fifth the size of whole cells (Fig. 3.2B). This fraction contained up to 5% whole cells; however, by limiting the number of cells applied to enucleation gradient, cytoplast preparations could be obtained which contained less than 1% of contaminated whole cells. The denser layer, designated cell + nucleoplast fraction, was more heterogeneous and contained some whole cells and cells from which a varying proportion of cytoplasm was removed (Fig. 3.2C).

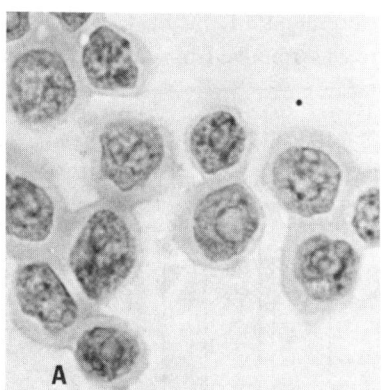
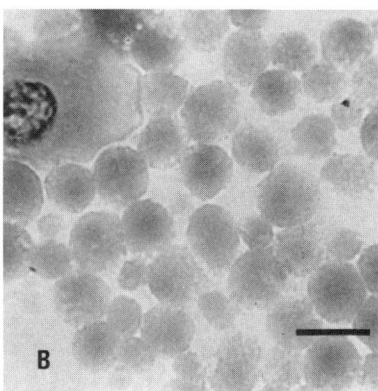

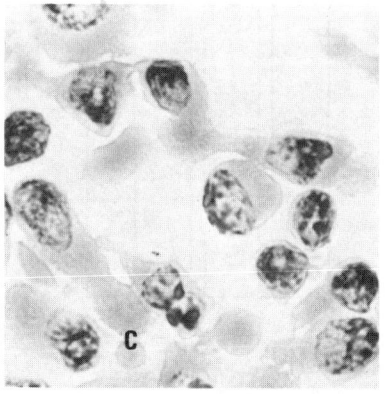

Figure 3.2. Whole GH$_3$ cells (A), cytoplasts (B), and cells + nucleoplasts (C). Bar is 10 μm. (From Welshons et al. 1984.)

B. RECEPTOR STUDIES IN WHOLE CELLS, CYTOPLASTS, AND
CELLS + NUCLEOPLASTS

The classic theory would predict that the concentration of receptor will be highest in the cytoplast fraction. In fact, we found just the opposite distribution. It can be seen in Figure 3.3 that receptor per protein is lowest in cytoplasts and slightly higher in cells + nucleoplasts, compared to whole cells, whereas receptor per DNA is similar in all cell fractions. In an experiment detailed in Table 3.1, in which the cytoplast fraction contained fewer than 1% whole cells, the concentration of receptor per protein was reduced more than 10-fold compared to whole cells. The recovery of protein, DNA, and estrogen receptor was essentially complete (Table 3.2), indicating that receptors were not selectively lost from cytoplasts during enucleation.

Since on the basis of protein measurements (Table 3.1), a fraction average of only 20% of the cytoplasm was removed by enucleation, it

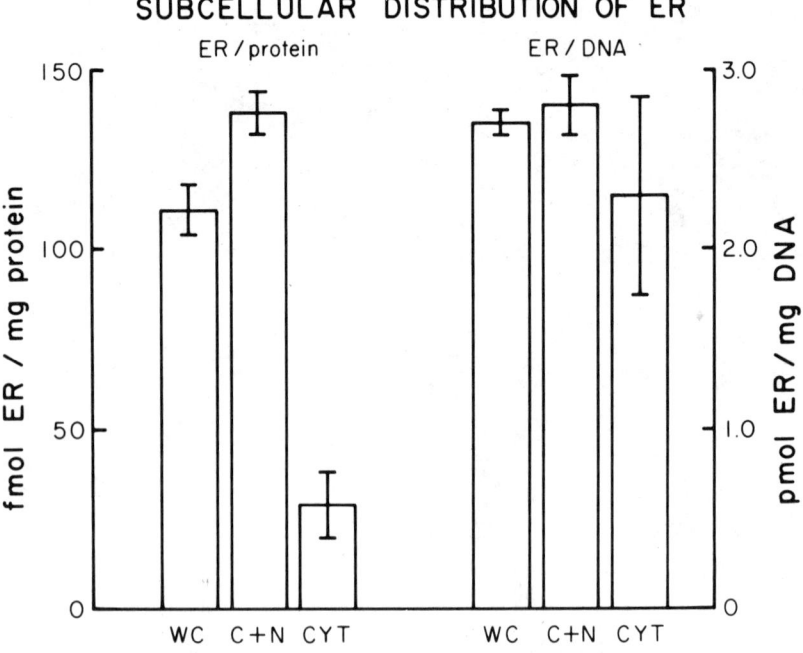

SUBCELLULAR DISTRIBUTION OF ER

Figure 3.3. Intracellular distribution of estrogen receptor (ER), in GH_3 cells. Estrogen receptor, protein, and DNA were measured in untreated density-selected whole cells (WC), in the cell + nucleoplast fraction (C+N) and the cytoplast fraction (CYT) after enucleation. (From Welshons et al. 1984.)

Table 3.1. Estrogen receptor in enucleated cells[a]

	ER/ protein (fmol/mg)	ER/ DNA (pmol/mg)	Protein/ cell (pg)	DNA/ protein (μg/mg)	ER/cell equivalent (molecules)
Whole cells	113	2.7	363	42	25,000
Cells + nucleoplasts	146	2.9	336	50	30,000
Cytoplasts	10	1.4	69	7.5	2,100[b]

From Welshons et al. 1984.
[a]Estrogen receptor per protein, per DNA, and per cell (by hemocytometer) in whole cells and enucleated cells. The cytoplast fraction contained fewer than 1% whole cells.
[b]Number of molecules per five cytoplasts, since cytoplasts are approximately one-fifth the size of whole cells.

might be argued that most of the receptor may be associated with the cytoplasm surrounding the nucleoplast. Two lines of evidence argue against this. First, by microscopic examination, it could be seen that the nucleoplast fraction contained some cells from which a much larger part of the cytoplasm was removed (Fig. 3.2C). Second, when the cell + nucleoplast fraction was subjected to further separation to obtain cells from which increasingly larger proportions of cytoplasm were removed, we found that as the density of the cells increased, so did the concentration of receptor per protein increase (Fig. 3.4). In the densest fraction (i.e., the cells containing the least amount of cytoplasm), receptor per protein had more than doubled, whereas receptor per DNA remained constant (Fig. 3.4). Thus, there was no evidence that removing most of the cytoplasm from the cells removed any unoccupied receptor.

The enucleation procedure did not appear to damage the cells. Dye-

Table 3.2. Recovery of estrogen binding, protein, and DNA after enucleation

	Total applied or recovered		
	Estrogen binding (pmol)	Protein (mg)	DNA (μg)
Before enucleation			
Whole cells	2.10	18.5	785
After enucleation			
Cells + nucleoplasts	2.26	15.5	777
Cytoplasts	0.024	2.3	18
Recovery	109%	96%	101%

From Shull et al. 1985.

DISTRIBUTION OF ESTROGEN RECEPTOR

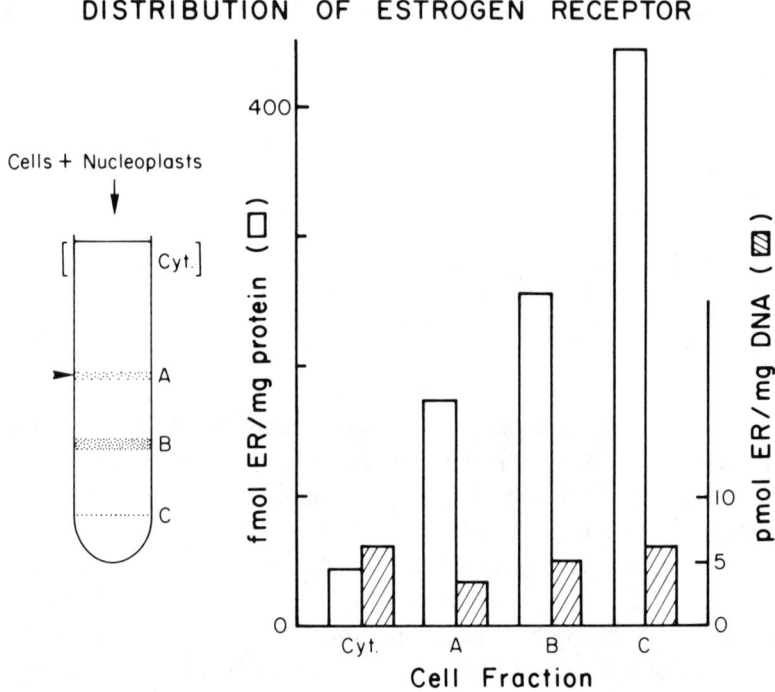

Figure 3.4. After enucleation, the cytoplasts were saved separately while the cell + nucleoplast layer was further fractionated on a density step gradient. The arrowhead at A indicates where the density-selected whole cells would have been found before enucleation, and the position that the cytoplasts would have occupied is indicated in brackets. Estrogen receptor, DNA, and protein were measured in each fraction. (From Welshons et al. 1984.)

exclusion remained high throughout the experimental period (Table 3.3), and the various cell fractions incorporated [³H]leucine into TCA-precipitable material and immunoprecipitable prolactin (Table 3.4). Cytochalasin B had no effect on the uptake of estradiol (Table 3.5), and the receptor in the cell + nucleoplast fraction was extractable into the cytosol after homogenization (Welshons et al. 1985). This confirms earlier studies with intact uteri in which cytochalasin had no effect on the uptake of estradiol, the binding, or the distribution of bound receptors in homogenized tissue (Gorski and Raker 1973).

The estrogen receptor was measured in these studies by uptake of [³H]estradiol into intact, live cells or cell fractions in order to avoid losses of receptor that would have been encountered during homogenization with the low quantity of material used. The specific uptake of estradiol was

Table 3.3. Dye exclusion of cells and fractions

	Percent excluding dye[a]	
	Initial	Final
Whole cells	97 ± 1	95 ± 1
Cells + nucleoplasts	98 ± 1	93 ± 1
Cytoplasts	98 ± 1	73 ± 4

From Shull et al. 1985.
[a]Trypan blue exclusion just after enucleation (Initial) and after measuring the receptor content by whole cell uptake at 37°C (Final). Mean ± SE, n's of 6–9.

Table 3.4. Prolactin synthesis by GH$_3$ cells and fractions[a]

	Leucine incorporation: $10^{-6} \times$ DPM/10^6 cells or equivalent	Prolactin synthesis: percent total protein synthesis
Whole cells	6.2	1.2 ± 0.02
Cells + nucleoplasts	5.7	1.3 ± 0.06
Cytoplasts	3.0[b]	3.4 ± 0.2

From Shull et al. 1985.
[a]Cells, cells + nucleoplasts, or cytoplasts were incubated with [^{3}H]leucine to measure general protein synthesis by TCA-precipitable leucine incorporation, and to measure prolactin synthesis using precipitation with antiprolactin antibody.
[b]Assuming five cytoplasts per whole cell equivalent.

Table 3.5. Effect of incubation of cells in enucleation medium on receptor content[a]

	Untreated	After incubation
Whole cell uptake	102 ± 2	98 ± 1

From Shull et al. 1985.
[a]Estrogen receptor content was measured in untreated cells and in cells incubated at 37°C for 2 hours in cytochalasin B plus solvent DMSO in Percoll. Receptor content was not significantly affected. Mean ± SE, n = 2.

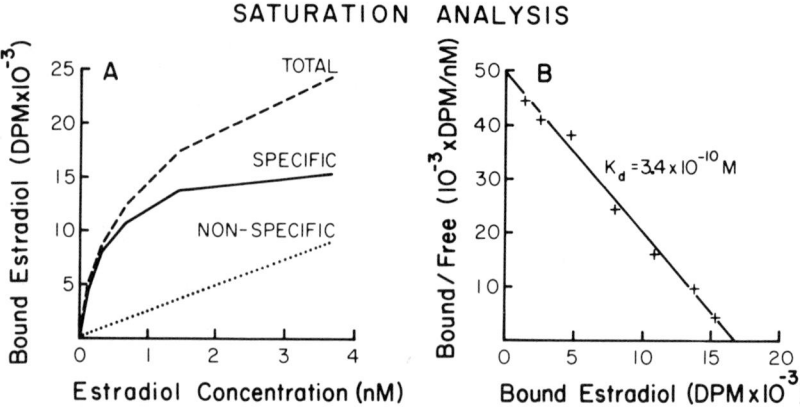

Figure 3.5. Saturation analysis of the whole cell uptake of [³H]estradiol at 37°C by GH₃ cells. (From Shull et al. 1985.)

saturable with a K_d of 3.4 × 10^{-10} M by Scatchard analysis (Fig. 3.5), and there were approximately 25,000 binding sites per cell. The linearity of the Scatchard plot in intact cells contrasts with the cooperative binding that is seen in extracts when receptor concentration is above 1 nM, as it is in intact cells (Notides et al. 1981; Sakai and Gorski 1984). We have interpreted this to suggest that in intact cells, the receptor may always be bound to some nuclear component (Gorski et al. 1984), since a soluble receptor would be expected to exhibit cooperative binding, whereas estrogen receptor immobilized on hydroxylapatite, like the receptor in intact cells, does not show this cooperativity (Sakai and Gorski 1984).

Nuclear localization of the estrogen receptor has been recently demonstrated by King and Greene (1984) and McClellan et al. (1984) by immunocytochemistry in a variety of target tissues and cells. Our data in the context of the literature cited above suggests that the unoccupied estrogen receptor is predominantly nuclear in the intact cell. We conclude that the cytosolic estrogen receptor represents a methodological artifact and that the translocation hypothesis is in error. Whether this conclusion will be applicable to other steroid hormone receptor systems remains to be established.

Acknowledgments

This work was supported by NIH grants AM-25694 (M.E.L.), 5F32-HD06008 (W.V.W.) and HD-08192 (J.G.).

References

Bossart, W., H. Loeffler and K. Bienz. 1975. Enucleation of cells by density gradient centrifugation. *Experimental Cell Research* 96:360–366.

Edwards, D. P., P. M. Martin, K. B. Horwitz, G. C. Chamness, and W. L. McGuire. 1980. Subcellular compartmentalization of estrogen receptors in human breast cancer cells. *Experimental Cell Research* 127:197–213.

Gorski, J., and B. Raker. 1973. The effects of cytochalasin B on estrogen binding and 2-deoxyglucose metabolism in the rat uterus. *Endocrinology* 93:1212–1216.

Gorski, J., D. Toft, G. Shyamala, D. Smith, and A. Notides. 1968. Hormone receptors: studies on the interaction of estrogen with the uterus. *Recent Progress in Hormone Research* 24:45–80.

Gorski, J., W. Welshons, and D. Sakai. 1984. Remodeling the estrogen receptor model. *Molecular and Cellular Endocrinology* 36:11–15.

Haug, E., O. Naess, and K. M. Gautvik. 1978. Receptors for 17β-estradiol in prolactin-secreting rat pituitary cells. *Molecular and Cellular Endocrinology* 12:81–95.

Herrick, G., B. B. Spear, and G. Veomett. 1976. Intracellular localization of mouse DNA polymerase-α. *Proceedings of the National Academy of Sciences* 73:1136–1139.

Jensen, E. V., T. Suzuki, T. Kawashima, W. E. Stumpf, P. W. Jungblut, and E. DeSombre. 1968. A two-step mechanism for the interaction of estradiol with rat uterus. *Proceedings of the National Academy of Sciences* 59:632–638.

King, W. J., and G. L. Greene. 1984. Monoclonal antibodies localize oestrogen receptor in the nuclei of target cells. *Nature* (London) 307:745–747.

Liao, S., and S. Fang. 1969. Receptor-proteins for androgens and the mode of action of androgens on gene transcription in ventral prostate. *Vitamins and Hormones* 27:17–90.

Linkie, D. M., and P. K. Siiteri. 1978. A re-examination of the interaction of estradiol with target cell receptors. *Journal of Steroid Biochemistry* 9:1071–1078.

Martin, P. M., and P. J. Sheridan. 1982. Towards a new model for the mechanism of action of steroids. *Journal of Steroid Biochemistry* 16:215–229.

McClellan, M. C., N. B. West, D. E. Tacha, G. L. Greene, and R. M. Brenner. 1984. Immunocytochemical localization of estrogen receptors in the macaque reproductive tract with monoclonal antiestrophilins. *Endocrinology* 114:2002–2014.

McCormack, S. A., and S. R. Glasser. 1980. Differential response of individual uterine cell types from immature rats treated with estradiol. *Endocrinology* 106:1634–1649.

Noteboom, W. D., J. B. Durham, and R. Mitra. 1982. Variations in the levels of estrogen receptors in prolactin producing pituitary tumor cells. *Journal of Steroid Biochemistry* 16:633–638.

Notides, A. C., N. Lerner, and D. E. Hamilton. 1981. Positive cooperativity of the estrogen receptor. *Proceedings of the National Academy of Sciences* 78:4926–4930.

O'Malley, B. W., M. R. Sherman, and D. O. Toft. 1970. Progesterone "receptors" in the cytoplasm and nucleus of chick oviduct target tissue. *Proceedings of the National Academy of Sciences* 67:501–508.

Oppenheimer, J. H., H. L. Schwartz, M. I. Surks, D. Koerner, and W. H. Dillman. 1976. Nuclear receptors and the initiation of thyroid hormone action. *Recent Progress in Hormone Research* 32:529–565.

Pietras, R. J., and C. N. Szego. 1979. Estrogen receptors in uterine plasma membrane. *Journal of Steroid Biochemistry* 11:1471–1483.

Poste, G. 1973. Anucleate mammalian cells: applications in cell biology and virology. *Methods in Cell Biology* 7:211–249.

Sakai, D., and J. Gorski. 1984. Estrogen receptor transformation to a high-affinity state without subunit-subunit interactions. *Biochemistry* 23:3541–3547.

Samuels, H. H., and J. S. Tsai. 1973. Thyroid hormone action in cell culture: demonstration of nuclear receptors in intact cells and isolated nuclei. *Proceedings of the National Academy of Sciences.* 70:3488–3492.

Sheridan, P. J., J. M. Buchanan, V. C. Anselmo, and P. M. Martin. 1979. Equilibrium: the intracellular distribution of steroid receptors. *Nature* (London) 282:579–582.

Shull, J. D., W. V. Welshons, M. E. Lieberman, and J. Gorski. 1985. The rat pituitary estrogen receptor: role of the nuclear receptor in the regulation of transcription of the prolactin gene and the nuclear localization of the unoccupied receptor. In *Molecular mechanisms of hormone action: recent advances*, ed. V. K. Moudgil, 539–562. Berlin: Walter de Gruyter.

Siiteri, P. K., B. E. Schwartz, I. Moriyama, R. Ashby, D. Linkie, and P. C. MacDonald. 1973. Estrogen binding in the rat and human. *Advances in Experimental Medicine and Biology* 36:97–112.

Stumpf, W. E. 1968. Subcellular distribution of ^{3}H-estradiol in rat uterus by quantitative autoradiography: a comparison between ^{3}H-estradiol and ^{3}H-norethynodrel. *Endocrinology* 83:777–782.

Tashjian, A. H., Jr., F. C. Bancroft, and L. Levine. 1970. Production of both prolactin and growth hormone by clonal strains of rat pituitary tumor cells: differential effects of hydrocortisone and tissue extracts. *Journal of Cell Biology* 47:61–70.

Tate, A. C., M. E. Lieberman, and V. C. Jordan. 1984. The inhibition of prolactin synthesis in GH$_3$ rat pituitary tumor cells by monohydroxytamoxifen is associated with changes in the properties of the estrogen receptor. *Journal of Steroid Biochemistry* 20:391–395.

Toft, D. O., and J. Gorski. 1966. A receptor molecule for estrogens: isolation from the rat uterus and preliminary characterizations. *Proceedings of the National Academy of Sciences* 55:1574–1581.

Toft, D., G. Shyamala, and J. Gorski. 1967. A receptor molecule for estrogens: studies using a cell-free system. *Proceedings of the National Academy of Sciences* 57:1740–1743.

Veomett, G., D. M. Prescott, J. Shay, and K. R. Porter. 1974. Reconstruction of mammalian cells from nuclear and cytoplasmic components separated by treatment with cytochalasin B. *Proceedings of the National Academy of Sciences* 71:1999–2002.

Walters, M. R., W. Hunziker, and A. W. Norman. 1980. Unoccupied 1,25-dihydroxyvitamin D$_3$ receptors: nuclear/cytosol ratio depends on ionic strength. *Journal of Biological Chemistry* 255:6799–6805.

Welshons, W. V., M. E. Lieberman, and J. Gorski. 1984. Nuclear localization of unoccupied oestrogen receptors. *Nature* (London) 307:747–749.

Welshons, W. V., B. M. Krummel, and J. Gorski. 1985. Nuclear localization of unoccupied receptors for glucocorticoids, estrogens and progesterone in GH$_3$ cells. *Endocrinology* 117:2140–2147.

Wilson, J. D., and E. R. Gloyna. 1970. The intranuclear metabolism of testosterone in the accessory organs of reproduction. *Recent Progress in Hormone Research* 26:309–336.

Yund, M. A., D. S. King, and J. W. Fristrom. 1978. Ecdysteroid receptors in imaginal discs of *Drosophilia melanogaster*. *Proceedings of the National Academy of Sciences* 75:6039–6043.

Zava, D. T., and W. L. McGuire. 1977. Estrogen receptor: unoccupied sites in nuclei of a breast tumor cell line. *Journal of Biological Chemistry* 252:3703–3708.

4

Multiple Binding Sites for Estrogen in Target Tissues

Barry M. Markaverich, James H. Clark, R. R. Roberts, and M. A. Alejandro

I.	Introduction	56
II.	Detection and Measurement of Inhibitor Activity	56
III.	Chromatography of Uterine Cytosol Inhibitor Activity	61
IV.	Comparison of LH-20 Elution Profiles of Inhibitor Activity from Normal and Malignant Tissues	63
V.	Purification and Characterization of the Endogenous Inhibitor	64
VI.	Discussion and Conclusions	67
	References	71

I. Introduction

Estrogen administration to immature or mature ovariectomized rats sets in motion a number of biochemical events associated with the stimulation of true uterine growth. These events include hormone binding to the estrogen receptor (type I sites), translocation of receptor-estrogen complexes to the nucleus (Shyamala and Gorski 1967; Jensen et al. 1971), and the stimulation or activation of nuclear type II sites (Markaverich and Clark 1979; Markaverich et al. 1981a,b,c) The precise role of type I or type II sites in estrogen action is unknown. However, we have demonstrated that antagonism of uterotrophic responses to estrogen is associated with the inhibition of the nuclear type II sites. This is the case for steroid antagonists such as dexamethasone and progesterone (Markaverich et al. 1981a) and triphenylethylene derivatives such as nafoxidine and clomiphene (Markaverich et al. 1981b).

In this chapter we summarize our recent work (Markaverich et al. 1983) which demonstrates the presence of an endogenous inhibitor of [^{3}H]estradiol binding to nuclear type II sites. We will show that this inhibitor is specific for nuclear type II sites and does not interfere with [^{3}H]estradiol binding to cytoplasmic or nuclear estrogen receptors. This material has been purified by high-performance liquid chromatography (HPLC) and analyzed by gas-liquid chromatography–mass spectrometry. On the basis of two derivatization procedures, we feel the activity is phenanthrenelike in nature with a molecular weight of approximately 300.

II. Detection and Measurement of Inhibitor Activity

The presence of an inhibitor for the binding of [^{3}H]estradiol to type II sites was first considered when we observed that the quantity of type II measured by [^{3}H]estradiol exchange sites increased as uterine nuclear fractions were diluted (Fig. 4.1 and Markaverich et al. 1983). These data show that with dilution (40 mg/ml to 10 mg/ml), specific [^{3}H]estradiol binding to nuclear type II sites increases even though the quantity of nuclei in the incubation mixture is decreased 2- to 4-fold. Expression of the data on a per uterine basis demonstrates that the quantities of nuclear type II

56

sites measured at the lower nuclear concentrations (10 and 20 mg/ml) are at least 3- to 4-fold greater than levels measured at 40 mg/ml. Although these binding curves appear to show that type I sites (0.4–8.0 nm [³H]estradiol) are also increased concurrently with dilution, we will show later that this is not the case. These apparent increases in receptor estimates are due only to an increasing influence of the type II site on the assay of type I sites, as we have described previously (Markaverich et al. 1981c).

These results suggest that the increased quantities of type II sites measured in more dilute nuclear fractions may result from dilution of a specific inhibitor of binding of [³H]estradiol to nuclear type II sites. To examine this possibility further, various dilutions of cytosol or equivalent

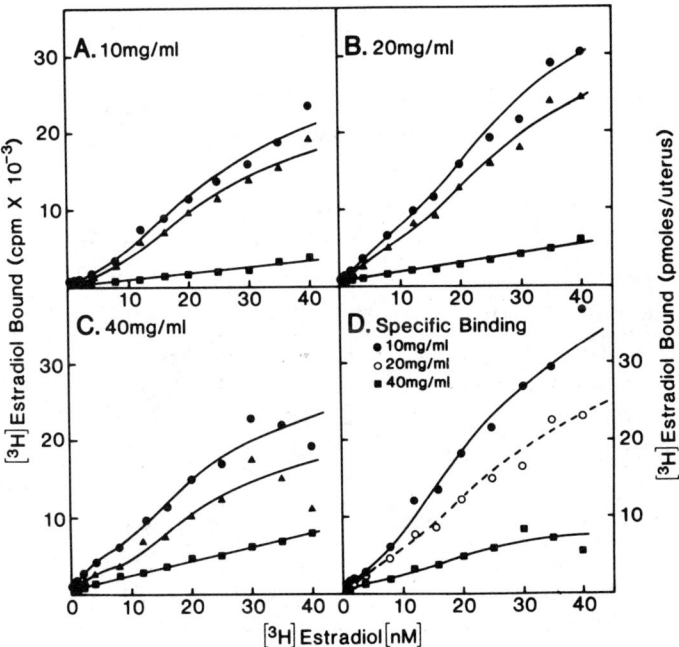

Figure 4.1. Effect of dilution on [³H]estradiol binding in uterine nuclear fractions from 17β-estradiol implanted (4 mg × 96 hrs) adult ovariectomized rats. Specific binding (▲; A–C) was determined by subtraction of nonspecific binding (■; A–C; noncompetable with 300-fold excess diethylstibestrol) from the total quantity (●; A–C) of [³H]estradiol bound. Panel D represents the specific binding measured at 10, 20, or 40 mg nuclear equivalents per ml (A–C) corrected for the dilution effect (pmols/uterus). See Markaverich et al. (1983) for details.

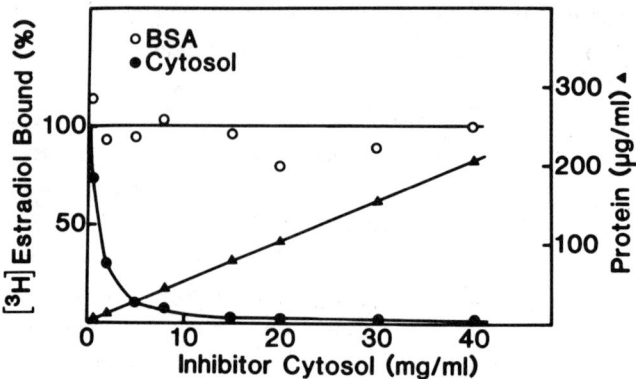

Figure 4.2. Effects of bovine serum albumin (O; BSA) and uterine cytosol (●) on [³H]estradiol binding to nuclear type II sites. Dilute (10 mg/ml) uterine nuclear fractions from estradiol-implanted rats (see legend to Fig. 4.1) were mixed with the indicated concentration of BSA or uterine cytosol. [³H]Estradiol binding to nuclear type II sites was determined by [³H]estradiol exchange (40 nM [³H]estradiol ± DES) at 4°C × 60′.

concentrations of bovine serum albumin (BSA) were incubated with uterine nuclei from estradiol-implanted rats containing large quantities of type II sites. The results of these experiments demonstrate (Fig. 4.2) that the addition of increasing concentrations of cytosol to the nuclear suspension decreases, in a hyperbolic fashion, the specific binding of [³H]estradiol to nuclear type II sites. Under these assay conditions (4°C × 60′) the type I site is not measured, since these sites are occupied by endogenous estrogen released by the beeswax pellet implant (Markaverich and Clark 1979) and [³H]estradiol exchange does not occur at 4°C. Even when diluted 20-fold (2 mg/ml), uterine cytosol reduced [³H]estradiol binding to nuclear type II sites by 70%, and 100% inhibition was observed with concentrations of cytosol above 15 mg/ml. The inhibition was not directly related to protein concentration, which decreased linearly with dilution, as would be expected. In addition, concentrations of BSA which were identical to the protein concentration measured in cytosol (200 μg/ml) did not inhibit [³H]estradiol binding to nuclear type II sites. These results suggest that uterine cytosol contains a specific inhibitor of [³H]estradiol binding to nuclear type II, and on the basis of the data presented in Figure 4.3, we feel this inhibition is probably of a competitive nature. However, since type II sites appear to bind [³H]estradiol in a cooperative manner (Fig. 4.1; sigmoidal saturation curve), interpretation of these competitive experiments is very complex. It is therefore also possible that estradiol and

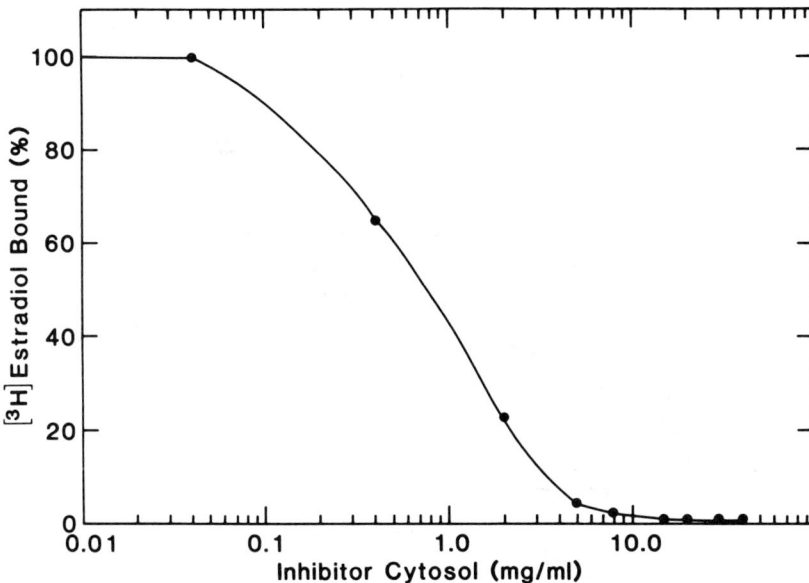

Figure 4.3. Semilogarithmic plot of cytosol (●) inhibition data in Figure 4.2.

the inhibitor molecule are binding to separate sites on the type II molecule.

The data presented in Figure 4.4 show the effects of dilution on the measurement of cytoplasmic and nuclear type I sites and suggest that the inhibitor does not interact with the estrogen receptor. Regardless of the dilution of these components in the exchange assays, identical quantities of cytoplasmic and nuclear estrogen receptors were measured when the data were corrected (pmols/uterus) for dilution. More direct evidence was provided by experiments in which cytoplasmic or nuclear type I sites were measured in the presence of various dilutions (1–1000-fold) of cytosol (0.04–40 mg/ml) containing this inhibitor activity (Fig. 4.4C). These experiments demonstrate that the addition of cytosol, which contains inhibitor activity for nuclear type II sites, to preparations of cytoplasmic or nuclear type I sites did not inhibit [³H]estradiol binding to the estrogen receptor. However, this same inhibitor preparation completely blocked estradiol binding to nuclear type II sites (Fig. 4.4C: △).

To determine whether cytoplasmic levels of inhibitor activity are modulated by estrogen, we prepared cytosol from ovariectomized controls (○) or estradiol-implanted rats (4 mg for 96 hours; ●) or ovariectomized-

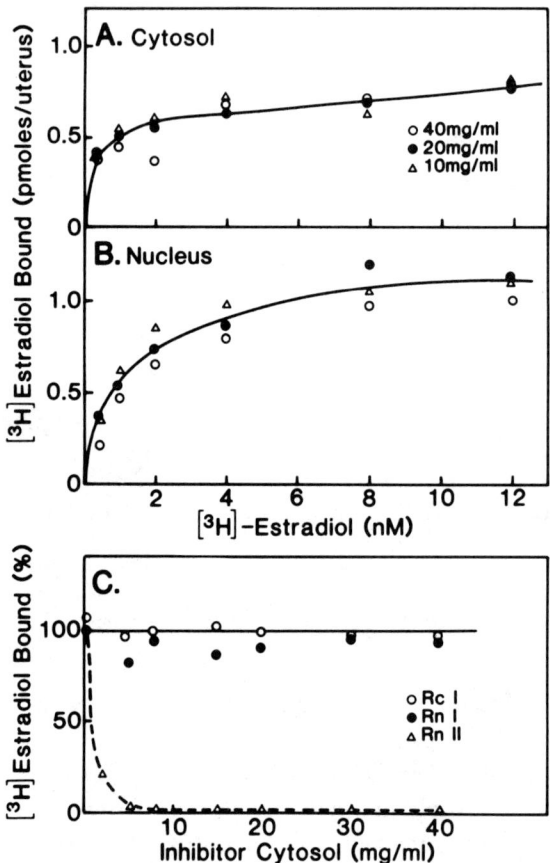

Figure 4.4. Effects of dilution (A and B) and cytosol inhibitor preparations (C) on [³H]estradiol binding to cytoplasmic and nuclear estrogen receptor (type I sites). Binding assays were performed as described in Figure 4.1 and in Markaverich et al. (1983).

adrenalectomized animals (△), diluted these cytosols to equivalent concentrations (mg fresh tissue/ml), and assayed them for inhibitor activity (Fig. 4.5). The results show that the inhibition curves for all three preparations were very similar and suggest that estradiol treatment does not change cytoplasmic levels of inhibitor activity. Likewise, the experiments with uterine cytosol from ovariectomized or adrenalectomized-ovariectomized rats (Fig. 4.5), or animals treated with progesterone or dexamethasone (not shown), as previously described (Markaverich et al. 1981a), suggest that cytoplasmic inhibitor levels are not modulated by ovarian or adrenal steroids.

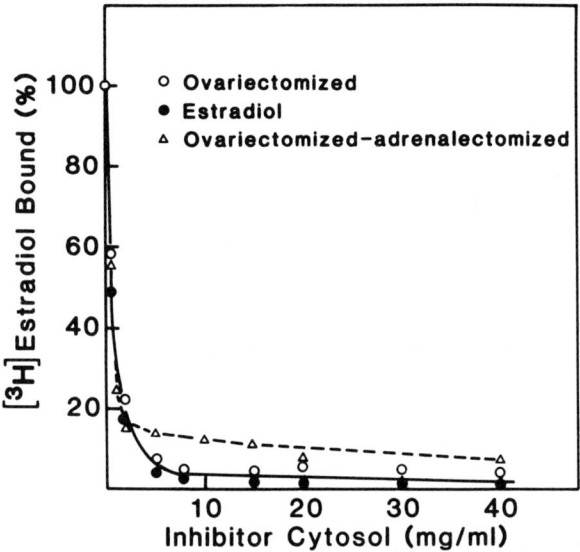

Figure 4.5. Effects of uterine cytosol inhibitor preparations from ovariectomized controls (○) or 96-hour 4 mg estradiol-implanted rats (●) or ovariectomized-adrenalectomized (△) animals (7–10 days) on [³H]estradiol binding to nuclear type II sites.

III. *Chromatography of Uterine Cytosol Inhibitor Activity*

Chromatography of boiled-acid precipitated cytosol from adult ovariectomized rat uteri on Sephadex G-25 revealed two major peaks of inhibitor activity, which we designated α and β (Fig. 4.6). This activity was measured in the column fractions by their ability to inhibit the binding of [³H]estradiol to nuclear type II sites. A minor peak of activity was also seen in the void volume of the column, which is apparently associated with protein, since there was a significant OD_{280} reading in these fractions. In addition, incubation of the cytosol inhibitor preparation with 0.4 KCl for 60 minutes at 4°C prior to chromatography on Sephadex G-25 (Tris-EDTA [TE] buffer containing 0.4 M KCl) dissociated the inhibitor activity from the void volume fractions (data not shown).

On the basis of sizing experiments using tryptophan (mol wt 204.2) and ATP (mol wt 507.2) as markers, we estimated that the molecular weight of the α and β inhibitor components is in the range of 300–400. Surprisingly, chromatography of an aliquot of this same cytosol preparation on LH-20 (Fig. 4.6B) shows that the two components are more clearly resolved. To determine if the order of elution of the α and β peaks

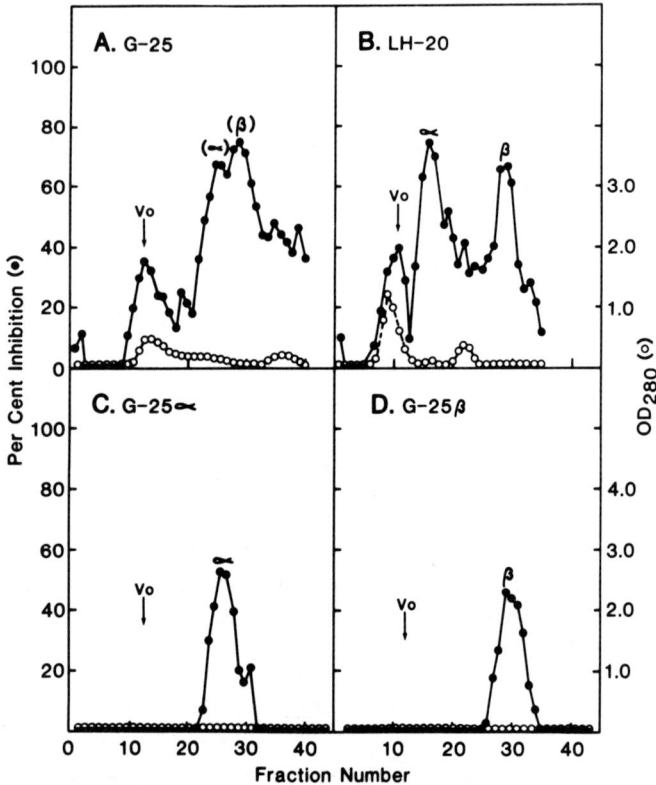

Figure 4.6. Chromatography of rat uterine cytosol inhibitor preparations on Sephadex G-25 (A, C, D) or LH-20 columns. See Markaverich et al. (1983) for details.

on LH-20 chromatography was analagous to their behavior on Sephadex G-25, we collected the individual α and β peak fractions from LH-20 and rechromatographed these fractions on the Sephadex G-25 column (Fig. 4.6C, D). The results demonstrate that the α and β peaks eluted from LH-20 columns correspond to the α and β peak material on Sephadex G-25. Chromatography of cytosol preparations on larger preparative LH-20 columns facilitates complete separation of the α and β peak fraction due to the selective retention of the β material and this has greatly facilitated purification of this inhibitor activity (see Section V).

IV. Comparison of LH-20 Elution Profiles of Inhibitor Activity from Normal and Malignant Tissues

Since nuclear type II sites may be involved in the mechanisms by which estrogens cause cell growth (Markaverich and Clark 1979; Markaverich et al. 1981a), we reasoned that perhaps this inhibitor may play a role in modulating these cellular responses. If this were the case, then rapidly proliferating neoplastic tissues which respond to estrogen might show deficiencies in inhibitor activity. To examine this possibility we prepared boiled-acid precipitated cytosol from rat uterus, normal lactating rat mammary gland, and estrogen-induced rat mammary tumors, and then chromatographed aliquots of these cytosols on LH-20. Individual fractions were assayed for inhibitor activity. These data show that the larger LH-20 column (1.0 × 50 cm; 75 ml bed volume) used for these experiments clearly separated the α and β inhibitor peaks (Fig. 4.7) in rat uterine cytosol (○). Furthermore, although rat mammary tumor cytosol contained approximately equivalent quantities of the α peak material, the tumors contained little of the β component (Fig. 4.7) and in some cases the β inhibitor component was nonmeasurable. This was in sharp contrast to the inhibitor preparations from normal lactating rat mammary glands (Fig. 4.8), which contained the α and particularly high qualities of the β peak inhibitor material.

This observation has also been extended to mouse mammary tumors and human breast cancer (Markaverich et al. 1984). Detailed studies by dilution analysis (Figs. 4.1–4.3) and LH-20 chromatography showed that mouse mammary gland contained 20-fold more inhibitor activity than mammary tumors in the same strain of animals. This difference in activity appears to result from a primary deficiency in the β inhibitor peak material (Markaverich et al. 1984). In addition, we have completed a series of mixing experiments where cytosol inhibitor preparations from uterus and tumor (Fig. 4.7) were mixed prior to LH-20 chromatography. The results of these experiments demonstrated that the β inhibitor component in uterine cytosol was quantitatively recovered (data not shown) following chromatography. These results suggest that the tumor cytosol is indeed deficient in the β inhibitor component, and the low levels of this molecule in tumor cytosol (as compared to uterus) is not due to some intrinsic degradation during the preparation. At present we do not know whether there is a precursor-product relationship between α and β inhibitor peaks (since

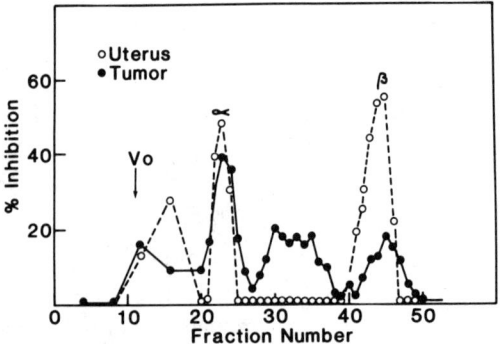

Figure 4.7. Comparison of LH-20 elution profiles from acid-precipitated-boiled cytosol preparations (100 fresh tissue equivalents mg/ml) from rat uterus (○) or an estrogen-induced rat mammary tumor (●). See Markaverich (1984) for details.

they are of very similar molecular weight) (Fig. 4.6C, D) and the tumor cannot readily form the β material (compare Fig. 4.7 and 4.8), or if perhaps the tumors metabolize this β inhibitor component. Certainly the inhibitor activity in fractions 28–38 (Fig. 4.7) suggests that there is an altered form of inhibitor in tumors which is not observed in the uterus. Whether this activity (fractions 28–38) represents an altered or metabolized form of the β peak material in tumors (Fig. 4.7) remains to be resolved. However, preliminary experiments indicate that the presence of the β peak material in crude inhibitor preparations is associated with biological activity. Acid-precipitated-boiled cytosol inhibitor preparations from rat uterus of liver (containing α and β inhibitor components) inhibit the growth of rat mammary tumor cells and MCF-7 human breast cancer in culture by approximately 80–90% in 16 hours. Conversely, inhibitor preparations from rat mammary tumors (contain α but lack the β inhibitor component) had no significant effect on cell growth in identical experiments continued for 3–4 weeks. These results suggest that the absence of the β inhibitor peak material in tumors is correlated with rapid cell proliferation in these populations.

V. Purification and Characterization of the Endogenous Inhibitor

As stated earlier, positive structural identification of the inhibitor activity (LH-20 β peak component) remains to be established. However HPLC analysis (Fig. 4.9) showed that a major peak of inhibitor activity can be eluted from the silica column. This experiment has been repeated a num-

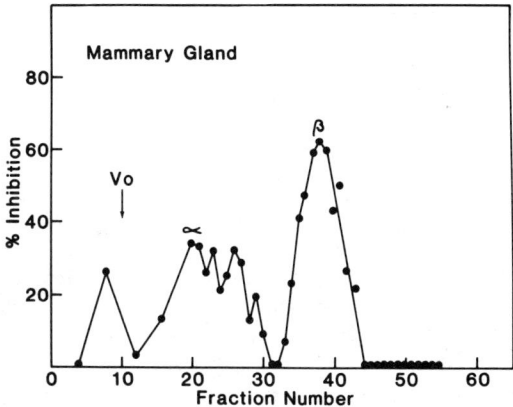

Figure 4.8. LH-20 elution profile of inhibitor activity from normal lactating mammary gland (day 2, postpartum).

ber of times on 3–4 separate liver preparations and the activity consistently elutes 5–6 minutes following injection. The samples at this point are very clean, since we observe a single peak of UV absorbance at 254 nM that is coincident with the inhibitor activity. As shown in Figure 4.9, the peak is somewhat broad and appears to have shoulders, suggesting multiple inhibitor components which are not separated. To date we have tried a number of HPLC procedures to separate these components (various elution conditions; reinjection of peak fractions) and we cannot further separate these components on a straight phase column.

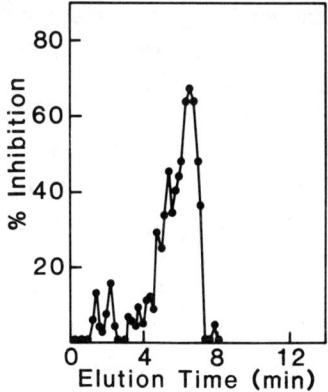

Figure 4.9. HPLC of a purified preparation of the β-inhibitor component from rat liver. Purified inhibitor (Markaverich et al. 1983) was chromatographed on a silica gel column using hexane:isopropanol (30:70) containing 0.5% acetonitrile as an eluent at a flow rate of 1 ml per minute. Fractions (0.2 minute) were collected, dried under nitrogen, and aliquots (1/10) assayed for inhibitor activity.

I. Chemistry and Biochemistry

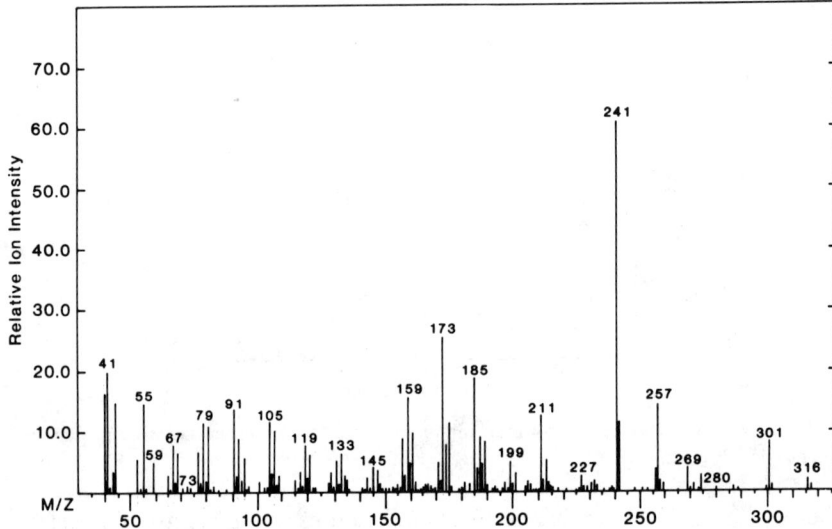

Figure 4.10. Mass spectrum of putative inhibitor molecule. An aliquot of the pooled diazomethane derivatized HPLC fractions of inhibitor activity (Fig. 4.9) was injected into a Finnegin 400 series GC-MS containing a silica capillary column (25 meter) coated with SE-54 utilizing helium (10 ml/min) as a carrier gas using a temperature program (100–280°C/minute).

This heterogeneity of putative inhibitor molecules was supported by gas chromatography–mass spectrometry (GC-MS) analysis. The GC-MS analysis of the pooled HPLC fractions (5.4–5.8 minutes; Fig. 4.9) positively identified a number of fatty acids as major components in the sample inhibitor preparations. However, these are unlikely candidates for the inhibitor, since the authentic compounds did not inhibit [³H]estradiol binding to type II sites over a wide range of concentrations (0.001 nM to 100 μM). The putative inhibitor activity appears to be associated with two remaining components in the sample. The mass spectrum for the major one of these components is shown in Figure 4.10. The molecular weight of this putative inhibitor molecule is 302 (molecular ion = 316 minus 14, due to methylation) when the mass of the diazomethane (14 atomic mass units [AMU]) is accounted for. Similarly, the spectrum for the remaining component was identical to that shown in Figure 4.10, except that the molecular ion was 318 AMU, suggesting molecular weight of this component to be 304. Comparison of sample spectra (Fig. 4.10) to those of known compounds in the National Institutes of Health bureau of standards library suggests that the inhibitor is very similar to phenanthrenelike molecules. We are currently working to improve the HPLC separation (gradient elution) in order to eliminate the fatty acid contaminants and obtain a homogeneous inhibitor preparation. Once this is accomplished, GC-MS analysis of diazomethane and trimethylsilane (Tmsi) derivatives will be compared to data obtained from direct probe insertion mass spectrometry (chemistry ionization; electron impact) and nuclear magnetic resonance studies for structural confirmation. Confirmation of identical molecular weights by probe insertion techniques and GC-MS data will also verify that we are observing the inhibitor molecule on GC-MS, since it is possible—although unlikely—that the molecule may not volatilize under the present conditions. However, it is likely that the phenanthrenelike diazomethane-derivatized molecule is the inhibitor, since we observed that diazomethane derivatization of the inhibitor preparation also destroys its biological activity (inhibition of [³H]estradiol binding to nuclear type II sites; data not shown).

VI. Discussion and Conclusions

These experiments demonstrate that the adult ovariectomized rat uterus and a variety of rat tissues contain an inhibitor which interferes with [³H]estradiol binding to type II sites in uterine nuclei. This inhibitor is specific for nuclear type II sites and does not interfere with estrogen binding to cytoplasmic or nuclear estrogen receptor (Fig. 4.3). Consequently, if this inhibitor is involved in the modulation of estrogenic response in target tissues, its effects are expressed through an interaction with nuclear type II sites. We currently feel that this molecule represents an endogenous ligand for type II sites (Markaverich et al. 1983, 1984).

Preliminary characterization of this inhibitor in rat uterine cytosol demonstrates that this molecule(s) is stable to heat (100°C × 60'), and 0.1 N HCl, and therefore it is unlikely to be protein in nature. In addition, trypsin and proteinase K do not destroy its activity (data not shown), and the inhibitor activity chromatographs on Sephadex G-25 or LH-20 (Fig. 4.7) as two major peaks with an estimated molecular weight of ~ 350. We have purified the β peak material from rat liver (which appears identical to that seen in the uterus) by thin-layer chromatography and HPLC, and it appears to consist of two nearly identical phenanthrenelike compounds with molecular weights on the basis of mass spectrometry of 302 and 304 (Fig. 4.10). Proof that these are in fact the inhibitor molecules awaits purification to homogeneity, structural identification, and demonstration that the "identified" material has equivalent biological activity. At the present time we feel these phenanthrene derivatives are good candidates for the inhibitor activity, since the only other measurable compounds in the sample preparation (free fatty acids) did not inhibit [³H]estradiol binding to nuclear type II sites. Although one could argue that if the putative inhibitor competes for [³H]estradiol binding to nuclear type II sites it should also compete for [³H]estradiol binding to the estrogen receptor, this is not necessarily the case. Nuclear type II sites do not bind triphenylethylene derivatives (antiestrogens) even though these compounds bind to the estrogen receptor (Markaverich et al. 1981c). Likewise, nuclear type II sites also appear to bind this inhibitor with amazing specifity, whereas we have been unable to show that this inhibitor interacts with the estrogen receptor (Fig. 4.3). Certainly, if the inhibitor were associated with the estrogen receptor *in vivo* we would have observed a dilution effect on binding (Fig. 4.3A) or direct inhibition of [³H]estradiol binding to type I sites in the direct competition experiments (Markaverich et al. 1981a). It is also possible that if we were able to obtain milligram amounts of the inhibitor, competition for [³H]estradiol binding to type I sites would be observed with pharmacological concentrations (mM). Our data demonstrate that at physiological concentrations (Fig. 4.3) this interaction is unlikely.

Since we have not been able to assess the effects of this inhibitor activity directly *in vivo*, it is very difficult at this early time to describe any direct role for this compound in estrogen action. These experiments await chemical identification of the inhibitor. Once a positive identification has been made, determination of its biological significance *in vivo* should be straightforward. Preliminary experiments *in vitro*, however, are very promising. It appears that there is a deficiency in the β inhibitor component in rat mammary tumor cytosol (Fig. 4.7) as compared to normal uterus (Fig. 4.7) and lactating mammary gland (Fig. 4.8). In experiments to be presented elsewhere, we have observed that inhibitor preparations from rat mammary tumors (Fig. 4.8) which were deficient in the β peak material did not inhibit growth of uterine stromal and myometrial cells, rat mammary tumor cells, and MCF-7 human breast cancer in culture. In contrast, inhibitor preparations from uterus or liver which contain the β peak material reduced cell numbers by 95% following 4–16 hours of treatment. Whether or not this inhibition of cell growth in culture results from an acceleration of cell death, or an inhibition of cell division, or both, remains to be resolved. We are currently initiating more definitive experiments with the HPLC-purified β peak material to answer these questions.

Although the physiological significance of this inhibitor remains to be resolved, we speculate at this time that the inhibitor may act to modify or regulate uterotrophic responses to estrogen or perhaps act in a "protective" capacity in cases of hyperestrogenization. Such hypotheses are consistent with our current knowledge concerning a possible role for nuclear type II sites in estrogen action. We have shown that these secondary nuclear estrogen binding sites are activated or stimulated in the nucleus only under conditions which cause uterine hypertrophy, hyperplasia, and DNA synthesis (Markaverich and Clark 1979; Markaverich et al. 1981a,b,c). Furthermore, dexamethasone and progesterone antagonism of uterine growth in the rat is associated with an inhibition of estrogen stimulation of nuclear type II sites (Markaverich et al 1981a) and these antagonists do not affect the normal functions of the estrogen receptor. On the basis of these experiments we have suggested that nuclear type II sites may be involved in estrogen action. Since nuclear type II estrogen binding sites appear to be localized on the nuclear matrix (Clark and Markaverich 1982), which has been implicated in DNA replication (Pardoll et al. 1980), we feel this inhibitor activity may modulate or block estrogen-induced DNA synthesis by inhibiting estrogen stimulation of these secondary nuclear estrogen binding sites. Structural identification of the inhibitor molecule will aid in the determination of the precise function of type II sites in estrogen action. These studies, it is hoped, will lead to an understanding of the intracellular mechanisms by which endogenous substances may modulate estrogenic responses in estrogen target tissues.

Perhaps the failure of estrogen to stimulate cell growth (hyperplasia; DNA synthesis) in estrogen target tissues such as the pituitary and hypothalamus (Kelner and Peck 1981) is related to the inability of estrogen to modulate the activity of this inhibitor in these tissues. Certainly, the failure of estrogen to stimulate nuclear type II sites in these estrogen target organs makes this a tenable hypothesis. Our findings that rat (Fig. 4.7) and mouse mammary tumors and human breast cancer (Markaverich et al. 1984) contain significantly lower levels ($\sim$ 15–20-fold) of this inhibitor activity, which is correlated with a deficiency in the β peak component (Fig. 4.7), is consistent with this hypothesis. Likewise, nuclear type II sites appear to be permanently activated in ovarian-dependent (Watson and Clark 1980) or independent (Watson et al. 1980; Markaverich et al. 1984) mouse mammary tumors and human breast cancer (Syne et al. 1982a, b) regardless of the endocrine status. Therefore these higher levels of nuclear type II sites in malignant tissues are correlated with this inhibitor deficiency.

Also, we have measured basal levels of nuclear type II sites in a variety of tissues which do not normally respond to estrogen via hypertrophy and hyperplasia (diaphragm, spleen, liver) and these tissues do contain significant quantities of inhibitor activity (Markaverich et al. 1983). Therefore our hypothesis is that this inhibitor may be a component of all tissues, as are nuclear type II sites. In tissues which do not normally respond to estrogen in a proliferative manner, type II sites are complexed with this inhibitor and the functions of these sites are consequently not expressed. Conversely, in tissues which do respond to estrogens, the association of the receptor-estrogen complex with target cell nuclei may result in a dissociation of the inhibitor from nuclear type II sites. Under these conditions cellular hypertrophy and hyperplasia are observed. Consistent with this hypothesis is our observation that in estrogen-treated nuclei (Fig. 4.1) additional nuclear type II sites are observed following dilution. Since this effect is not observed in uterine nuclei from ovariectomized animals (controls; not shown), we feel that this dissociation of the inhibitor from nuclear type II sites is estrogen dependent. Obviously, the lower levels of inhibitor activity in neoplastic tissues are consistent with the elevated levels of type II sites measured in tumors and the rapid proliferation rate in these cell populations. Although it is only tentative at this time, we feel that this is a reasonable model for potential regulation of cell proliferation by this nuclear type II binding inhibitor.

The precise intracellular mechanism(s) regulating the interaction of the inhibitor molecule(s) with nuclear type II sites in the rat uterus is unknown. However, we suspect that such regulation may involve the type II estrogen binding sites we have described for cytosol preparations of rat uterus (Eriksson et al. 1978) and mouse mammary tumors (Watson and Clark 1980; Watson et al. 1980). Cytosol type II sites appear very similar to nuclear type II sites in many respects in terms of estrogen inducibility, target tissue specificity, and hormone specificity (to be published elsewhere). One perplexing but interesting aspect of cytosol type II sites is that they are not depleted from the cytosol following estrogen treatment (Eriksson et al. 1978), but instead, these sites appear to increase continuously in the cytoplasmic compartment. In fact, the level of cytosol type II sites at all times (0.5–96 hours) following estrogenic stimulation precedes and exceeds the level of nuclear type II sites by 25–35%, suggesting a cause-and-effect relationship (Markaverich et al. 1986). In addition, experiments analogous to those shown in Figures 4.1–4.4 for nuclear type II sites have demonstrated that cytosol type II sites also bind this endogenous inhibitor. These results would suggest that cytosol type II sites may function as a compartmentalized "inhibitor binding protein" (IBP), which is estrogen inducible. The hypothetical function of this IBP may be to bind the endogenous inhibitor in such a way that the "free levels" of the compound in estrogen target cells are decreased. Consequently the intracellular level of free inhibitor available for interacting with the nuclear type II sites would also be decreased. Under these circumstances the function of nuclear type II sites would be expressed and one would observe cellular hypertrophy and hyperplasia.

Acknowledgments

The authors would like to thank Lynn Williams for technical assistance, Georgietta Brown for typing the manuscript, and David Scarff for the illustrations. Supported by NIH grants HD-08436, CA-20605, and CA-35480.

References

Clark, J. H., and B. M. Markaverich. 1982. Heterogeneity of estrogen-binding sites and the nuclear matrix. In *The nuclear envelope and the nuclear matrix*, ed. G. G. Maul, 260–269. New York: Alan R. Liss.

Eriksson, H. A., S. Upchurch, J. W. Hardin, E. J. Peck, Jr., and J. H. Clark. 1978. Heterogeneity of estrogen receptors in the cytosol and nuclear fractions of the rat uterus. *Biochemical and Biophysical Research Communications* 81:1–7.

Jensen, E. V., M. Numata, P. I. Brecher, and E. R. DeSombre. 1971. Hormone-receptor interaction as a guide to biochemical mechanisms. In *The biochemistry of steroid hormone action*, ed. R. M. S. Smellie, 133–159. London: Academic Press.

Kelner, K. L., and E. J. Peck, Jr. 1981. Resolution of estrogen binding species in hypothalamus and pituitary. *Journal of Receptor Research* 2:47–62.

Markaverich, B. M., and J. H. Clark. 1979. Two binding sites for estradiol in rat uterine nuclei: relationship to uterotropic response. *Endocrinology* 105:1458–1462.

Markaverich, B. M., S. Upchurch, and J. H. Clark, 1981a. Progesterone and dexamethasone antagonism of uterine growth: a role for a second nuclear binding site for estradiol in estrogen action. *Journal of Steroid Biochemistry* 14:125–132.

Markaverich, B. M., S. Upchurch, S. McCormack, S. R. Glasser, and J. H. Clark. 1981b. Differential stimulation of uterine cells by nafoxidene and clomiphene: relationship between nuclear estrogen receptors and type II estrogen binding sites and cellular growth. *Biology of Reproduction* 24:171–181.

Markaverich, B. M., M. Williams, S. Upchurch, and J. H. Clark. 1981c. Heterogeneity of nuclear estrogen-binding sites in the rat uterus: a simple method for the quantitation of type I and type II sites by [³H]estradiol exchange. *Endocrinology* 109: 62–69.

Markaverich, B. M., R. R. Roberts, R. W. Finney, and J. H. Clark. 1983. Preliminary characterization of an endogenous inhibitor of [³H]estradiol binding in rat uterine nuclei. *Journal of Biological Chemistry* 258:11663–11671.

Markaverich, B. M., R. R. Roberts, M. A. Alejandro, and J. H. Clark. 1984. An endogenous inhibitor of [³H]estradiol binding to nuclear type II estrogen binding sites in normal and malignant tissues. *Cancer Research* 44:1515–1519.

Markaverich, B. M., R. R. Roberts, M. A. Alejandro, and J. H. Clark. 1986. Cytosol type II sites in the rat uterus: interaction with an endogenous ligand. *Endocrinology* (in press).

Pardoll, D. M., B. Vogelstein, and D. S. Coffey. 1980. A fixed site of DNA replication in eucaryotic cells. *Cell* 19:527–536.

Shyamala, G., and J. Gorski. 1967. Estrogen receptors in the rat uterus. *Journal of Biological Chemistry* 244:1097–1103.

Syne, J. S., B. M. Markaverich, J. H. Clark, and W. B. Panko. 1982a. Estrogen binding sites in the nucleus of normal and malignant human tissue: optimization of an exchange assay for the measurement of specific binding. *Cancer Research* 42:4443–4448.

Syne, J. S., B. M. Markaverich, J. H. Clark, and W. B. Panko. 1982b. Estrogen binding sites in the nucleus of normal and malignant human tissue: characteristics of the multiple nuclear binding sites. *Cancer Research* 42:4449–4454.

Watson, C. S., and J. H. Clark. 1980. Heterogeneity of estrogen binding sites in mouse mammary cancer. *Journal of Receptor Research* 1:91–111.

Watson, C. S., D. Medina, and J. H. Clark. 1980. Characterization of progesterone receptors, estrogen receptors and estrogen (type II) binding sites in the hormone independent variant of the MXT-3590 mouse mammary tumor. *Endocrinology* 107:1432–1437.

5

Radiolabeled Antiestrogens and Other Probes for the Estrogen Receptor

John A. Katzenellenbogen

I.   Introduction   74
II. Radiolabeled Antiestrogens   74
     A. Synthesis of Tritium-Labeled Antiestrogens   74
     B. Use of Radiolabeled Antiestrogens to Probe Receptor
         Mechanisms   74
III. Other Probes for the Estrogen Receptor   83
     A. Gamma-Emitting Ligands as Imaging Agents for Receptor-
         Positive Breast Tumors   83
     B. Fluorescent Estrogens for the Assay of Estrogen
         Receptors in Single Cells   85
IV. Conclusion   87
     References   87

73

I. Introduction

T HE high affinity interaction between the estrogen receptor and estrogens or antiestrogens provides diverse opportunities for the development of "probes" that can be used to study the physicochemical characteristics of the receptor itself and the intracellular distribution and dynamics of receptor complexes, as well as the metabolic fate of the ligands *in vivo* or *in vitro*. In addition, this interaction can form the basis for novel diagnostic modalities. This chapter gives a brief review of our development and use of radiolabeled antiestrogens and other probes for the estrogen receptor.

II. Radiolabeled Antiestrogens

A. SYNTHESIS OF TRITIUM-LABELED ANTIESTROGENS

We have reported the synthesis of several antiestrogens in tritium-labeled form: U 23,469 (Fig. 5.1, 1a) (Tatee et al. 1979), CI 628 (Fig. 5.1, 2a) (Katzenellenbogen et al. 1978), and tamoxifen (Fig. 5.1, 3a) (Robertson and Katzenellenbogen 1982) and their hydroxylated analogs (Fig. 5.1, 1b, 2b, and 3b) (Katzenellenbogen et al. 1981b). U 23,469 and U 23,469M (Fig. 5.1) were labeled by saturation of a double bond with carrier-free tritium gas, the remainder by a tritium-halogen exchange reaction. In all cases, materials with high radiochemical and chemical purity and high specific activities were obtained, and in the case of tamoxifen and hydroxytamoxifen, both *cis* and *trans* isomers were prepared and separated. We have also prepared tamoxifen aziridine (Fig. 5.1, 4), an affinity label for the estrogen receptor, in tritium-labeled form (Katzenellenbogen et al. 1983).

B. USE OF RADIOLABELED ANTIESTROGENS TO PROBE RECEPTOR MECHANISMS

1. *In Vivo* Studies of Metabolism and Receptor Dynamics

The action of estrogens and antiestrogens is thought to be mediated by their interaction with the estrogen receptor in the nucleus of target cells. Indeed, after the treatment of immature female rats with antiestrogens

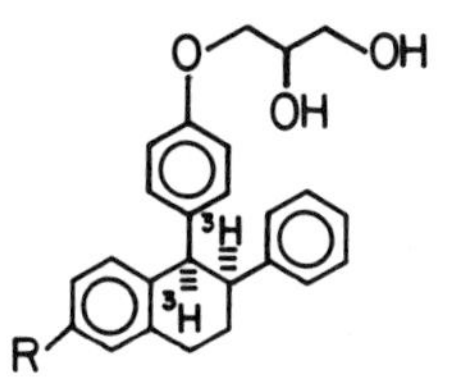

Ia U 23, 469 (R=OCH$_3$)

Ib U 23, 469M (R=OH)

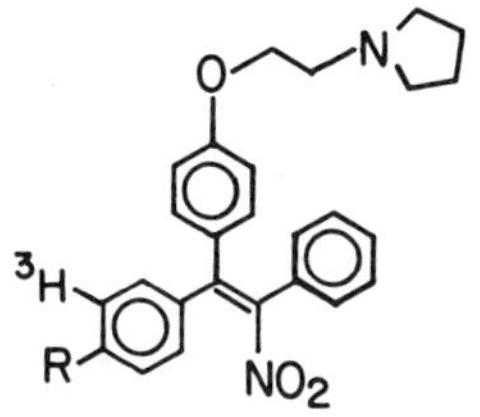

2a CI 628 (R=OCH$_3$)

2b CI 628M (R=OH)

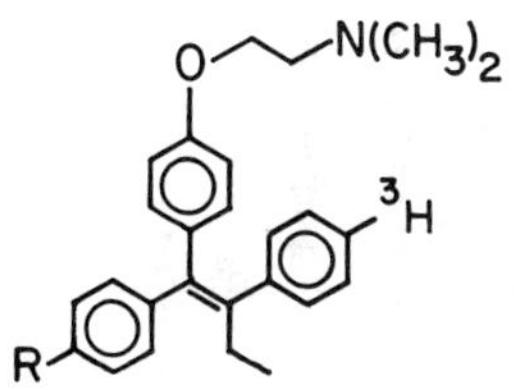

3a tamoxifen (R=H)

3b hydroxytamoxifen (R=OH)

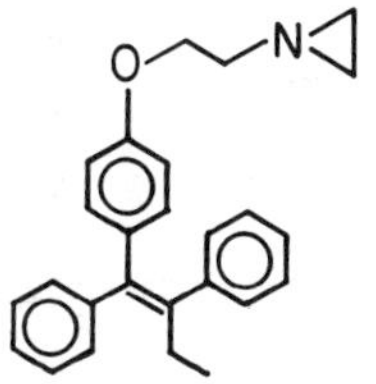

4 tamoxifen aziridine

Figure 5.1. Structures of tritium-labeled antiestrogens.

such as U 23,469, CI 628, and tamoxifen, the estrogen receptor is found in the nuclear fraction, occupied by a ligand and resistant to extraction by hypotonic buffers. The use of radiolabeled antiestrogens reveals interesting dynamic and metabolic details of this process.

Whereas the estrogen receptor appears initially to be associated with the form of the antiestrogen administered to the animal, with time there is a rapid accumulation of more polar metabolites in the nuclear receptor fraction. Since the quantity of antiestrogen associated with receptor is too minute to permit identification by direct chemical or spectroscopic analysis, its structure must be inferred by indirect methods: exhaustive chromatographic comparisons of the receptor-associated, radiolabeled metabolites generated *in vivo,* with authentic samples of candidate metabolites prepared by unambiguous synthetic procedures. By this approach, we have identified the demethylated analogs of U 23,469 and CI 628 (U 23,469M and CI 628M) (Katzenellenbogen et al. 1978; Tatee et al. 1979) and the hydroxylated analog of tamoxifen (hydroxytamoxifen) (Robertson

trans-Tamoxifen

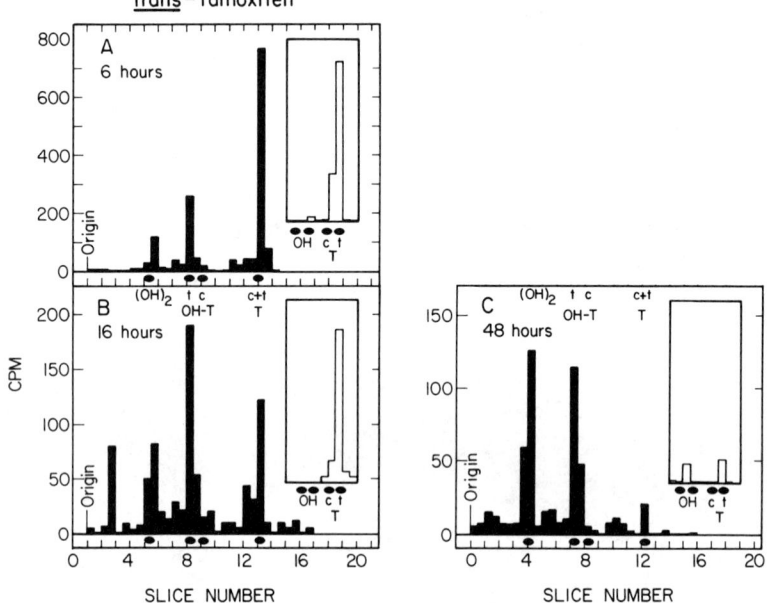

Figure 5.2. Chromatographic analysis of the metabolites of [^{3}H]*trans*-tamoxifen in uterine nuclear extracts. Immature rats were injected with [^{3}H]*trans*-tamoxifen (5 μg; 165 μCi), and at 6, 16, or 48 hours after injection, ethanol extracts of uterine nuclear fractions were prepared and analyzed by thin-layer chromatography in benzene-piperidine (9:1, v/v) or benzene-triethylamine (9:1, v/v, inserts only). The mobility of chromatographic standards is indicated by the darkened ellipses below each chromatogram: c- and t-T, *cis*- and *trans*-tamoxifen; c- and t-OH-T, *cis*- and *trans*-hydroxytamoxifen; OH, the monophenol isomers obtained by removal of the dimethylaminoethyl side chain of the tamoxifen isomer; (OH)$_2$, the bisphenol obtained by removal of the basic side chain from hydroxytamoxifen. (From Robertson et al. 1982.)

et al. 1982) as the principal metabolites of the parent antiestrogens found associated with receptor within a few hours after injection. These analogs have been prepared and shown to have far greater affinity for the estrogen receptor than the parent antiestrogens (Tatee et al. 1979; Hayes et al. 1981; Katzenellenbogen et al. 1981, 1984).

A most intriguing aspect of these studies is the demonstration of "metabolite selection" by receptor: although many different compounds are being produced by metabolism of the administered antiestrogen, the estrogen receptor selectively sequesters only those metabolites showing the highest affinity binding. This sequestration is seen both in terms of time and with respect to target tissue.

An example of sequestration with time is evident in Figure 5.2, where the polar, high affinity metabolities of tamoxifen (OH-T, plus a yet more polar component) progressively accumulate in the nuclear fraction with time (Robertson et al. 1982). By sequestration with respect to target tissue, we mean that a particular high affinity metabolite, which may be present only as a minor component in serum or nontarget tissues, so as not to be noticed, may be much more prominent in the whole target tissue, or especially in the nuclear estrogen receptor fraction. An example of this phenomenon is seen in Figure 5.3, in which the more polar metabolite of U 23,469, barely discernible in serum at 1 hour (panel B), is clearly evident in uterine nuclei at this time (panel D); at 13 hours, when the polar metabolite accounts for half of the serum activity (panel A), it is almost the only species evident in the nucleus (panel C) (Tatee et al. 1979).

Such a "receptor-driven" approach to the study of metabolism *in vivo* is applicable not only to antiestrogens, but to all drugs and hormones. Its cardinal advantage is that it provides a means for selective observation of those metabolites of an administered compound that are potentially of greatest biological significance. In this regard, it is of note that at longer times after administration of tamoxifen to rats there appears a third, yet more polar metabolite that is associated with receptor (cf. Fig. 5.2C; Robertson et al. 1982). The nature of this intriguing metabolite has not yet been adequately investigated.

2. *In Vitro* Studies of Receptor-Antiestrogen Complexes

a. *The Nature of Estrogen Receptor Complexes with Estrogens vs Antiestrogens*

Since the metabolites of antiestrogens found associated with receptor *in vivo* are, most likely, the forms responsible for the *in vivo* activity of these compounds, it is appropriate that detailed studies on the physico-chemical characteristics of estrogen receptor complexes with estrogens vs antiestrogens focus on complexes with these biopotent forms of the antiestrogens. It was with this aim in mind that the high affinity, hydroxylated forms of the antiestrogens (U 23,469M, CI 628M, and hydroxytamoxifen) were prepared in tritium-labeled form.

Interesting differences in the state of receptor association, depending upon whether it is liganded with an estrogen or an antiestrogen, have been found, with the receptor-antiestrogen complex having a greater tendency to be found in a 5S form (which may be a receptor dimer) and the receptor-estrogen complex having a greater tendency to be found in a 4S (monomer) form (Katzenellenbogen et al. 1981; Miller et al. 1984). The

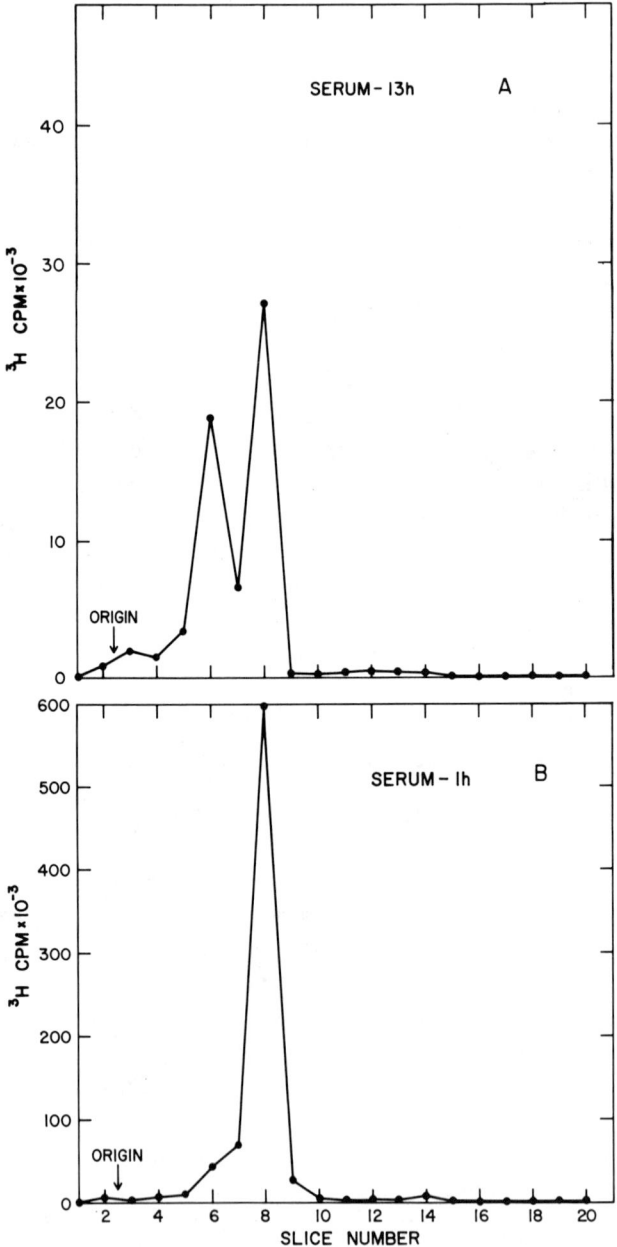

Figure 5.3. Thin-layer chromatographic profiles of the antiestrogen [³H]U 23,469 and its metabolites generated *in vivo*. Immature rats were injected with [³H]U 23,469 (25 μg sc/rat), and at 1 and 13 hours after injection, serum was prepared and extracted with ethyl acetate. At the same time, uteri were excised and homogenized, and the three-times-washed

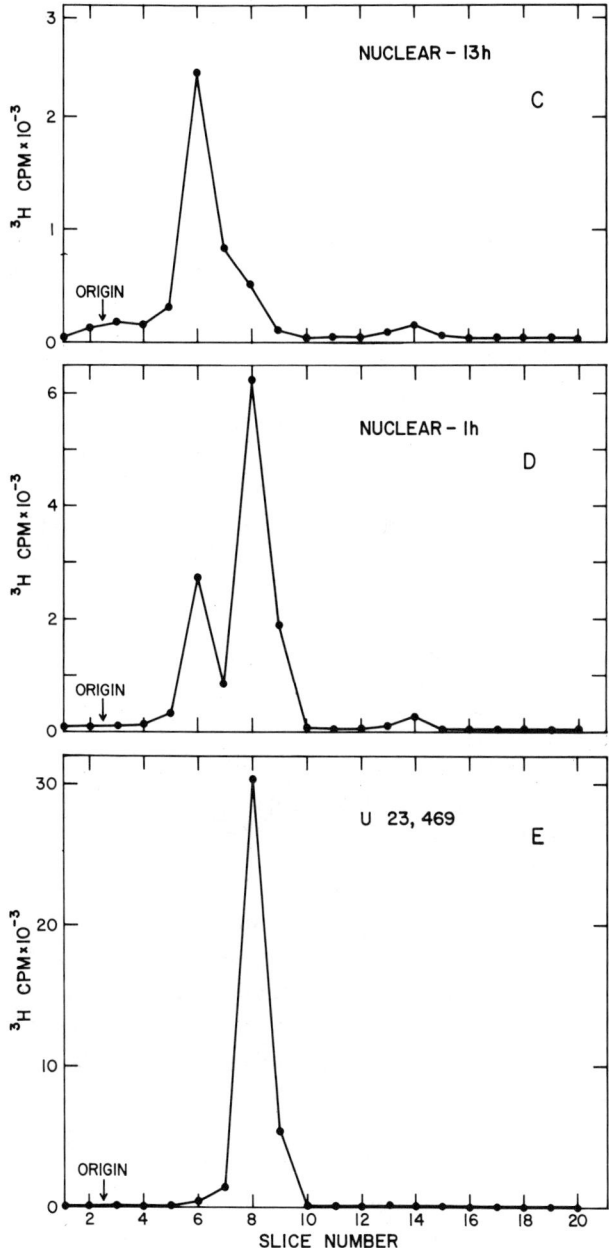

nuclear pellet was then ethanol-extracted. The extracts were concentrated and analyzed on thin-layer silica gel plates developed in ether-ethanol (98:2). In this system U 23,469 moves in fraction 8, and the polar metabolite (des-O-methyl U 23,469) moves in fraction 6. (From Tatee et al. 1979.)

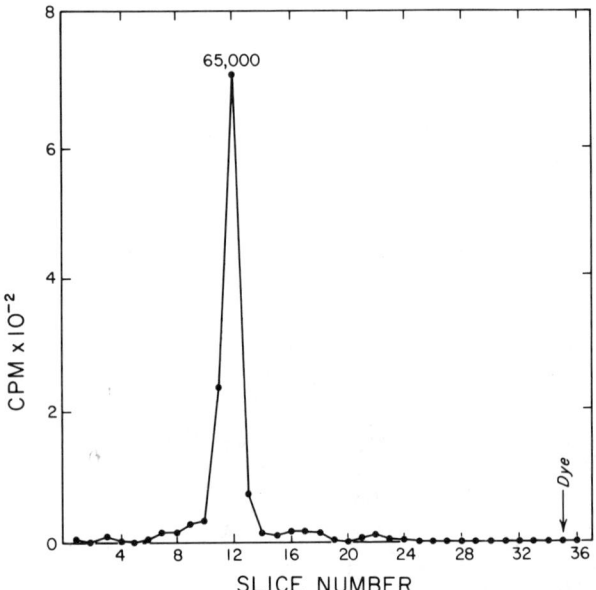

Figure 5.4. SDS-polyacrylamide gel electrophoresis of nuclear estrogen receptor from MCF-7 cells. An 0.6 M KCl extract of nuclear estrogen receptor from cells treated with 20 nM of [³H]tamoxifen aziridine was analyzed on SDS-polyacrylamide gels, after purification over an antireceptor immunoadsorbent column. (Adapted from Monsma et al. 1984.)

results of these studies are reported in greater detail in Miller et al., Chapter 8 in this volume.

b. Studies with Covalently Labeling Antiestrogens

Tamoxifen aziridine, a covalently labeling antiestrogen, can be used to characterize estrogen receptors in detail, under denaturing conditions. This compound, which is now commercially available, has been used to label estrogen receptors in cell-free cytosol preparations and in whole cells in culture; the labeling is selective and efficient (Katzenellenbogen et al. 1983).

Analysis of covalently labeled receptor by SDS-polyacrylamide gel electrophoresis indicates that the highest molecular weight form is 65,000 (Fig. 5.4). Vigorous attempts to see larger forms in whole cells, by direct lysis of labeled cells in hot SDS sample buffer, have failed to show any labeled species larger than 65,000 (Monsma et al. 1984). Covalently labeled estrogen receptor from human and rat sources also appears indistinguishable on the basis of electrophoretic mobility on SDS gels (Katzenellenbogen et al. 1983; Monsma et al. 1984).

The estrogen receptors in MCF-7 cells can be pulse labeled, and the fate of the labeled receptor followed, thereafter, with time (Monsma et al. 1984). In such experiments, the 65,000 molecular weight species disappears with a half-life of about 3–4 hours, and there is very little evidence of the formation of stable species of intermediate size. The rate of turnover of receptor covalently labeled with tamoxifen aziridine is similar to that determined by the heavy amino acid–density shift method (Eckert et al. 1984; Monsma et al. 1984). In contrast to the "clean" degradation of tamoxifen aziridine-labeled receptor in whole cells, labeled receptor in cytosol preparations shows progressive proteolysis to intermediate forms with molecular weights of about 53,000 and 37,000 (Monsma et al. 1984).

c. Studies on Hydroxytamoxifen Isomerization

In uterotrophic and cell growth studies, the isomers of tamoxifen have distinctly different potencies and activities: the *trans* isomer is a potent antagonist (or partial antagonist), whereas the *cis* isomer is a weak, though pure, agonist. Therefore, we were intrigued to find that in cell culture studies, *cis*-hydroxytamoxifen was a reasonably potent antagonist of cell growth (Katzenellenbogen et al. 1984).

In order to investigate the possibility that the *cis* isomer was being converted to the more potent *trans* isomer under the conditions of the cell growth assay, parallel incubations with each hydroxytamoxifen isomer in tritium-labeled form were monitored over the 2-day assay period (Katzenellenbogen et al. 1985). In each case, conversion to the opposite isomer had progressed to the extent of about 20% after 2 days (cf. Fig. 5.5B, where 17% *trans*-hydroxytamoxifen has been generated from pure *cis*-hydroxytamoxifen after a 2-day incubation in the media). However, since the *trans* isomer has so much higher affinity for the estrogen receptor, the receptor-associated form was found to be almost exclusively the *trans* isomer, even in the case where the *cis* isomer was added to the cell culture (Fig. 5.5C). The isomerization process appears to involve radical intermediates, since it can be inhibited by antioxidants.

These findings serve to highlight an important caveat in studies of biological activity: when the biological activity of a particular compound is being investigated, it is essential to determine the chemical nature of the species bound to the receptor that is mediating the observed effect, before

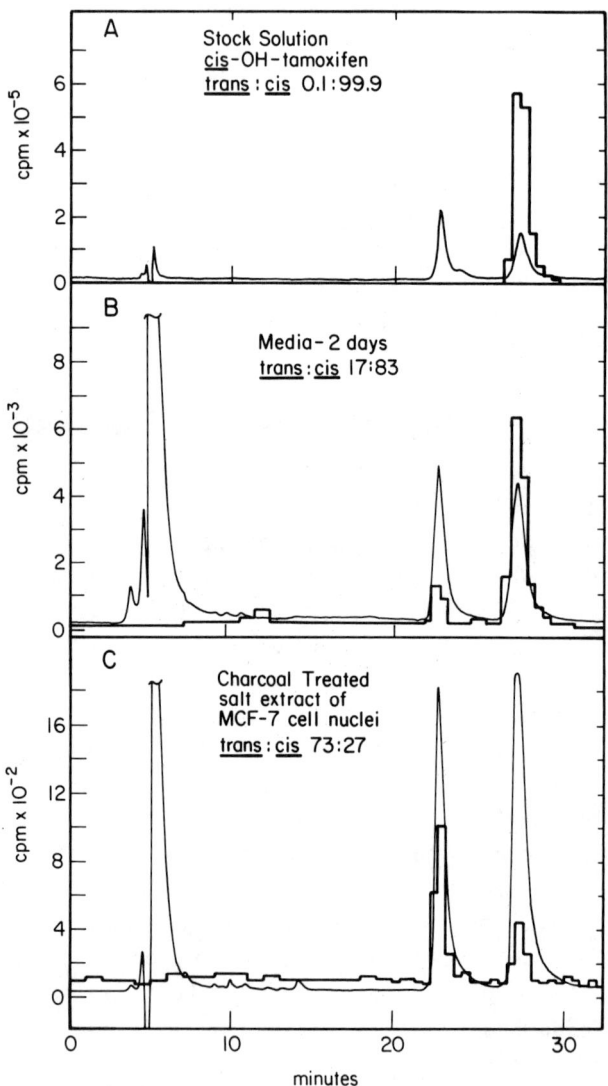

Figure 5.5. High-performance liquid chromatography (HPLC) analysis of the isomerization of *cis*-hydroxytamoxifen to *trans*-hydroxytamoxifen. Freshly purified [³H]*cis*-hydroxytamoxifen (panel A) was added to MCF-7 cells in MEM medium containing 5% charcoal-dextran-treated calf serum. After 2 days at 37°C, the composition of the media (panel B) and the charcoal-treated salt extract of the cell nuclei (panel C) were analyzed by HPLC after the addition of carrier *cis*- and *trans*-hydroxytamoxifen (73% methanol, 27% 0.25 M diethylammonium phosphate pH 9.0, at 0.8 ml/min on C-8 reversed-phase column, Supelco DB-8 25 × 0.46 cm).

one can ascribe an observed biological effect to the particular compound; it is possible that isomerization or biotransformation has produced a new compound (that may be more potent than the one administered) and that receptor occupancy by this new compound is producing the observed effect.

III. Other Probes for the Estrogen Receptor

A. GAMMA-EMITTING LIGANDS AS IMAGING AGENTS FOR RECEPTOR-POSITIVE BREAST TUMORS

The presence of estrogen receptors in the majority of human breast tumors provides a potential mechanism for the selective uptake of an estrogenic ligand by the tumor tissue. If such an agent were suitably labeled with a gamma-emitting radionuclide, it might be useful as an imaging agent for the tumor.

Two factors are of paramount importance in developing such breast tumor imaging agents—the specific activity of the agent and its binding selectivity (Katzenellenbogen et al. 1982a). Since the receptor system is of limited capacity, agents of high specific activity (~ 1000 Ci/mmol) are needed to ensure that adequate activity is taken up within the capacity of the receptor system; in order for receptor-mediated uptake to be detectable above background binding, the affinity of these agents for the estrogen receptor not only needs to be high, but the nonspecific binding must also be low.

We have developed several gamma-emitting estrogens (Fig. 5.6, 5–7) as potential breast tumor imaging agents. The first set was labeled with the single photon-emitter bromine-77 (Fig. 5.6, 5) (Katzenellenbogen et al. 1981a, 1982b; McElvany et al. 1982a; Senderoff et al. 1982). Although these compounds demonstrated adequate specific activities and

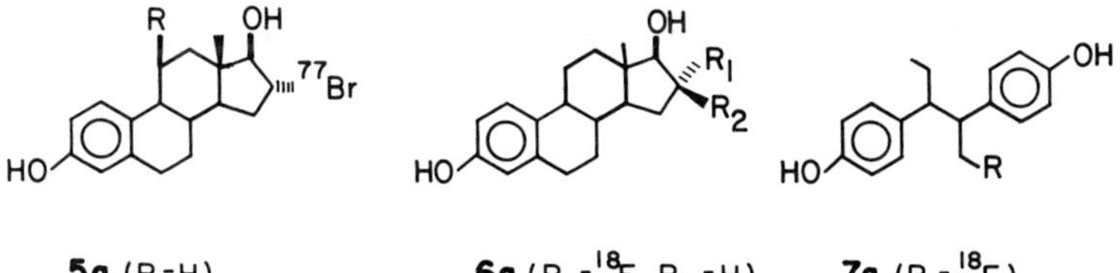

5a (R=H) **6a** (R$_1$ = ^{18}F, R$_2$ =H) **7a** (R = ^{18}F)

5b (R=OCH$_3$) **6b** (R$_1$=H, R$_2$ = ^{18}F) **7b** (R =CH$_2$^{18}F)

Figure 5.6. Structures of gamma-emitting estrogens.

Table 5.1. Uptake of 16α-[^{18}F]fluoroestradiol in the immature rat[a]

	Tissue-to-blood ratios		
	0.5 hr	1.0 hr	2.0 hr
Uterus	30.4	33.4	85.8
Ovaries	10.1	11.4	22.5
Liver	13.1	9.2	12.6
Kidney	7.6	5.8	5.7
Muscle	1.3	1.2	1.8
Spleen	0.9	0.8	1.7
Esophagus	1.1	1.6	2.2
Lung	1.5	1.2	1.7
Bone	1.1	1.2	2.6

[a]Five 21-day (50 g) immature female Sprague-Dawley rats were injected with 5 μCi of $16\alpha - $[^{18}F]fluoroestradiol in saline. The radioactivity per gram of each organ was determined by gamma counting
at the indicated times and is expressed as a ratio with the activity in
the blood at the same time. (Data adapted from Kiesewetter et al.
1984b.)

good binding selectivities, the high levels of scattering associated with the
energetic gamma emission of Br-77 precluded most applications of imaging in humans (McElvany et al. 1982b). More recently, we have prepared
steroidal (Fig. 5.6, 6) and nonsteroidal (Fig. 5.6, 7) estrogens labeled
with the positron-emitter flourine-18 (Landvatter et al. 1983; Kiesewetter
et al. 1984a). These compounds demonstrate very favorable binding characteristics, and very high uptake selectivities are found in experimental
animals *in vivo* (Landvatter et al. 1983; Kiesewetter et al. 1984b). We are
currently developing 16α-fluoroestradiol (Fig. 5.6, 6a) as an imaging
agent for humans. From the results shown in Table 5.1, it is evident that
this compound shows very high selectivity for uptake by target tissues in
the rat.

Whereas one might think that gamma-emitting antiestrogens would be
as useful as estrogens as imaging agents for breast tumors, the presence
of nonreceptor binding sites for these basic compounds (antiestrogen-
specific sites) (Sutherland et al. 1980; Kon 1983; Sudo et al. 1983) will,
most likely, result in reduced uptake selectivity by target tissues and
receptor-positive tumors. In fact, the pattern of *in vivo* uptake of tritium-
labeled hydroxytamoxifen, an antiestrogen with very high receptor binding affinity, showed less selectivity for estrogen target tissues than estradiol does, presumably because of its binding to the antiestrogen-specific
binding sites (Jordan and Bowser-Finn 1982).

B. FLUORESCENT ESTROGENS FOR THE ASSAY OF ESTROGEN RECEPTORS IN SINGLE CELLS

It would be extremely useful to have a method for assaying estrogen receptors in single cells, in order to evaluate the homogeneity of receptor distribution (and hence potential hormone responsiveness) of cells in breast tumors. Although such determinations can be done, in principle, by autoradiography, the process is tedious. Recently developed immuno-cytochemical methods, based on monoclonal antibodies to the estrogen receptor, appear very promising in this application (King and Greene 1984).

An alternative approach under active investigation in many laboratories is the use of fluorescent estrogens. Because of the low concentrations of estrogen receptors in cells, this application is at the sensitivity limit of fluorescence methodology and will require either image-intensified fluorescence microscopy or very careful flow cytometry (Martin et al. 1983). Many reports of successful fluorescence-based receptor assays may well be artifactual (Chamness et al. 1980; McCarty et al. 1981).

We are working on the development of three types of fluorescent estrogens: estrogen-fluorophore conjugates, fluorescent ligands, and photofluorogenic ligands (Fig. 5.7). The first type (I) consists simply of an estrogenic ligand (nonfluorescent) chemically coupled to a fluorophore (e.g., Fig. 5.7, 8) (J. E. Lloyd, T. L. Fevig, and J. A. Katzenellenbogen, unpublished observations). Many reagents of this type have been prepared by other workers; however, although the fluorophore may have good spectroscopic characteristics, the conjugates generally are large species, with low affinity for receptor and questionable chemical stability. The second type of agent (II) is exemplified by 12-oxo-9(11)-dehydroestradiol (Fig. 5.7, 9), a compound that differs from estradiol only by inclusion of a C-ring enone system (Martin et al. 1983). Although such agents may have good affinity for receptor, their fluorescence properties are often suboptimal.

In an attempt to develop agents that have both very high receptor binding affinity and excellent fluorescence properties, we have begun a systematic investigation of photofluorogenic systems (III). Such behavior is exemplified by the antiestrogen analog desmethylnafoxidine (Fig. 5.7, 10). This compound, a diaryldihydronaphthalene, binds to the estrogen receptor with high affinity, but it is nonfluorescent. However, brief irradiation in the short ultraviolet results in a photocyclization-oxidation reaction that converts the *cis*-stilbene system of the diaryldihydronaphthalene into

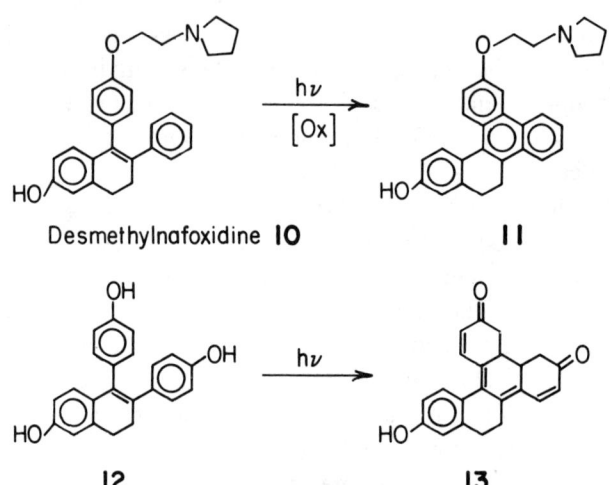

Figure 5.7. Examples of the three types of fluorescent estrogens.

a phenanthrene (Fig. 5.7, 11), which is fluorescent (Bindal and Katzenel-lenbogen, 1985). Whereas the fluorophore produced by photocyclization-oxidation of desmethylnafoxidine does not have exceptional spectroscopic characteristics, the photoproduct from the triphenol (Fig. 5.7, 12) is a hydroxyphenyltetraenedione (Fig. 5.7, 13) that had fluorescence charac-teristics very similar to those of fluorescein (R. D. Bindal and J. A. Katz-enellenbogen, unpublished observations).

Photofluorogenic compounds enable the conversion of a high affinity ligand for receptor into a good fluorophore, by an efficient photochemical process, thus uniting two characteristics that are difficult to combine in a single molecule. However, in developing methods to utilize these agents in receptor assays, it will be important to avoid conditions that result in the dissociation of ligand receptor complexes, since the photoproducts have only low affinity for the receptor (Bindal and Katzenellenbogen, 1985). Ultimately, it may be possible to develop photofluorogenic estrogens that will attach to receptor covalently, as does tamoxifen aziridine.

IV. *Conclusion*

By utilizing the high affinity interaction between the estrogen receptor and estrogenic and antiestrogenic ligands, we have been able to prepare a variety of derivatives that can be used as probes for the receptor. These agents have proven useful in studies of antiestrogen metabolism and the dynamics of these metabolites *in vitro* and *in vivo,* the nature of the receptor complex with estrogens and antiestrogens, and the physicochemical properties of the receptor. We are also developing gamma-emitting and fluorescent agents to be used for diagnostic purposes *in vivo* and *in vitro.* These applications are indicative of the utility of specific probes for the estrogen receptor.

References

Bindal, R. D., and J. A. Katzenellenbogen. 1985. 1,2-Diaryl-3,4-dihydronaphthalenes: photofluorogenic ligands for the estrogen receptor. *Journal of Steroid Biochemistry* 23:929–937.

Chamness, G. C., W. D. Mercer, and W. L. McGuire. 1980. Are histochemical methods for oestrogen receptor valid? *Journal of Histochemistry and Cytochemistry* 28:792–798.

Eckert, R. L., A. Mullick, E. A. Rorke, and B. S. Katzenellenbogen. 1984. Estrogen receptor synthesis and turnover in MCF-7 breast cancer cells measured by a density shift technique. *Endocrinology* 114:629–637.

Hayes, J. R., E. A. Rorke, D. W. Robertson, B. S. Katzenellenbogen, and J. A. Katzenellenbogen. 1981. Biological potency and uterine estrogen receptor interactions of the metabolites of the antiestrogens CI-628 and U23,469. *Endocrinology* 108:164–172.

Jordan, V. C., and R. A. Bowser-Finn. 1982. Binding of [³H]monohydroxytamoxifen by immature rat tissue *in vivo. Endocrinology* 110:1281–1288.

Katzenellenbogen, B. S., J. A. Katzenellenbogen, E. F. Ferguson, and N. Krauthammer. 1978. Antiestrogen interaction with uterine estrogen receptors: studies with a radiolabeled antiestrogen (CI-628). *Journal of Biological Chemistry* 253:697–708.

Katzenellenbogen, B. S., E. J. Pavlik, D. W. Robertson, and J. A. Katzenellenbogen. 1981. Interaction of a high affinity antiestrogen (α-[4-pyrrolidinoethoxy]phenyl-4-

hydroxy-α'-nitrostilbene, CI-628M) with uterine estrogen receptors. *Journal of Biological Chemistry* 256:2908–2915.

Katzenellenbogen, B. S., M. J. Norman, R. L. Eckert, S. W. Pletz, and W. F. Mangel. 1984. Bioactivities, estrogen receptor interactions, and plasminogen activator-inducing activities of tamoxifen and hydroxy-tamoxifen isomers in MCF-7 human breast cancer cells. *Cancer Research* 44:112–119.

Katzenellenbogen, J. A., S. G. Senderoff, K. D. McElvany, H. A. O'Brien, Jr., and M. J. Welch. 1981a. [^{77}Br]-16α-bromoestradiol-17β: a high specific activity gamma-emitting estrogen that shows selective, receptor-mediated uptake by uterus and DMBA-induced mammary tumors in rats. *Journal of Nuclear Medicine* 22:42–77.

Katzenellenbogen, J. A., T. Tatee, and D. W. Robertson. 1981b. Preparation of tritium-labeled 4-hydroxy-α-[p-(2-(N-pyrrolidino)ethoxy)phenyl]-α'-nitrostilbene (CN-928), a biologically-important metabolite of the antiestrogen CI-628. *Journal of Labeled Compounds and Radiopharmaceuticals* 18:865–879.

Katzenellenbogen, J. A., D. F. Heiman, K. E. Carlson, and J. E. Lloyd. 1982a. *In vivo* and *in vitro* steroid receptor assays in the design of estrogen pharmaceuticals. In *Receptor binding radiotracers*, vol. 1, ed. W. C. Eckelman, 93–126. Boca Raton, Fla.: CRC Press.

Katzenellenbogen, J. A., K. D. McElvany, S. G. Senderoff, K. E. Carlson, S. W. Landvatter, and M. J. Welch. 1982b. 16α-[^{77}Br]-bromo-11β-methoxyestradiol-17β. A gamma emitting estrogen imaging agent with high uptake and retention by target organs. *Journal of Nuclear Medicine* 23:411–419.

Katzenellenbogen, J. A., K. E. Carlson, D. F. Heiman, D. W. Robertson, and B. S. Katzenellenbogen. 1983. Efficient and highly selective covalent labeling of the estrogen receptor with [^{3}H]tamoxifen aziridine. *Journal of Biological Chemistry* 258:3487–3495.

Katzenellenbogen, J. A., K. E. Carlson, and B. S. Katzenellenbogen. 1985. Facile geometric isomerization of phenolic non-steroidal estrogens and antiestrogens: limitations to the interpretation of experiments characterizing the activity of individual isomers. *Journal of Steroid Biochemistry* 22:589–596.

Kiesewetter, D. O., J. A. Katzenellenbogen, M. R. Kilbourn, and M. J. Welch. 1984a. The synthesis of 16-fluoroestrogens by unusually facile fluoride ion displacement reactions: prospects for the preparation of fluorine-18 labeled estrogens. *Journal of Organic Chemistry* 49:4900–4905.

Kiesewetter, D. O., M. R. Kilbourn, S. W. Landvatter, D. F. Heiman, J. A. Katzenellenbogen, and M. J. Welch. 1984b. Preparation and target tissue-selective uptake of four fluorine-18 labeled estrogens in immature rats. *Journal of Nuclear Medicine* 25:1212–1221.

King, W. J., and G. L. Greene. 1984. Monoclonal antibodies localize oestrogen receptor in the nuclei of target cells. *Nature* (London) 307:745–747.

Kon, O. L. 1983. An antiestrogen-binding protein in human tissues. *Journal of Biological Chemistry* 258:3173–3177.

Landvatter, S. W., D. O. Kiesewetter, M. R. Kilbourn, J. A. Katzenellenbogen, and M. J. Welch. 1983. (2R*,3S*)-1-[^{18}F]fluoro-2,3-bis(4-hydroxyphenyl)pentane ([^{18}F] fluoronorhexestrol) a positron-emitting estrogen that shows highly-selective, receptor mediated uptake by target tissues in vivo. *Life Sciences* 33:1933–1938.

Martin, P., H. Magdelenat, B. Benyahia, O. Rigaud, and J. A. Katzenellenbogen. 1983. A new approach for visualizing estrogen receptors in target tissues using inherently fluorescent ligands and image intensification. *Cancer Research* 43:4956–4565.

McCarty, K. S., Jr., D. S. Reitgen, H. F. Seigler, and K. S. McCarty, Sr. 1981. Cytochemistry of steroid receptors: a critique. *Breast Cancer Research and Treatment* 1:315–325.

McElvany, K. D., K. E. Carlson, M. J. Welch, S. G. Senderoff, and J. A. Katzenellenbogen. 1982a. In vivo comparison of 16α-[^{77}Br]-bromoestradiol-17β and 16α-[^{125}I]-iodoestradiol-17β. *Journal of Nuclear Medicine* 23:420–424.

McElvany, K. D., J. A. Katzenellenbogen, K. E. Shafer, B. A. Siegel, S. G. Senderoff, and M. J. Welch. 1982b. 16α-[^{77}Br]-bromoestradiol-17β: dosimetry and preliminary clinical studies. *Journal of Nuclear Medicine* 23:425–430.

Miller, M. A., G. L. Greene, and B. S. Katzenellenbogen. 1984. Estrogen receptor transformation in MCF-7 breast cancer cells: characterization by immunochemical and sedimentation analyses. *Endocrinology* 114:296–298.

Monsma, F. J., Jr., B. S. Katzenellenbogen, M. A. Miller, Y. S. Ziegler, and J. A. Katzenellenbogen. 1984. Characterization of the estrogen receptor and its dynamics in MCF-7 human breast cancer cells using a covalently attaching antiestrogen. *Endocrinology* 115:143–153.

Robertson, D. W., and J. A. Katzenellenbogen. 1982. The synthesis of the *E* and *Z* isomers of the antiestrogen tamoxifen and its metabolite, monohydroxytamoxifen, in tritium-labeled form. *Journal of Organic Chemistry* 47:2387–2392.

Robertson, D. W., J. A. Katzenellenbogen, D. J. Long, E. A. Rorke, and B. S. Katzenellenbogen. 1982. A comparison of the activity, pharmacokinetics, and metabolic activation of the *cis* and *trans* isomers of tamoxifen. *Journal of Steroid Biochemistry* 16:1–13.

Senderoff, S. G., K. D. McElvany, K. E. Carlson, D. F. Heiman, J. A. Katzenellenbogen, and M. J. Welch. 1982. Synthetic methodology for the preparation of 16α-[^{77}Br]-bromoestradiol-17β and 16α-[^{77}Br]-bromo-11β-methoxyestradiol-17β. Two high specific activity estrogen receptor-binding radiopharmaceuticals. *International Journal of Applied Radiation and Isotopes* 33:545–551.

Sudo, K., F. J. Monsma, Jr., and B. S. Katzenellenbogen. 1983. Antiestrogen binding sites distinct from the estrogen receptor: subcellular localization, ligand specificity, and distribution in tissues of the rat. *Endocrinology* 112:425–434.

Sutherland, R. L., M. S. Foo, M. D. Greene, A. M. Waybourne, and Z. S. Krozowski. 1980. High affinity antiestrogen binding site distinct from the estrogen receptor. *Nature* (London) 288:273–275.

Tatee, T., K. E. Carlson, J. A. Katzenellenbogen, D. W. Robertson, and B. S. Katzenellenbogen. 1979. Antiestrogens and antiestrogen metabolites: preparation of tritium-labeled (+)-*cis*[p-(1,2,3,4-tetrahydro-6-methoxy-2-phenyl-1-naphthyl)-phenoxy]-1,2-propanediol and characterization and synthesis of a biologically important metabolite. *Journal of Medicinal Chemistry* 22:1509–1517.

II

Antiestrogen Binding Sites

6

Properties of
High Affinity Intracellular
Binding Sites for Antiestrogens

COLIN K. W. WATTS, LEIGH C. MURPHY,
AND ROBERT L. SUTHERLAND

I. INTRODUCTION 94
II. PROPERTIES OF ANTIESTROGEN BINDING SITES 94
    A. SUBCELLULAR AND TISSUE DISTRIBUTION 94
    B. BINDING PROPERTIES 98
    C. BINDING SPECIFICITY 99
    D. MOLECULAR PROPERTIES OF MICROSOMAL AEBS 104
    E. MOLECULAR PROPERTIES OF DETERGENT-SOLUBILIZED AEBS 104
III. PUTATIVE FUNCTION OF ANTIESTROGEN BINDING SITES 109
IV. CONCLUSION 111
    REFERENCES 111

I. Introduction

THE interactions of synthetic nonsteroidal antiestrogens, such as tamoxifen (TAM), with the estrogen receptor (ER) system of estrogen target cells have been described in numerous studies (Sutherland and Jordan 1981). The experimental data from these studies indicate that many of the biological actions of these compounds (which include estrogen antagonistic and agonistic effects, antifertility properties, cell-cycle effects, and antitumor activities) are mediated by the ER system, although by mechanisms not yet fully defined. Some properties, such as the species and tissue variations in drug action (Martin 1981; Sutherland 1981; Sutherland and Jordan 1981) and the estrogen-irreversible (ER-independent?) cytotoxic effects of TAM which have been observed *in vivo* in rat uterine glandular epithelial cells (Martin 1981) and *in vitro* in MCF-7 human breast cancer cells (Murphy and Sutherland 1983, 1985; Reddel et al. 1983; Sutherland et al. 1983), are difficult to explain solely in terms of ER-mediated events.

The availability of radiolabeled nonsteroidal antiestrogens in recent years and their use in saturation and competition studies made possible the initial identification of high affinity binding sites for nonsteroidal antiestrogens, distinct from ER, which have no affinity for estradiol and other steroids (Sutherland and Foo 1979; Faye et al. 1980; Gulino and Pasqualini 1980; Sutherland and Murphy 1980; Sutherland et al. 1980). Interest in the physiological function of these antiestrogen binding sites (AEBS) and their role as possible mediators of drug action has stimulated research in this area by several workers. In this chapter we review some of our more recent experimental data on the AEBS.

II. *Properties of Antiestrogen Binding Sites*

A. SUBCELLULAR AND TISSUE DISTRIBUTION

Although the AEBS was first detected in cytosol, the inability of some workers to detect significant quantities of AEBS in such preparations (Borgna and Rochefort 1980; Katzenellenbogen et al. 1981; Eckert and Katzenellenbogen 1982) was subsequently shown to be due to the loss of the majority of AEBS to the high-speed pellet. Subcellular fractionation studies in MCF-7 cells (Murphy et al. 1983; Watts et al. 1984), rat uterus (Sudo et al. 1983), and rat liver (Watts and Sutherland 1984) showed the AEBS to be concentrated within the microsomal fraction. Figure 6.1 shows that the distribution of AEBS between subcellular fractions of rat

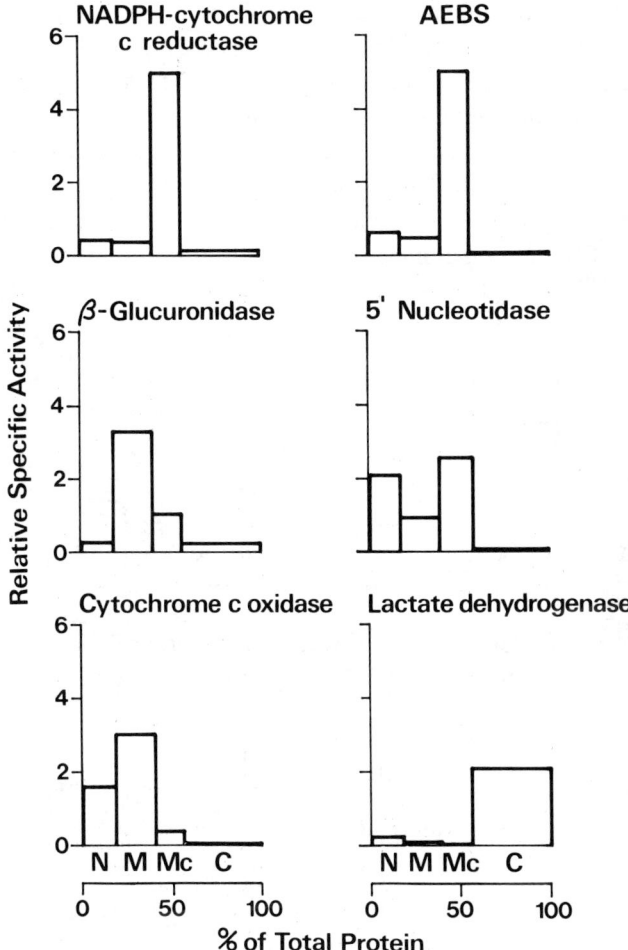

Figure 6.1. Subcellular localization of AEBS in rat liver. Rat liver homogenates were separated by differential centrifugation into nuclear (N), mitochondrial (M), microsomal (Mc), and cytosol (C) fractions. The distribution of marker enzymes for plasma membranes (5′nucleotidase), endoplasmic reticulum (NADPH cytochrome c reductase), lysosomes (β-glucuronidase), mitochondria (cytochrome c oxidase), and cytosol (lactate dehydrogenase) and the distribution of AEBS in each fraction are shown. (From Watts and Sutherland 1984.)

liver parallels the distribution of NADPH cytochrome c reductase, a marker enzyme for the endoplasmic reticulum, the major component of rat liver microsomes. The AEBS present in nuclear, mitochondrial, and soluble (cytosol) fractions can be accounted for by microsomal contamination of these fractions. Figure 6.2 illustrates the higher specific activity of the AEBS in rough endoplasmic reticulum compared with smooth endoplasmic reticulum. The site appeared to be associated with the membrane rather than the ribosomal component of the rough endoplasmic reticulum (Watts and Sutherland 1984).

The concentration of AEBS in rat tissues and in several estrogen receptor–positive (ER +) and estrogen receptor–negative (ER −) human breast tumors and cell lines is shown in Tables 6.1 and 6.2. The data show that the AEBS is ubiquitous, is not confined to classic estrogen target

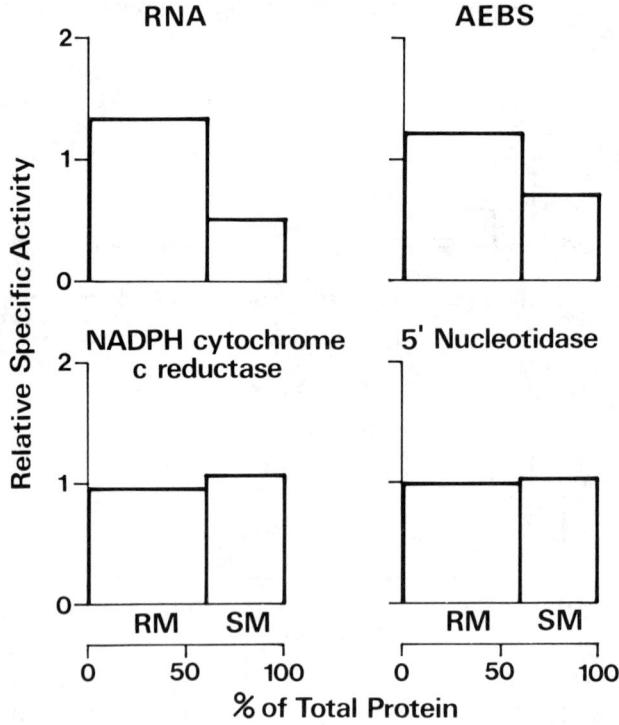

Figure 6.2. Distribution of AEBS between subfractions of rat liver microsomes. Microsomes were separated on a discontinuous sucrose gradient containing CsC1 into rough membrane (RM) and smooth membrane (SM) fractions. The distribution of marker enzymes for plasma membranes and endoplasmic reticulum and the distribution of AEBS and RNA are shown. (From Watts and Sutherland 1984.)

Table 6.1. Tissue distribution of AEBS in microsomal fractions of rat tissues

Tissue	Concentration (fmol/mg microsomal protein)	K_d (nM)
Liver	30,500	0.9
Colon	1,060	2.9
Stomach	870	1.3
Ovary	820	2.3
Uterus	730	1.6
Kidney	650	1.6
Esophagus	530	2.1
Spleen	390	1.2
Lung	100	4.9
Heart	0	—
Skeletal muscle	0	—
Small intestine	0	—

tissues or to ER+ tumors or cell lines, and that the rat liver is a concentrated and convenient source of AEBS for biochemical studies. Many researchers (Gulino and Pasqualini 1982; Sutherland et al. 1982; Kon 1983; Miller and Katzenellenbogen 1983; Sudo et al. 1983; Winneker and Clark 1983; Winneker et al. 1983) have presented similar data on the tissue distribution of AEBS in various species.

Several groups have suggested that AEBS concentration is under hormonal control. Faye et al. (1980) showed variations in AEBS in rat uterine cytosol during the estrous cycle and lowered levels in castrated animals. Gulino and Pasqualini (1983) produced increases in neonatal guinea pig uterine AEBS by estradiol administration. This effect was antagonized by simultaneous administration of progesterone. Winneker and Clark (1983) have extended the study of the estrogenic regulation of rat uterine and liver AEBS to show that AEBS levels increased with age, especially at the time of puberty in female animals, and that treatment of ovariectomized animals with physiological amounts of estradiol also produced significant increases in AEBS. Our own data (Table 6.2) show that the AEBS is present in significantly higher concentrations in a series of ER+ breast cancer cell lines when compared with ER− lines (236,600 ± 29,000 vs 66,600 ± 16,800 sites/cell respectively). However, when human breast tumor biopsies were studied, AEBS was present in significantly higher concentrations in ER− tumors, i.e., those containing < 10 fmol ER/mg cytosol protein (Table 6.2). This difference between AEBS concentrations

Table 6.2. AEBS in human breast cell lines and tumor biopsies

	Concentration $(10^{-5} \times$ sites/cell)	K_d (nM)
ER + cell lines		
MCF-7	1.41 ± 0.20	0.97 ± 0.15
	(4500 fmol/mg microsomal protein)	
ZR-75-1	3.29 ± 0.51	1.30 ± 0.06
MDA-MB-134	3.12	0.93
MDA-MB-361	2.23 ± 0.27	1.30 ± 0.15
T47D	0.99 ± 0.21	1.07 ± 0.15
BT-474	2.14	0.96
ER − cell lines		
BT-20	1.08	0.75
Hs0578T	0.26 ± 0.15	0.88
MDA-MB-330	0.90 ± 0.22	0.95 ± 0.22
HBL-100	0.27	0.71
MDA-MB-231	0.82	0.65
ER + breast tumors	31.42 ± 4.45 (fmol/mg tissue)	2.22 ± 0.14
ER − breast tumors	64.71 ± 12.75 (fmol/mg tissue)	2.40 ± 0.33

in ER + and ER − tumors was apparent only when the concentration was expressed as fmol/mg tissue and did not hold when data were expressed as fmol/mg microsomal protein.

B. BINDING PROPERTIES

Scatchard analysis of the binding of [³H]TAM to the microsomal AEBS shows a single class of noninteracting binding sites of high affinity, e.g., K_d = 0.97 ± 0.15 nM in MCF-7 cells (Watts et al. 1984), K_d = 0.92 ± 0.05 nM in rat liver (Watts and Sutherland 1984), and K_d = 1.8 − 2.1 nM in rat uterus (Sudo et al. 1983). Somewhat lower affinity binding was seen in a series of human tumors (Table 6.2) (K_d = 2.27 ± 0.14 nM, n = 57) (Sutherland and Watts, unpublished observations) and in some rat tissues (Table 6.1 and Sudo et al. 1983).

At 4°C the affinity of TAM for the AEBS is somewhat higher than for ER (Gulino and Pasqualini 1980; Murphy and Sutherland 1981a; Gulino and Pasqualini 1982; Faye et al. 1983). Murphy and Sutherland (1981a) found, for example, K_d values of 1.2 ± 0.3 nM and 2.9 ± 0.3 nM for tamoxifen binding to AEBS and ER, respectively, when assayed under identical conditions. The K_d of the TAM-AEBS interaction remains constant between 4°C and 37°C (Watts et al. 1984), whereas that of the TAM-

ER interaction increases because of a relative increase of the dissociation rate constant (Gulino and Pasqualini 1982). Because of the rapid association rate at higher temperatures and the thermal stability of AEBS (Sudo et al. 1983; Watts et al. 1984), binding assays can be carried out rapidly at 20–30°C.

C. BINDING SPECIFICITY

1. Competition Studies

The structural requirements for binding to the AEBS have been extensively studied (Sutherland et al. 1980; Murphy and Sutherland 1981b; Murphy et al. 1981; Murphy et al. 1983; Sudo et al. 1983; Watts et al. 1984). To summarize these studies, high affinity binding requires the presence of both a hydrophilic basic aminoether side chain and a hydrophobic aromatic ring structure (usually di- or tricyclic). Structural modifications to either influence binding affinity. Figure 6.3 shows the generalized structure of triphenylethylene derivatives, and Figure 6.4 shows the competitive binding of several TAM and clomiphene analogs to rat liver microsomal AEBS. Tables 6.3 and 6.4 report the relative binding affinities (RBA) of these analogs and other compounds. The influence of side chain structure is complex. For example, changes to side chains which produce different hydrocarbon backbone lengths (TAM vs 47108) or variations in the structure of the terminal basic nitrogen-containing group (TAM vs N-desmethyl-TAM, clomiphene vs 9599, TAM vs Compound 13) can affect binding affinity. Sudo et al. (1983) have observed that the basicity of the terminal basic amino group *per se* does not appear to determine binding affinity for AEBS.

Compounds including TAM and clomiphene analogs, which lack side

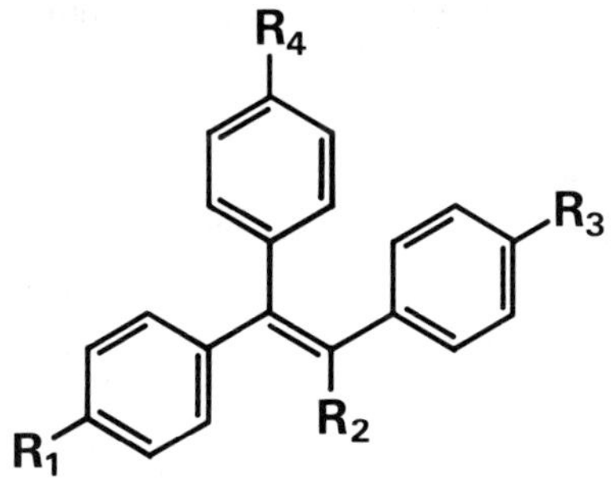

Figure 6.3. Generalized structure of triphenylethylene derivatives.

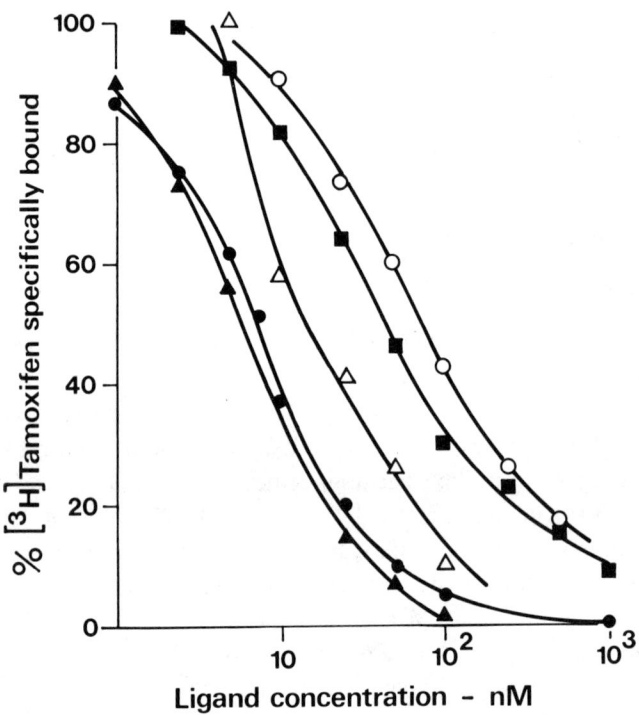

Figure 6.4. Binding of antiestrogens to rat liver microsomes. Competition of antiestrogens for [³H]TAM binding to AEBS in rat liver microsomes. Tamoxifen (●), N-desmethyltamoxifen (○), 4-hydroxytamoxifen (■), enclomiphene (▲), 9599 (△). The relative binding affinities are given in Table 6.3. (From Watts and Sutherland 1984.)

chains (TAM vs metabolite E) or which have nonbasic side chains (TAM vs 145680), have no affinity for AEBS. Natural and synthetic steroids also have no affinity. The cholesterol derivative 5-cholestene-3β-ol-7-one (7-ketocholesterol) (C. Lazier, personal communication) is the only compound tested that has no basic side chain and also binds to AEBS with any detectable affinity.

That the presence of a basic amino side chain is not sufficient for high affinity binding of antiestrogens is illustrated by the RBA of LY 117018, showing that aromatic ring structure and substitution are important. Hence hydroxylation of TAM at a position corresponding to the 3-phenolic hydroxy position of estradiol reduces RBA (4-hydroxy-TAM vs TAM). Both LY 117018 (Sutherland et al. 1984) and 4-hydroxy-TAM (Reddel et al. 1983) have much higher affinities for ER than TAM and this emphasizes

Table 6.3. Relative binding affinities (RBA) of some tamoxifen and enclomiphene derivatives for ER and microsomal AEBS of rat liver and MCF-7 cells

Compound	R_1^a	R_2^a	R_4^a	AEBS[b] (Rat liver)	AEBS[c] (MCF-7)	ER[d,e] (MCF-7)
Tamoxifen (*trans*)	H	C_2H_5	$OCH_2CH_2N(CH_3)_2$	100	100	1.3 ± 0.3
4-Hydroxytamoxifen	OH	C_2H_5	$OCH_2CH_2N(CH_3)_2$	17	80 ± 4	41 ± 3
N-Desmethyltamoxifen	H	C_2H_5	$OCH_2CH_2NHCH_3$	11	19 ± 2	2 ± 1
Enclomiphene	H	Cl	$OCH_2CH_2N(C_2H_5)_2$	136	142 ± 5	2
F6599	H	Cl	$OCH_2CH_2NHC_2H_5$	46	37 ± 2	0.7

R_1–R_4 refer to Figure 6.3; R_3 = H in all cases.
[b] Watts and Sutherland 1984.
[c] Watts et al. 1984.
[d] Sutherland et al. 1984.
[e] Estradiol has a RBA for ER of 100.

the very different binding specificities of AEBS and ER (Murphy et al. 1981, 1983; Sutherland et al. 1984).

Among a miscellaneous group of compounds having basic amino ether side chains (Table 6.4), some, such as the local anesthetic agents tetracaine, procaine, benzocaine, and lignocaine, have little or no binding affinity for AEBS, whereas others, such as propranalol and the cytochrome P_{450} inhibitor SKF-525A and its analogs, can bind with relatively high affinity.

2. Tissue Differences in Specificity

Some tissue and species variations in RBA are apparent in Table 6.3, and in particular a 4-fold difference in RBA for 4-hydroxy-TAM is seen between rat liver and MCF-7 AEBS. Whether AEBS derived from different sources has distinct properties or whether RBA is influenced by other tissue components is unknown.

3. Natural Ligands

The existence of an endogenous ligand for the AEBS is suggested by findings that charcoal extraction of cytosol and nuclear extracts prior to the measurement of [³H]TAM binding can produce several-fold increases in apparent AEBS concentration (Fishman 1983; Murphy et al. 1984). We have found that pretreatment of rat liver microsomes with charcoal (2.5% w/v for 2 hours at 0°C) resulted in a 40% increase in [³H]TAM binding.

Table 6.4. Relative binding affinities (RBA) of TAM derivatives and miscellaneous compounds for microsomal AEBS

Compound	Side chain structure[a]	RBA	Tissue	Reference
Tamoxifen derivatives				
TAM (*trans*)	$O(CH_2)_2N(CH_3)_2$	100	MCF-7	Watts et al. 1984
TAM (*cis*)	$O(CH_2)_2N(CH_3)_2$	98 ± 9	MCF-7	Watts et al. 1984
Metabolite E	OH	0	MCF-7	Sutherland et al. 1984
47108	$O(CH_2)_3N(CH_3)_2$	36 ± 1	MCF-7	Watts et al. 1984
145680	$OCH_2CHOHCHCH_3OH$	0	MCF-7	Watts et al. 1984
Compound 13	$O(CH_2)_2\text{-c-}N(CH_2CH_2)_2O$	1174 ± 424	Rat uterus	Sudo et al. 1983
Compound 14	$O(CH_2)_2\text{-c-}NC_4H_4$	0	Rat uterus	Sudo et al. 1983
Miscellaneous compounds				
LY 117018	$O(CH_2)_2\text{-c-}NC_4H_8$	2	MCF-7	Sutherland and Watts, unpub. obs.
U 23469	$OCH_2CHOHCH_2OH$	0	MCF-7	Sutherland and Watts, unpub. obs.
Tetracaine	$COO(CH_2)_2N(CH_3)_2$	< 0.1	MCF-7	Watts et al. 1984
Propranolol	$OCH_2CHOHCH_2NHCH(CH_3)_2$	1.4	Rat uterus	Sudo et al. 1983
5 cholestene-3β-ol-7-one	—	1	Rat liver	Sutherland and Watts, unpub. obs.
SKF-525A	$CO(CH_2)_2N(C_2H_5)_2$	11.5 ± 1.32	Rat liver	Sutherland and Watts, unpub. obs.

[a]R_4 in Figure 6.3 for the TAM derivatives.

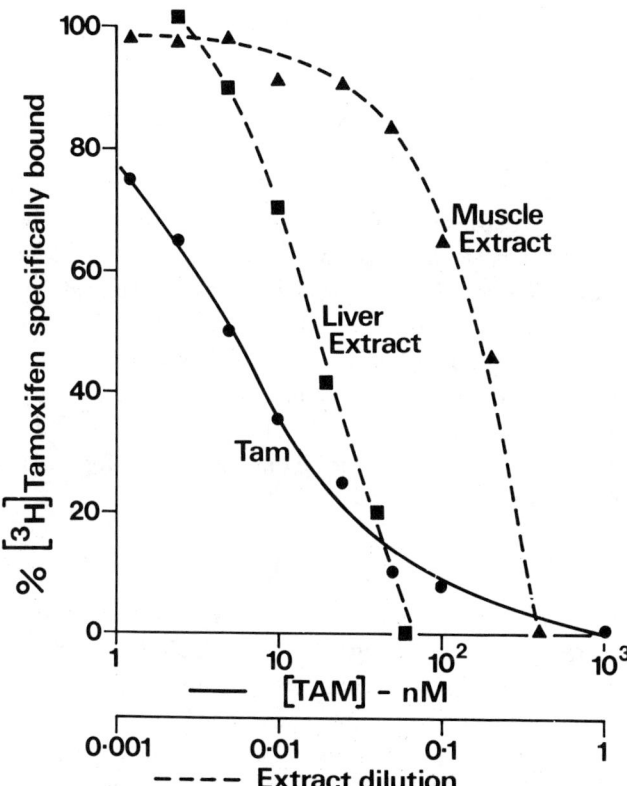

Figure 6.5. Inhibition of [³H]TAM binding to AEBS by ethanol extracts of rat tissues. Equal wet weights of liver and muscle from mature male rats were extracted with boiling ethanol for 1 hour. The extracts were filtered and diluted and after drying down under nitrogen used in competitive binding assays with [³H]TAM and rat liver microsomal AEBS.

Clark et al. (1983) and Murphy et al. (1984) have detected, in solvent extracts of serum and tissues, components which act as competitive inhibitors of the binding of [³H]TAM to AEBS. We have confirmed these findings, and Figure 6.5 shows the ability of ethanol extracts of rat liver and skeletal muscle to inhibit [³H]TAM binding to rat liver microsomal AEBS. It is not known whether such inhibitors are true natural ligands for AEBS and what roles these ligands play in normal cellular physiology.

D. MOLECULAR PROPERTIES OF MICROSOMAL AEBS

1. Enzyme Susceptibility

AEBS binding activity has been reported to be destroyed by protease treatment (Sutherland et al. 1980; Faye et al. 1983; Kon 1983; Sudo et al. 1983), although we have found that high protease concentrations are needed to affect AEBS in MCF-7 microsomal preparations. The AEBS in cytosol preparations is not susceptible to lipase, ribonuclease, deoxyribonuclease, phospholipase, amylase, or neuraminidase (Sutherland et al. 1980; Gulino and Pasqualini 1982; Faye et al. 1983; Kon 1983) but in MCF-7 microsomes the AEBS is sensitive to lipase and phospholipase C. Pretreatment with these enzymes enhanced susceptibility to trypsin (Fig. 6.6). These results indicate that the AEBS is partly protein in nature but may require lipid as a cofactor for binding activity or for maintenance of structural integrity.

2. Other Factors Influencing Binding

Microsomes extracted with 1 M KCl or low concentrations of sodium deoxycholate retain AEBS, suggesting that AEBS is neither a loosely adsorbed or extrinsic membrane protein nor a luminal (i.e., newly synthesized) protein of the microsomal vesicles (Watts and Sutherland 1984).

Low concentrations of Ca^{2+} or Mg^{2+} (< 10 mM) appear to inhibit binding of [³H]TAM to AEBS. However, this effect results from divalent cation-induced aggregation of microsomal vesicles, which are subsequently pelleted when dextran-charcoal suspensions are centrifuged during AEBS assay. AEBS activity is retained by these aggregates and Ca^{2+} has little effect when added to detergent-solubilized microsomes. Binding activity is unaffected by 10 mM EDTA or EGTA.

AEBS binding activity is reduced by 20 ± 4% in the presence of 1 mM dithiothreitol, suggesting that disulphide bonds play a role in maintaining the structural conformation of the AEBS.

A narrow pH optimum around pH 7.5 for the binding of [³H]TAM to the AEBS has been observed (Sudo et al. 1983; Watts et al. 1984).

E. MOLECULAR PROPERTIES OF DETERGENT-SOLUBILIZED AEBS

As an initial step in AEBS purification we have studied the solubilization of AEBS from rat liver microsomes by a range of detergents. Some detergents with very low critical micelle concentrations, such as Triton X-

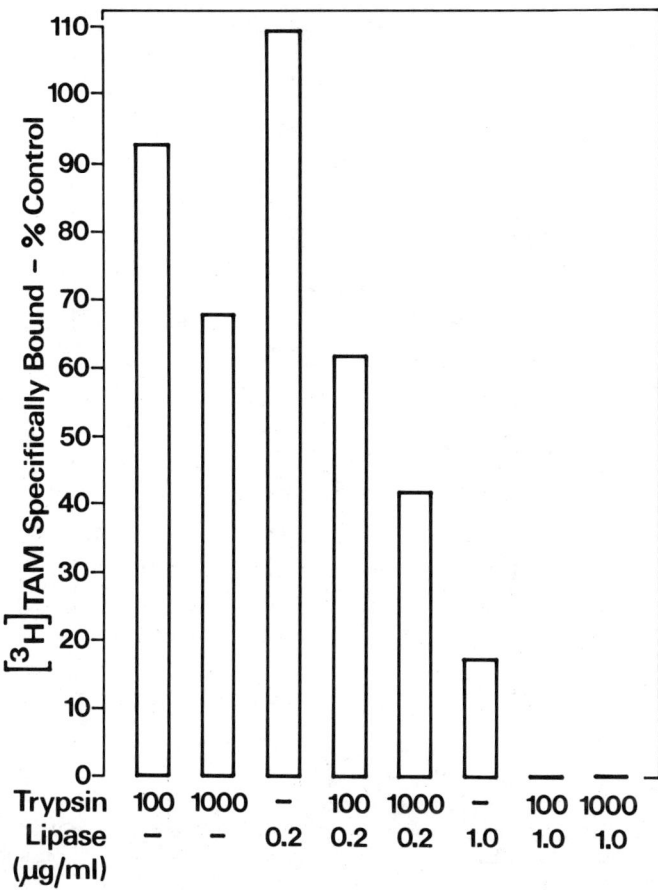

Trypsin	100	1000	–	100	1000	–	100	1000
Lipase	–	–	0.2	0.2	0.2	1.0	1.0	1.0
(µg/ml)								

Figure 6.6. Effect of enzyme pretreatment on the ability of MCF-7 microsomes to bind [³H]TAM. Enzymes, at the final concentrations shown, were incubated with MCF-7 microsomal preparations for 1 hour at 37°C, except when lipase and trypsin were both added, in which case a 30-minute incubation with lipase was followed by addition of trypsin and a further 30-minute incubation period.

100, were unsuitable because of their interference with dextran-charcoal removal of free ligand during assay of AEBS. Other detergents solubilized microsomal material but inactivated AEBS (e.g., CHAPS, CHAPSO, β-D-octyl glucoside). Sodium deoxycholate solubilized AEBS in low yield but solubilized material was unstable, whereas sodium cholate at high concentrations (> 1% w/v) was effective in producing a relatively stable form of soluble AEBS in high yield. Solubilization was more effective in the presence of 1 M NaCl (Fig. 6.7). Binding affinity for [³H]TAM is

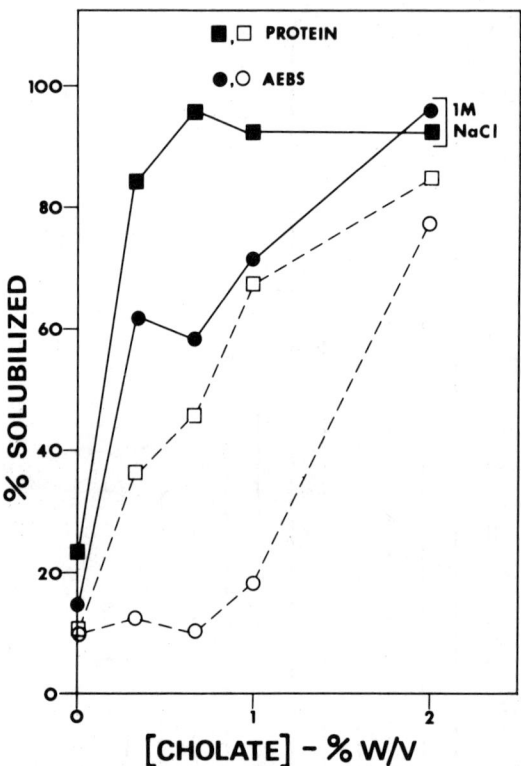

Figure 6.7. Detergent solubilization of rat liver microsomal AEBS. Sodium cholate was added in increasing concentrations to rat liver microsomes, in the presence or absence of 1 M NaCl. Solubilized AEBS and protein were assayed in the supernatant after centrifugation at 130,000 g_{av} for 1 hour.

reduced in the presence of sodium cholate. Thus in the solubilized state and at cholate concentrations greater than 1% w/v, the AEBS has no affinity for [^{3}H]TAM. Binding activity is restored by detergent dilution which allows reconstitution of protein-lipid vesicles.

Gel filtration chromatography of solubilized rat liver microsomes (Fig. 6.8) showed a relatively broad peak of binding activity with an apparent molecular weight of 440,000–490,000. Whether this peak of activity represents the native AEBS or a complex with other undissociated lipid or protein components is unknown. Gel filtration of whole rat liver microsomes or postmitochondrial supernatants (cytosol + microsomes) on the same columns showed that AEBS activity was present only at the column

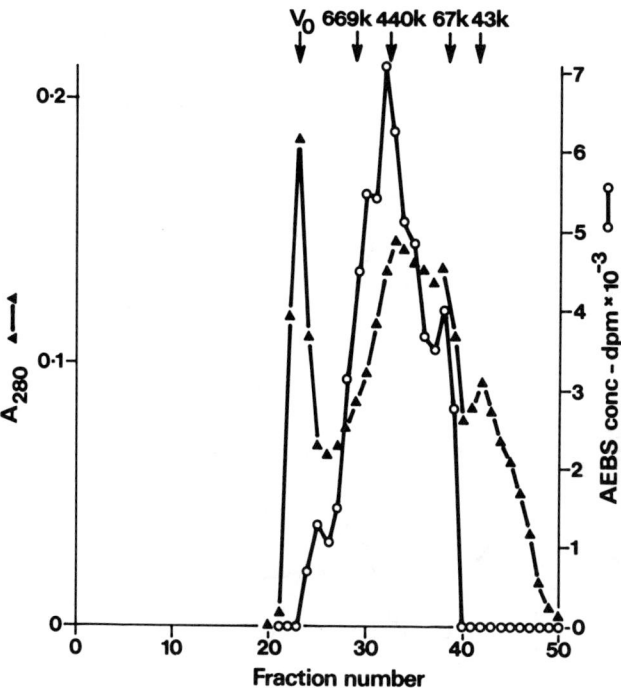

Figure 6.8. Gel filtration of detergent solubilized AEBS. Rat liver microsomes were solubilized in a 10 mM Tris-HCl buffer (pH 7.4) containing 25 mM KCl, 0.25 M sucrose, 1% w/v sodium cholate, and 1 M NaCl, and then chromatographed using the same buffer on a Fractogel TSK 65F column (fractionation range 50–5,000 kilodaltons). After dilution, fractions were assayed for AEBS activity. V_0 represents the void volume and calibration proteins, fractionated separately on the same column, were thyroglobulin (669 K), ferritin (440 K), bovine serum albumin (67 K) and ovalbumin (43 K).

void volume (exclusion limit of approximately 5,000 kilodaltons), as would be expected for a membrane-bound component.

Solubilized AEBS was not bound by a variety of lectin-agaroses (concanavalin-A-, castor bean-, lentil-, and wheat germ-agarose) but appeared to be progressively bound when passed over hydrophobic gels of increasing chain length (agarose-$NH(CH_2)_nCH_3$ and agarose-$NH(CH_2)_nNH_2$, Fig. 6.9A, B). Although hydrophobic interaction chromatography is a promising purification step, as yet we have had no success in eluting AEBS from these gels in an active form.

Selective polyethylene glycol protein precipitation of AEBS from solubilized microsomes results in precipitation of 50% and 100% of AEBS

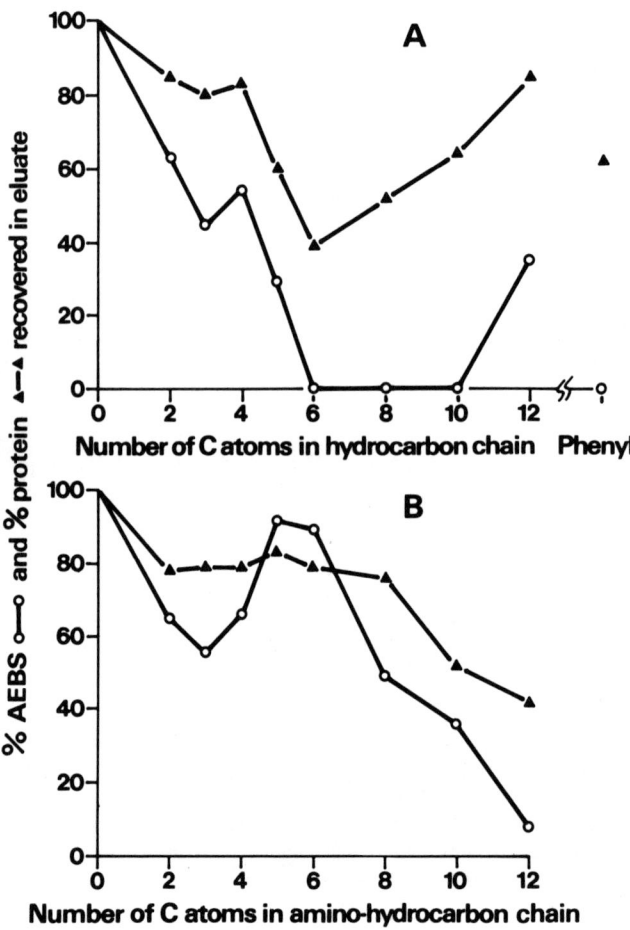

Figure 6.9. Hydrophobic chromatography of detergent solubilized AEBS. Aliquots of solubilized rat liver microsomes (see legend to Fig. 6.8) were passed through columns containing hydrophobic gels of increasing chain length: agarose-NH(CH$_2$)$_n$CH$_3$ and phenyl-agarose (panel A) or agarose-NH(CH$_2$)$_n$NH$_2$ (panel B). For the latter series of gels the applied sample was adjusted to 4 M NaCl. After a washing step the eluates were assayed for AEBS and protein concentration.

by 10% and 18% w/v PEG 6000, respectively. Precipitated AEBS retains binding activity and can be resolubilized in detergent solutions but is prone to reaggregation upon detergent dilution, preventing use of dextran-charcoal assay techniques.

III. *Putative Function of Antiestrogen Binding Sites*

"The affinity and concentration of this specific antiestrogen binding site are such that it may play a significant role in the intracellular binding of nonsteroidal antiestrogens and may regulate the amount of antiestrogen available for estrogen receptor binding." Although this hypothesis was advanced in the first published report of the AEBS (Sutherland and Foo 1979), there is, as yet, no direct evidence for a functional role for the AEBS either as a mediator of drug action or in the normal physiology of the cell.

Even though removal of basic side chains from nonsteroidal antiestrogenic compounds usually results in both loss of affinity for AEBS and loss of antiestrogenic properties, antiestrogenicity in general parallels affinity for ER rather than affinity for AEBS. This is shown by the estrogen-reversible inhibition of breast cancer cell proliferation *in vitro* (Coezy et al. 1982; Murphy and Sutherland 1983, 1985; Sutherland et al. 1984; Reddel et al. 1985) and by antiuterotrophic potencies *in vivo* in the rat (Jordan et al. 1977; Robertson et al. 1982). As assessed by antiuterotrophic assay, some compounds which have nonbasic side chains and have no affinity for AEBS (e.g., U 23,469, Sudo et al. 1983) are nevertheless antiestrogenic (Hayes et al. 1981), whereas others such as *cis*-TAM (ICI 47,699) and zuclomiphene (*cis*-clomiphene) have high affinity for AEBS but act as estrogen agonists (Jordan et al. 1978). These findings indicate a lack of involvement of the AEBS in the antiestrogenic properties of nonsteroidal compounds. However, the above observations are complicated by several unexplained features of antiestrogenic action. For example, in the chick oviduct Sutherland (1981) found that antiestrogenic potency *in vivo* could not be correlated with affinity for ER, and also that ICI 47,699 and zuclomiphene had no agonistic activity and seemed to act as weak antagonists. Also, studies of the effects on MCF-7 cell proliferation of derivatives of clomiphene (Murphy and Sutherland 1983) and TAM (Murphy and Sutherland 1985) showed unexplained differences in potency between compounds having the same affinities for ER. Enhanced potency was accompanied by an enhanced affinity for AEBS. However, whether in examples such as these the interaction of nonsteroidal antiestrogens with the AEBS contributes to their antiestrogenic properties remains undefined.

Murphy and Sutherland (1983, 1985) have been able to correlate the affinities of some nonsteroidal compounds for AEBS with their activities in estradiol-irreversible growth inhibition and cytotoxicity in MCF-7 cells. Affinity for AEBS was essential for the expression of cytotoxicity. However, such effects are only observed at high extracellular drug concentrations, i.e., > 2.5 μM. If similar intracellular concentrations were achieved, they would be far in excess of those required to saturate the AEBS, so it is uncertain how the AEBS could mediate these drug activities. Lam (1984) has reported that TAM can act as a potent competitive inhibitor of the activation by calmodulin of cAMP phosphodiesterase (IC_{50} = 2 μM). We do not know whether the inhibition of such calmodulin-dependent cellular processes is responsible for the growth inhibition and cytotoxicity of TAM at high concentrations or whether the AEBS is involved in these effects.

Other evidence that the AEBS might play a role in some aspects of triphenylethylene drug action has been provided by Faye et al. (1983), who have described a TAM-resistant MCF-7 cell line, RTx6, which had low concentrations of AEBS but unchanged ER levels and in which TAM had little effect on cell growth or thymidine incorporation compared to wild-type MCF-7 cells.

The high concentration of AEBS in the liver (a major site of TAM metabolism) and in the endoplasmic reticulum, and the relatively high affinity of AEBS for SKF-525A analogs (Sutherland and Watts, unpublished observations), which bind tightly to and inhibit cytochrome P_{450}, suggest that the AEBS may be a binding site on P_{450}. However, unlike P_{450}, the AEBS in rat liver is neither induced by phenobarbital treatment nor reduced by cobalt-heme treatment *in vivo*. P_{450} and AEBS have different submicrosomal distributions and do not copurify upon detergent extraction (Watts, unpublished observations). Direct but low affinity interactions of TAM and clomiphene with P_{450} have been reported (Ruenitz and Toledo 1980), and in rat liver microsomes this interaction results in potent inhibition of the mixed function oxidase system by TAM and its metabolites N-desmethyl-TAM and 4-hydroxy-TAM (Meltzer et al. 1984). Other components of this system may be potential locations for the AEBS which might also contribute to inhibition of drug metabolism. Interestingly, despite high concentrations of AEBS in the MCF-7 line, these cells do not metabolize TAM (Horwitz et al. 1978; Borgna and Rochefort 1981).

That the AEBS may be important in the normal physiology of the cell is suggested by the estrogen regulation of AEBS (Section II.A) and by the possible existence of endogenous ligands (Section II.C). Proposed roles for the ligand-AEBS system have included involvement in the control of cholesterol metabolism (Clark et al. 1983) and in regulation of estrogen action (Fishman 1983).

IV. Conclusion

The existence of the AEBS, a microsomal binding site, distinct from the ER, which has high affinity for the triphenylethylene series of nonsteroidal antiestrogens and several other structurally related compounds, has been confirmed by several groups since its first documentation in this laboratory. Although the molecular properties of the AEBS have been described in some detail, no function has yet been identified. There is, however, evidence that the AEBS may be involved in aspects of the pharmacology of triphenylethylene derivatives and that a natural ligand may exist. There will no doubt be continued interest in further understanding the functional significance of the AEBS.

References

Borgna, J. L., and H. Rochefort. 1980. High-affinity binding to the estrogen receptor of [³H]4-hydroxytamoxifen, an active antiestrogen metabolite. *Molecular and Cellular Endocrinology* 20:71–86.

Borgna, J. L., and H. Rochefort. 1981. Hydroxylated metabolites of tamoxifen are formed *in vivo* and bound to estrogen receptor in target tissues. *Journal of Biological Chemistry* 256:859–868.

Clark, J. H., R. C. Winneker, S. C. Guthrie, and B. M. Markaverich. 1983. An endogenous ligand for the triphenylethylene antiestrogen binding site. *Endocrinology* 113:1167–1169.

Coezy, E., J. L. Borgna, and H. Rochefort. 1982. Tamoxifen and metabolites in MCF-7 cells: correlation between binding to estrogen receptor and inhibition of cell growth. *Cancer Research* 42:317–323.

Eckert, R. L., and B. S. Katzenellenbogen. 1982. Physical properties of estrogen receptor complexes in MCF-7 human breast cancer cells: differences with antiestrogen and estrogen. *Journal of Biological Chemistry* 257:8840–8846.

Faye, J. C., B. Lasserre, and F. Bayard. 1980. Antiestrogen specific, high affinity, saturable binding sites in rat uterine cytosol. *Biochemical and Biophysical Research Communications* 93:1225–1231.

Faye, J. C., S. Jozan, G. Redeuilh, E. E. Baulieu, and F. Bayard. 1983. Physicochemical and genetic evidence for specific antiestrogen binding sites. *Proceedings of the National Academy of Sciences* 80:3158–3162.

Fishman, J. H. 1983. Estradiol and tamoxifen interaction at receptor sites at 37°C. *Endocrinology* 113:1164–1166.

Gulino, A., and J. R. Pasqualini. 1980. Specific binding and biological response of antiestrogens in the fetal uterus of the guinea pig. *Cancer Research* 40:3821–3826.

Gulino, A., and J. R. Pasqualini. 1982. Heterogeneity of binding sites for tamoxifen and tamoxifen derivatives in estrogen target and nontarget fetal organs of guinea pig. *Cancer Research* 42:1913–1921.

Gulino, A., and J. R. Pasqualini. 1983. Modulation of tamoxifen-specific binding sites and estrogen receptors by estradiol and progesterone in the neonatal uterus of guinea pig. *Endocrinology* 112:1871–1873.

Hayes, J. R., E. A. Rorke, B. S. Katzenellenbogen, D. W. Robertson, and J. A. Katzenellenbogen. 1981. Biological potency and uterine estrogen receptor interactions of the metabolites of the antiestrogens CI628 and U23,469. *Endocrinology* 108:164–172.

Horwitz, K. B., Y. Koseki, and W. L. McGuire. 1978. Estrogen control of progesterone receptor in human breast cancer: role of estradiol and antiestrogen. *Endocrinology* 103:1742–1751.

Jordan, V. C., M. M. Collins, L. Rowsby, and G. Prestwich. 1977. A monohydroxylated metabolite of tamoxifen with potent antioestrogenic activity. *Journal of Endocrinology* 75:305–316.

Jordan, V. C., C. J. Dix, K. E. Naylor, G. Prestwich, and L. Rowsby. 1978. Nonsteroidal antiestrogens: their biological effects and potential mechanisms of action. *Journal of Toxicology and Environmental Health* 4:363–390.

Katzenellenbogen, B. S., E. J. Pavlik, D. W. Robertson, and J. A. Katzenellenbogen. 1981. Interaction of a high affinity antiestrogen (a-[4-pyrrolidinoethoxy]phenyl-4-hydroxy-a8-nitrostilbene, CI628M) with uterine estrogen receptors. *Journal of Biological Chemistry* 256:2908–2915.

Kon, O. L. 1983. An antiestrogen-binding protein in human tissues. *Journal of Biological Chemistry* 258:3173–3177.

Lam, H-Y. P. 1984. Tamoxifen is a calmodulin antagonist in the activation of cAMP phosphodiesterase. *Biochemical and Biophysical Research Communications* 118:27–32.

Martin, L. 1981. Effects of antioestrogens on cell proliferation in the rodent reproductive tract. In *Non-steroidal antioestrogens: molecular pharmacology and antitumour activity*, ed. R. L. Sutherland and V. C. Jordan, 143–163. Sydney: Academic Press.

Meltzer, N. M., P. Stang, L. A. Sternson, and A. E. Wade. 1984. Influence of tamoxifen and its N-desmethyl and 4-hydroxy metabolites on rat liver microsomal enzymes. *Biochemical Pharmacology* 33:115–123.

Miller, M. A., and B. S. Katzenellenbogen. 1983. Characterization and quantitation of antiestrogen binding sites in estrogen receptor-positive and -negative human breast cancer cell lines. *Cancer Research* 43:3094–3100.

Murphy, L. C., and R. L. Sutherland. 1981a. A high affinity binding site for the antioestrogens, tamoxifen and CI 628, in immature rat uterine cytosol which is distinct from the oestrogen receptor. *Journal of Endocrinology* 91:155–161.

Murphy, L. C., and R. L. Sutherland. 1981b. Modifications in the aminoether side chain of clomiphene influence affinity for a specific antiestrogen binding site in MCF-7 cell cytosol. *Biochemical and Biophysical Research Communications* 100:1353–1360.

Murphy, L. C., and R. L. Sutherland. 1983. Anti-tumor activity of clomiphene analogs *in vitro:* relationship to affinity for the estrogen receptor and another high affinity antiestrogen-binding site. *Journal of Clinical Endocrinology and Metabolism* 57:373–379.

Murphy, L. C., and R. L. Sutherland. 1985. Differential effects of tamoxifen and analogs with nonbasic sidechains on cell proliferation *in vitro. Endocrinology* 116:1071–1078.

Murphy, L. C., M. S. Foo, M. D. Green, B. K. Milthorpe, A. M. Whybourne, Z. S. Krozowski, and R. L. Sutherland. 1981. Binding of non-steroidal antioestrogens to saturable binding sites distinct from the oestrogen receptor in normal and neoplastic tissues. In *Non-steroidal antioestrogens: molecular pharmacology and antitumour activity*, ed. R. L. Sutherland and V. C. Jordan, 317–337. Sydney: Academic Press.

Murphy, L. C., C. K. W. Watts, and R. L. Sutherland. 1983. Structural requirements for binding of antiestrogens to a specific high affinity site in MCF-7 human mammary carcinoma cells: correlation with antitumor activity *in vitro*. *Rational basis for chemotherapy*, ed. B. A. Chabner, 195–210. *UCLA Symposia on Molecular and Cellular Biology*, vol. 4. New York: Alan R. Liss.

Murphy, P. R., C. Butts, and C. B. Lazier. 1984. Triphenylethylene antiestrogen-binding sites in cockerel liver nuclei: evidence for an endogenous ligand. *Endocrinology* 115:420–426.

Reddel, R. R., L. C. Murphy, and R. L. Sutherland. 1983. Effects of biologically active metabolites of tamoxifen on the proliferation kinetics of MCF-7 human breast cancer cells *in vitro*. *Cancer Research* 43:4618–4624.

Reddel, R. R., L. C. Murphy, R. E. Hall, and R. L. Sutherland. 1985. Differential sensitivity of human breast cancer cell lines to the growth inhibitory effects of tamoxifen. *Cancer Research* 45:1525–1531.

Robertson, D. W., J. A. Katzenellenbogen, J. R. Hayes, and B. S. Katzenellenbogen. 1982. Antiestrogen basicity-activity relationships: A comparison of the estrogen receptor binding and antiuterotrophic potencies of several analogues of (Z)-1,2-diphenyl-1-[4-[2-(dimethylamino)ethoxy]phenyl]-1-butene (Tamoxifen, Nolvadex) having altered basicity. *Journal of Medicinal Chemistry* 25:167–171.

Ruenitz, P. C., and M. M. Toledo. 1980. Inhibition of rabbit liver microsomal oxidative metabolism and substrate binding by tamoxifen and the geometric isomers of clomiphene. *Biochemical Pharmacology* 29:1583–1587.

Sudo, K., F. J. Monsma, and B. S. Katzenellenbogen. 1983. Antiestrogen-binding sites distinct from the estrogen receptor: sub-cellular localization, ligand specificity, and distribution in tissues of the rat. *Endocrinology* 112:425–434.

Sutherland, R. L. 1981. Estrogen antagonists in chick oviduct. Antagonist activity of eight synthetic triphenylethylene derivatives and their interactions with cytoplasmic and nuclear estrogen receptors. *Endocrinology* 109:2061–2068.

Sutherland, R. L., and M. S. Foo. 1979. Differential binding of antiestrogens by rat uterine and chick oviduct cytosol. *Biochemical and Biophysical Research Communications* 91:183–191.

Sutherland, R. L., and V. C. Jordan (eds.). 1981. *Non-steroidal antioestrogens: molecular pharmacology and antitumour activity*. Sydney: Academic Press.

Sutherland, R. L., and L. C. Murphy. 1980. The binding of tamoxifen to human mammary carcinoma cytosol. *European Journal of Cancer* 16:1141–1148.

Sutherland, R. L., L. C. Murphy, M. S. Foo, M. D. Green, A. M. Whybourne, and Z. S. Krozowski. 1980. High-affinity anti-oestrogen binding site distinct from the oestrogen receptor. *Nature* (London) 288:273–275.

Sutherland, R. L., C. K. W. Watts, and L. C. Murphy. 1982. Binding properties and ligand specificity of an intracellular binding site with specificity for synthetic oestrogen antagonists of the triphenylethylene series. In *Hormone antagonists*, ed. M. K. Agarwal, 147–161. Berlin: Walter de Gruyter.

Sutherland, R. L., R. E. Hall, and I. W. Taylor. 1983. Cell proliferation kinetics of MCF-7 human mammary carcinoma cells in culture and effects of tamoxifen on exponentially growing and plateau-phase cells. *Cancer Research* 43:3998–4006.

Sutherland, R. L., L. C. Murphy, R. E. Hall, R. R. Reddel, C. K. W. Watts, and I. W. Taylor. 1984. Effects of antioestrogens on human breast cancer cells *in vitro*. Interaction with high affinity intracellular binding sites and effects on cell proliferation kinetics. In *Hormones and cancer 2. Progress in cancer research and therapy*, vol. 31, ed. F. Bresciani, R. J. B. King, M. E. Lippman, M. Namer, and J. P. Raynaud, 193–212. New York: Raven Press.

Watts, C. K. W., and R. L. Sutherland. 1984. High affinity specific antiestrogen binding sites are concentrated in rough microsomal membranes of rat liver. *Biochemical and Biophysical Research Communications* 120:109–115.

Watts, C. K. W., L. C. Murphy, and R. L. Sutherland. 1984. Microsomal binding sites for nonsteroidal antiestrogens in MCF-7 human mammary carcinoma cells. Demonstration of high affinity and narrow specificity for basic ether derivatives of triphenylethylene. *Journal of Biological Chemistry* 259:4223–4229.

Winneker, R. C., and J. H. Clark. 1983. Estrogenic stimulation of the antiestrogen specific binding site in rat uterus and liver. *Endocrinology* 112:1910–1915.

Winneker, R. C., S. C. Guthrie, and J. H. Clark. 1983. Characterization of a triphenylethylene-antiestrogen-binding site on rat serum low density lipoprotein. *Endocrinology* 112:1823–1827.

7

Antiestrogen Action and Antiestrogen Binding Sites

JAMES H. CLARK, BARRY M. MARKAVERICH,
S. C. GUTHRIE, AND R. C. WINNEKER

I. INTRODUCTION 116
II. THE AGONISTIC/ANTAGONISTIC ACTIONS OF ANTIESTROGENS 116
III. SPECIFIC BINDING SITES FOR TRIPHENYLETHYLENE ANTIESTROGENS 119
IV. TRIPHENYLETHYLENE BINDING SITES AND LOW DENSITY LIPOPROTEINS 120
V. AN ENDOGENOUS LIGAND FOR THE TRIPHENYLETHYLENE
ANTIESTROGEN BINDING SITES (TABS) 123
REFERENCES 125

I. Introduction

ANTIESTROGENS, such as clomiphene and tamoxifen, are triphenylethylene derivatives which are used to induce ovulation and treat hormone-
dependent breast cancer (for review see Clark and Markaverich 1982; Furr
and Jordan 1984). Although they have been used effectively for years,
their mechanism of action remains unknown. Most investigators believe
antiestrogens interfere with the action of estrogen at the receptor level;
however, as we describe below, the picture is complex and may involve
indirect actions which do not result from estrogen receptor interactions.

II. The Agonistic/Antagonistic Actions of Antiestrogens

Antiestrogens are thought to interfere with estrogen action by competing
for estrogen receptor sites and thereby reducing the number of active
receptor-estrogen complexes. The receptor-antiestrogen complexes are
thought to be inactive or partially active. Indeed, this explanation does
appear to have validity in experiments done with cells *in vitro* (Lieberman
et al. 1983), but the concept does not seem to apply to the *in vivo* situation. When rats are given estradiol by pellet implant or nafoxidine by
injection, the response profiles observed for nuclear binding of the estrogen receptor and RNA polymerase activity are essentially identical (Fig.
7.1; Hardin et al. 1976; Clark and Peck 1979; Padykula et al. 1981). This
also occurs when the two compounds are administered simultaneously and
is true for other triphenylethylene antiestrogens (Clark and Markaverich
1982). Thus, with respect to these three parameters of estrogen action,
triphenylethylene drugs are agonistic, not antagonistic. Antagonism is observed, however, when uterine weight and histology are examined. The
data in Figure 7.2 show that, by 72 hours after exposure to the hormones,
the uteri of estradiol-treated animals are approximately twice the size of
those of the rats treated with nafoxidine or nafoxidine plus estradiol. This
difference in size is attributable to the ability of estradiol to stimulate cellular hypertrophy and hyperplasia in all of the tissue layers of the uterus,
whereas nafoxidine and other triphenylethylene antiestrogens only partially stimulate these tissues (Clark and Markaverich 1982; Furr and Jor-

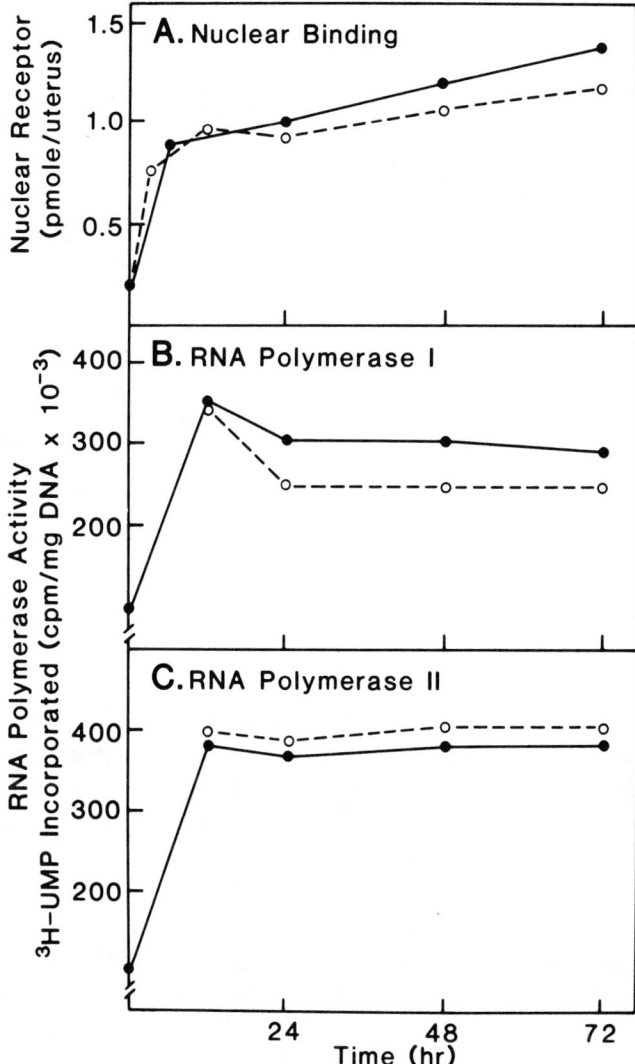

Figure 7.1. Effect of estradiol or nafoxidine on nuclear receptor levels and RNA polymerase activity. Estradiol (●) was administered by pellet implant in order to provide continuous occupancy of nuclear estrogen receptors. Nafoxidine or nafoxidine plus estradiol (○) was given by a single subcutaneous injection, which also causes continuous occupancy of nuclear estrogen receptors. See Padykula et al. (1981) for details.

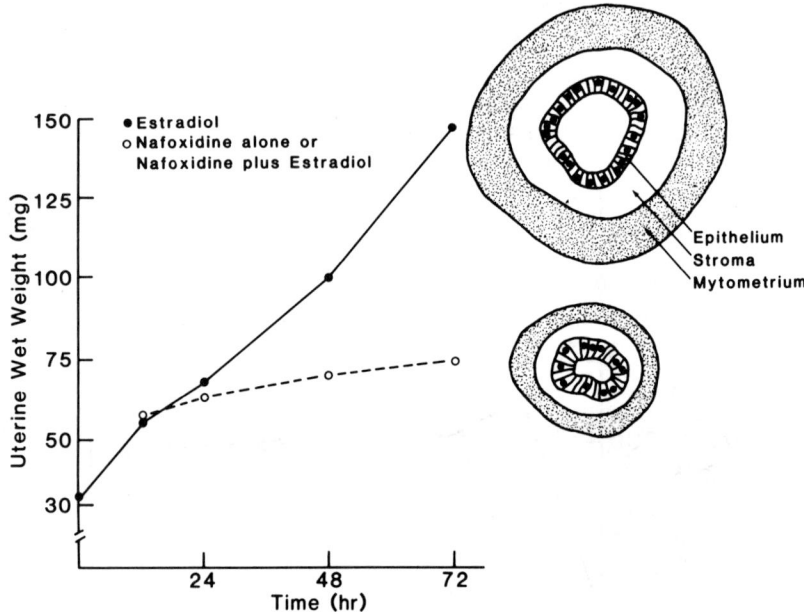

Figure 7.2. Effect of estradiol or nafoxidine on uterine growth.

dan 1984). This failure of antiestrogens to fully stimulate cellular growth is difficult to understand in light of the previous data (Fig. 7.1), which show that triphenylethylene drugs are estrogenic. At least part of the explanation must lie in the divergence in growth that occurs at 20–24 hours after hormonal exposure. During the first 20–24 hours the weight and histology of the uteri of both groups are identical. This is also true for most of the uterotrophic responses that have been measured (Hardin et al. 1976; Lan and Katzenellenbogen 1976; Mairesse and Galand 1979). Therefore, both compounds are acting as agonists. This first 24-hour period is also the time during which DNA synthesis is taking place in preparation for subsequent cell division (Kaye et al. 1972; Kirkland et al. 1979). Both estrogens and antiestrogens increase DNA synthesis and mitotic activity in all three tissue layers of the uterus (Makku et al. 1981); however, DNA synthesis apparently ceases in the antiestrogen-treated uterus but continues under the influence of estradiol. Thus, at the end of a 3-day period of treatment the estrogen-treated uterus contains twice as much DNA as the antiestrogen-treated uterus (Markaverich et al. 1981). Apparently, during the first 24 hours all biosynthetic systems are functioning as though they had received an estrogen signal, and at later times this estrogen signal is being inhibited in some fashion in the antiestrogen-treated animals. These considerations imply that triphenylethylene drugs are acting as estrogenic compounds and that antiestrogenicity is being expressed in some indirect and delayed fashion. Such an indirect mechanism may involve the antiestrogen binding sites, which are discussed in the following sections.

III. Specific Binding Sites for Triphenylethylene Antiestrogens

Sutherland et al. (1980) showed that there are antiestrogen-specific binding sites in various tissues and suggested that these sites might be receptors for antiestrogens. The presence of these sites has been confirmed by several investigators (Faye et al. 1980; Gulino and Pasqualini 1980; Kon 1983; Sudo et al. 1983). Our interest in these sites arose from the possibility that there might be an endogenous ligand for these sites that might represent an endogenous antiestrogen.

In order to test the possibility of an endogenous ligand we first examined the characteristics of the triphenylethylene antiestrogen binding site (TABS). These sites are found in the low-speed cytosol of several different tissues, and they appear to be associated with the particulate components of the homogenate, since they can be cleared from the cytosol by high-speed centrifugation (Sudo et al. 1983).

TABS have some properties in common with receptors, and others which are not. There are a limited number of sites/cell which have a high affinity (K_d, 2 nM) for the binding of triphenylethylene drugs (Fig. 7.3). These sites are very specific for the binding of triphenylethylene drugs and do not recognize estrogens or any of the other steroids (Watts et al. 1984). They are found in several tissues of the body and are not restricted to estrogen target tissues (Kon 1983; Sudo et al. 1983). This distribution makes it unlikely that TABS are antiestrogen receptors *per se* but does not rule out an indirect role in estrogen antagonism.

The possible involvement of TABS in the mechanism of action of antiestrogens is suggested by the observation that estrogen administration and the physiological state of the ovary have effects on the level of TABS in both liver and uterus (Winneker and Clark 1983). At the time of puberty, the liver TABS concentration increases significantly in the female in comparison to both mature males or immature females. TABS levels in the rat uterine cytosol increase significantly in mature females in compar-

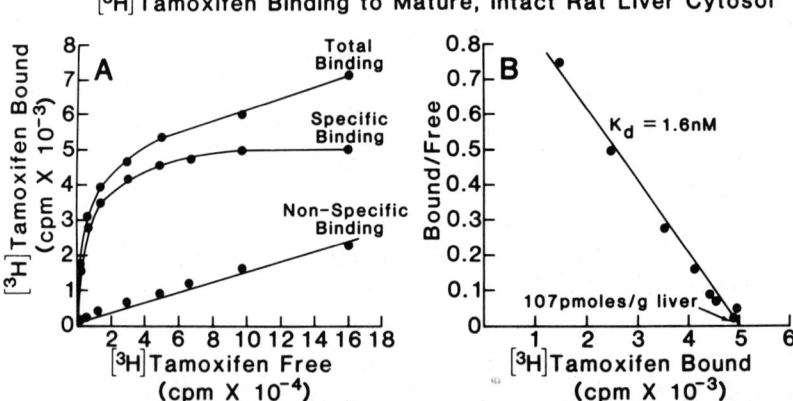

Figure 7.3. Saturation (A) and Scatchard (B) analysis of [³H]tamoxifen binding to rat liver cytosol. Samples of liver cytosol were exposed to different concentrations of [³H]tamoxifen for 1 hour at 30°C, followed by dextran-charcoal separation. A 200-fold excess of diethylstilbestrol (DES) was added to all assay tubes to inhibit [³H]tamoxifen estrogen receptor interactions. Only specific binding data were used for Scatchard plots.

ison to either castrated or younger animals. In addition, both uterine and liver TABS levels fluctuate throughout the estrous cycle and reach a peak approximately on the day of estrus. Treatment of ovariectomized rats with physiological amounts of estradiol causes a 2-fold increase in TABS levels in the uterus, thus mimicking the midcycle peak of TABS (Fig. 7.4). A similar elevation in TABS occurs in the liver following estrogen treatment. Recently, Gulino and Pasqualini (1983) have shown that the level of TABS is modulated in the guinea pig uterus by estradiol and progesterone.

These results indicate that TABS are being regulated by ovarian steroids, primarily estrogens. If TABS were involved in antiestrogen action, it might be expected that estrogens would regulate or modify the level of these sites. That is, one can speculate that one of the estrogenic responses of target tissues is to produce TABS, which may in some way modify the ability of the tissue to respond to estrogen.

IV. Triphenylethylene Binding Sites and Low Density Lipoproteins

During the course of the studies discussed above we also examined rat serum for the presence of TABS and were surprised to find substantial

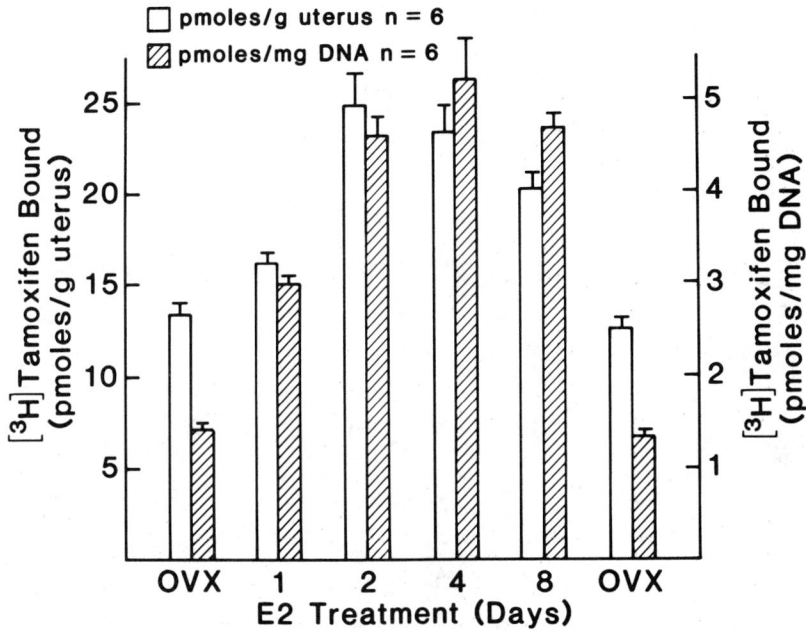

Figure 7.4. The effect of estradiol treatment on rat uterine cytosol TABS. Ovariectomized rats implanted with beeswax pellets containing 20 μg of estradiol were killed 1, 2, 4, and 8 days later. Control animals were killed on days 1 and 8 only. The concentration of TABS normalized per g liver and mg DNA are shown.

quantities of sites resembling but not identical to the sites found in the liver and uterus (Winneker et al. 1983). The serum TABS has a lower affinity for triphenylethylene drugs (K_d, 28 nM) but the hormonal specificity is similar. Since there were high concentrations of this site present in serum we decided to characterize this site. Preliminary studies using A 1.5 M agarose columns indicated that the molecular weight of TABS was greater than 10^6 daltons. Since serum lipoproteins are found in these large molecular weight classes, we examined the possibility that these lipoproteins contained the TABS.

When serum is separated into its lipoprotein fractions, by flotation sucrose density gradient centrifugation, specific binding of [^{3}H]tamoxifen can be found in the gradient fraction containing low density lipoproteins (LDL; Fig. 7.5). These LDL-TABS sites have the same binding characteristics and hormone specificity as the serum TABS. They are destroyed

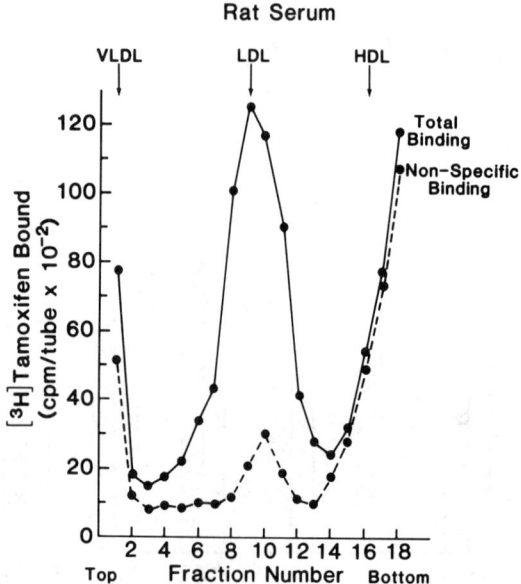

Figure 7.5. Potassium bromide density gradient centrifugation profile illustrating the fractionation of rat serum lipoproteins (VLDL, very low density lipoprotein; LDL, low density lipoprotein; HDL, high density lipoprotein) and the binding of [³H]tamoxifen to these fractions. Note that the TABS (tamoxifen-specific binding site) resides under the LDL marker.

by exposure to protease enzymes and not by DNAse or RNAse; therefore, they are probably associated with the protein component of the LDL.

The physiological significance of our findings is not known; however, it has been recognized for some time that triphenylethylene drugs inhibit cholesterol synthesis (for a review of this topic see Clark and Markaverich 1982). In addition, since cellular cholesterol synthesis is thought to be controlled by LDL-cholesterol (Goldstein and Brown 1979), it is possible that triphenylethylene drugs are involved in this process. Also, it has been demonstrated that treatment with hyperphysiological levels of estrogen decreases serum LDL levels in the rat (Hay et al. 1971) and increases the uptake of LDL by the rat liver (Kovanen et al. 1979). We have recently observed that physiological levels of estradiol will also decrease LDL-TABS in ovariectomized rats (unpublished observations). These effects of estrogen may be related to the observations discussed in the previous section that estradiol treatment increases the number of intracellular TABS in the liver and uterus.

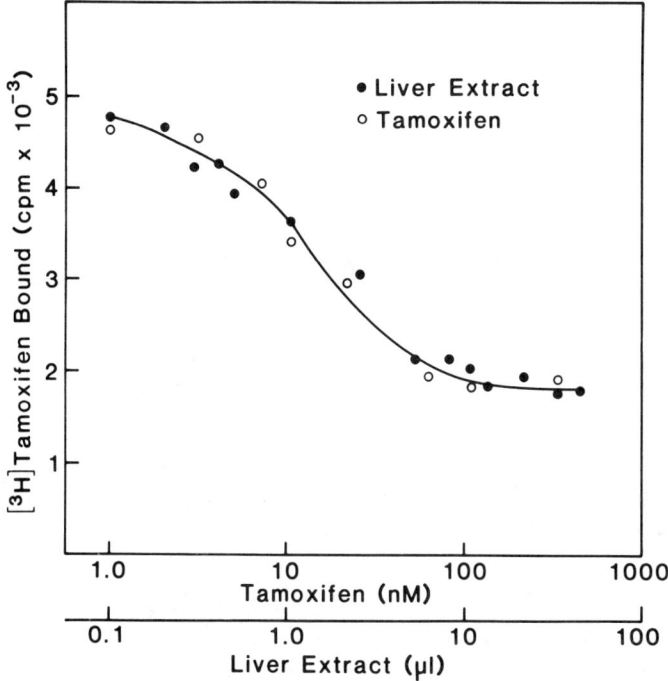

Figure 7.6. Inhibition of the binding of [³H]tamoxifen to liver TABS by nonlabeled tamoxifen and rat liver extract.

V. An Endogenous Ligand for the Triphenylethylene Antiestrogen Binding Sites (TABS)

The presence of specific binding sites for triphenylethylene in various tissues and in the LDL fraction of rat serum opens the possibility that the activity of these sites is regulated by an endogenous ligand. We examined this possibility by extracting liver tissue in boiling ethanol and fractionating the extract by silica gel column chromatography. Each fraction was assayed for its ability to inhibit the binding of [³H]tamoxifen to liver TABS and these were collected and used in a competitive binding assay (Fig. 7.6) (Clark et al. 1983). These data show that various dilutions of the endogenous ligand inhibit the binding of [³H]tamoxifen to TABS in a fashion similar to that of nonlabeled tamoxifen.

The ability of the endogenous ligand to inhibit the binding of [³H]tamoxifen to serum LDL fractions was also tested. The data in Figure

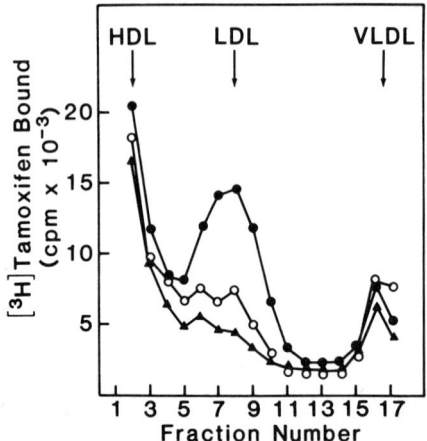

Figure 7.7. Density gradient profiles of serum lipoproteins labeled with [³H]tamoxifen alone (●); [³H]tamoxifen plus 100-fold excess of nonlabeled tamoxifen (▲) or [³H]tamoxifen plus 100 μl of endogenous ligand (○).

7.7 show that [³H]tamoxifen binds to HDL, LDL, and VLDL fractions; however, inhibition of binding by 100-fold excess of nonlabeled tamoxifen or 100 μl of endogenous ligand is observed only in the fractions containing LDL.

These data suggest that an endogenous ligand is present in the ethanol extracts of rat liver which acts as a competitive inhibitor of the binding of [³H]tamoxifen to TABS in liver cytosol and serum LDL. The presence of such a ligand implies that it may be an endogenous antiestrogen; however, the binding of triphenylethylene antiestrogens to TABS has not been shown to be involved in antiestrogen action. Therefore, the term *endogenous antiestrogen* is used with reservation and is an operational term rather than a functional one.

The significance of TABS associated with LDL is not known; however, as mentioned previously, LDL is involved in the control of cholesterol metabolism (Goldstein and Brown 1979), and triphenylethylene drugs inhibit these pathways (for review of this topic see Clark and Markaverich 1982). Therefore, it seems possible that LDL-TABS and the endogenous ligand may be involved in the control of cholesterol metabolism. If such were the case, it is possible to suggest a mechanism of indirect estrogen antagonism by triphenylethylene drugs. The binding interactions of estrogens with target tissues stimulate the biosynthetic processes, culminating in cell growth and proliferation, which occurs between 24 and 72 hours after exposure to estrogens. Triphenylethylene antiestrogens may interfere with the uptake or proper utilization of cholesterol during this 24–72-hour period and thus block the ability of cells to synthesize new membranes necessary for growth. It is well known, as explained earlier, that antiestrogens act as agonists during the period prior to 24 hours and act as antagonists after this time. Thus, it is possible that these compounds block the full expression of estrogen action by interfering with the delivery or utilization of cholesterol by target tissue cells. In nontarget tissues, which also contain TABS, estrogens are not active as stimulators of cell growth and hence no dramatic effect would be expected. However, triphenylethylene drugs are known to have effects on many tissues other than those of the reproductive tract, and it is possible that these effects occur via the TABS system.

Acknowledgments

We thank G. Brown for typing this manuscript and D. Scarf for drawing the figures. This work was supported by NIH grant HD-08436.

References

Clark, J. H., and B. M. Markaverich. 1982. The agonistic-antagonistic properties of clomiphene: a review. *Pharmacology and Therapeutics* 15:467.

Clark, J. H., and E. J. Peck, Jr. 1979. *Female sex steroids: receptors and function. Monographs on endocrinology*, vol. 14. Berlin: Springer-Verlag.

Clark, J. H., R. C. Winneker, S. C. Guthrie, and B. M. Markaverich. 1983. An endogenous ligand for the triphenylethylene antiestrogen binding site. *Endocrinology* 113:1167–1169.

Faye, J-C., B. Lasserre, and F. Bayard. 1980. Antiestrogen specific, high affinity saturable binding sites in rat uterine cytosol. *Biochemical and Biophysical Research Communications* 93:1225–1231.

Furr, B. J. A., and V. C. Jordan. 1984. The pharmacology and clinical uses of tamoxifen [Nolvadex]. *Pharmacology and Therapeutics* 25:127–205.

Gulino, A., and J. R. Pasqualini. 1980. Specific binding and biological response of antiestrogens in the fetal uterus of the guinea pig. *Cancer Research* 40:3821–3826.

Gulino, A., and J. R. Pasqualini. 1983. Modulation of the tamoxifen-specific binding sites and estrogen receptors by estradiol and progesterone in the neonatal uterus of guinea pig. *Endocrinology* 112:1871–1873.

Goldstein, J. L., and M. S. Brown. 1979. The LDL receptor locus and the genetics of familial hypercholesterolemia. *Annual Review of Genetics* 13:259–291.

Hardin, J. W., J. H. Clark, S. R. Glasser, and E. J. Peck, Jr. 1976. Estrogen receptor binding by uterine nuclei: relationship to endogenous nuclear RNA polymerase activity. *Biochemistry* 15:1370–1374.

126   *II. Antiestrogen Binding Sites*

Hay, R. V., L. A. Potenger, A. L. Reingold, G. S. Getz, and R. W. Wissler. 1971. Degradation of [^{125}I]-labelled serum low density lipoprotein in normal and estrogentreated male rats. *Biochemical and Biophysical Research Communications* 44:1471–1476.

Kaye, A. M., D. Sheratzky, and H. R. Lindner. 1972. Kinetics of DNA synthesis in immature rat uterus: age dependence and estradiol stimulation. *Biochimica et Biophysica Acta* 261:475–486.

Kirkland, J. L., L. B. LaPointe, E. Justin, and G. M. Stancel. 1979. Effects of estrogen on mitosis in individual cell types of the immature rat uterus. *Biology of Reproduction* 21:269–272.

Kon, O. L. 1983. An antiestrogen binding protein in human tissues. *Journal of Biological Chemistry* 258:3173–3177.

Kovanen, P. T., M. S. Brown, and J. L. Goldstein. 1979. Increased binding of low density lipoprotein to liver membranes from rats treated with 17 α-ethinyl estradiol. *Journal of Biological Chemistry* 254:11367–11373.

Lan, N. C., and B. S. Katzenellenbogen. 1976. Temporal relationships between hormone receptor binding and biological responses in the uterus: studies with short- and longacting derivatives of estriol. *Endocrinology* 98:220–227.

Lieberman, M. E., V. C. Jordan, M. Fritsch, M. A. Santos and J. Gorski. 1983. Direct and reversible inhibition of estradiol-stimulated prolactin synthesis by antiestrogens *in vitro*. *Journal of Biological Chemistry* 258:4734–4740.

Mairesse, N., and P. Galand. 1979. Comparison between the action of estradiol and that of the antiestrogen U-11,100A on the induction in the rat uterus of a specific protein (the induced protein). *Endocrinology* 105:1248–1253.

Makku, V. R., J. L. Kirkland, M. Hardy, and G. M. Stancel. 1981. Stimulatory and inhibitory effects of estrogen and antiestrogen on uterine cell division. *Endocrinology* 109:1005–1010.

Markaverich, B. M., S. Upchurch, S. A. McCormack, S. R. Glasser, and J. H. Clark. 1981. Differential stimulation of uterine cells by nafoxidine and clomiphene: relationship between nuclear estrogen receptors and type II estrogen binding sites and cellular growth. *Biology of Reproduction* 24:171–181.

Padykula, H. A., M. Fitzgerald, J. H. Clark and J. W. Hardin. 1981. Nuclear bodies as structural indicators of estrogenic stimulation in uterine luminal epithelial cells. *Anatomical Record* 201:679–696.

Sudo, K., F. J. Monsma, Jr., and B. S. Katzenellenbogen. 1983. Antiestrogen-binding sites distinct from the estrogen receptor: subcellular localization, ligand specificity, and distribution in tissues of the rat. *Endocrinology* 112:425–434.

Sutherland, R. L., L. C. Murphy, M. S. Foo, M. D. Green, and A. M. Whybourne. 1980. High affinity anti-oestrogen binding site distinct from the estrogen receptor. *Nature* (London) 228:273.

Watts, C. K. W., L. C. Murphy, and R. L. Sutherland. 1984. Microsomal binding sites for non-steroidal anti-estrogens in MCF7 human mammary carcinoma cells. *Journal of Biological Chemistry* 259:4223–4229.

Winneker, R. C., and J. H. Clark. 1983. Estrogenic stimulation of the antiestrogen specific binding site in rat uterus and liver. *Endocrinology* 112:1910–1915.

Winneker, R. C., S. C. Guthrie, and J. H. Clark. 1983. Characterization of a triphenylethylene-antiestrogen-binding site on rat serum low density lipoprotein. *Endocrinology* 112:1823–1827.

8

Antiestrogen Binding to Estrogen Receptors and Additional Antiestrogen Binding Sites in Human Breast Cancer Cells

MARGARET ANN MILLER, YHUN YHONG SHEEN,
ALAKA MULLICK, AND
BENITA S. KATZENELLENBOGEN

I. INTRODUCTION   128
II. EFFECTS OF ANTIESTROGENS ON BREAST CANCER CELL PROLIFERATION   129
III. INTERACTION OF ANTIESTROGENS WITH ESTROGEN-NONCOMPETABLE
     ANTIESTROGEN BINDING SITES   130
IV. ANTIESTROGEN BINDING TO THE ESTROGEN RECEPTOR   136
     A. IN VIVO BIOACTIVATION AND BINDING AFFINITIES OF
         ANTIESTROGENS FOR THE ESTROGEN RECEPTOR   136
     B. PHYSICOCHEMICAL ANALYSES OF ESTROGEN- AND ANTIESTROGEN-
         RECEPTOR COMPLEXES   136
     C. CHARACTERIZATION OF AFFINITY-LABELED ESTROGEN RECEPTOR
         COMPLEXES   139
     D. ESTROGEN RECEPTOR TURNOVER IN BREAST CANCER CELLS   140
V. CONCLUSIONS   144
     REFERENCES   145

I. Introduction

NONSTEROIDAL triphenylethylene-derived antiestrogens have become commonly used drugs in the treatment of hormone-responsive breast cancer. With antiestrogens, one can achieve noninvasively the same tumor-suppressive effects that normally follow more drastic endocrine-ablative surgeries (Tormey et al. 1976; McGuire 1979). The ability of these compounds to antagonize estrogen-stimulated cell growth and to suppress the growth of estrogen receptor–positive human breast cancer cells explains the clinical utility of these compounds and the tremendous interest in understanding their pharmacology and mechanism of action (Horwitz and McGuire 1978a; McGuire 1979; Coezy et al. 1982; Katzenellenbogen et al. 1984b).

Although the mechanism by which antiestrogens evoke their antagonistic activity is incompletely understood, most experimental data support the hypothesis that antiestrogens act via the estrogen receptor system of target cells (Lippman et al. 1976; Horwitz and McGuire 1978a; Katzenellenbogen et al. 1979, 1981, 1984a,b; Rochefort and Borgna 1981; Coezy et al. 1982). In target cells, estrogens exert their biological activity by binding to an intranuclear receptor protein (Sheridan et al. 1979; King and Greene 1984; Welshons et al. 1984). Ligand-free estrogen receptors are weakly associated with nuclear components. Following ligand binding, receptor complexes become tightly associated with specific nuclear components, and this association produces changes in gene expression (Jensen et al. 1975; Gorski and Gannon 1976; Katzenellenbogen 1980). Triphenylethylene-derived antiestrogens also bind directly to the estrogen receptor (Coezy et al. 1982; Eckert and Katzenellenbogen 1982a,b). These antiestrogen receptor complexes also become tightly associated with chromatin but presumably inhibit the events which promote cell growth. Clinically, the efficacy of antiestrogen therapy is highly correlated with the presence of a functional estrogen receptor system in tumor cells (Horwitz and McGuire 1978a; McGuire 1979).

In addition to binding to the estrogen receptors, triphenylethylene compounds bind to saturable binding sites present in human breast cancer cell lines and other estrogen target and many estrogen nontarget tissues (Sutherland and Foo 1979; Sutherland and Murphy 1980; Sutherland et al. 1980; Miller and Katzenellenbogen 1983; Sudo et al. 1983). These sites are distinguishable from estrogen receptor by the fact that they bind triphenylethylene antiestrogens but not steroidal or nonsteroidal estrogens. These sites have been termed "antiestrogen-specific" or "estrogen-noncompetable" binding sites.

In this chapter, we examine the effect of estrogens and antiestrogens on the growth of human breast cancer cells and relate it to the binding of these compounds to estrogen receptors and to antiestrogen binding sites. Our results indicate that antiestrogens act primarily by binding to the estrogen receptor. This binding evokes a conformational change in the receptor, which makes the antiestrogen receptor complexes distinguishable from estradiol-occupied receptor complexes and which may be important in mediating the antagonistic action of antiestrogens.

II. *Effects of Antiestrogens on Breast Cancer Cell Proliferation*

Studies with cultured human breast cancer cells which differ in their estrogen receptor levels demonstrate that antiestrogens selectively inhibit the proliferation of estrogen receptor–containing breast cancer cells (Fig. 8.1). MCF-7 cells contain high levels of estrogen receptor and their growth is inhibited markedly by the antiestrogen tamoxifen. T47D cells contain low levels of estrogen receptor and their growth is inhibited weakly by tamoxifen. MDA-MB-231 cells contain no detectable estrogen receptors and their growth is unaffected by tamoxifen. Thus, the effects of antiestrogens on the proliferation of three human breast cancer cell lines that differ in their estrogen receptor content show that the sensitivity to growth supression by antiestrogens such as tamoxifen correlates well with their cellular estrogen receptor levels. This finding is similar to the results with human breast cancer patients, where tumors that have substantial quantities of estrogen receptor are most sensitive to antiestrogen treatment (McGuire 1979; DeSombre and Jensen 1980). The suppression of cell growth by antiestrogens is reversed by estradiol (Lippman et al. 1976; Sheen et al. 1985a). Analyses of cell cycle kinetics have indicated that antiestrogens arrest cells in the G_0–G_1 stage of the cell cycle and this arrest is also reversed by estradiol (Sutherland et al. 1983; Osborne et al. 1984). Thus, it appears that antiestrogens exert their growth-suppressive effects by binding to the estrogen receptor.

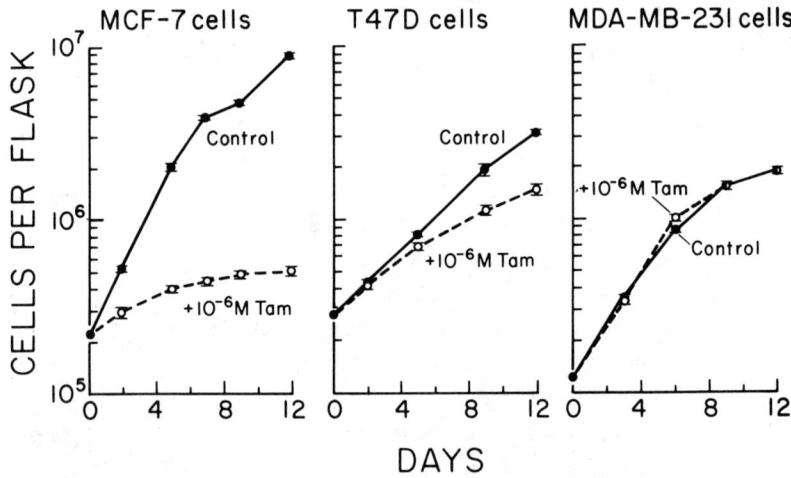

Figure 8.1. Effect of tamoxifen (Tam; 10^{-6} M) on the proliferation of MCF-7, T47D, and MDA-MB-231 human breast cancer cells. Cells were grown in the continuous presence of tamoxifen, and media with fresh tamoxifen were renewed every other day. On the days indicated, triplicate flasks of cells were counted. Values are the means of the triplicate determinations. Bars represent SE. (From Miller and Katzenellenbogen 1983.)

III. *Interaction of Antiestrogens with Estrogen-Noncompetable Antiestrogen Binding Sites*

In addition to binding directly to the estrogen receptor, antiestrogens interact with binding sites that are estrogen-noncompetable (AEBS). Since the initial observation by Robert Sutherland's laboratory (1979, 1980a), there has been considerable interest in determining the properties and nature of these binders and whether antiestrogen interaction with these sites mediates or modulates the antagonistic effects of these compounds. In contrast to the estrogen receptor which is present only in estrogen target cells, AEBS are present in a wide variety of tissues from the several species examined—rat, mouse, guinea pig, and human (Gulino and Pasqualini 1982; Kon 1983; Sudo et al. 1983). As seen in Table 8.1, AEBS are most highly concentrated in the liver, which shows levels 10 times those found in uterus, esophagus, ovary, brain, and kidney; lower levels are found in lung and spleen and negligible levels are found in muscle and heart. Hence, the AEBS are not localized exclusively or primarily in estrogen target tissues, and their level does not parallel that of the estrogen receptor, which is high only in uterus and ovary, with lower levels in liver and kidney.

Table 8.1. Antiestrogen binding sites (AEBS) in different tissues in the rat

Tissue	R_o (fmol/mg prot)	K_d (nM)	Protein concentration (mg/ml)[a]	R_o (nM)[b]
Uterus	98 (94–103)[c]	1.9 (1.8–2.1)[c]	4.1[d]	0.40[d]
Ovary	70 (55–85)	1.0 (0.5–1.5)	3.7	0.25
Esophagus	124 (100–47)	3.0 (2.2–3.8)	2.7	0.34
Kidney	76 (64–87)	2.2 (1.2–3.2)	6.6	0.50
Spleen	24 (20–28)	1.8 (1.8–1.9)	7.5	0.18
Brain	91 (70–112)	2.4 (1.3–3.5)	3.6	0.34
Lung	38 (26–50)	2.5 (1.6–3.3)	3.9	0.15
Liver[e]	882 (730–1033)	8.0 (4–12)	6.8	6.00
Muscle	14 (12–16)	1.1 (0.8–1.3)	3.0	0.043
Heart	13 (11–15)	2.0 (1.4–2.5)	4.0	0.053

From Sudo et al. 1983.
[a]Protein concentration in the 12,000 × g × 30 minutes supernatant. Protein content of the microsomal pellet is approximately one-eighth that present in this supernatant fraction.
[b]Concentration of AEBS in the tissue extract, 12,000 × g × 30 minutes supernatant.
[c]Mean and range of determinations in two separate experiments.
[d]Mean of two determinations from separate experiments.
[e]Value and site concentration are affected by protein concentration in the binding assay.

An examination of AEBS in three human breast cancer cell lines, MCF-7, T47D, and MDA-MB-231, which differ markedly in their estrogen receptor content and sensitivity to growth suppression by tamoxifen (Fig. 8.1), indicated that the concentration of AEBS was similar in these three cell lines and, likewise, the affinity of the AEBS for tamoxifen was the same in all three cell lines (Fig. 8.2).

Fractionation of cells by differential centrifugation and characterization of cell fractions with marker enzymes demonstrated that AEBS were membrane associated (Miller and Katzenellenbogen 1983; Sudo et al. 1983). When tamoxifen binding was investigated in homogenates of MCF-7 cells centrifuged at different speeds for various periods of time, "antiestrogen-specific" binding sites (AEBS) were present in the 800 and 12,000 × g for 30-minute low-speed supernatants of cell homogenates, but they were pelleted upon centrifugation at 100,000 or 180,000 × g for 60 minutes (Fig. 8.3). Figure 8.3 shows the results of assays in which a trace amount of tritiated tamoxifen (1.5 nM) was incubated in the presence of increasing concentrations of unlabeled estradiol or unlabeled tamoxifen (after a 30-minute pretreatment with 10^{-6} M estradiol to occupy estrogen receptors fully). The difference between the estradiol curve and the tamoxifen plus 10^{-6} M estradiol curve is considered to represent the estrogen-

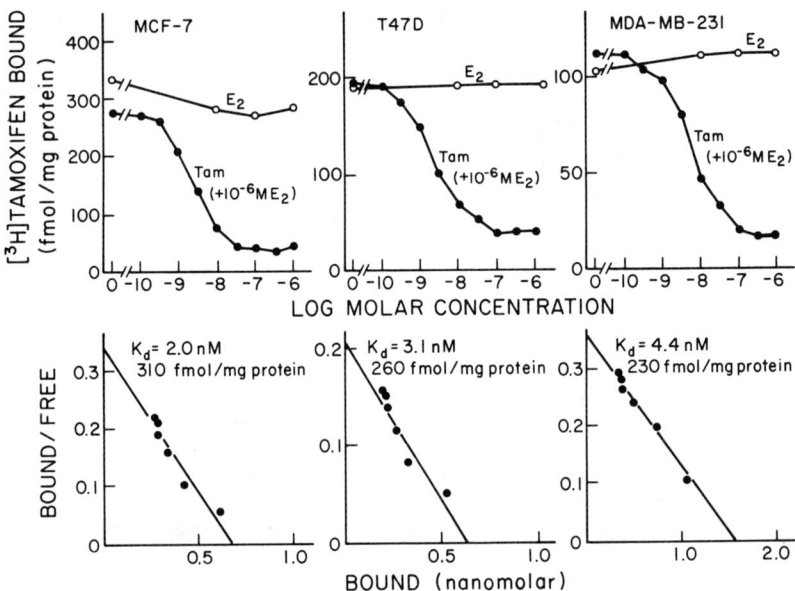

Figure 8.2. Evaluation of the levels of estrogen-noncompetable antiestrogen binding sites (AEBS) and their affinity for tamoxifen in three different human breast cancer cell lines. MCF-7, T47D, and MDA-MB-231 cells were homogenized and the 30-minute, 12,000 × g supernatant was incubated with 1.5 nM[^{3}H]tamoxifen alone ($\bigcirc$), [^{3}H]tamoxifen with increasing (10^{-8}–10^{-6} M) concentrations of estradiol (E_2; $\bigcirc$), or [^{3}H]tamoxifen plus 10^{-6} M estradiol for 30 minutes at 0°C to fill estrogen receptor sites ($\bullet$) prior to addition of tamoxifen (Tam; 10^{-10}–10^{-6} M; $\bullet$). Incubations were maintained for 18 hours at 0°C prior to charcoal-dextran treatment. Values for [^{3}H]tamoxifen-bound radioactivity were normalized for protein concentration of the cell supernatants (all ~ 1.2–1.6 mg protein/ml) and are expressed as fmol [^{3}H]tamoxifen bound/mg protein. In the lower panels, data on antiestrogen binding are analyzed by Scatchard plot analysis from which the K_d and number of sites were calculated. (From Miller and Katzenellenbogen 1983.)

noncompetable, but antiestrogen-competable ("antiestrogen-specific") binding sites. The subcellular fractionation pattern for AEBS differs from that of the estrogen receptor (Fig. 8.3, right of each panel), which remained soluble at all centrifugation speeds. However, the 100,000 and 180,000 × g supernatants contain approximately 50–70% of the estrogen receptors in the 800 and 12,000 × g supernatant fractions and, therefore, some estrogen receptors may be pelleted at higher centrifugation speeds. It is important to note that, since the different subcellular fractions contain a different proportion of AEBS and estrogen receptor sites, the distribution of the tritiated tamoxifen among these sites varies in the different supernatant preparations. Hence, the apparent increase in effectiveness of estra-

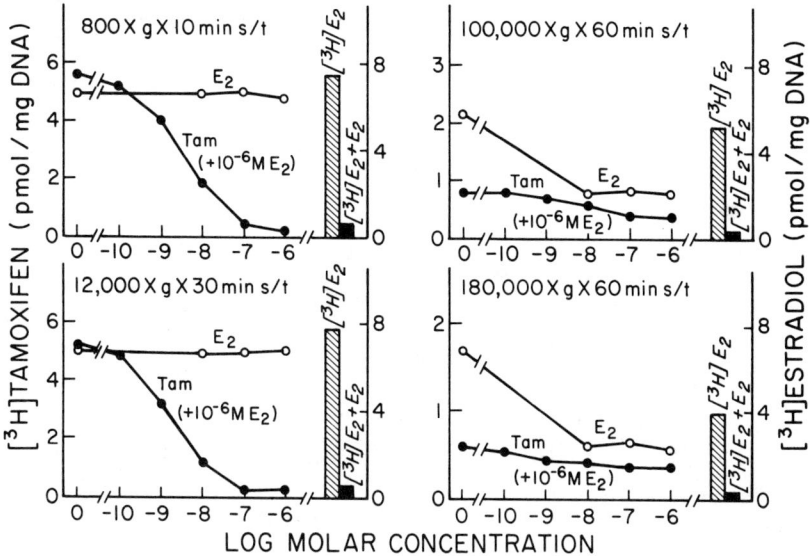

Figure 8.3. Subcellular fractionation of antiestrogen binding sites and estrogen receptors from MCF-7 cells. Cells were homogenized, and the homogenate was centrifuged at the different speeds for the times indicated. After centrifugation, the supernatants (s/t) were incubated with [³H]tamoxifen (1.5 nM) alone (○), [³H]tamoxifen with increasing (10^{-8}–10^{-6} M) concentrations of estradiol (E_2;○), or [³H]tamoxifen plus 10^{-6} M estradiol for 30 minutes at 0°C to fill estrogen receptor sites (●) prior to addition of tamoxifen (Tam; 10^{-10}–10^{-6} M; ●). Incubations were maintained for 18 hours at 0°C prior to charcoal-dextran treatment. Additional aliquots of the supernatants from each centrifugal fraction were incubated with [³H]estradiol (10 nM) in the absence and presence of 10^{-6} M unlabeled estradiol to monitor estrogen receptor levels (▨; ■). Values are expressed as pmol [³H]tamoxifen bound/mg cell DNA (left ordinate) and as pmol [³H]estradiol bound/mg cell DNA (right ordinate). Note that the scale for antiestrogen binding sites is expanded for clarity in the 100,000 × g and 180,000 × g fractions. (From Miller and Katzenellenbogen 1983.)

diol in competing for tritiated tamoxifen binding (estradiol curves) in the 100,000 and 180,000 × g supernatant preparations is most probably attributable to the relative increase in estrogen receptor content versus AEBS and nonspecific binding, and not to an increase in the affinity of tamoxifen for the receptor.

Further fractionation studies were carried out on rat liver, the richest source of AEBS, using the method of Adelman et al. (1974). As seen in Table 8.2, more than half of the microsomal AEBS were associated with the rough endoplasmic reticulum. Smaller amounts are present in the smooth endoplasmic reticulum, which may represent some rough endo-

Table 8.2. Microsomal antiestrogen binding sites

Fraction[a]	Percentage distribution (mean ± range)
Rough endoplasmic reticulum	55 ± 4
"Smooth endoplasmic reticulum"[b]	32 ± 21
Ribosomes	13 ± 11

[a]Microsomes from female (day 23) rat liver were prepared and fractionated by the method of Adelman et al. (1974). Values are the mean ± range from two separate experiments.
[b]This smooth endoplasmic reticulum fraction is also contaminated to some extent with rough endoplasmic reticulum.

plasmic reticulum contamination. Very few AEBS are associated with the ribosomes. Therefore, the majority of the microsomal AEBS appear to be associated with the membrane component of the rough endoplasmic reticulum. This finding agrees with another recent study, which used a slightly different microsomal fractionation procedure (Watts and Sutherland 1984). Our data and those of Watts and Sutherland (1984) suggest that almost all of the intracellular AEBS are associated with microsomes, although these binders can be relocated to the cytosol fraction as a consequence of certain homogenization procedures (Sutherland and Foo 1979). The AEBS are destroyed upon treatment with proteases and their membrane association is confirmed by their rapid sedimentation on sucrose gradients (Sudo et al. 1983; Watts et al. 1984).

In order to gain greater insight into the role of these AEBS in the actions of antiestrogens, we and others have examined the biopotency of different antiestrogens and correlated their effectiveness as estrogen antagonists with their affinity for estrogen receptors and AEBS (Murphy and Sutherland 1981; Miller and Katzenellenbogen 1983; Sudo et al. 1983). The order of affinities of different antiestrogens for the AEBS is CI 628 > tamoxifen > *trans*-hydroxytamoxifen > CI 628M > H 1285 > LY 117018. As seen in Table 8.3, this order of affinities parallels neither the affinity of these compounds for the estrogen receptor nor their potency as antiestrogens. Indeed, compounds with the highest affinity for the estrogen receptor and the greatest antiestrogenic potency have low affinities for these AEBS. Antiestrogenic potency correlates best with estrogen receptor affinity and not with affinity for AEBS (i.e., high ER:AEBS ratio, Table 8.3). It is worth noting that *cis*-tamoxifen has an affinity for the AEBS equal to that of *trans*-tamoxifen and that *cis*-

Table 8.3. Affinity of compounds for estrogen receptor and antiestrogen binding sites and their potencies in growth inhibition

	Binding affinity			Growth inhibition potency[c]
	ER[a]	AEBS[b]	ER:AEBS	
LY 117018	160	5	32.0	+5
H 1285	120	13	9.2	+5
CI 628M	90	18	5.0	+5
trans-OH-TAM	185	38	4.9	+5
Tamoxifen	2	100	0.02	+3
CI 628	3	156	0.02	+3
BPEA	0	6	0	0

[a]Affinity for estrogen receptor (ER) where the affinity of estradiol is set at 100. Values are from Eckert and Katzenellenbogen 1982a,b; Robertson et al. 1982; Miller and Katzenellenbogen 1983; Sudo et al. 1983; Katzenellenbogen et al. 1984b; Sheen et al. 1985a,b; and unpublished observations.
[b]Affinity for estrogen-noncompetable antiestrogen binding sites (AEBS) where the affinity of tamoxifen is set at 100. Values are from Miller and Katzenellenbogen 1983; Sudo et al. 1983; Sheen et al. 1985a,b; and unpublished observations.
[c]Potency in inhibiting the growth of MCF-7 cells *in vitro*. Values are from Katzenellenbogen et al. 1984b; Sheen et al. 1985a,b; and unpublished observations.

tamoxifen behaves as an estrogen in MCF-7 cells and in rat uterus (Robertson et al. 1982; Sudo et al. 1983; Katzenellenbogen et al. 1984b).

In addition, we have synthesized and studied the properties of t-butylphenoxyethyl diethylamine (BPEA), a compound incorporating the features important in binding to AEBS, i.e., an aromatic ring system and an amine side chain, but lacking the features required for binding to the estrogen receptor. As seen in Table 8.3, BPEA has a relative binding affinity for AEBS 6% that of tamoxifen, but has no affinity (less than 0.0003% that of estradiol) for the estrogen receptor. We find that this compound has no effect, either stimulatory or inhibitory, on proliferation of MCF-7 cells over a wide range of concentrations (from 10^{-11} M to 10^{-5} M). At these high concentrations, we would expect this compound to fully occupy the antiestrogen binding sites (Katzenellenbogen et al. 1984a). In addition, this compound exhibits no uterotrophic activity and no antiuterotrophic activity when assayed in immature female rats. Therefore, occupancy of the antiestrogen binding site, at least by BPEA, does not result in growth suppression (Sheen et al. 1985b).

As mentioned earlier, these AEBS are present in many nontarget tissues which are not growth suppressed by antiestrogens, and these sites are present in equal amounts in three breast cancer cell lines (MCF-7, T47D, and MDA-MB-231) that differ markedly in their estrogen receptor content and in their sensitivity to growth suppression by antiestrogens. In addition, AEBS are present in equal amounts in MCF-7 cells and in two variant MCF-7 clones designated R27 and R3-98, which are no longer growth inhibited by antiestrogens (Miller et al. 1984b). Therefore, the AEBS do not appear to mediate directly the antagonistic action of antiestrogens. At present, their function is unknown.

IV. Antiestrogen Binding to the Estrogen Receptor

A. IN VIVO BIOACTIVATION AND BINDING AFFINITIES OF ANTIESTROGENS FOR THE ESTROGEN RECEPTOR

Studies with antiestrogens *in vivo* have shown that the biological activity of these compounds represents a composite of the activities of the parent antiestrogen and its metabolites. The antiestrogens tamoxifen, CI 628, and U 23,469 are metabolized to more polar metabolites having a higher affinity for the estrogen receptor. For the antiestrogens CI 628 and U 23,469, bioactivation corresponds to demethylation, whereas tamoxifen is hydroxylated at the 4-position (reviewed in B. S. Katzenellenbogen et al. 1983). These three compounds, which now have phenolic hydroxyl groups, have a markedly increased affinity for the estrogen receptor (Table 8.2). Tamoxifen also undergoes additional metabolism to generate several compounds; the major metabolite in humans appears to be N-desmethyl tamoxifen (Adam 1981), which has an affinity for the estrogen receptor similar to that of tamoxifen itself ($\sim$ 2% that of estradiol; Robertson et al. 1982). The bioactivation and metabolism of the antiestrogens *in vivo* occurs largely in the liver, and it is not observed in breast cancer cells in culture. Therefore, although metabolic activation of antiestrogens is an important aspect of the pharmacology of these compounds *in vivo*, metabolism of antiestrogens is not required to elicit their biological activity.

B. PHYSICOCHEMICAL ANALYSES OF ESTROGEN- AND ANTIESTROGEN-RECEPTOR COMPLEXES

Antiestrogens are known to compete with estrogen for binding to estrogen receptor sites and the antiestrogen-occupied complexes localize in the cell nucleus (Horwitz and McGuire 1978a,b,c; Katzenellenbogen et al. 1979). The nuclear antiestrogen receptor complex, however, appears to be only partially active in promoting specific biological responses, and is effective in blocking the actions of estrogen. Early studies on the molecular mechanism of antiestrogen action using indirect exchange assays, and direct binding assays with low affinity radiolabeled antiestrogens, were hindered by the dissociation of the antiestrogen receptor complex during characterization due to the low affinity of many antiestrogens for estrogen receptor.

Since the demethylated form of CI 628 (designated CI 628M) and the hydroxylated form of tamoxifen, *trans*-4-hydroxytamoxifen, have substantially enhanced affinities for the estrogen receptor, these two antiestrogens were synthesized in high specific activity tritium-labeled form (Katzenellenbogen et al. 1981; Robertson and Katzenellenbogen 1982; Robertson et al. 1982) and used to study directly the receptor interactions of these high affinity compounds. Use of these high affinity antiestrogens as well as the related hydroxylated antiestrogen, H 1285, permitted the accurate characterization of the direct interactions of antiestrogen with the estrogen receptor. Saturation binding analyses have indicated that these antiestrogens bind with high affinity to the estrogen receptor of MCF-7 cells with a K_d of 1.3×10^{-10} M for tritiated estradiol, 1.4×10^{-10} M for tritiated *trans*-4-hydroxytamoxifen, 2.2×10^{-10} M for tritiated CI 628M, and 1.2×10^{-10} M for tritiated H 1285 (Eckert and Katzenellenbogen 1982a; Sheen et al. 1985a).

Our studies with high affinity radiolabeled antiestrogens in MCF-7 and ZR-75 human breast cancer cells indicate that these antiestrogens all favor maintenance of a 5.5S form of the estrogen receptor complex. When breast cancer cells are incubated with tritiated estradiol or tritiated antiestrogen and nuclear salt-extracted receptor complexes are analyzed on high salt sucrose gradients containing a phosphate-thioglycerol-glycerol buffer, the estradiol receptor complex sedimented as a 4S species, whereas the antiestrogen receptor complex is predominantly a 5.5S form (Fig. 8.4). On Sephadex G-200 column chromatography, the antiestrogen receptor complex also showed a larger Stokes radius than did the estrogen receptor complex. Estimation of the molecular weight of the receptor complexes based on sedimentation coefficients and Stokes radii gave an estimated molecular weight of 140,000 for the antiestrogen receptor complex and 75,000 for the estradiol receptor complex (Eckert and Katzenellenbogen 1982a).

Interestingly, these differences in the physical properties of nuclear estrogen and antiestrogen receptor complexes were obliterated in the pres-

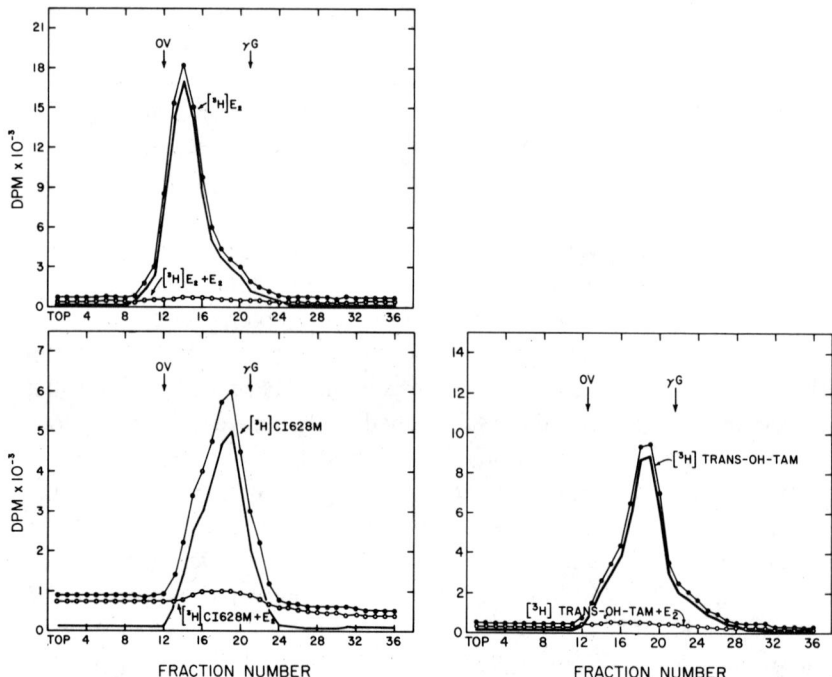

FRACTION NUMBER   FRACTION NUMBER

Figure 8.4. High salt sucrose gradient analysis of salt-extracted nuclear receptor after incubation of MCF-7 cells at 37°C with radiolabeled estradiol, CI 628M, or *trans*-hydroxytamoxifen. Cells were incubated for 0.5 hour with 10 nM [³H]estradiol or for 1 hour with 20 nM [³H]CI 628M or [³H]*trans*-hydroxytamoxifen. Parallel flasks were incubated with the indicated concentration of radiolabeled compound plus 100-fold excess of radioinert estradiol (E_2). The cells were harvested, washed, and the nuclear salt extract prepared and charcoal-dextran treated. A 300 μl aliquot was sedimented on 5–20% sucrose gradients containing 0.4 M KCl (15 hours at 4°C at 357,000 g). ¹⁴C-ovalbumin (OV, 3.5S) and ¹⁴C-gamma globulin (γG, 6.6S) were included in all gradients as markers and their positions are designated by arrows. The heavy curve represents the difference between total binding (●) and nonspecific binding (○). (From Eckert and Katzenellenbogen 1982a.)

ence of 3 M urea, where the 75 kilodalton form is seen. This result suggests that the nuclear 5S antiestrogen receptor complex represents an estrogen receptor molecule which is associated with an additional protein (Eckert and Katzenellenbogen 1982a). Upon further analyses, we have demonstrated that the estradiol-labeled receptor complex from MCF-7 cells sediments as a 5.5S form under certain defined conditions (Miller et al. 1984a). Thus, the sedimentation profile of the nuclear receptor complex with estradiol was found to vary with the buffer composition of the sucrose gradients, being 4.1S in phosphate-thioglycerol-glycerol buffered gradients and predominantly 5.5S in Tris-EDTA buffered gradients. In contrast, the receptor complex with antiestrogen (radiolabeled CI 628M, *trans*-hydroxytamoxifen, or H 1285) always showed the same sedimentation profile (5.5S) regardless of the buffer composition (Miller et al. 1984a; Sheen et al. 1985a).

The 5S estrogen receptor with antiestrogen appears to be conformationally different from the 5S estrogen receptor with estradiol. Hence, although the complexes are similar in terms of their reaction with the estrogen receptor monoclonal antibody D547 Spγ (Miller et al. 1984a,c), the 5S antiestrogen receptor complex is more stable, i.e., it tends not to dissociate to the 4S monomeric form as readily as does the 5S estrogen receptor complex. This difference in receptor complex stability may alter the interaction of receptor with chromatin and therefore be important in mediating the antagonistic activity of antiestrogens. The basis for the difference in the stability of the 5S receptor complex with antiestrogen versus estradiol remains under intensive investigation. These differences may reflect a difference in sensitivity to proteolysis, differences in phosphorylation, or other ligand-induced changes.

C. Characterization of Affinity-Labeled Estrogen Receptor Complexes

Our analysis of the structure and dynamics of estrogen receptor complexes was aided greatly by our ability to specifically label estrogen receptors in cells in culture with the covalently attaching compound [³H]tamoxifen aziridine (TA) (J. A. Katzenellenbogen et al. 1983; Monsma et al. 1984). When MCF-7 cells were exposed to 20 nM [³H]TA for 1 hour, TA covalently labeled all the receptors, and these receptors were found to be firmly localized in the nucleus. The salt-extracted nuclear [³H]TA-labeled receptor has an apparent molecular weight of approximately 65,000 on sodium dodecyl sulfate (SDS)-polyacrylamide gels and a predominant isoelectric point (pI) of 5.7 by gel isoelectric focusing in the presence of 8 M urea. The molecular weight and pI of the cytosol receptor labeled with [³H]TA was identical to that of the nuclear receptor (Monsma et al. 1984).

Under disaggregating and denaturing conditions, the TA-labeled receptor is a monomeric protein which sediments as a 4S complex on sucrose gradients and has a molecular weight of approximately 65,000. Further characterization of the 5S antiestrogen receptor complex labeled with [³H]TA and chemically crosslinked with the reversible crosslinker, 2-

iminothiolane, showed that these crosslinked complexes sediment as a 5.5S species on disaggregating sucrose gradients and have a molecular weight of approximately 130,000 on SDS-polyacrylamide gels (Miller et al. 1984c, 1985). Therefore, the 5S antiestrogen receptor complexes appear to be composed of two subunits of approximately the same molecular weight, and the molecular weight of these subunits is similar to the 4S monomeric receptor complex. These results suggest that the 5S antiestrogen receptor complex is a homodimer of two 4S, $M_r \sim 65,000$ monomers. In other target tissues, the 5S estrogen receptor complex also appears to be a homodimer of two 4S monomers. Our crosslinking studies suggest that the 5S estradiol receptor complex of MCF-7 cells is also a homodimer and further studies are under way in our laboratory to confirm this hypothesis. We believe that both antiestrogens and estrogens promote the formation of a 5S homodimer of estrogen receptor monomers but that the antiestrogens induce a conformational change in the receptor that is reflected in their enhanced propensity to remain in a 5S dimeric form. Further characterization of such conformational changes will reveal whether they are important in mediating the antagonistic action of antiestrogens.

D. Estrogen Receptor Turnover in Breast Cancer Cells

There has been considerable interest in evaluating whether antiestrogens alter estrogen receptor synthesis or degradation. This question has arisen, in particular, because in *in vivo* studies in animals and in studies in breast cancer cells *in vitro* it has been observed that antiestrogens maintain elevated levels of nuclear estrogen receptors firmly associated with chromatin for a prolonged period of time (Horwitz and McGuire 1978a,b,c; Katzenellenbogen et al. 1979; Eckert and Katzenellenbogen 1982b). Hence, there has been considerable interest in evaluating whether antiestrogens may perturb the turnover of the estrogen receptor, possibly preventing turnover such that receptors would become fixed or locked in the nucleus in an unproductive manner.

To determine the turnover rate of the estrogen receptor in intact cells, MCF-7 cells were incubated with [³H]TA for 1 hour, which covalently labels all the estrogen receptors. Examination of the salt-extracted nuclear estrogen receptor on SDS gels (Fig. 8.5A) reveals that the receptor migrates as a 65,000 molecular weight species. Following the 1 hour pulse labeling with tritiated tamoxifen aziridine, the cells are washed free of tamoxifen aziridine and exposed to a chase of unlabeled estradiol so that any newly synthesized receptors will become occupied by radioinert estra-

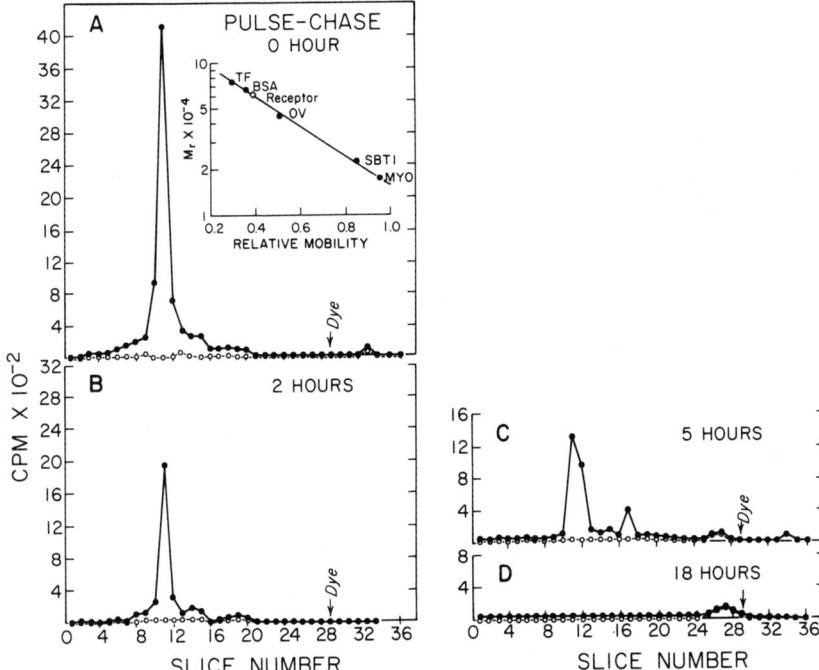

Figure 8.5. Sodium dodecyl sulfate–polyacrylamide gel electrophoretic analysis of the MCF-7 nuclear receptor; pulse-chase experiment. Flasks of cells were labeled with 20 nM tritiated tamoxifen aziridine with or without 2 μM estradiol for 1 hour at 37°C and then chased with 10^{-6} M estradiol for various time periods ranging from 0 hour (no chase) to 18 hours. Panel A, 1-hour tritiated tamoxifen aziridine label, no chase; panels B, C, and D, 1-hour tritiated tamoxifen aziridine label and then respectively, 2-, 5-, or 18-hour chase with estradiol. After the indicated chase period, nuclear salt extracts were prepared and analyzed on SDS-polyacrylamide gels. The inset of panel A shows the mobility of protein standards and receptor relative to the bromophenol blue dye band. The protein standards were transferrin (TF; mol wt 74,000), bovine serum albumin (BSA; mol wt 67,000), ovalbumin (OV; mol wt 43,000), soybean trypsin inhibitor (SBTI; mol wt 20,000), and myoglobin (MYO; mol wt 17,000). (From Monsma et al. 1984.)

diol. Analyses of nuclear receptor by SDS gels revealed that the tritiated tamoxifen aziridine labeled receptor disappeared with a half-life of about 3–4 hour. By 2 hours, there was already a noticeable decrease in the amount of the 65,000 molecular weight labeled species (Fig. 8.5B); by 5 hours, less than half of the original tritiated tamoxifen aziridine labeled receptor was seen (Fig. 8.5C); and by 18 hours, none of the original pulse-labeled receptor remained (Fig. 8.5D). Figure 8.6 summarizes data from several of such pulse-chase studies. The loss of tritiated tamoxifen aziri-

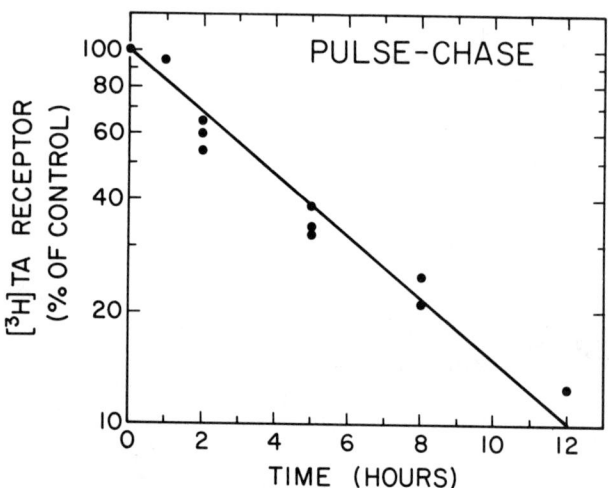

Figure 8.6. Rate of degradation of nuclear receptor in MCF-7 cells covalently labelled with tritiated tamoxifen aziridine, determined from pulse-chase experiments and SDS-gel electrophoretic analysis. Pulse-chase experiments were performed exactly as described in Figure 8.5. Cells were harvested after the indicated time of chase with 10^{-6} M estradiol, and data are presented as the percentage of tritiated tamoxifen aziridine-labeled receptor present after 1 hour of tritiated tamoxifen aziridine exposure and no chase (i.e., 0 hour chase). Each point represents data obtained in duplicate from one T-150 flask of cells. (From Monsma et al. 1984.)

dine labeled receptor appeared to be first order with a half-life of approximately 4 hours. It is of note (Fig. 8.5) that the loss of the tritiated tamoxifen aziridine labeled nuclear receptor reflects simply a decrease in the 65,000 molecular weight receptor species with time; no significant accumulation of smaller tamoxifen aziridine labeled fragments was seen in the nuclear extract or in the cytosol fraction that was also analyzed (not shown) (Monsma et al. 1984). Hence, the receptor in these cells is rapidly turning over.

To further examine the effect of receptor occupancy on the intracellular dynamics of the receptor, we have used dense amino acids (^{2}H^{13}C^{15}N amino acids) to follow the synthesis and degradation of estrogen receptors in MCF-7 breast cancer cells (Eckert et al. 1984). For these studies, cells were grown for various time periods in dense amino acid–containing medium with estradiol, antiestrogens, or control vehicle; and receptor turnover was analyzed by monitoring the shift from "old-light" (pre-existing) to "new-dense" (newly synthesized) receptors by velocity sedimentation on sucrose gradients prepared in buffered deuterium oxide. The results of

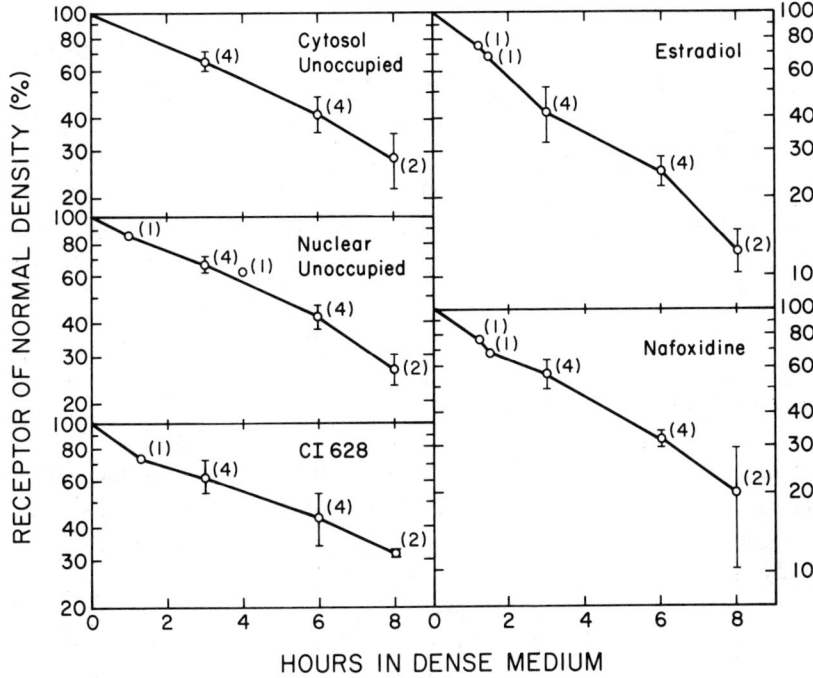

Figure 8.7. Half-life of the estrogen receptor in MCF-7 cells determined by dense amino acid labeling and density shift experiments. MCF-7 cells were cultured for periods up to 8 hours in dense amino acid medium in the absence of hormone, unoccupied cytosol receptor sites and unoccupied nuclear receptor sites were analyzed on sucrose gradients, and the proportions of normal and dense forms of the estrogen receptor were quantitated. Cells were also exposed to 10 nM E_2, 200 nM nafoxidine, or 200 nM CI 628 for 3 hours in normal medium before replacement of normal medium with dense amino acid medium containing E_2, nafoxidine, or CI 628 for the times indicated (1–8 hours) before harvesting the cells. Dense and normal receptors were separated on sucrose gradients and quantitated. Values represent the mean ± SEM, with the number of separate determinations indicated in parentheses. (From Eckert et al. 1984.)

these experiments are summarized in Figure 8.7. The half-life of the estrogen receptor in control cells and in cells exposed to estradiol or the antiestrogens nafoxidine or CI 628 was determined from these semilogarithmic plots of the amount of receptor of normal density as a percentage of the total receptor in cells cultured for up to 8 hours in dense amino acid medium. The half-life of unoccupied receptors in control cells was about 4–4.5 hours. Although receptor half-life was significantly shorter in cells exposed to estradiol (~ 3 hours), it is of note that receptor half-lives were similar to the control in cells exposed to the antiestrogens.

Hence, we found that antiestrogens did not prevent estrogen receptor synthesis and they did not either accelerate or block estrogen receptor degradation. Therefore, although antiestrogens evoke a change in receptor conformation, this does not alter estrogen receptor synthesis or turnover rates in breast cancer cells. The apparent prolonged maintenance of antiestrogen-occupied receptors firmly associated with the nucleus most likely reflects the long biological half-lives of the antiestrogen compounds in serum, tissues, and cells so that new receptors are continuously exposed to ligand.

V. Conclusions

Triphenylethylene-type antiestrogens bind with high affinity to the estrogen receptor and to additional microsomal binding sites which do not bind estrogens. These latter sites, called antiestrogen binding sites (AEBS), are present in equal concentrations in estrogen receptor–positive and receptor–negative breast cancer cells and are present in a number of estrogen target and nontarget tissues. The antagonistic potency of antiestrogens correlates with their affinity for estrogen receptor and not with their affinity for AEBS. Studies with t-butylphenoxyethyl diethylamine, which binds to AEBS but not to estrogen receptor, indicate that occupancy exclusively of the AEBS, at least by this compound, does not antagonize cell growth. Our findings raise serious doubts about the role of AEBS in mediating the growth-suppressive actions of antiestrogens and suggest that the binding of antiestrogens to the estrogen receptor is most likely the mechanism underlying the growth-inhibitory effects of antiestrogens.

Analyses of estrogen receptor synthesis and turnover using a covalently attaching antiestrogen (tamoxifen aziridine) or dense amino acid labeling reveal that unoccupied and antiestrogen-occupied receptors turn over rapidly with similar half-lives of about 4 hours. Therefore, antiestrogens do not prevent estrogen receptor synthesis nor do they accelerate or block estrogen receptor degradation.

Antiestrogens undergo metabolism *in vivo* and some of the resulting metabolites have a greater biopotency and enhanced affinity for the estrogen receptor. Studies with radiolabeled antiestrogens having a high affinity for the estrogen receptor indicate that these compounds cause a conformational change in receptor which promotes the maintenance of a 5S receptor complex. The antiestrogen-induced conformational changes in receptors may cause a difference in receptor-chromatin interaction which results ultimately in altered protein synthesis and cell proliferation.

Acknowledgments

These studies were supported by NIH grants CA-18119 and CA-31870 (to B.S.K.) from the National Cancer Institute. We thank the Eli Lilly Company, ICI Americas, Parke-Davis and Company, and the Upjohn Company for supplies of antiestrogens and Drs. John Katzenellenbogen and David Robertson for providing radiolabeled antiestrogens.

References

Adam, H. K. 1981. A review of the pharmacokinetics and metabolism of "Nolvadex" (tamoxifen). In *Non-steroidal antioestrogens: molecular pharmacology and antitumour activity,* ed. R. L. Sutherland and V. C. Jordan, 59–74. Sydney: Academic Press.

Adelman, M. R., G. Blobel, and D. D. Sabatini. 1974. Nondestructive separation of rat liver rough microsomes into ribosomal and membranous components. *Methods in Enzymology* 31:201–215.

Coezy, E., J-L Borgna, and H. Rochefort. 1982. Tamoxifen and metabolites in MCF-7 cells: correlation between binding to estrogen receptor and inhibition of cell growth. *Cancer Research* 42:317–323.

DeSombre, E. R., and E. V. Jensen. 1980. Estrophilin assays in breast cancer: quantitative features and application to the mastectomy specimen. *Cancer* (Philadelphia) 46: 2783–2790.

Eckert, R. L., and B. S. Katzenellenbogen. 1982a. Physical properties of estrogen receptor complexes in MCF-7 human breast cancer cells: differences with antiestrogen and estrogen. *Journal of Biological Chemistry* 257:8840–8846.

Eckert, R. L., and B. S. Katzenellenbogen. 1982b. Effects of estrogens and antiestrogens on estrogen receptor dynamics and the induction of progesterone receptor in MCF-7 human breast cancer cells. *Cancer Research* 42:139–144.

Eckert, R. L., A. Mullick, E. A. Rorke, and B. S. Katzenellenbogen. 1984. Estrogen receptor synthesis and turnover in MCF-7 breast cancer cells measured by a density shift technique. *Endocrinology* 114:629–637.

Gorski, J., and F. Gannon. 1976. Current models of steroid hormone action: a critique. *Annual Review of Physiology* 38:425.

Gulino, A., and J. R. Pasqualini. 1982. Heterogeneity of binding sites for tamoxifen and tamoxifen derivatives in estrogen target and nontarget fetal organs of guinea pig. *Cancer Research* 42:1913–1921.

Horwitz, K. B., and W. L. McGuire. 1978a. Antiestrogens: mechanism of action and effects in breast cancer. In *Breast cancer: advances in research and treatment.* Vol. 2: *Experimental biology,* ed. W. L. McGuire, 155. New York: Plenum Press.

Horwitz, K. B., and W. L. McGuire. 1978b. Estrogen control of progesterone receptor in human breast cancer. *Journal of Biological Chemistry* 253:2223–2228.

Horwitz, K. B., and W. L. McGuire. 1978c. Nuclear mechanisms of estrogen action. Effects of estradiol and antiestrogens on estrogen receptors and nuclear receptor processing. *Journal of Biological Chemistry* 253:8185–8191.

Jensen, E. V., P. I. Brecher, M. Numata, S. Smith, and E. R. DeSombre. 1975. Estrogen interaction with target tissues: two-step transfer of receptor to the nucleus. *Methods in Enzymology* 36:267.

Katzenellenbogen, B. S. 1980. Dynamics of steroid hormone receptor action. *Annual Review of Physiology* 42:17.

Katzenellenbogen, B. S., H. S. Bhakoo, E. R. Ferguson, N. C. Lan, T. Tatee, T. L. Tsai, and J. A. Katzenellenbogen. 1979. Estrogen and antiestrogen action in reproduction tissues and tumors. *Recent Progress in Hormone Research* 35:259–300.

Katzenellenbogen, B. S., M. A. Miller, R. L. Eckert and K. Sudo. 1983. Antiestrogen pharmacology and mechanism of action. *Journal of Steroid Biochemistry* 19:59–68.

Katzenellenbogen, B. S., M. A. Miller, A. Mullick, and Y. Y. Sheen. 1984a. Antiestrogen binding proteins. In *Endocrinology*, ed. F. Labrie and L. Proulx, 537–540. *Proceedings of the Seventh International Congress of Endocrinology*, Excerpta Medica International Congress Series 655. Amsterdam: Elsevier.

Katzenellenbogen, B. S., M. J. Norman, R. E. Eckert, S. W. Peltz, and W. F. Mangel. 1984b. Bioactivities, estrogen receptor interactions and plasminogen activator-inducing activities of tamoxifen and hydroxy-tamoxifen isomers in MCF-7 human breast cancer cells. *Cancer Research* 44:112–119.

Katzenellenbogen, J. A., T. Tatee, and D. W. Robertson. 1981. Preparation of tritium-labeled 4-hydroxy-α-[p-(2-(N-pyrrolidino)ethoxy)phenyl]-α'-nitrostilbene (CN-928), a biologically-important metabolite of the antiestrogen CI-628. *Journal of Labeled Compounds and Radiopharmaceuticals* 18:865–879.

Katzenellenbogen, J. A., K. E. Carlson, D. F. Heiman, D. W. Robertson, L. L. Wei, and B. S. Katzenellenbogen. 1983. Efficient and highly selective covalent labeling of the estrogen receptor with [³H]tamoxifen aziridine. *Journal of Biological Chemistry* 258:3487–3495.

King, W. J., and G. L. Greene. 1984. Monoclonal antibodies localize oestrogen receptor in nuclei of target cells. *Nature* (London) 307:745–747.

Kon, O. L. 1983. An antiestrogen-binding protein in human tissues. *Journal of Biological Chemistry* 258:3173–3177.

Lippman, M., G. Bolan, and K. Huff. 1976. The effects of estrogens and antiestrogens on hormone-responsive human breast cancer in long-term tissue culture. *Cancer Research* 36:4595–4601.

McGuire, W. L. 1979. Steroid receptor sites in cancer therapy. *Advances in Internal Medicine* 24:127–140.

Miller, M. A., and B. S. Katzenellenbogen. 1983. Characterization and quantitation of antiestrogen binding sites in estrogen receptor-positive and -negative human breast cancer cell lines. *Cancer Research* 43:3094–3100.

Miller, M. A., G. L. Greene, and B. S. Katzenellenbogen. 1984a. Estrogen receptor transformation in MCF-7 breast cancer cells: characterization by immunochemical and sedimentation analyses. *Endocrinology* 114:296–298.

Miller, M. A., M. E. Lippman, and B. S. Katzenellenbogen. 1984b. Antiestrogen binding in antiestrogen growth-resistant estrogen-responsive clonal variants of MCF-7 human breast cancer cells. *Cancer Research* 44:5038–5045.

Miller, M. A., A. Mullick, and B. S. Katzenellenbogen. 1984c. Crosslinking and density shift experiments to study the subunit nature of the 5S nuclear estrogen receptor complex in MCF-7 breast cancer cells. *Proceedings of the Seventh International Congress of Endocrinology*, Quebec. Abstract 1599, p. 1060.

Miller, M. A., A. Mullick, G. L. Greene, and B. S. Katzenellenbogen. 1985. Characterization of the subunit nature of nuclear estrogen receptors by chemical cross-linking and dense amino acid labeling. *Endocrinology* 117:515–522.

Monsma, F. J., Jr., B. S. Katzenellenbogen, M. A. Miller, Y. S. Ziegler, and J. A. Katzenellenbogen. 1984. Characterization of the estrogen receptor and its dynamics in MCF-7 human breast cancer cells using a covalently-attaching antiestrogen. *Endocrinology* 115:143–153.

Murphy, L. C., and R. L. Sutherland. 1981. Modifications in the aminoether side chain of clomiphene influence affinity for a specific antiestrogen binding site in MCF-7 cell cytosol. *Biochemical and Biophysical Research Communications* 100:1353–1369.

Osborne, C. K., D. H. Boldt, and P. Estrada. 1984. Human breast cancer cell cycle synchronization by estrogens and antiestrogens in culture. *Cancer Research* 44:1433–1439.

Robertson, D. W., and J. A. Katzenellenbogen. 1982. Synthesis of the E and Z isomers of the antiestrogen tamoxifen and its metabolite, hydroxytamoxifen, in tritium-labeled form. *Journal of Organic Chemistry* 47:2387–2393.

Robertson, D. W., J. A. Katzenellenbogen, D. J. Long, E. A. Rorke, and B. S. Katzenellenbogen. 1982. A comparison of the activity, pharmacokinetics, and metabolic activation of the *cis* and *trans* isomers of tamoxifen. *Journal of Steroid Biochemistry* 16:1–13.

Rochefort, H., and J. L. Borgna. 1981. Differences between the activation of the oestrogen receptor by oestrogen and by antioestrogen. *Nature* (London) 292:257–259.

Sheen, Y. Y., T. S. Ruh, W. F. Mangel, and B. S. Katzenellenbogen. 1985a. Antiestrogenic potency and binding characteristics of the triphenylethylene H1285 in MCF-7 human breast cancer cells. *Cancer Research* 45:4192–4199.

Sheen, Y. Y., D. M. Simpson, and B. S. Katzenellenbogen. 1985b. An evaluation of the role of antiestrogen-binding sites in mediating the growth modulatory effects of antiestrogens: studies using t-butylphenoxyethyl diethylamine, a compound lacking affinity for the estrogen receptor. *Endocrinology* 117:561–564.

Sheridan, P. J., J. M. Buchanan, V. C. Anselmo, and P. M. Martin. 1979. Equilibrium: the intracellular distribution of steroid receptors. *Nature* (London) 282:579–581.

Sudo, K., F. J. Monsma, Jr., and B. S. Katzenellenbogen. 1983. Antiestrogen binding sites distinct from the estrogen receptor: subcellular localization, ligand specificity, and distribution in tissues of the rat. *Endocrinology* 112:425–434.

Sutherland, R. L., and M. S. Foo. 1979. Differential binding of antiestrogens by rat uterine and chick oviduct cytosol. *Biochemical and Biophysical Research Communications* 91:183–191.

Sutherland, R. L., and L. C. Murphy. 1980. The binding of tamoxifen to human mammary carcinoma cytosol. *European Journal of Cancer* 16:1141–1148.

Sutherland, R. L., M. S. Foo, M. D. Green, A. M. Waybourne, and Z. S. Krozowski. 1980. High affinity antiestrogen binding site distinct from the estrogen receptor. *Nature* (London) 288:273–275.

Sutherland, R. L., M. D. Green, R. E. Hall, R. R. Reddel, and I. W. Taylor. 1983. Tamoxifen induces accumulation of MCF-7 human mammary carcinoma cells in the G_0–G_1 phase of the cell cycle. *European Journal of Cancer and Clinical Oncology* 19:615–621.

Tormey, D. C., R. M. Simon, M. E. Lippman, J. M. Bull, and C. E. Meyers. 1976. Evaluation of tamoxifen dose in advanced breast cancer: a progress report. *Cancer Treatment Reports* 60:1451–1459.

Watts, C. K. W., and R. L. Sutherland. 1984. High affinity specific antiestrogen binding sites are concentrated in rough microsomal membranes of rat liver. *Biochemical and Biophysical Research Communications* 120:109–115.

Watts, C. K. W., L. C. Murphy, and R. L. Sutherland. 1984. Microsomal binding sites for nonsteroidal antiestrogens in MCF-7 human mammary carcinoma cells. Demonstration of high affinity and narrow specificity for basic ether derivatives of triphenylethylene. *Journal of Biological Chemistry* 259:4223–4229.

Welshons, W. V., M. E. Lieberman, and J. Gorski. 1984. Nuclear localization of unoccupied oestrogen receptors. *Nature* (London) 307:747–749.

III

Pharmacology

9

The Progesterone Receptor as a Marker for Estrogen and Antiestrogen Activity in Vivo and in Vitro

Carolyn A. Campen, V. Craig Jordan,
and Jack Gorski

I. Introduction 152
II. The Progesterone Receptor as a Marker for Estrogen Action 153
III. Antiestrogen Activity *in Vivo* 154
   A. Rabbits and Hamsters 154
   B. Rats 156
   C. Other Studies 156
   D. Structure-Function Studies 157
IV. Antiestrogen Activity *in Vitro* 157
   A. The MCF-7 Human Breast Cancer Cell Line 157
   B. Primary Uterine Cell Cultures 159
V. Summary 165
References 166

I. *Introduction*

The female sex steroid 17β-estradiol (E_2) produces a pleiotropic effect upon its target tissues, usually resulting in growth and differentiation (Gorski and Gannon 1976; Katzenellenbogen et al. 1979; Katzenellenbogen 1980). How steroid hormones such as estradiol produce their effect has been the subject of intensive investigation by a number of laboratories. It is generally accepted that estradiol produces its effect through receptor proteins that are present only in target tissues and which bind to the steroid with high affinity and precise specificity. Estrogenic compounds, upon binding to the receptor *in vivo*, somehow alter the receptor's biological function and hence its ability to interact with cellular components such as chromatin and DNA (O'Malley et al. 1972; Katzenellenbogen and Gorski 1975; Grody et al. 1982). These new properties presumably allow the receptor to alter gene expression in that target tissue. However, the mechanism by which the estrogen–estrogen receptor complex mediates these and other cellular changes remains poorly understood.

One way of analyzing receptor-mediated events is to understand not only the structural requirements necessary for a ligand to bind to the receptor, but also those necessary for the receptor to achieve its full biologically active state. Antiestrogens are nonsteroidal, synthetic analogs of estrogens that bind competitively and reversibly to the estrogen receptor (Katzenellenbogen et al. 1979). Several compounds, with different structures (Table 9.1), have been used as tools to understand the mode of action of estrogens via the estrogen receptor.

Antiestrogens are able to prevent estradiol from exerting its full effect upon the target tissue (McGuire et al. 1978; Katzenellenbogen et al. 1979; Sutherland and Murphy 1982). However, they are not pure antagonists, since they exhibit varying degrees of estrogenic activity *in vivo* depending upon the species, tissue, estrogenic endpoint used for assay, and chemical nature of the compound. This review focuses upon the use of antiestrogens as probes of estrogen action in mammalian cells both *in vivo* and *in vitro* in terms of their ability to induce a specific estrogen endpoint—the progesterone receptor.

Table 9.1. Name and structure of commonly used estrogens and antiestrogens

Name	Structure	Name	Structure
17β-Estradiol (E$_2$)		ICI 77,949	
16α-Estradiol		Bisphenol	
Estriol		LY 117018	
Diethylstilbestrol (DES)		Nafoxidine (U 11,100A)	
MER 25		U 23,469	
Tamoxifen (*trans*)		CI 628	
4-Hydroxytamoxifen (*trans*)		TACE	
ICI 47,699 (*cis*-Tamoxifen)			

II. The Progesterone Receptor as a Marker for Estrogen Action

The use of the progesterone receptor (PgR) as an estrogenic endpoint has significant physiological relevance. Estradiol is responsible for what was termed "priming" in the uterus of various species (Milgrom et al. 1973; Rao et al. 1973; Sar and Stumpf 1973, 1974; Leavitt et al. 1978). Priming insured a responsiveness to the other female sex steroid, progesterone (Pg), which is secreted by the corpus luteum during the luteal phase of the estrus cycle. This sensitivity to Pg was found to be mediated by a progesterone-specific receptor (PgR). The increase in PgR content is in turn dependent upon the presence of estradiol secreted during the previous follicular phase of the cycle. This "priming" effect of estrogen, then, is the ability of E_2 to induce an increase in PgR content. This increase is probably due to increased synthesis of PgR but the evidence for this is limited. This effect of estradiol can easily be seen during the cyclical changes which occur in the intact female animal (Vu Hai et al. 1977). Therefore, the expression of PgR is a relevant marker for the biologically active form of the estrogen receptor in normal tissue. Other tissues that show an increase in PgR in response to estradiol are the mammary glands, oviduct, anterior pituitary, vagina, and hypothalamus (Faber et al. 1972; Feil et al. 1972; Horwitz and McGuire 1978a). Most of these tissues have been used as model systems to study the activity of estrogens and antiestrogens as probes to the estrogen receptor. There does exist at least one system, the T47D breast cancer cell line, in which the increase in PgR is independent of any estrogen, estrogen receptor–mediated process (Horwitz et al. 1982, 1983). It is not known how the synthesis of PgR is regulated in this cell line.

III. *Antiestrogen Activity* in Vivo

A. RABBITS AND HAMSTERS

The first nonsteroidal antiestrogen to be described, MER 25 (Lerner et al. 1958), inhibits the estrogen priming of immature rabbit uteri (Lerner 1958, 1981). However, MER 25 alone is able to prime as efficiently as estradiol (Lerner et al. 1958). Many nonsteroidal compounds have been synthesized subsequently and have been shown to possess competitive and reversible binding to the estrogen receptor (Sutherland and Murphy 1982; Jordan et al. 1984). Contrary to their name, however, many of these "antiestrogens" can serve as priming agents like MER 25. Leavitt and coworkers were the first to demonstrate that antiestrogens can directly stimulate the production of PgR *in vivo* (Leavitt et al. 1977). Their studies showed that nafoxidine, CI 628, TACE (a nonsteroidal estrogen), and both isomers of clomiphene all stimulated PgR production in the adult ovariectomized female golden hamster. Nafoxidine, enclomiphene, and CI 628 were slightly less estrogenic than zuclomiphene (an estrogen). One inconsistency with previous findings was that MER 25 was inactive in stimulating the production of PgR, perhaps because of a species difference in activity. There was a fair correlation between binding affinity and biological activity (i.e., PgR production) of the ligand. Discrepancies were attributed to metabolism, biological half-life of the drug, or differences in nuclear retention time of the antiestrogen receptor complex.

At this point, it is necessary to clarify current receptor terminology. For the past 20 years, most investigators believed that the unoccupied estrogen receptor was located in the cytoplasm of target tissues (Gorski et al. 1968; Jensen et al. 1968) because it appeared in the cytosolic fraction of target tissue homogenates. Recent evidence suggests that the unoccupied estrogen receptor is nuclear in localization (King and Greene 1984; Welshons et al. 1984). However, it is still true that the unoccupied estrogen receptor (whether nuclear or not) typically has different extraction and sedimentation properties from those of the nuclear, occupied receptor (for review, see Grody et al. 1982). Therefore, to be consistent with previous work, "ER_c" and "cytosolic" will be used to denote the unoccupied, nontransformed form of the estrogen receptor. After exposure to estrogens or antiestrogens, this cytosolic form of the estrogen receptor (ER_c) is depleted and the nuclear form (ER_n) increases, presumably as a result of ligand binding and transformation. The "nuclear retention time" would then be defined as the period during which the estrogen receptor remains in the ER_n form. It follows that a compound causing a long nuclear retention time of the estrogen receptor would also inhibit replenishment of ER_c.

One early theory of antiestrogen action was based on the observation that antiestrogens inhibited ER_c replenishment, presumably because they caused a prolonged nuclear retention time of the estrogen receptor (Clark et al. 1973; Clark and Peck 1976; Katzenellenbogen et al. 1979). Since antiestrogens both stimulated the production of PgR and blocked replenishment of ER_c, it was predicted that the PgR:ER ratio would be dramatically increased. Subsequent exposure to Pg, which was shown to inhibit ER_c replenishment (Hsueh et al. 1976), would further block the target cells' ability to respond to estrogen. It was therefore postulated that the prolonged nuclear retention of ER_n and the production of PgR were each important parts of the mechanism of action of antiestrogens. However, these actions probably are only a result of the long biological half-life of antiestrogens (they are retained by the body for a longer time than estradiol) and are not characteristic of antiestrogens (Jordan et al. 1978a). That is, if the biological half-life of a drug is long, then any replenished ER_c would immediately be bound with ligand and become ER_n. Therefore, one could not distinguish easily between a long biological half-life of a compound and an inhibition of replenishment caused by a real increase in the nuclear retention time of the estrogen receptor.

B. RATS

As in hamsters, many antiestrogens can stimulate the production of PgR in the rat. For example, a single injection of tamoxifen increases PgR content in the uterus of an ovariectomized, adrenalectomized adult female rat (Koseki et al. 1977a). However, Pg failed to reduce either ER_c or ER_n in tamoxifen-"primed" animals in this system, which was interpreted by the workers as a failure of Pg to inhibit ER_c replenishment. This result, along with the finding that some antiestrogens actually stimulate the synthesis of ER (Capony and Rochefort 1975; Koseki et al. 1977b), suggests that the induction of PgR by antiestrogens in $vivo$ is not part of the cause of estrogen antagonism.

Tamoxifen, 4-hydroxytamoxifen, and the Lilly compound LY 117018 also stimulate PgR production in immature female rat uteri to varying degrees (Jordan and Prestwich 1978; Jordan and Dix 1979; Dix and Jordan 1980a,b; Jordan et al. 1980; Jordan and Gosden 1983; Campen et al. 1985). Nafoxidine derivatives (Allen and Jordan 1980) and trioxifene (Jordan and Gosden 1982) stimulate PgR induction in $vivo$ as well. Dix and Jordan (1980b) correlated the induction of PgR with ER_n "processing." Processing is the term applied to the apparent loss of estrogen binding capacity usually seen after exposure to estradiol. Processing has been proposed by some investigators (Horwitz and McGuire 1978b) to be linked to consequent gene expression, e.g., PgR induction (for review, see Kassis and Gorski 1983). The finding that 4-hydroxytamoxifen stimulated PgR induction and that the antiestrogen–nuclear receptor complexes were processed led Dix and Jordan (1980b) to suggest that antiestrogen-ER_n as well as estrogen-ER_n complexes were in an active, "dynamic," state. This indicated that it was solely the long biological half-life of antiestrogens (Jordan et al. 1978b; Katzenellenbogen et al. 1978) and not simply a long nuclear retention time that was responsible for the apparent delay in replenishment of ER_c.

C. OTHER STUDIES

There are other systems in $vivo$ in which antiestrogens have been shown to stimulate PgR production. They are: (1) DMBA (dimethylbenzanthracene)-induced rat mammary tumors (Horwitz and McGuire 1977; Kelly et al. 1977; Tsai and Katzenellenbogen 1977), (2) mammalian brain tissue (Roy et al. 1979; Wilcox and Feder 1983), and (3) fetal guinea pig uterus (Gulino and Pasqualini 1980). Enclomiphene increased nuclear progestin receptor levels in the guinea pig brain, and CI 628 was a partial agonist with antagonistic properties for PgR induction in the adult female rat brain. Tamoxifen was a partial agonist of PgR induction in the fetal guinea pig uterus.

D. STRUCTURE-FUNCTION STUDIES

Structural requirements necessary for the agonistic or antagonistic properties of the antiestrogen ligand have also been explored in the immature rat uterine model, using PgR induction as the estrogenic endpoint. For example, removal of the side chain from tamoxifen, which is a partial agonist with antagonistic properties, produces ICI 77,949, a full agonist of PgR induction (Jordan and Gosden 1982). This was a clear demonstration of the pharmacological necessity for the alkylaminoethyl side chain for antiestrogenic activity of a ligand.

A unifying model for the structure-activity relationships for antiestrogens at this point is difficult to formulate, as most of the antiestrogens switched on PgR induction *in vivo* to some extent, and as this phenomenon seemed unrelated to the actual antagonism of estrogen. The estrogenicity of some of these compounds may have been due to metabolism, biological half-life of the compound, or other pharmacological parameters encountered *in vivo*. Researchers have therefore turned to *in vitro* systems, which are assumed to be free of these problems, in order to directly ascertain the biological activity of antiestrogens.

IV. *Antiestrogen Activity* in Vitro

Several cell or tissue cultures that respond to estrogen by an increase in PgR content have been used to study antiestrogens. The MCF-7 cell culture system, perhaps the most widely used, and the ZR-75-1 cell culture system represent permanent transformed cell lines. Primary cultures of rat uterine cells are nontransformed and also respond to estrogen by an increase in PgR content.

A. THE MCF-7 HUMAN BREAST CANCER CELL LINE

The MCF-7 human breast cancer cell line was derived from a patient with metastatic breast cancer (Soule et al. 1973). This cell line exhibits estrogen-dependent PgR synthesis (Horwitz and McGuire 1978a). Tamoxifen at 1 μM both inhibits cell growth and prevents the induction of PgR by 0.1 nM E_2. This effect is completely reversible with increasing concentrations of E_2. However, at lower concentrations, tamoxifen stimulated PgR induction (Horwitz et al. 1978). (This "biphasic" nature of tamoxifen activity was apparently not due to metabolism.) A different antiestrogen, nafoxidine, did not stimulate the induction of PgR over a wide concentration range, although it inhibited cell growth. The stimulatory effect on PgR production by tamoxifen has not always been reproducible. Katzenellenbogen and coworkers (1984) reported that tamoxifen in the MCF-7 cells showed almost negligible estrogenicity up to 0.1 μM, and only slight estrogenicity at concentrations over that. Additionally, tamoxifen (10^{-6}– 10^{-8}) showed no ability to induce PgR in the estrogen-sensitive ZR-75-1 human breast cancer cell line (Allegra et al. 1981). The fact that the ZR-75-1 cell line was grown in serum-free defined media whereas the MCF-7 cells are grown in 5–15% serum may have affected the activity of tamoxifen in these cultures.

Nuclear receptor processing initially appeared to be correlated with the induction of PgR in MCF-7 cells, because decreased ER levels preceded PgR appearance and, upon withdrawal of E_2, the restoration to control levels of ER paralleled the fall in PgR (Horwitz and McGuire 1978b). Nuclear receptor processing was impaired partially with tamoxifen and completely with nafoxidine. Tamoxifen induced PgR, whereas nafoxidine did not. This has been supported by the findings of Nawata and coworkers (1981) in which there is no estrogen-dependent PgR induction and no processing of the ER. However, the extent of estrogen receptor processing does not always correlate well with the induction of PgR. Processed levels of ER are greater when the MCF-7 cells are exposed to estradiol than when they are exposed to tamoxifen (70% vs 26% decrease in total binding), yet PgR induction is greater with tamoxifen than with E_2. Moreover, other workers have found a similar lack of correlation between processing and PgR stimulation, using antiestrogens that are structurally related to nafoxidine and tamoxifen (Eckert and Katzenellenbogen 1982; Katzenellenbogen et al. 1984).

It has been proposed that extended nuclear retention time of occupied estrogen receptor is required for hormone response (Anderson et al. 1973; Anderson et al. 1975; Ferguson and Katzenellenbogen 1977). In the MCF-7 cell culture system, however, the nuclear retention times of antiestrogens (nafoxidine > tamoxifen > E_2) do not correlate well with PgR induction by the antiestrogens (tamoxifen > E_2 >> nafoxidine = 0). Although nafoxidine does not stimulate processing or PgR induction, it apparently has some affect on the nuclear form of the estrogen receptor, as it sensitizes ER_n to subsequent stimulation by E_2 (Horwitz et al. 1981).

1. Structure-Function Studies in MCF-7 Cell Lines

The structure of antiestrogens has been correlated with their biological activity as inducers of PgR in MCF-7 cells (Katzenellenbogen et al. 1984). The *cis* isomer of tamoxifen was a full agonist of PgR induction, whereas the *trans* isomer was an extremely weak inducer. The concentration of *cis*-tamoxifen needed to elicit a full response reflects its weaker affinity for the estrogen receptor. Demethylating the 3′ phenolic hydroxyl group of either CI 628 or U 23,469 increased their affinity for the estrogen receptor and also greatly increased their potency in stimulating the induction of PgR (Eckert and Katzenellenbogen 1982). Thus, estrogenicity and the affinity for ER are related in this cell line.

B. PRIMARY UTERINE CELL CULTURES

Recently, a primary cell culture system derived from immature rat uteri was found to contain ER and to be estrogen responsive (Kassis et al. 1984a). These cell cultures are thought to be mainly myometrial in origin. The ER content in these cells is sensitive to changes in the medium but can be maintained by certain feeding schedules (Kassis et al. 1984b). Progesterone receptors can be induced in a concentration-dependent manner by 17β-estradiol. Interestingly, the induction of PgR in this system is unrelated to processing, since no apparent decrease in estrogen binding capacity occurred during the induction of PgR (Kassis et al. 1986).

1. Structure-Function Studies

The primary uterine cell culture system has been used to analyze the structure-function relationship of various estrogens and antiestrogens based on their ability to induce PgR (Campen et al. 1985). Figure 9.1 shows the effect of 16α-estradiol and estriol on the induction of PgR. Both 16α-estradiol and estriol were full agonists of the response but at higher concentrations than is necessary for estradiol, reflecting their decreased affinity for ER. Tamoxifen, 4-hydroxytamoxifen, and LY 117018 were all nonagonists of the response, in contradiction to previous findings *in vivo* and *in vitro* (Fig. 9.2). The *cis* isomer of tamoxifen and ICI 77,949 were both full agonists of the response but at concentrations reflecting their decreased binding affinity to the ER (Fig. 9.3). Bisphenol was found to

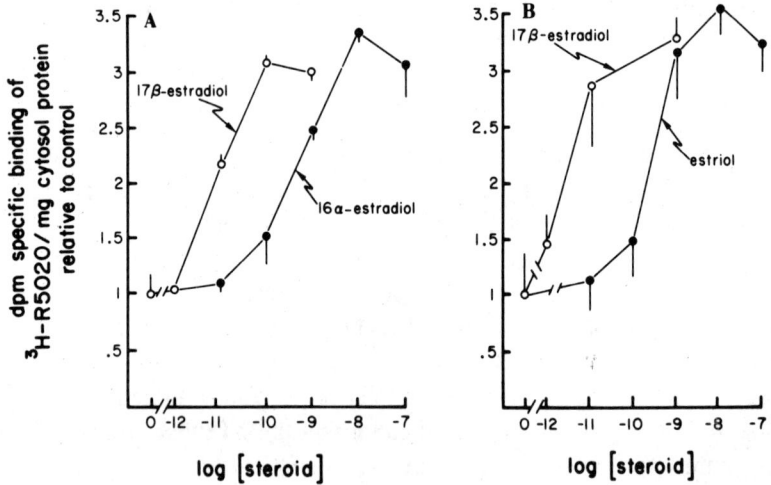

Figure 9.1. Comparison of the effects of E_2, 16α-estradiol (A), and estriol (B) on the level of cytosolic progesterone receptor in primary rat uterine cell cultures.

be a partial agonist/partial antagonist (Figs. 9.3B, 9.4). Tamoxifen, 4-hydroxytamoxifen, and LY 117018 were found to be full antagonists of the estrogen-induced PgR response (Fig. 9.5). This antagonistic effect was competitive and reversible with increasing concentrations of estradiol. A model of antiestrogen action can be derived in this system by correlating the structures of these compounds with their agonistic and/or antagonistic activity (Fig. 9.6). As found *in vivo* (Jordan and Gosden 1982), the side chain is necessary for antiestrogenic activity of a ligand. The presence of a 3′ phenolic hydroxyl group increases the biological potency of a ligand, for either estrogenic or antiestrogenic compounds. The necessity for proper geometric conformation is exemplified by the opposing bioactivity of the *cis/trans* isomers of tamoxifen.

However, the primary uterine cell culture is not without its problems. The cultured cells are only of one cell type (myometrial fibroblasts), whereas the uterus is composed of three cell types—luminal epithelium, stroma, and myometrium. It is known that antiestrogens have varying degrees of activity in these different cell types (Clark et al. 1978; Dix and Jordan 1980a).

Other questions arise from this study. In mice, antiestrogens are full agonists *in vivo*, whereas in rats *in vivo* they are partial agonists (Jordan

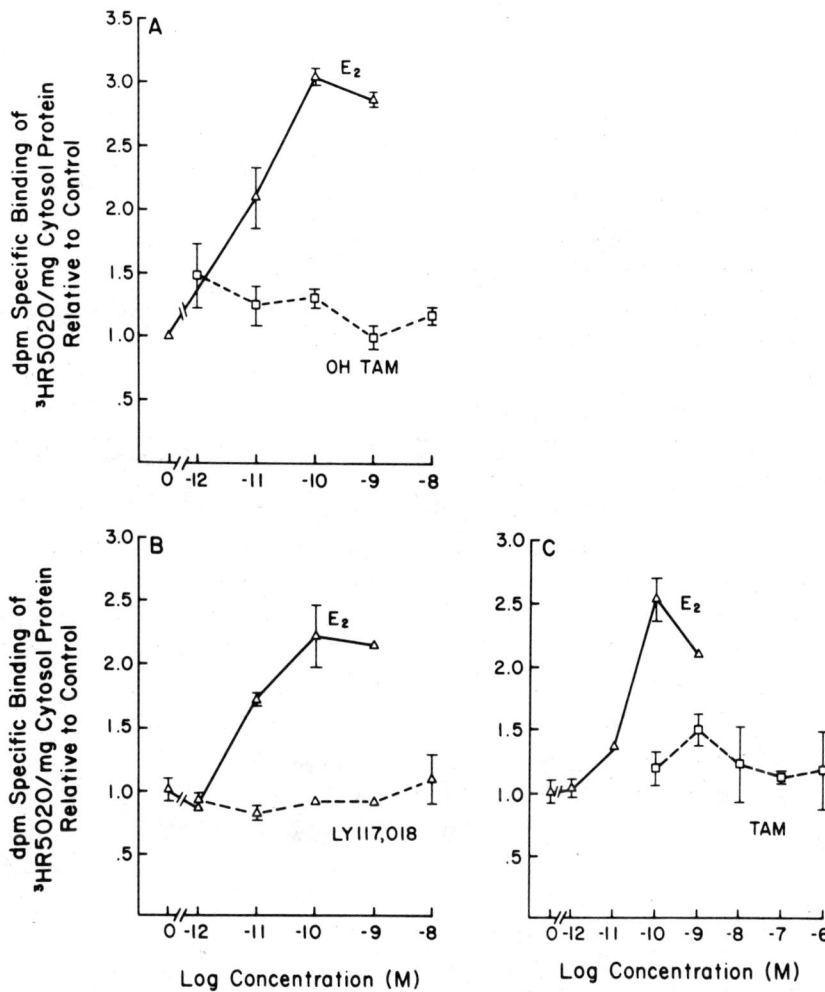

Figure 9.2. Comparison of the effects of E_2, 4-hydroxytamoxifen (A), LY 117018 (B), and tamoxifen (C) on the level of cytosolic progesterone receptor in primary rat uterine cell cultures. (From Campen et al. [1985] with the permission of the editor.)

et al. 1978b; Campen et al. 1985). It might be inferred therefore that antiestrogens might exhibit some estrogenic potential *in vitro*. Mouse uterine cell cultures were developed to specifically address this point. Estradiol stimulates the production of PgR in these cultures (Fig. 9.7A). However, 4-hydroxytamoxifen was still a nonagonist of PgR induction with full antagonistic properties (Fig. 9.7B).

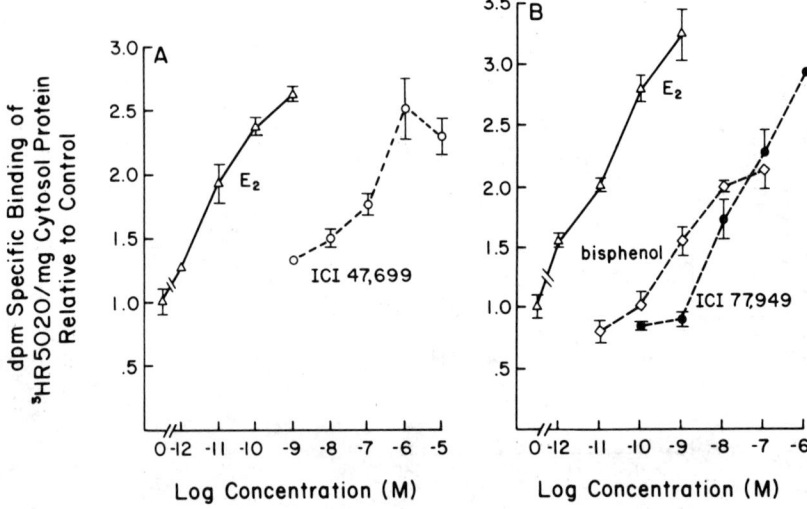

Figure 9.3. Comparison of the effects of E_2, ICI 47,699 (A), bisphenol, and ICI 77,949 (B) on the level of cytosolic progesterone receptor in primary rat uterine cell cultures. (From Campen et al. [1985] with the permission of the editor.)

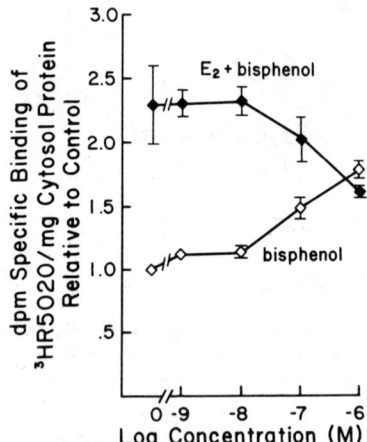

Figure 9.4. Effect of bisphenol on the E_2-induced increase in cytosolic progesterone receptors in primary rat uterine cell cultures. (From Campen et al. [1985] with the permission of the editor.)

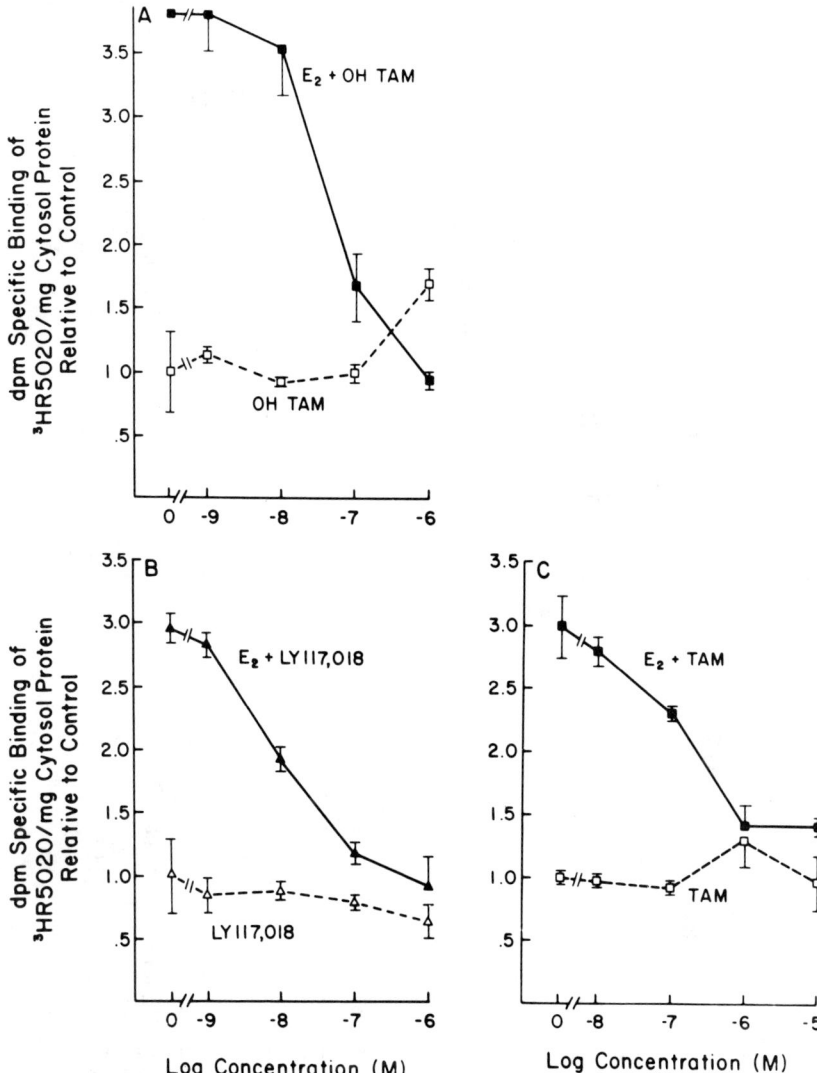

Figure 9.5. Effect of 4-hydroxytamoxifen (A), LY 117018 (B), and tamoxifen (C) on the E₂-induced increase in cytosolic progesterone receptors in primary rat uterine cell cultures. (From Campen et al. [1985] with the permission of the editor.)

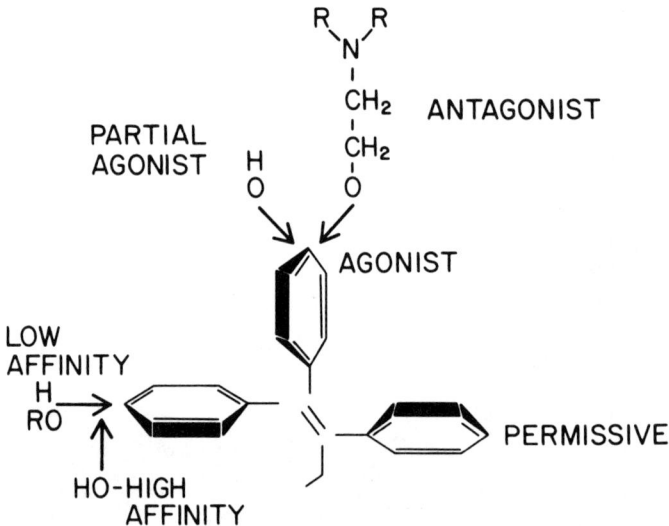

Figure 9.6. Specific substitutions on a triphenylethylene which affect its biological activity and potency *in vitro*. (From Campen et al. [1985] with the permission of the editor.)

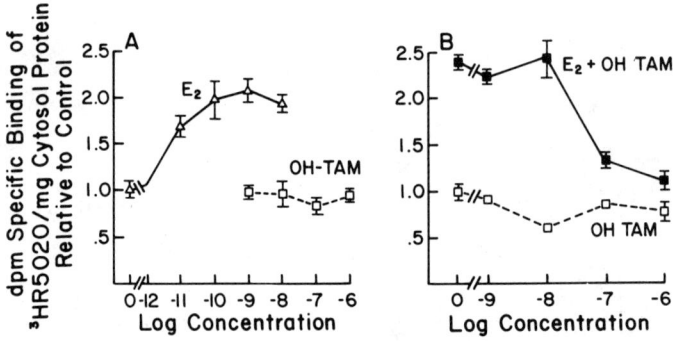

Figure 9.7. Comparison of the effects of E_2 and 4-hydroxytamoxifen on the level of cytosolic progesterone receptor in primary mouse uterine cell cultures (A); effect of 4-hydroxytamoxifen on the E_2-induced increase in cytosolic progesterone receptors in primary mouse uterine cell cultures (B). (From Campen et al. [1985] with the permission of the editor.)

V. *Summary*

A model for the action of antiestrogens *in vitro* is shown in Figure 9.6. This model is also consistent with results in primary pituitary cultures in which prolactin was the measured estrogenic endpoint (Lieberman et al. 1983). This strengthens the model because the same results were obtained from two different cell types measuring two separate, yet classic, estrogenic endpoints.

This model of ligand structure incorporates the characteristics of both potency and activity of antiestrogens. Potency is related to the relative binding affinity of a compound, which is clearly dependent on the presence of a correctly positioned phenolic hydroxyl group. For example, 4-hydroxytamoxifen is more potent than tamoxifen, and bisphenol is more potent than ICI 77,949. Similarly, the methylated analogs of CI 628 and U 23,469 are much less potent than their demethylated counterparts (Eckert and Katzenellenbogen 1982). Yet increased potency alone does not determine activity. According to the model, activity is determined by a correctly positioned aminoethoxy side chain. For example, addition of a dimethylaminoethoxy side chain to the agonist ICI 77,949 produces the antagonist tamoxifen. One explanation of this is that a properly oriented side chain would perturb the conformation of the estrogen receptor such that the intrinsic activity of the complex is zero (Jordan et al. 1984). The agonistic activity of *cis*-tamoxifen can be explained by the preference of the estrogen receptor for a planar, *trans,* configuration. The *cis* isomer can approximate this by rotating its side chain away from the receptor and use its ether oxygen to bind to the receptor's phenolic binding site. This would, of course, have an effect on the potency of *cis*-tamoxifen. Bisphenol, being a partial agonist, is by definition a partial antagonist and so does not need the side chain to possess antiestrogenic activity.

This model only describes antiestrogenic activity *in vitro*. The model cannot explain the typical increase in estrogenic activity of these compounds when measured *in vivo*. It may be that other factors are present *in vivo* that are not *in vitro*. In addition, the absence or presence of specific cell types in the primary cultures may affect the activity of the compounds, as previously mentioned. However limited, this model is a useful beginning for the development of other synthetic estrogen receptor ligands for both research tools and possible therapeutic agents.

References

Allegra, J. C., O. Korat, H. M. T. Do, and M. Lippman. 1981. The regulation of progesterone receptor by 17β-estradiol and tamoxifen in the ZR-75-1 human breast cancer cell line in defined medium. *Journal of Receptor Research* 2:17–27.

Allen, K. E., and V. C. Jordan. 1980. Antioestrogenic derivatives of nafoxidine stimulate progesterone receptor synthesis *in vivo*. *British Journal of Pharmacology* 68:156–157.

Anderson, J. N., E. J. Peck, Jr., and J. H. Clark. 1973. Nuclear receptor estrogen complex: relationship between concentration and early uterotrophic responses. *Endocrinology* 92:1488–1495.

Anderson, J. N., E. J. Peck, Jr., and J. H. Clark. 1974. Nuclear receptor estradiol complex: a requirement for uterotrophic responses. *Endocrinology* 95:174–178.

Anderson, J. N., E. J. Peck, Jr., and J. H. Clark. 1975. Estrogen-induced uterine responses and growth: relationship to receptor estrogen binding by uterine nuclei. *Endocrinology* 96:160–167.

Campen, C. A., V. C. Jordan, and J. Gorski. 1985. Opposing biological actions of antiestrogens *in vitro* and *in vivo:* induction of progesterone receptor in the rat and mouse uterus. *Endocrinology* 116:2327–2336.

Capony, F., and H. Rochefort. 1975. *In vivo* effect of anti-oestrogens on the localisation and replenishment of oestrogen receptor. *Molecular and Cellular Endocrinology* 3:233–251.

Clark, J. H., and E. J. Peck, Jr. 1976. Nuclear retention of receptor-oestrogen complex and nuclear acceptor sites. *Nature* (London) 260:635–637.

Clark, J. H., J. N. Anderson, and E. J. Peck, Jr. 1973. Oestrogen receptor anti-oestrogen complex—atypical binding by uterine nuclei and effects on uterine growth. *Steroids* 22:707–718.

Clark, J. H., J. W. Hardin, S. A. McCormack, and H. A. Padykula. 1978. Mechanism of action of estrogen antagonist: relationship to estrogen receptor binding and hyperestrogenization. In *Hormones, receptors, and breast cancer. Progress in cancer research and therapy*, vol. 10, ed. W. L. McGuire, 107–133. New York: Raven Press.

Dix, C. J., and V. C. Jordan. 1980a. Subcellular effects of monohydroxytamoxifen in the rat uterus: steroid receptors and mitosis. *Journal of Endocrinology* 85:393–404.

Dix, C. J., and V. C. Jordan. 1980b. Modulation of rat uterine steroid hormone receptors by estrogen and antiestrogen. *Endocrinology* 107:2011–2020.

Eckert, R. L., and B. S. Katzenellenbogen. 1982. Effects of estrogens and antiestrogens on estrogen receptor dynamics and the induction of progesterone receptor in MCF-7 human breast cancer cells. *Cancer Research* 42:139–144.

Faber, L. E., M. L. Sandmann, and H. E. Stavely. 1972. Progesterone-binding proteins of rat and rabbit uterus. *Journal of Biological Chemistry* 247:5648–5649.

Feil, P. D., S. R. Glasser, D. O. Toft, and B. W. O'Malley. 1972. Progesterone binding in the mouse and rat uterus. *Endocrinology* 91:738–746.

Ferguson, E. R., and B. S. Katzenellenbogen. 1977. A comparative study of antiestrogen action: temporal patterns of antagonism of estrogen stimulated uterine growth and effects on estrogen receptor levels. *Endocrinology* 100:1242–1251.

Gorski, J., and F. Gannon. 1976. Current models of steroid hormone action: a critique. *Annual Review of Physiology* 38:425–450.

Gorski, J., D. Toft, G. Shyamala, D. Smith, and A. Notides. 1968. Hormone receptors: Studies on the interaction of estrogen with the uterus. *Recent Progress in Hormone Research* 24:45–80.

Grody, W. W., W. T. Schrader, and B. W. O'Malley. 1982. Activation, transformation, and subunit structure of steroid hormone receptors. *Endocrine Reviews* 3:141–163.

Gulino, A., and J. R. Pasqualini. 1980. Specific binding and biological response of antiestrogens in the fetal uterus of the guinea pig. *Cancer Research* 40:3821–3826.

Horwitz, K. B., and W. L. McGuire. 1977. Progesterone and progesterone receptors in experimental breast cancer. *Cancer Research* 37:1733–1738.

Horwitz, K. B., and W. L. McGuire. 1978a. Estrogen control of progesterone receptor in human breast cancer. *Journal of Biological Chemistry* 253:2223–2228.

Horwitz, K. B., and W. L. McGuire. 1978b. Nuclear mechanisms of estrogen action: effects of estradiol and antiestrogens on estrogen receptors and nuclear receptor processing. *Journal of Biological Chemistry* 253:8185–8191.

Horwitz, K. B., Y. Koseki, and W. L. McGuire. 1978. Estrogen control of progesterone receptor in human breast cancer: role of estradiol and antiestrogen. *Endocrinology* 103:1742–1751.

Horwitz, K. B., P. Aiginger, F. Kuttenn, and W. L. McGuire. 1981. Nuclear estrogen receptor release from antiestrogen suppression: amplified induction of progesterone receptor in MCF-7 human breast cancer cells. *Endocrinology* 108:1703–1709.

Horwitz, K. B., M. B. Mockus, and B. A. Lessey. 1982. Variant T47D human breast cancer cells with high progesterone receptor levels despite estrogen and antiestrogen resistance. *Cell* 28:633–642.

Horwitz, K. B., M. B. Mockus, A. W. Pike, P. V. Fennessey, and R. L. Sheridan. 1983. Progesterone receptor replenishment in T47D human breast cancer cells: role of protein synthesis and hormone metabolism. *Journal of Biological Chemistry* 258:7603–7610.

Hsueh, A. J. W., E. J. Peck, Jr., and J. H. Clark. 1976. Control of uterine estrogen receptor levels by progesterone. *Endocrinology* 98:438–444.

Jensen, E. V., T. Suzuki, T. Kawashima, W. E. Stumpf, P. W. Jungblut, and E. R. DeSombre. 1968. A two-step mechanism for the interaction of estradiol with rat uterus. *Proceedings of the National Academy of Sciences* 59:632–638.

Jordan, V. C., and C. J. Dix. 1979. Effect of oestradiol benzoate, tamoxifen and monohydroxytamoxifen on immature rat uterine progesterone receptor synthesis and endometrial cell division. *Journal of Steroid Biochemistry* 11:285–291.

Jordan, V. C., and B. Gosden. 1982. Importance of the alkylaminoethoxy side chain for the estrogenic and antiestrogenic actions of tamoxifen and trioxifene in the immature rat uterus. *Molecular and Cellular Endocrinology* 27:291–306.

Jordan, V. C., and B. Gosden. 1983. Differential antiestrogen action in the immature rat uterus: a comparison of hydroxylated antiestrogens with high affinity for the estrogen receptor. *Journal of Steroid Biochemistry* 19:1249–1258.

Jordan, V. C., and G. Prestwich. 1978. Effect of non-steroidal antioestrogens on the concentration of rat uterine progesterone receptors. *Journal of Endocrinology* 76:363–364.

Jordan, V. C., C. J. Dix, K. E. Naylor, G. Prestwich, and L. Rowsby. 1978a. Nonsteroidal antiestrogens: their biological effects and potential mechanism of action. *Journal of Toxicology and Environmental Health* 4:363–390.

Jordan, V. C., L. Rowsby, C. J. Dix, and G. Prestwich. 1978b. Dose-related effects of non-steroidal antioestrogens and oestrogens on the measurement of cytoplasmic oestrogen receptors in the rat and mouse uterus. *Journal of Endocrinology* 78:71–81.

Jordan, V. C., G. Prestwich, C. J. Dix, and E. R. Clark. 1980. Binding of antioestrogens to the estrogen receptor, the first step in antiestrogen action. In *Pharmacological modulation of steroid action*, ed. E. Genazzani, F. DiCarlo, and W. I. P. Mainwaring, 81–98. New York: Raven Press.

Jordan, V. C., M. E. Lieberman, E. Courmier, R. Koch, J. R. Bagley, and J. C. Ruenitz. 1984. Structural requirements for the pharmacological activity of nonsteroidal antiestrogens *in vitro*. *Molecular Pharmacology* 26:272–278.

Kassis, J. A., and J. Gorski. 1983. On the mechanism of estrogen receptor replenishment: recycling, resynthesis and/or processing. *Molecular and Cellular Biochemistry* 52:27–36.

Kassis, J. A., D. Sakai, J. H. Walent, and J. Gorski. 1984a. Primary cultures of estrogen-responsive cells from rat uteri: induction of progesterone receptors and a secreted protein. *Endocrinology* 114:1558–1566.

Kassis, J. A., J. H. Walent, and J. Gorski. 1984b. Estrogen receptors in rat uterine cell cultures: effects of media on receptor concentration. *Endocrinology* 115:762–769.

Kassis, J. A., J. H. Walent, and J. Gorski. 1986. Estrogen receptors in cultured rat uterine cells: induction of progesterone receptors in the absence of estrogen receptor processing. *Endocrinology* 118:603–608.

Katzenellenbogen, B. S. 1980. Dynamics of steroid hormone receptor action. *Annual Review of Physiology* 42:17–35.

Katzenellenbogen, B. S., and J. Gorski. 1975. Estrogen actions on syntheses of macromolecules in target cells. In *Biochemical action of hormones*, vol. 3, ed. G. Litwack, 187–243. New York: Academic Press.

Katzenellenbogen, B. S., J. A. Katzenellenbogen, E. R. Ferguson, and N. Kranthammer. 1978. Antiestrogen interaction with uterine estrogen receptors: studies with a radiolabelled antiestrogen (CI628). *Journal of Biological Chemistry* 253:697–707.

Katzenellenbogen, B. S., H. S. Bhakoo, E. R. Ferguson, N. C. Lan, T. Tatee, T.-L. S. Tsai, and J. A. Katzenellenbogen. 1979. Estrogen and antiestrogen action in reproductive tissues and tumors. *Recent Progress in Hormone Research* 35:259–300.

Katzenellenbogen, B. S., M. J. Norman, R. L. Eckert, S. W. Peltz, and W. F. Mangel. 1984. Bioactivities, estrogen receptor interactions and plasminogen activator-inducing activities of tamoxifen and hydroxytamoxifen isomers in MCF-7 human breast cancer cells. *Cancer Research* 44:112–119.

Kelly, P. A., J. Asselin, M. G. Caron, F. Labrie, and J. P. Raynaud. 1977. Potent inhibitory effect of a new antiestrogen (RU 16117) on the growth of 7,12-dimethylbenz(a)-anthracene–induced rat mammary tumors. *Journal of the National Cancer Institute* 58:623–628.

King, W. J., and G. L. Greene. 1984. Monoclonal antibodies localize oestrogen receptor in the nuclei of target cells. *Nature* (London) 307:745–747.

Koseki, Y., D. T. Zava, G. C. Chamness, and W. L. McGuire. 1977a. Progesterone interaction with estrogen and antiestrogen in the rat uterus: receptor effects. *Steroids* 30:169–177.

Koseki, Y., D. T. Zava, G. C. Chamness, and W. L. McGuire. 1977b. Estrogen-receptor translocation and replenishment by the antiestrogen tamoxifen. *Endocrinology* 101:1104–1110.

Leavitt, W. W., T. J. Chen, T. C. Allen, and J. O. Johnston. 1977. Regulation of progesterone receptor formation by estrogen action. *Annals of the New York Academy of Sciences* 286:210–225.

Leavitt, W. W., T. J. Chen. Y. S. Do, B. D. Carlton, and T. C. Allen. 1978. Biology of progesterone receptors. In *Receptors and hormone action*, vol. 2, B. W. O'Malley and L. Birnbaumer, 157–188. New York: Academic Press.

Lerner, L. J. 1958. Estrogen antagonistic activity of 1-(p-2-diethylaminoethoxyphenyl)-1-phenyl-2-p-anisylethanol (MER 25). *Federation Proceedings of the American Societies for Experimental Biology* 17:388.

Lerner, L. J. 1981. The first non-steroidal antioestrogen—MER 25. In *Non-steroidal antioestrogens: molecular pharmacology and antitumour activity,* ed. R. L. Sutherland and V. C. Jordan, 1–16. Sydney: Academic Press.

Lerner, L. J., J. F. Holthaus, and C. R. Thompson. 1958. A nonsteroidal estrogen antagonist 1-(p-2-diethylaminoethoxyphenyl)-2-phenyl-2-p-methoxyphenylethanol. *Endocrinology* 63:295–318.

Lieberman, M. E., J. Gorski, and V. C. Jordan. 1983. An estrogen receptor model to describe the regulation of prolactin synthesis by antiestrogens *in vitro. Journal of Biological Chemistry* 258:4741–4745.

McGuire, W. L., K. B. Horwitz, D. T. Zava, R. E. Garola, and G. C. Chamness. 1978. Hormones and breast cancer—update. *Metabolism* 27:487–501.

Milgrom, E., L. Thi, M. Atger, and E. E. Baulieu. 1973. Mechanism regulating the concentration and the conformation of progesterone receptor(s) in the uterus. *Journal of Biological Chemistry* 248:6366–6374.

Nawata, H., M. T. Chong, D. Bronzert, and M. E. Lippman. 1981. Estradiol-independent growth of a subline of MCF-7 human breast cancer cells in culture. *Journal of Biological Chemistry* 256:6895–6902.

O'Malley, B. W., T. C. Spelsberg, W. T. Schrader, F. Chytil, and A. W. Steggles. 1972. Mechanisms of interaction of a hormone receptor complex with the genome of a eukaryotic target cell. *Nature* (London) 235:141.

Rao, B. R., W. G. Wiest, and W. B. Allen. 1973. Progesterone receptor in rabbit uterus. I. Characterization and estradiol-17β augmentation. *Endocrinology* 92:1229–1240.

Roy, E. J., N. J. MacLusky, and B. S. McEwen. 1979. Antiestrogen inhibits the induction of progestin receptors by estradiol in the hypothalamus-preoptic area and pituitary. *Endocrinology* 104:1333–1336.

Sar, M., and W. E. Stumpf. 1973. Neurons of hypothalamus concentrate ^{3}H-progesterone or its metabolites. *Science* 182:1266–1268.

Sar, M., and W. E. Stumpf. 1974. Cellular and subcellular localization of [^{3}H]-progesterone or its metabolites in the oviduct, uterus, vagina, and liver of the guinea pig. *Endocrinology* 94:1116–1125.

Soule, H. D., J. Vasquez, A. Long, S. Albert, and M. J. Brennan. 1973. A human cell line from a pleural effusion derived from a breast carcinoma. *Journal of the National Cancer Institute* 51:1409–1416.

Sutherland, R. L., and L. C. Murphy. 1982. Mechanisms of oestrogen antagonism by nonsteroidal antiestrogens. *Molecular and Cellular Endocrinology* 25:5–23.

Tsai, T. L., and B. S. Katzenellenbogen. 1977. Antagonism of development and growth of 7,12-dimethylbenzanthracene–induced rat mammary tumors by the antiestrogen U 23,469 and effects on estrogen and progesterone receptors. *Cancer Research* 37:1537–1543.

Vu Hai, M. T., F. Logeat, M. Warembourg, and E. Milgrom. 1977. Hormonal control of progesterone receptors. *Annals of the New York Academy of Sciences* 286:199–209.

Welshons, W. V., M. E. Lieberman, and J. Gorski. 1984. Nuclear localization of unoccupied oestrogen receptors. *Nature* (London) 307:747–749.

Wilcox, J. N., and H. H. Feder. 1983. Long term priming with a low dosage of estradiol benzoate or an antiestrogen (enclomiphene) increases nuclear progestin receptor levels in the brain. *Brain Research* 266:243–251.

10

Antiestrogen Action in the Chicken

C. B. Lazier and P. R. Murphy

I. Estrogen Action in the Chicken   172
II. Metabolism and Pharmacokinetics of the Antiestrogens   173
III. Antiestrogens and the Chick Liver   174
    A. Agonistic Actions   174
    B. Antagonistic Actions   174
    C. Binding to Hepatic Estrogen Receptors   175
    D. Antiestrogen Binding Sites   177
    E. AEBS Inhibitory Activity: The Question of Endogenous
       Ligands   180
IV. Antiestrogens and the Chick Oviduct   182
    A. Antagonistic Actions of Tamoxifen and the Absence of
       Agonistic Action   182
    B. Paradoxical Effects of Tamoxifen Combined with
       Progesterone or Glucocorticoids   183
    C. Interaction with Estrogen Receptors   184
    D. Antiestrogen Binding Sites   185
V. Summary   185
    References   187

I. *Estrogen Action in the Chicken*

T HE chicken has been a very useful model for the study of the mechanism of estrogen action. The initial impetus for the work came not so much from particular interest in the animal *per se,* but because of the impressive magnitude of the response to estrogen in the oviduct. This enabled the isolation of ovalbumin mRNA and pioneering work in the molecular biology of eukaryotic gene expression (O'Malley et al. 1979; Chambon et al. 1984). In oviduct, estrogen stimulates pronounced differentiation and growth of the tissue and induction of large amounts of egg white proteins such as ovalbumin, conalbumin, and lysozyme. In chick liver, however, the hormone induces synthesis of the egg yolk protein precursor vitellogenin and of the apolipoproteins of very low density lipoprotein (VLDL), apo VLDL II, and apo VLDL B. The liver effect appears to be direct and highly specific for estradiol and can take place without the necessity for massive differentiation and growth (Shapiro 1982). In differentiated oviduct other classes of steroids, including progestins, glucocorticoids, and androgens, can also regulate egg white protein synthesis. Within a given target tissue there are differences in kinetics and dose responsiveness of individual loci, suggesting further subtleties in modes of steroid regulation (Palmiter et al. 1981). Thus, the chicken, with two such distinctive estrogen targets, makes an excellent subject for the study of differential gene regulation and tissue specificity. Both tissues contain estrogen receptors, but each tissue responds according to its unique developmental program.

If we assume, somewhat tentatively, that estrogen receptors are similar in different target tissues of an animal, then control of specificity must lie at the level of the chromatin. Presumably unoccupied receptor (in cytosol, or loosely bound in nuclei and entering cytosol upon homogenization) binds hormone, and the resulting receptor-hormone complex undergoes a conformational alteration (activation) that enables it to bind to discrete sites in chromatin and to stimulate specific transcriptional activity. The nature and regulation of the chromatin sites is of fundamental importance and is just now becoming open to experimental analysis. Preferential binding of steroid receptors to known sequences of DNA and transfection experiments with fusion genes have helped define DNA sequences in promoter regions, which are important for steroid regulation of genes expressed in oviduct (Dean et al. 1984; Renkawitz et al. 1984) and in liver (Jost et al. 1984).

Because triphenylethylene antiestrogens in the chicken appear to be uniquely antagonistic (Sutherland et al. 1977; Lazier et al. 1981), they should be invaluable probes of the mechanism of estrogen action in such studies as those discussed above. The following sections detail current knowledge on antiestrogen pharmacokinetics in chicks and on their estrogen-antagonistic and possible estrogen-independent actions.

II. *Metabolism and Pharmacokinetics of the Antiestrogens*

Rigorous interpretation of the actions of any drug requires knowledge of its metabolism and pharmacokinetics, especially when the reported studies involve *in vivo* administration of the drug along with a hormone. Tamoxifen injected intramuscularly in propylene glycol into chicks is cleared slowly from the circulation. Binart et al. (1979) have reported that the half-life of a dose of tamoxifen of 10 mg/kg is about 20 hours. An active dose of estrogen (1 mg/kg of estradiol benzoate) is cleared much more rapidly. The ratio of tamoxifen to estrogen thus changes with time after injection; this could affect the proportion of estrogen receptors occupied by antiestrogen ligand. The availability of estrogen and antiestrogen to receptor sites might also be influenced by the binding of either ligand to nonreceptor entities such as antiestrogen binding sites (AEBS), plasma, or tissue steroid binding proteins (Lazier 1979; Lazier and Jordan 1982; Taylor and Smith 1982).

Metabolism of tamoxifen in the chicken has been studied to the extent that it appears that 4-hydroxytamoxifen and possibly also more polar compounds such as the 3,4-dihydroxy derivative are produced (Borgna and Rochefort 1980, 1981). [³H]4-Hydroxytamoxifen is concentrated in fractions of liver nuclei both after *in vivo* injection or *in vitro* exposure of liver slices to [³H]tamoxifen. According to one report (Borgna and Rochefort 1981), the oviduct accumulates and is capable of producing 4-hydroxytamoxifen; however, in another report such activities were not detected (Binart et al. 1979). This metabolic transformation is of particular importance because of the pronounced effect of 4-hydroxylation on the affinity of tamoxifen for AEBS and for estrogen receptor, both in oviduct and liver (Sections III.C, D, and IV.C, D).

III. Antiestrogens and the Chick Liver

A. AGONISTIC ACTIONS

Experimental data dealing with the actions of antiestrogens in chick liver as known before 1980 have been summarized in two review articles (Lazier 1979; Lazier et al. 1981). Briefly, the principal findings were that high doses of nafoxidine, tamoxifen, or CI 628 had no apparent agonistic action with regard to induction of vitellogenin or the VLDL apoproteins. The methods used were electrophoretic or phosphoprotein analysis of serum, or specific immunoprecipitation of fractions of liver tissue labeled with [^{3}H]amino acids in vitro. More recently, Blue and Williams (1981) have reported that highly sensitive radioimmunoassay techniques permitted detection of very low levels of apo VLDL II and vitellogenin in sera from nonestrogenized roosters. Tamoxifen (30 mg/kg) raised the basal level of serum apo VLDL II about 50-fold and of vitellogenin about 15-fold. The basal levels reported were in the range of 1–40 ng/ml for apo VLDL II and 4–8 ng/ml for vitellogenin. The maximum agonistic activity of tamoxifen is still no more than 0.1% of the maximum response to estradiol. Thus tamoxifen, if not a pure antagonist, is an exceedingly weak partial agonist, and these agonistic actions are much less pronounced than those seen in other species. It is worth noting that the dose-response relationship for the tamoxifen effect on apo VLDL II synthesis was biphasic, with optimum effects noted at a dose of 9 mg/kg and a lower response at higher doses. This could mean that agonistic actions could be missed unless a wide dose range was investigated.

B. ANTAGONISTIC ACTIONS

The early studies with nafoxidine and CI 628 on vitellogenin and apo VLDL II synthesis in avian liver uniformly showed that the triphenylethylene compounds were extremely potent antagonists of estrogen action (Gschwendt 1975; Lazier 1975; Chan et al. 1977; Lazier and Alford 1977). Nafoxidine (50 mg/kg) given with estradiol in a molar dose ratio of 1.2:1 resulted in the complete suppression of the vitellogenin response at 48 hours. In addition, the estrogen stimulation of apo VLDL B synthesis is very sensitive to inhibition by tamoxifen, even when the drug is administered 2–8 hours after estradiol (Capony and Williams 1980, 1981). This suggests that, despite depletion of cytosol estrogen receptor levels (Lazier and Haggarty 1979), the antagonist is able to enter the nucleus and disrupt the functioning of the estrogen receptor complex, possibly by exchanging for the hormone. A corollary is that the antiestrogen does not require cytosol receptor for transport to the nucleus.

Most studies on tamoxifen antagonism in chick liver have been carried out at the level of protein synthesis. Recently, Gschwendt et al. (1983) have reported that vitellogenin synthesis after tamoxifen treatment is proportional to the level of hepatic vitellogenin mRNA as measured by Northern blot analysis. Further work on antiestrogen action on transcription of specific liver genes would be very useful, especially to interpret experiments such as those on tamoxifen reversal mentioned above.

C. Binding to Hepatic Estrogen Receptors

The importance of hepatic metabolism in generating forms of antiestrogens which bind to estrogen receptor with very high affinity has only recently been realized. The initial reports showed that the affinities of nafoxidine and CI 628 for chick liver nuclear estrogen receptor were less than 5% that for estradiol (Gschwendt 1975; Lazier and Alford 1977). Lazier and Jordan (1982) subsequently found that tamoxifen exhibited a K_i of 2.6 nM for the chick liver salt-soluble nuclear estrogen receptor, whereas that for 4-hydroxytamoxifen was 0.1 nM and the K_d for estradiol was 0.7 nM. The very high affinity of 4-hydroxytamoxifen for the receptor has since been confirmed directly, using the [^{3}H]-labeled compound (C. B. Lazier, unpublished observations). This observation raises the possibility that 4-hydroxytamoxifen bound to the nuclear estrogen receptor may be very difficult to exchange in conventional assays (Gschwendt et al. 1982; Lazier and Jordan 1982) and indicates that it is incumbent upon an experimentalist to demonstrate that exchange can occur in assays attempting to analyze the effects of antiestrogen treatment on the concentration of nuclear estrogen receptor. Indeed, both aforementioned groups have shown that salt-soluble nuclear receptor occupied by 4-hydroxytamoxifen shows only limited exchange for [^{3}H]estradiol under the usual conditions. Optimizing conditions by pretreatment of the antiestrogen–estrogen receptor complexes with 1.7% charcoal at 37°C for 15 minutes permits exchange of some 60–70% of the bound antiestrogen (Lazier and Jordan 1982). Taking this into account, it can be shown that tamoxifen treatment of chicks does result in increased levels of salt-soluble nuclear estrogen receptor (Fig. 10.1). The extent of the increase and its time course probably depend on pharmacokinetic considerations as well as on the efficacy of the antiestrogen–estrogen receptor complex in the mechanisms leading to nuclear accumulation of the receptor.

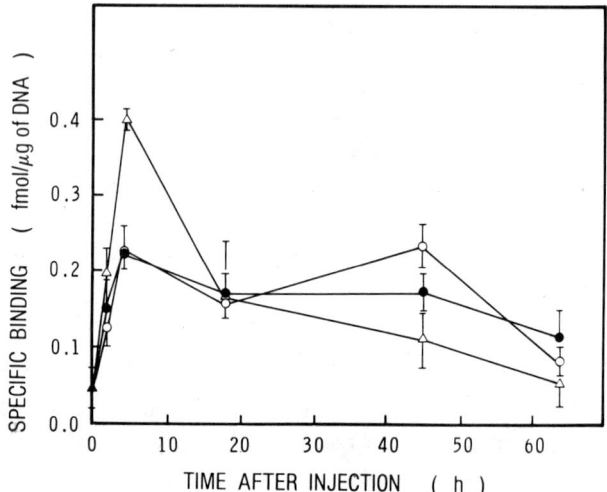

Figure 10.1. Time course of the effect of tamoxifen and 4-hydroxytamoxifen treatment *in vivo* on the salt-soluble nuclear estrogen receptor. Chicks were injected with estradiol (△, 3 mg/kg) or with tamoxifen (●), or 4-hydroxytamoxifen (○) (each 6 mg/kg). The salt extracts of nuclei were pretreated with 1.7% charcoal suspension at 37°C for 15 minutes before [³H]estradiol binding assay. The exchange efficiency for 4-hydroxytamoxifen is 60–70%; therefore the receptor concentrations in the antiestrogen-treated chicks could be 30–40% low, depending in the case of tamoxifen upon the degree of metabolite hydroxylation. (From Lazier and Jordan 1982. Reprinted by permission from *The Biochemical Journal*, vol. 206, pp. 387–394; copyright © 1982 The Biochemical Society, London.)

The effect of prior antiestrogen treatment on the levels of estrogen receptor in intact nuclei and in nuclear matrix preparations has also been investigated. In contrast to the increased levels of receptor seen in charcoal-pretreated salt extracts of nuclei, little or no increase in receptor is seen on assay of intact nuclei under conventional exchange conditions (Lazier et al. 1981; Lazier and Jordan 1982; Simmen et al. 1984). In addition, no increase in nuclear matrix–associated estrogen receptor was found 4 hours after tamoxifen treatment (Simmen et al. 1984).

Injection of antiestrogens with estrogen, followed by assay of estrogen receptor in intact nuclei or nuclear matrix over the next 48 hours results in a marked decrease in estrogen receptor compared to that seen if estrogen is injected alone (Lazier et al. 1981; Lazier and Jordan 1982; Simmen et al. 1984). However, in view of the assay difficulties mentioned above, it has not been possible to establish whether the decrease reflects actual loss or mere masking of the receptor sites.

Another problem with assays of estrogen receptor in intact nuclei is

Table 10.1. Relative binding affinities of antiestrogens and estradiol for the estrogen receptor in salt extracts and intact nuclei from chick liver[a]

	Relative binding affinities[b]	
	Salt extracts	Nuclei
Estradiol	100	100
Tamoxifen	9	1
4-Hydroxytamoxifen	440	140
N-Desmethyltamoxifen	28	< 1

Adapted from Lazier and Jordan 1982.
[a]Nuclei or nuclear salt extracts from liver of estrogen-treated chicks were incubated at 30°C with 8 nM [^{3}H]estradiol in the presence or absence of various concentrations of competitors.
[b]Relative binding affinity is the ratio of the IC_{50} for estradiol to that for the antiestrogen × 100. The IC_{50} for estradiol in both cases was 7 nM.

illustrated by the observation that the relative binding affinities of tamoxifen and two derivatives for nuclear receptor are considerably less when measured using intact nuclei as compared to salt extracts (Table 10.1). In other words, a much higher concentration of antiestrogen is required to give 50% inhibition of [^{3}H]estradiol binding in intact nuclei than in salt extracts. This suggests that the nuclei contain antiestrogen-specific sites which in effect lower the amount of drug available for binding to the estrogen receptor. Such sites could also lead to concentration of antiestrogens in nuclei *in vivo,* with subsequent dissociation and interference with the estrogen receptor assay *in vitro.*

D. ANTIESTROGEN BINDING SITES

The recent availability of high specific activity [^{3}H]-labeled tamoxifen has permitted direct analysis of interactions of the drug in various tissues. Sutherland et al. (1980), in their important article surveying specific AEBS in a variety of tissues and species, reported detection of high affinity AEBS in chick liver cytosol. Our primary interest in nuclear estrogen receptors led us first to investigate AEBS in that cellular compartment (Lazier et al. 1984a; Murphy et al. 1984). Salt extracts of purified nuclei from liver contain specific AEBS which exhibit binding characteristics typical of AEBS reported by others in different tissues; that is, nafoxidine

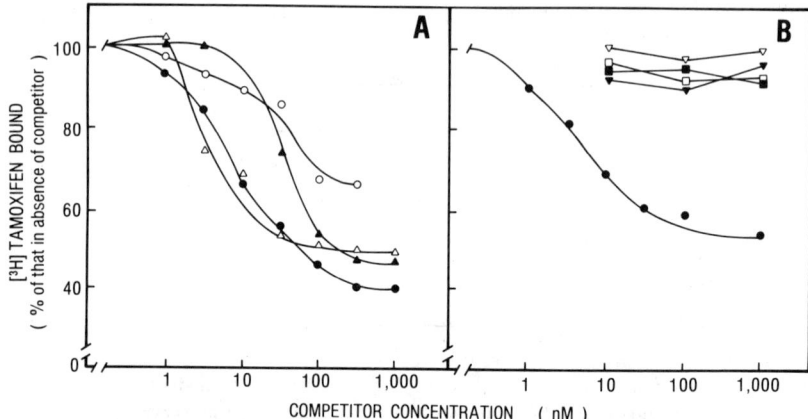

Figure 10.2. Ligand specificity of cockerel liver nuclear AEBS. Nuclear salt extract was incubated with 8 nM [³H]tamoxifen and increasing concentrations of various antiestrogens (A) or DES or various steroids (B). Tamoxifen, ●; nafoxidine, △; N-desmethyltamoxifen, ▲; 4-hydroxytamoxifen, ○; diethylstilbestrol (DES), □; estradiol, ■; estrone, ▼; and cholesterol, ▽. (From Murphy et al. [1984] with the permission of the editor.)

exhibits high affinity about equivalent to [³H]tamoxifen, and 4-hydroxy-tamoxifen binds considerably less avidly (Gulino and Pasqualini 1982; Sudo et al. 1983) (Fig. 10.2). This is in marked contrast to the liver estrogen receptor (Lazier and Alford 1977; Lazier and Jordan 1982). The nuclear AEBS concentration in cockerel liver is 30-fold higher than the estrogen receptor concentration (Murphy et al. 1984) and is not altered by estrogen treatment (P. R. Murphy and C. B. Lazier, unpublished observations).

Our initial preparation of subcellular fractions of AEBS involved homogenization of liver in the same glycerol-containing buffers used for purification of nuclei (Snow et al. 1978). The intracellular distribution of the AEBS under these conditions is shown in Table 10.2. The estimates of the AEBS concentration in cytoplasmic fractions are considerably higher than those reported earlier (Sutherland et al. 1980; Lazier et al. 1984a). This is probably due to two effects: first, that the AEBS assay is very subject to inhibitory effects of high protein concentrations, and second, that divalent cations inhibit AEBS (Lazier et al. 1984b).

Linearity of [³H]tamoxifen binding with increasing liver fraction volume is seen over only a limited range, especially with the lower speed supernatant fractions. Under the homogenization and assay conditions used (Table 10.2), this range was about 2–30 μl per 0.3 ml reaction vol-

Table 10.2. Intracellular distribution of cockerel liver AEBS[a]

Liver fraction	AEBS activity (pmol/g liver)
5000 × g supernatant	862
pellet	244
33,000 × g supernatant	777
pellet	150
100,000 × g supernatant	296
pellet	372

[a]Liver was homogenized in 10 volumes of glycerol containing buffer (10 mM Tris, 1.5 mM MgCl$_2$, 10 mM thioglycerol, 50% glycerol v/ v, pH 7.5 at 25°C). After centrifugation at 5000 × g for 20 minutes, a portion of the supernatant fraction was centrifuged at 100,000 × g for 1 hour. For assay, 10 μl of the supernatant or of the pellet resuspended in the original volume of homogenization buffer were incubated with 10 nM [^{3}H]tamoxifen, 0.275 ml of TE buffer (10 mM Tes, 1.5 mM EDTA, 10 mM thioglycerol, pH 7.4) in a total volume of 0.3 ml. Nonspecific binding was measured in the presence of 100× excess of radioinert tamoxifen. Diethylstilbestrol (1 μM) was added to all tubes to saturate any estrogen receptor present. Incubation was for 30 minutes at 30°C, followed by charcoal treatment and liquid scintillation counting as described by Murphy et al. (1984).

ume for the 5000 × g and 33,000 × g supernatant fractions, and wider for the 100,000 × g fraction. High concentrations of Mg^{++} or Ca^{++} (> 1.0 mM) inhibit the AEBS assay. In the assay shown here, the final Mg^{++} concentration is very low (0.05 mM) and is balanced by excess EDTA.

The revised estimates for the concentration of AEBS in cockerel liver cytoplasmic fractions suggest that the overall contribution by nuclear AEBS is quite low. It seems likely that, as for other species, the AEBS is primarily concentrated in the microsomal fraction (Sudo et al. 1983; Watts et al. 1984). Indeed, homogenization of cockerel liver in Tes-EDTA buffer results in the bulk of the AEBS sedimenting on centrifugation at 100,000 × g (C. B. Lazier, unpublished observations). For routine preparation of AEBS, however, the glycerol homogenization technique for preparation of the 100,000 × g supernatant fraction has several advantages, particularly convenience of storage in the fluid form at −20°C and much superior stability. Sucrose gradient analysis of this cytosol shows the AEBS associated with material sedimenting at 10–30S.

The ligand specificity of the liver cytosol AEBS is very similar to that reported for the nuclear fractions (Murphy et al. 1984). In addition we have found that although cholesterol shows no inhibition of AEBS at concentrations up to the limits of solubility, two cholesterol metabolites, namely 7-ketocholesterol and Δ4-cholestene-3-one, do exhibit measurable affinity for the sites (Murphy et al. 1985). The relative binding affinity for the 7-keto derivative is about 1% that of tamoxifen. Although this is small, it could be of consequence, considering that serum or tissue concentrations might well be within this range.

E. AEBS INHIBITORY ACTIVITY: THE QUESTION OF ENDOGENOUS LIGANDS

The first report of a possible endogenous ligand for AEBS came from the laboratory of Clark et al. (1983). Boiling-ethanol extracts of rat liver were shown to inhibit [³H]tamoxifen binding to AEBS in rat liver and serum low density lipoprotein. We also reported AEBS inhibitory activity in ether extracts of chick serum and liver nuclei (Fig. 10.3). These observations, together with the finding that charcoal pretreatment of liver nuclear AEBS significantly enhanced subsequent binding of [³H]tamoxifen, led us to propose that the AEBS were occupied by an "endogenous ligand" *in vivo* (Murphy et al. 1984). We have since screened various chick tissues for AEBS inhibitory activity and found highest concentrations in liver cytosol and microsomes; but we also found moderately high concentrations in kidney and oviduct. The distribution shows no obvious connection with estrogen target tissues or even with the tissue concentration of AEBS.

Human serum also contains ether-soluble AEBS inhibitory activity, as assayed using chick liver or human breast tumor AEBS preparations (C. B. Lazier, P. R. Murphy, and S. Hutchison, unpublished observations). The human serum extracts contain at least two chromatographically distinct classes of AEBS inhibitory activity. These can be separated by sterol isolation techniques such as hexane and digitonin precipitation (Murphy et al. 1985). Further, the "sterol" fraction contains two chromatographically separable activities, one of which appears on gas liquid chromatography to contain 7-ketocholesterol in sufficient concentration to be inhibitory (Murphy et al. 1985). The nonsterol-soluble fraction remaining after hexane and digitonin precipitation behaves like a fatty acid ester. Much more work, however, appears to be necessary for purification or definitive identification of the inhibitory compounds.

The scope of the problem in identifying putative "endogenous ligands" by isolation from serum can be illustrated by a simple calculation based on the observed IC_{50} for inhibition of [³H]tamoxifen binding to the AEBS.

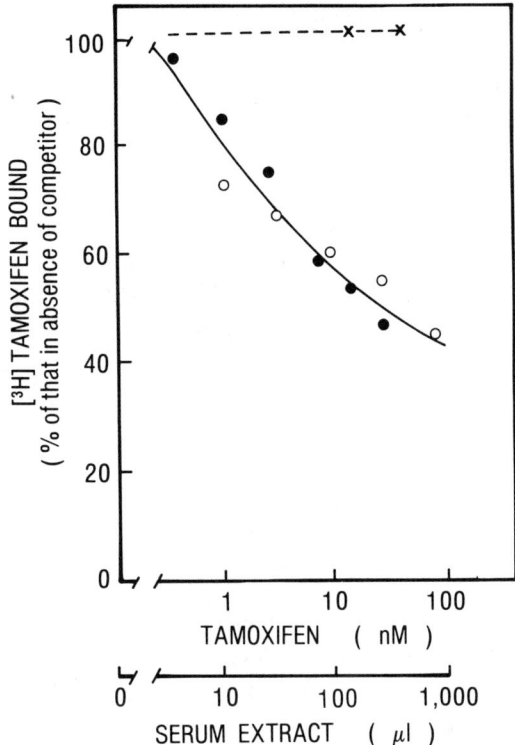

Figure 10.3. Inhibition of [³H]tamoxifen binding to liver nuclear AEBS by tamoxifen (○), chick serum ether extract (●), or the ether vehicle alone (x). The ether was evaporated prior to addition of the other components of the incubation mixture. (From Murphy et al. [1984] with the permission of the editor.)

With the chick serum extract, for example (Murphy et al. 1984), ether extract equivalent to 28 μl of serum gives 50% inhibition in a 0.3 ml incubation mixture containing 6 nM [³H]tamoxifen. Thus for straight-forward competition by a compound of equal affinity to tamoxifen, a liter of serum should contain about 65 nmol of inhibitor. The serum extracts, however, appear to be quite heterogeneous and most likely contain compounds with a range of affinities for the AEBS. Further, the distribution in serum of ether-soluble compounds in lipoprotein particles and protein-bound forms must also be considered. It must be admitted that the prospect of identification of physiologically relevant ligands by this approach is somewhat daunting. However, knowledge of the general classes of ether-soluble compounds in serum which have AEBS inhibitory potential should be helpful in formulating hypotheses on the possible function of these distinctive but mysterious binding sites.

Structure-function studies in breast cancer cell lines suggest that the triphenylethylene antiestrogens may have some estrogen-independent actions in inhibition of cell growth (Murphy and Sutherland 1985), but no such correlations have been drawn in the chick system. Some recent studies with hen granulosa cells do suggest, however, that clomiphene and tamoxifen may inhibit progesterone synthesis at a site distinct from that affected by estrogen (Sgarlata et al. 1984). Whether or not these actions are mediated by AEBS remains to be seen.

IV. *Antiestrogens and the Chick Oviduct*

A. ANTAGONISTIC ACTIONS OF TAMOXIFEN AND THE ABSENCE OF AGONISTIC ACTION

The virtual absence of agonistic effects of tamoxifen and 4-hydroxy-tamoxifen given alone has been noted in numerous studies on oviduct growth and differentiation and on the synthesis or activity of particular estrogen-induced oviduct proteins (Sutherland et al. 1977; Binart et al. 1979; Catelli et al. 1980; Mester et al. 1981; Sutherland 1981; Binart et al. 1982; Gravanis et al. 1984). Parameters examined include tissue weight, DNA content, histological differentiation, ovalbumin and conalbumin synthesis, and the activities of ornithine decarboxylase and DNA polymerase α. Most studies have been conducted in estrogen-withdrawn chicks, that is, in young birds in which primary oviduct differentiation has been stimulated by a series of estrogen injections in the first 2 weeks after hatch, following which the animals have been withdrawn from treatment for 4–6 weeks. In these animals, eight different antiestrogens have been tested in a wide dose range and in single and multiple injections, but in no case was any effect observed on any of the growth characteristics mentioned above (Sutherland 1981). The only study in which a possible agonistic effect of tamoxifen is apparent shows a small but statistically significant increase in the relative rate of conalbumin synthesis in tamoxifen-treated as compared to control chicks (from 0.83% to 1.20%) (Binart et al. 1982). This might be explained by interaction with endogenous glucocorticoids, as will be discussed below.

In immature oviduct, from chicks not previously exposed to estrogen, tamoxifen does not induce ovalbumin or conalbumin synthesis, nor does it promote any histologically detectable differentiation of the tissue (Binart et al. 1982).

The estrogen-antagonistic actions of tamoxifen in oviduct have been amply demonstrated with regard to all of the parameters mentioned in the above studies, in general using simultaneous administration of drug and hormone. In addition, inhibitory effects can also be observed upon delayed administration of tamoxifen relative to estradiol (Palmiter et al. 1977; Catelli et al. 1980; Mester et al. 1981). Antagonism is observed when tamoxifen is given up to 4 hours after estradiol benzoate, although different kinetics are found in the inhibition of conalbumin and ovalbumin synthesis. This may possibly be due to differences in the characteristics of receptor-genome interaction for the two loci (Palmiter et al. 1981). The reversal experiments underline the contention, also noted with apoprotein B synthesis in liver (Capony and Williams 1981), that tamoxifen administered after estrogen has access to nuclear estrogen receptor complexes, even though cytosol estrogen receptor levels are low. Presumably it is at the level of nuclear estrogen receptor that the antiestrogenic ligand displays its inhibitory properties, possibly by inducing inappropriate conformational changes.

B. Paradoxical Effects of Tamoxifen Combined with Progesterone or Glucocorticoids

Progesterone is well known as an inducer of egg white protein synthesis in the estrogen-withdrawn chick oviduct. Unlike estrogen however, it does not promote differentiation of the immature oviduct and in fact inhibits this action of estradiol (Palmiter and Wrenn 1971). Administration of progesterone (3 mg/chick) plus tamoxifen (10 mg/chick) to week-old chicks produces an "estrogenlike" increase in organ weight and in ovalbumin and conalbumin synthesis and induces cytodifferentiation of tubular gland cells (Binart et al. 1982). In estrogen-withdrawn chicks (~ 6 weeks old), the combined dose results in enhancement of the effect seen with progesterone alone. Thus, under these conditions, tamoxifen can be said to have some estrogenic activity. Similarly, administration of tamoxifen plus dexamethasone results in pronounced estrogenlike actions, much greater than seen with the glucocorticoid alone (Gravanis et al. 1984). No such effects of tamoxifen plus progesterone or dexamethasone have been observed on specific protein synthesis in chick liver (C. B. Lazier, unpublished observations). The molecular basis for the seemingly bizarre oviduct responses is quite unknown but may be the result of some interaction of the tamoxifen-bound estrogen receptor with the progesterone or gluco-corticoid receptors at nuclear sites.

C. INTERACTION WITH ESTROGEN RECEPTORS

Estrogen receptors in salt extracts of oviduct nuclei bind antiestrogens in a fashion similar to that reported for liver (K_d for estradiol: 0.36 nM; K_i for tamoxifen 2.6 nM; and K_i for 4-hydroxytamoxifen 0.2 nM) (Binart et al. 1979). In addition, Sutherland (1981) has investigated the binding of a series of eight triphenylethylene antiestrogens to both cytosol and salt-soluble nuclear estrogen receptor preparations from oviduct. The highest relative binding activities observed ranged from 10% to 24% compared to estradiol, and corresponded to the most potent antagonists screened (enclomiphene, CI 628, CI 680, tamoxifen, and nafoxidine). By contrast, weaker antagonists such as the *cis* isomers zuclomiphene, ICI 47,699, and U 23,469 exhibited comparatively lower affinity for oviduct estrogen receptor (0.2–1.4%). Overall, 4-hydroxytamoxifen has clearly the highest affinity for the estrogen receptor of any of the antiestrogens tested in the two studies.

Analysis of the dissociation kinetics of 4-hydroxytamoxifen bound to oviduct cytosol estrogen receptor shows distinctly lower rate constants than those observed with estradiol as ligand (Rochefort and Borgna 1981; Geynet et al. 1983). In addition, Rochefort and Borgna noted that although inhibition of receptor activation by molybdate gave the expected increased dissociation rate constant with bound estradiol, no change was observed with bound 4-hydroxytamoxifen. The proposed interpretation of these results is that receptor activation mediated by the antiestrogen is somehow defective. Further, Geynet et al. (1983) observed some differences in the sedimentation coefficients of heat-treated and untreated complexes prepared with the estrogen or antiestrogen as ligand, which is also consistent with defective receptor transformation or activation.

Defective activation or transformation could lead to impaired association of receptor with nuclear sites. Treatment of estrogen-withdrawn chicks with 4-hydroxytamoxifen or tamoxifen results in an increase in the concentration of nuclear salt-soluble estrogen receptor, although not quite to the extent seen upon estrogen treatment (Sutherland et al. 1977; Binart et al. 1979). Analysis of chromatin fractions, however, gives another story, and it appears that injection of 4-hydroxytamoxifen itself (1 mg/kg) results in little or no increase in estrogen receptor in soluble chromatin or in discrete chromatin fractions isolated by micrococcal nuclease treatment and sucrose gradient centrifugation (Lebeau et al. 1982). Injection of 4-

hydroxytamoxifen with estradiol benzoate (1 mg/kg) antagonizes the increase in estrogen receptor in the 13–14S and 7–8S chromatin fractions normally seen with the hormone alone. The inhibitory effects of the antiestrogen cannot be explained by a lack of exchange in the assay, since considerable dissociation of prebound [^{3}H]4-hydroxytamoxifen was demonstrated under similar incubation conditions. It is possible that chromatin 4-hydroxytamoxifen–estrogen receptor complexes are comparatively labile, or that they are unable to associate correctly with the particular chromatin sites solubilized by the nuclease.

D. ANTIESTROGEN BINDING SITES

The first suggestion of triphenylethylene antiestrogen-specific high affinity binding sites arose from work with the estrogen-withdrawn chick oviduct (Sutherland and Foo 1979; Murphy et al. 1981). The ratio in cytosol of tamoxifen to estrogen binding sites was over 3, thus making the detection of the sites in this tissue easier than in immature rat uterus where the ratio was only 1 (Sutherland et al. 1980). The K_d for tamoxifen binding to oviduct AEBS appears to be somewhat higher than that found in other tissues (9.82 ± 1.96 nM); but for CI 628 the K_d is 1.90 ± .072 nM (Sutherland and Foo 1979). Apart from these studies, there appears to have been no further published characterization of the oviduct AEBS.

We have found (C. B. Lazier and K. Lonergan, unpublished observations) that homogenization of oviduct from estrogen-treated chicks in 0.25 M sucrose-containing buffer gives an AEBS concentration of about 300 pmol/g tissue in the 800 × g supernatant fraction. Centrifugation at 35,000 or 100,000 × g does not result in sedimentation of these sites, and under these conditions few AEBS are recovered in the microsomal fraction. About 3 pmol/g tissue are detectable in salt extracts from purified oviduct nuclei. These extracts also contain estrogen receptor at a concentration of about 900 fmol/g tissue.

It appears that, as in liver, oviduct contains high concentrations of AEBS. Apart from any possible physiological role, they probably are relevant in the pharmacokinetics of the antiestrogens.

V. Summary

After almost a decade of investigation by several groups, the conclusions still hold that the triphenylethylene antiestrogens are extremely potent antagonists of estrogen action in the chicken and that they display less agonistic activity than has been reported in any other animal model. The only exception to the case appears to be in oviduct when tamoxifen is given with progesterone or glucocorticoids, but the mechanisms involved are not yet understood.

Estrogen receptors in the chick oviduct and liver uniformly exhibit high affinity for binding 4-hydroxytamoxifen, higher even than for estradiol itself. It is not clear, however, whether metabolic hydroxylation of tamoxifen is a prerequisite for antagonistic action or even if it is always an advantage. It does appear that *trans* derivatives are more potent antagonists than the *cis* isomers.

In vivo administration of antiestrogens gives rise to increased levels of nuclear estrogen receptor, at least in the salt-soluble fraction. Intranuclear distribution of receptor, particularly in the matrix and in discrete chromatin fractions, may be altered. In addition, there is some evidence in oviduct that receptor activation may be abnormal in the presence of antiestrogens.

Antiestrogen binding sites (AEBS) with high affinity and distinctive specificity are present in many chick tissues and are particularly abundant in liver and oviduct. In addition, serum and many tissues contain ether-soluble compounds, which competitively inhibit [^{3}H]tamoxifen binding to AEBS. The inhibitory fraction from serum is chromatographically heterogeneous and appears to contain sterol-like compounds as well as fatty acid esters.

Obvious directions for future work in this field include investigation of the nature of the antiestrogen–estrogen receptor complex, its interaction with the genome, and the mechanisms of its effects on transcription. Another priority is investigation of estrogen-independent actions of tamoxifen, of the physiological function of AEBS, and of the identity of the AEBS inhibitory compounds.

Acknowledgments

Grant support for the chick liver work was from the Medical Research Council and the National Cancer Institute of Canada. Technical assistance by Kim Lonergan and Pauline Champion is gratefully acknowledged. Thanks are also due to Dr. Carl Breckenridge of the Lipoprotein Research Group, Dalhousie University, for helpful discussions.

References

Binart, N., M. G. Catelli, C. Geynet, V. Puri, R. Hahnel, J. Mester, and E.-E. Baulieu. 1979. Monohydroxytamoxifen an antioestrogen with high affinity for the chick oviduct oestrogen receptor. *Biochemical and Biophysical Research Communications* 91:812–818.

Binart, N., J. Mester, E.-E. Baulieu, and M.-G. Catelli. 1982. Combined effects of progesterone and tamoxifen in the chick oviduct. *Endocrinology* 111:7–16.

Blue, M. L., and D. L. Williams. 1981. Induction of avian serum lipoprotein II and vitellogenin by tamoxifen. *Biochemical and Biophysical Research Communications* 98:785–791.

Borgna, J. L., and H. Rochefort. 1980. High affinity binding to the estrogen receptor of [^{3}H]4-hydroxytamoxifen, an active antiestrogen metabolite. *Molecular and Cellular Endocrinology* 20:71–85.

Borgna, J. L., and H. Rochefort. 1981. Hydroxylated metabolites of tamoxifen are formed in vivo and bound to estrogen receptor in target tissues. *Journal of Biological Chemistry* 256:859–868.

Capony, F., and D. L. Williams. 1980. Apolipoprotein B of avian very low density lipoprotein: characteristics of its regulation in nonstimulated and estrogen-stimulated roosters. *Biochemistry* 19:2219–2226.

Capony, F., and D. L. Williams. 1981. Antiestrogen action in avian liver: the interaction of estrogens and antiestrogens in the regulation of apolipoprotein B synthesis. *Endocrinology* 108:1862–1868.

Catelli, M. G., N. Binart, F. Elkik, and E.-E. Baulieu. 1980. Effect of tamoxifen on oestradiol and progesterone-induced synthesis of ovalbumin and conalbumin in chick oviduct. *European Journal of Biochemistry* 107:165–172.

Chambon, P., A. Dierich, M. P. Gaub, S. Jakowlev, J. Jongstra, A. Krust, J.-P. LePennec, P. Oudet, and T. Reudelhuber. 1984. Promoter elements of genes coding for proteins and modulation of transcription by estrogens and progesterone. *Recent Progress in Hormone Research* 40:1–39.

Chan, L., R. L. Jackson, and A. R. Means. 1977. Female steroid hormones and lipoprotein synthesis in the cockerel: effects of progesterone and nafoxidine on the estrogenic stimulation of very low density lipoprotein (VLDL) synthesis. *Endocrinology* 100:1636–1643.

Clark, J. H., R. C. Winneka, S. C. Guthrie, and B. M. Markaverich. 1983. An endogenous ligand for the triphenylethylene binding site. *Endocrinology* 113:1167–1169.

Dean, D. C., R. Gope, B. J. Knoll, M. E. Riser, and B. W. O'Malley. 1984. A similar 5'-flanking region is required for estrogen and progesterone induction of ovalbumin gene expression. *Journal of Biological Chemistry* 259:9967–9970.

Geynet, C., G. Shyamala, and E.-E. Baulieu. 1983. Similarities and differences of the binding of estradiol and 4-hydroxytamoxifen (an antiestrogen) in the chicken oviduct cytosol. *Biochimica et Biophysica Acta* 756:349–353.

Gravanis, A., N. Binart, P. Robel, E.-E. Baulieu and M.-G. Catelli. 1984. Estrogen-like effects of combined dexamethasone and tamoxifen in chick oviduct. *Biochemical and Biophysical Research Communications* 124:57–62.

Gschwendt, M. 1975. The effect of antiestrogens on egg yolk protein synthesis and estrogen-binding to chromatin in the rooster liver. *Biochimica et Biophysica Acta* 399:395–402.

Gschwendt, M., G. Rincke, and T. Schuster. 1982. The estrogen-induced vitellogenin synthesis in chicken liver after estrogen withdrawal or antiestrogen treatment. *Molecular and Cellular Endocrinology* 26:231–242.

Gschwendt, M., G. Rincke, and T. Schuster. 1983. Inhibition of the estrogen-induced synthesis of vitellogenin mRNA in chick liver by tamoxifen. *Biochemical and Biophysical Research Communications* 112:425–430.

Gulino, A., and J. R. Pasqualini. 1982. Heterogeneity of binding sites for tamoxifen and tamoxifen derivatives in estrogen target and nontarget fetal organs of guinea pig. *Cancer Research* 42:1913–1921.

Jost, J.-P., M. Seldran, and M. Geiser. 1984. Preferential binding of estrogen-receptor complex to a region containing the estrogen-dependent hypomethylation site preceding the chicken vitellogenin II gene. *Proceedings of the National Academy of Sciences* 81:429–433.

Lazier, C. B. 1975. [³H]Estradiol binding by chick liver nuclear extracts: mechanism of increase in binding following estradiol injection. *Steroids* 26:281–298.

Lazier, C. B. 1979. Estrogen-binding proteins in avian liver: characteristics, regulation and ontogenesis. In *Ontogeny of receptors and reproductive hormone action,* ed. T. H. Hamilton, J. H. Clark, and W. A. Sedler, 353–370. New York: Raven Press.

Lazier, C. B., and W. S. Alford. 1977. Interaction of the anti-oestrogen nafoxidine hydrochloride, with the soluble nuclear oestradiol-binding protein in chick liver. *Biochemical Journal* 164:659–667.

Lazier, C. B., and A. J. Haggarty. 1979. A high-affinity oestrogen-binding protein in cockerel liver cytosol. *Biochemical Journal* 180:347–353.

Lazier, C. B., and V. C. Jordan. 1982. High affinity binding of anti-oestrogen to the chick liver nuclear oestrogen receptor. *Biochemical Journal* 206:387–394.

Lazier, C. B., F. Capony and D. L. Williams. 1981. Antioestrogen action in chick liver: effects on oestrogen receptors and oestrogen-induced proteins. In *Non-steroidal antioestrogens: molecular pharmacology and antitumor activity,* ed. R. L. Sutherland and V. C. Jordan, 215–230. Sydney: Academic Press.

Lazier, C. B., P. R. Murphy, C. Butts, A. Gillis, and K. Lonergan. 1984a. High affinity binding sites for triphenylethylene anti-estrogens in the chicken. *Proceedings of the Seventh International Congress of Endocrinology,* Quebec. Abstract 1323.

Lazier, C. B., P. R. Murphy, A. Gillis, and W. C. Breckenridge. 1984b. High affinity binding of the triphenylethylene antiestrogens in the chicken liver. *Seventh International Congress of Endocrinology Satellite Symposium: Workshop on Estrogen and Antiestrogen Action.* Abstract.

Lebeau, M. C., N. Massol, and E.-E. Baulieu. 1982. Oestrogen and progesterone receptors in chick oviduct chromatin after administration of oestradiol, progesterone or antioestrogen. *Biochemical Journal* 204:653–662.

Mešter, J., N. Binart, M. G. Catelli, C. Geynet, R. Hähnel, V. Puri, D. Seeley, R. L. Sutherland, and E. E. Baulieu. 1981. Mechanisms of oestrogen antagonism by tamoxifen and monohydroxytamoxifen in chick oviduct. In *Non-steroidal antioestrogens: molecular pharmacology and antitumor activity,* ed. R. L. Sutherland and V. C. Jordan, 177–194. Sydney: Academic Press.

Murphy, L. C., and R. L. Sutherland. 1985. Differential effects of tamoxifen and analogues with nonbasic sidechains on cell proliferation *in vitro. Endocrinology* 116:1071–1078.

Murphy, L. C., M. S. Foo, M. D. Green, B. K. Milthorpe, A. M. Whybourne, Z. S. Krozowski, and R. L. Sutherland. 1981. Binding of non-steroidal antioestrogens to saturable binding sites distinct from the oestrogen receptor in normal and neoplastic tissues. In *Non-steroidal antioestrogens: molecular pharmacology and antitumor activity,* ed. R. L. Sutherland and V. C. Jordan, 317–337. Sydney: Academic Press.

Murphy, P. R., C. Butts, and C. B. Lazier. 1984. Triphenylethylene antiestrogen-binding sites in cockerel liver nuclei: evidence for an endogenous ligand. *Endocrinology* 115:420–426.

Murphy, P. R., W. C. Breckenridge, and C. B. Lazier. 1985. Binding of oxygenated cholesterol metabolites to antiestrogen binding sites from chick liver. *Biochemical and Biophysical Research Communications* 127:786–792.

O'Malley, B. W., D. R. Roop, E. C. Lai, J. L. Nordstrom, J. F. Catteral, G. E. Swaneck, D. A. Colbert, M.-J. Tsai, A. Dugaiczyk, and S. L. C. Woo. 1979. The ovalbumin gene: organization, structure, transcription and regulation. *Recent Progress in Hormone Research* 35:1–42.

Palmiter, R. D., and J. T. Wrenn. 1971. Interaction of estrogen and progesterone in chick oviduct development. III. Tubular gland cell cytodifferentiation. *Journal of Cell Biology* 50:598–615.

Palmiter, R. D., E. R. Mulvihill, G. S. McKnight, and A. W. Senear. 1977. Regulation of gene expression in the chick oviduct by steroid hormones. *Cold Spring Harbor Symposia on Quantitative Biology* 42:639–649.

Palmiter, R. D., E. R. Mulvihill, J. H. Shepherd, and G. S. McKnight. 1981. Steroid hormone regulation of ovalbumin and conalbumin gene expression: a model based on multiple regulatory sites and intermediary proteins. *Journal of Biological Chemistry* 256:7910–7916.

Renkawitz, R., G. Schutz, D. von der Ahe, and M. Beato. 1984. Sequences in the promoter region of the chicken lysozyme gene required for steroid regulation and receptor binding. *Cell* 37:503–510.

Rochefort, H., and J. L. Borgna. 1981. Differences between oestrogen receptor activation by oestrogen and antioestrogen. *Nature* (London) 292:257–259.

Sgarlata, C. S., G. Mikhail, and F. Hertelendy. 1984. Clomiphene and tamoxifen inhibit progesterone synthesis in granulosa cells: comparison with estradiol. *Endocrinology* 114:2032–2038.

Shapiro, D. 1982. Steroid hormone regulation of vitellogenin gene expression. *CRC Critical Reviews in Biochemistry* 12:187–203.

Simmen, R. C., A. R. Means, and J. H. Clark. 1984. Estrogen modulation of nuclear matrix-associated steroid hormone binding. *Endocrinology* 115:1197–1202.

Snow, L. D., H. Erickkson, J. W. Hardin, L. Chan, R. L. Jackson, J. H. Clark, and A. R. Means. 1978. Nuclear estrogen receptor in the avian liver: correlation with biologic response. *Journal of Steroid Biochemistry* 9:1017–1023.

Sudo, K., F. J. Monsma, Jr., and B. S. Katzenellenbogen. 1983. Antiestrogen-binding sites distinct from the estrogen receptor: subcellular localization, ligand specificity and distribution in tissues of the rat. *Endocrinology* 112:425–434.

Sutherland, R. L. 1981. Estrogen antagonists in chick oviduct: Antagonist activity of eight synthetic triphenylethylene derivatives and their interactions with cytoplasmic and nuclear estrogen receptors. *Endocrinology* 109:2061–2068.

Sutherland, R. L., and M. S. Foo. 1979. Differential binding of antiestrogens by rat uterine and chick oviduct cytosol. *Biochemical and Biophysical Research Communications* 91:183–191.

Sutherland, R., J. Mester, and E.-E. Baulieu. 1977. Tamoxifen is a potent 'pure' antioestrogen in chick oviduct. *Nature* (London) 267:434–435.

Sutherland, R. L., L. C. Murphy, M. S. Foo, M. D. Green, A. M. Whybourne, and Z. S. Krozowski. 1980. High-affinity anti-oestrogen binding site distinct from the oestrogen receptor. *Nature* (London) 288:273–275.

Taylor, R. N., and R. C. Smith. 1982. Identification of a novel sex steroid binding protein. *Proceedings of the National Academy of Sciences* 79:1742–1746.

Watts, C. K. W., L. C. Murphy, and R. L. Sutherland. 1984. Microsomal binding sites for nonsteroidal antiestrogens in MCF-7 human mammary carcinoma cells. *Journal of Biological Chemistry* 259:4223–4229.

11

Metabolism of Nonsteroidal Antiestrogens

STEWART D. LYMAN AND V. CRAIG JORDAN

I.	INTRODUCTION	192
II.	METABOLITES OF TAMOXIFEN	193
III.	METABOLISM OF TAMOXIFEN BY LABORATORY ANIMALS *IN VIVO*	195
IV.	TAMOXIFEN METABOLISM *IN VITRO*	197
V.	TAMOXIFEN METABOLISM IN HUMANS	198
	A. SINGLE DOSES	198
	B. CHRONIC ADMINISTRATION	199
VI.	EFFECT OF TAMOXIFEN ON THE METABOLISM OF OTHER DRUGS	201
VII.	BIOLOGICAL PROPERTIES OF TAMOXIFEN METABOLITES	202
VIII.	ANALYTICAL MEASUREMENT OF TAMOXIFEN AND ITS METABOLITES	204
IX.	METABOLISM OF OTHER NONSTEROIDAL ANTIESTROGENS	207
	A. OVERVIEW	207
	B. ENCLOMIPHENE	210
	C. NITROMIPHENE (CI 628)	210
	D. U 23,469	211
	E. LN 1643	212
	F. CHLOROTRIANISENE	212
X.	DISCUSSION	213
	REFERENCES	215

I. Introduction

Iт is the goal of this review to draw together all of the studies involving the metabolism of the nonsteroidal antiestrogens, both *in vitro* and *in vivo*, with the hope of identifying those metabolic transformations that are common to compounds of this drug class. Metabolism of these antiestrogens appears to play an important role in mediating the biological potency of such compounds and may also affect their biological activity. This review is not intended to cover the general pharmacology of antiestrogens, which has been extensively reviewed (Lerner 1964; Dorfman 1968; Furr et al. 1979; Katzenellenbogen et al. 1979; Sutherland and Jordan 1981). Rather, we limit our discussion of the biology of these compounds to a comparison of the pharmacological properties of antiestrogen metabolites with the properties of the parent compounds. The pharmacokinetics of these compounds are also not discussed because the field has not changed significantly since this subject was last reviewed (Adam 1981). Most of the work described in this review has been done with the antiestrogen tamoxifen (ICI 46,474; Nolvadex), since this is the only antiestrogen in current use for the treatment of hormone-dependent breast cancer (Patterson 1981).

First, we briefly review a number of pharmacological variables that can influence whether a particular metabolite may be formed or detected in a given tissue and at what concentration it may be present. It is important to remember these variables when attempting to reconcile the sometimes conflicting results obtained by different investigators, since each of these factors has been shown to affect drug metabolism. These variables include: (1) use of different species; (2) use of different strains of the same species; (3) dose of compound administered; (4) route of drug administration; (5) solvent used to administer drug; (6) age of animal; (7) sex of animal; (8) choice of tissue (or cell fraction) for metabolite extraction; (9) preparation of tissue for extraction; (10) solvent used to extract tissue; (11) time of tissue sampling after drug administration; and (12) analytical methodology employed to detect metabolites. Where possible in this review, we will identify the factor or factors that may be responsible for the disparate results obtained by different workers.

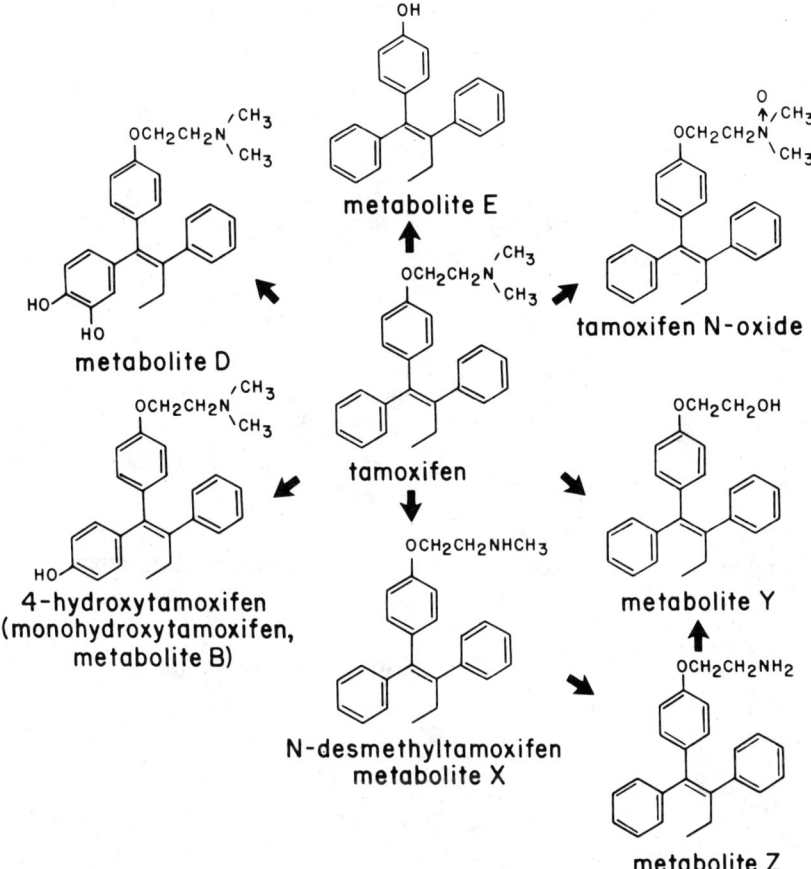

Figure 11.1. Structures of tamoxifen and its well-characterized metabolites.

II. *Metabolites of Tamoxifen*

Tamoxifen (ICI 46,474) is the only antiestrogen currently in clinical use for the treatment of hormone-dependent breast cancer. The metabolism of tamoxifen (Fig. 11.1) has therefore been studied more extensively than has the metabolism of other nonsteroidal antiestrogens. Because of this, the metabolism of tamoxifen will be described in some detail, since the general principles derived have been shown to apply to other antiestrogens with related structures.

The first report on tamoxifen metabolism was published by Fromson et al. (1973a). These workers administered [¹⁴C]tamoxifen to female mice, rats, beagles, and rhesus monkeys, extracted the radioactivity from blood, urine, feces, and bile, and analyzed the extracts by thin-layer chromatography (TLC) for the presence of metabolites. No effort was made to identify metabolites in any estrogen target tissues, such as the uterus, or in the liver, the primary organ for drug metabolism in the body. The levels of radioactivity in blood and urine were too low to allow these workers to identify and characterize any compounds; however, six metabolites, designated A through F, were isolated from bile and feces. The absolute structures of three of these metabolites (A, B, E) were established using gas chromatography–mass spectrometry (GC-MS); identification of the other compounds (C, D, F) was (and remains) tentative and they will not be discussed further. It must be pointed out before discussing the metabolites individually that most of the radioactivity extracted from the feces of each of these species was not associated with any of the six metabolites or with tamoxifen. This material, which remained at the point of application on the TLC plates, was presumed to be some unidentified polar metabolite(s) and sulfate and glucuronide conjugates of polar metabolites; in spite of their abundance, however, these materials were not further characterized.

Metabolite B (4-hydroxytamoxifen) was reported to be the major metabolite formed in all four species. This aromatic hydroxylation reaction has subsequently been shown to occur with a number of related triphenylethylene compounds and will be discussed elsewhere in this review. Metabolite A, which is formed as a result of the hydration of the ethylene double bond, was reported to be a minor metabolite in rhesus monkeys. However, it is possible that this metabolite was an artifact formed during the acid hydrolysis step used to isolate some of the metabolites, since this compound has never been detected in any subsequent metabolism studies. Metabolite E was found to be a minor metabolite in dog bile; this compound is formed by removal of the dimethylaminoethyl portion of the side chain.

Since the publication of the report by Fromson et al. (1973a), only four other tamoxifen metabolites have been identified either *in vitro* or *in vivo*. Adam et al. (1979) showed that the major metabolite of tamoxifen in the serum of breast cancer patients was N-desmethyltamoxifen (metabolite X), and not 4-hydroxytamoxifen, as was originally reported by Fromson et al. (1973b) (see Section V).

Foster et al. (1980) reported that rat liver microsomes prepared from phenobarbital-treated rats and cultured hepatocytes from these same animals (Bates et al. 1982) could convert tamoxifen into tamoxifen-N-oxide. This metabolite was characterized by mass spectrometry and was found to have the same chromatographic properties by high-performance liquid chromatography (HPLC) as a synthetic standard. These workers suggested that tamoxifen-N-oxide might have been present in the studies of Fromson et al. (1973a,b) because this metabolite, along with most of the radioactivity, does not migrate from the point of application in the TLC solvent system used in these early studies.

Bain and Jordan (1983) discovered a new tamoxifen metabolite, designated Y, in sera from patients receiving high-dose (150 mg twice a day) tamoxifen therapy. The structure of this compound, a deaminated derivative of tamoxifen, was established by mass spectrometry. Subsequent work showed (Jordan et al. 1983) that this metabolite was also present in sera from patients on low-dose (10 mg twice a day) tamoxifen therapy.

Kemp et al. (1983) also identified a new tamoxifen metabolite in the serum of patients on tamoxifen therapy. This compound, a didemethylated derivative of tamoxifen, was designated metabolite Z. The formation of metabolite Z is thought to be analogous to the formation of the didemethylated metabolite of imipramine, which has a side chain similar to tamoxifen's. Synthetic metabolite Z was found to cochromatograph by TLC with material isolated from sera in four solvent systems. However, the small amounts of this metabolite isolated from sera were insufficient to confirm the structure of this metabolite by GC-MS; therefore, the identification of metabolite Z as a didemethylated derivative of tamoxifen must be considered tentative.

III. *Metabolism of Tamoxifen by Laboratory Animals* in Vivo

The metabolism of tamoxifen in the mouse was first studied by Fromson et al. (1973a). Most of the radioactivity extracted from the feces of mice given [¹⁴C]tamoxifen was present as sulfate and glucuronide conjugates; the only nonconjugated metabolite detected was 4-hydroxytamoxifen. Similarly, Wilking et al. (1982) have shown that 4-hydroxytamoxifen was the principal metabolite in the livers of ovariectomized mice 4 hours after administration of [¹⁴C]tamoxifen. Work in our laboratory (Lyman and Jordan 1985) has shown that 4-hydroxytamoxifen is the major metabolite of tamoxifen in mouse liver and uterus 24 hours after tamoxifen administration.

The metabolism of tamoxifen in the rat has been studied by several groups. Fromson et al. (1973a) reported that 4-hydroxytamoxifen was the major metabolite extracted from rat feces. Similarly, Borgna and Rochefort (1981) found that 4-hydroxytamoxifen was the major tamoxifen metabolite extracted from uterine cytosol and nuclei following [³H]tamoxifen administration. Bowman et al. (1982) reported that 4-hydroxytamoxifen was the principal metabolite found in the serum of female rats given tamoxifen and that N-desmethyltamoxifen was not present at detectable levels. The metabolism of both the *trans* and *cis* isomers of tamoxifen in immature female rats was studied by Robertson et al. (1982). The principal metabolite of *trans*-tamoxifen in uterine nuclear extracts at 6 or 16 hours was 4-hydroxytamoxifen; however, by 48 hours the principal metabolite was an unidentified compound that was more polar than 4-hydroxytamoxifen. Although this material comigrated on thin-layer chromatography with a tamoxifen derivative known as bisphenol, the authors stated that this material was actually a mixture of several compounds. Metabolite E was not found as a *trans*-tamoxifen metabolite at any time. In contrast to the results of Bowman et al. (1982), Robertson et al. (1982) and Borgna and Rochefort (1981) found very little 4-hydroxytamoxifen in rat serum, with the principal metabolites being unidentified polar materials that were most likely sulfate and glucuronide conjugates of tamoxifen metabolites. This discrepancy may be due to differences in the solvents used to extract the serum; Bowman et al. (1982) used hexane:amyl alcohol (no extraction efficiency given), whereas Robertson et al. (1982) and Borgna and Rochefort (1981) used ethyl acetate (extraction efficiency only 30–60% at 16 hours). Borgna and Rochefort (1981) also reported a decreased efficiency of extraction of radioactivity from plasma with time (down to 25% at 72 hours) with ethyl acetate. Alternatively, these disparate findings may reflect the different doses of *trans*-tamoxifen administered by Bowman et al. (1982) and Robertson et al. (1982) (1750 μg/kg in the former study vs 100 μg/kg in the latter).

The principal metabolite of *cis*-tamoxifen in uterine nuclear extracts was unidentified, although it was suggested that this compound might be *cis*-N-desmethyltamoxifen. The principal metabolites extracted from the serum of *cis*-tamoxifen–treated rats were unidentified polar compounds that were probably sulfate and glucuronide conjugates. It should be noted that Robertson et al. found no interconversion of the *trans* and *cis* isomers of tamoxifen *in vivo*.

Fromson et al. (1973a) reported that most of the radioactivity found in the feces of dogs dosed with [^{14}C]tamoxifen was present as sulfate and glucuronide conjugates. This group also found metabolites B, C, and D in feces; metabolite B, as in the mouse, was the principal metabolite identified. Examination of dog bile revealed the presence of small amounts of metabolite E; this is the only species in which this metabolite has been identified. Fromson et al. (1973a) also studied tamoxifen metabolism in rhesus monkeys; as in the dog, most of the radioactivity appeared as conjugates, and metabolites B, C, and D were detected, with metabolite B being the principal metabolite present.

Borgna and Rochefort (1981) studied the metabolism of [^{3}H]tamoxifen in immature female chickens and found large amounts of 4-hydroxytamoxifen formed as virtually the only metabolite in plasma, oviduct, and liver. We have confirmed that 4-hydroxytamoxifen is the major metabolite formed by chicken liver *in vivo* (Lyman and Jordan 1985). Binart et al. (1979), who also studied the metabolism of [^{3}H]tamoxifen in the chicken, found, in contrast to the findings of Borgna and Rochefort (1981), no 4-hydroxytamoxifen in serum, although this metabolite did account for about 20% of the radioactivity extracted from bile. The failure of Binart et al. to measure 4-hydroxytamoxifen in serum may result from their using ether as the extraction solvent, since other workers (Golander and Sternson 1980) have reported the photochemical degradation of 4-hydroxytamoxifen in this solvent.

IV. *Tamoxifen Metabolism* in Vitro

Foster et al. (1980) incubated tamoxifen with liver microsomes prepared from phenobarbital-treated rats and found three metabolites formed: N-desmethyltamoxifen (20%), 4-hydroxytamoxifen (1.5%), and tamoxifen-N-oxide (6%). These same metabolites were also formed, although in slightly different amounts, when tamoxifen was incubated with hepatocytes isolated from phenobarbital-treated rats (Bates et al. 1982). The low levels of 4-hydroxytamoxifen found in these studies probably resulted from the use of ether as the extraction solvent (see above).

Robertson et al. (1982) studied the metabolism of both the *trans* and *cis* isomers of tamoxifen by rat liver microsomes. They found the N-desmethyl and 4-hydroxy derivatives of each of these isomers to be the major metabolites present; it is unclear if any N-oxides were formed, since these standards were not included in their thin-layer chromatography systems.

Borgna and Rochefort (1981) focused their studies *in vitro* on determining whether 4-hydroxytamoxifen could be formed from tamoxifen by different tissues of several species. They found that liver slices from rat, chicken, and frog could catalyze this transformation, as could lamb and sheep uteri and oviducts from immature chickens. In contrast to these results, Binart et al. (1979) did not see any 4-hydroxytamoxifen formed when tamoxifen was incubated with chicken magnum (the largest portion of the oviduct). This disparate finding was probably a result of the different assay conditions and tissue preparations used by the two groups.

Several groups (Horwitz et al. 1978; Binart et al. 1979) have reported that MCF-7 cells do not metabolize tamoxifen to a significant extent. However, in one of these reports (Horwitz et al. 1978) an unknown compound was observed to appear in the media. This compound was shown to be a breakdown product of tamoxifen, since its formation was detected in the absence of the MCF-7 cells. Unfortunately, this breakdown product was not identified.

V. *Tamoxifen Metabolism in Humans*

A. SINGLE DOSES

Fromson et al. (1973b) and Fromson and Sharp (1974) studied the metabolism of [^{14}C]tamoxifen in women who were being treated with tamoxifen for breast cancer or uterine bleeding. Radioactive drug was administered orally and was extracted later from serum and feces for analysis by TLC. Most of the radioactivity (52–67%) extracted from feces remained at the origin on the TLC plates; as in animals (Fromson et al. 1973a), this material is presumably polar metabolites and conjugates of polar metabolites. The only compounds identified in feces were tamoxifen, metabolite B, and metabolite F. The major portion of radioactivity extracted from serum also failed to migrate on TLC; tamoxifen accounted for only a small percentage of the serum radioactivity, and the principal metabolite was reported to be 4-hydroxytamoxifen. However, subsequent work (Adam et al. 1979) has shown that the actual major metabolite of tamoxifen in the serum of breast cancer patients is N-desmethyltamoxifen (metabolite X). The misidentification of N-desmethyltamoxifen as 4-

hydroxytamoxifen occurred because the single TLC solvent system employed by Fromson et al. (1973a,b) in their studies was not capable of separating these two metabolites. Adam et al. (1979) was able to distinguish metabolites B and X by the following criteria: (1) these metabolites could be separated by TLC using a different solvent system; (2) metabolite X could be differentially extracted from metabolite B in serum made basic with NaOH; and (3) treatment of these two metabolites with diazomethane altered the migration of metabolite B but not metabolite X on TLC. Other workers have subsequently shown (see below) that N-desmethyltamoxifen is the major tamoxifen metabolite in the sera of breast cancer patients.

Although Adam et al. (1979) demonstrated that N-desmethyltamoxifen is the major metabolite of tamoxifen in breast cancer patients, subsequent work has shown that 4-hydroxytamoxifen is also formed in these patients. Mendenhall et al. (1978) reported measuring both tamoxifen and 4-hydroxytamoxifen in sera from women given a single dose of 10 mg tamoxifen/m^2 body surface. It is not clear, however, that the metabolite formed was actually 4-hydroxytamoxifen, since no analytical data were presented to confirm the identity of these compounds. Levels of 4-hydroxytamoxifen in the sera of breast cancer patients are generally very low compared to the levels of tamoxifen and other metabolites (see Section V.B).

Adam et al. (1980a,b) measured the levels of tamoxifen in female breast cancer patients following the administration of either 10 or 20 mg of tamoxifen. Peak serum levels were found to be 26 and 42 ng/ml, respectively. No attempt was made to quantitate any metabolites in one study (Adam et al. 1980a); in the other (Adam et al. 1980b), N-desmethyltamoxifen levels peaked at a concentration of 12 ng/ml (29% of the peak tamoxifen level). This study (Adam et al. 1980b) also indicated that N-desmethyltamoxifen has a longer biological half-life than the parent compound; this observation was later confirmed by Patterson et al. (1980) in patients treated chronically with tamoxifen.

B. Chronic Administration

Daniel et al. (1979) measured tamoxifen and 4-hydroxytamoxifen levels in patients receiving 10 mg tamoxifen twice a day for breast cancer. Tamoxifen levels in plasma were in the range of 100–200 ng/ml, whereas 4-hydroxytamoxifen levels were 2–7 ng/ml. In comparison to these values, estradiol levels were 0.03 to 0.09 ng/ml, which is within the normal range reported for postmenopausal women. Thus, it is clear that even minor metabolites of tamoxifen will be present in much greater concentrations in plasma than estradiol. In subsequent studies from this same group (Daniel et al. 1981), the mean levels of tamoxifen, N-desmethyltamoxifen, and 4-hydroxytamoxifen in plasma of breast cancer patients given 20 mg tamoxifen twice a day were 300, 462, and 7 ng/ml respectively. Estradiol levels were reported to be 0.15 ng/ml. Similarly, N-desmethyltamoxifen levels were higher and 4-hydroxytamoxifen levels were lower than tamoxifen levels in homogenates prepared from breast tumor tissue obtained by biopsy (Daniel et al. 1981). However, interpatient variability was quite high; in one patient (J. C.) the tamoxifen:N-desmethyltamoxifen ratio in biopsy tissue was 1:19, whereas in another (E. St) this ratio was 1:0.5. Whether this variability reflects differential metabolism, uptake, or retention of tamoxifen or its metabolites by the tumor tissue is unknown.

Patterson et al. (1980) found that the levels of tamoxifen were 285 ± 19 ng/ml and N-desmethyltamoxifen levels were 477 ± 35 ng/ml in the serum of breast cancer patients receiving 20 mg tamoxifen twice a day. These levels were virtually identical to those reported by Daniel et al. (1981) (see above). Half-lives *in vivo* for tamoxifen and its N-desmethyltamoxifen were reported to be 7 and 14 days, respectively. Similar levels of tamoxifen and N-desmethyltamoxifen were found in responders and nonresponders to the tamoxifen therapy, and serum estradiol levels were also similar between these two groups (approximately 0.024 ng/ml serum).

The first report on the levels of metabolite Y of tamoxifen in human serum was published by Jordan et al. (1983). Tamoxifen, N-desmethyltamoxifen, and metabolite Y levels in patients taking 10 mg tamoxifen twice a day were in the ranges 78–189, 179–265, and 5–49 ng/ml of serum, respectively. Thus, even metabolite Y, which has a low binding affinity for estrogen receptors, might effectively compete with estradiol for receptors at these concentrations. Kemp et al. (1983) reported that the mean levels of tamoxifen, N-desmethyltamoxifen, and metabolite Y in sera of patients receiving 20 mg tamoxifen twice a day were 310, 481, and 49 ng/ml. Those values are about twice as high as those reported by Jordan et al. (1983), as would be expected because the dose was doubled. The results of Kemp et al. (1983) are also very similar to those reported by Patterson et al. (1980), which is not surprising, since many of the same patients were used in both studies. Kemp et al. (1983) also reported finding a new tamoxifen metabolite, designated Z, which was tentatively identified as a didemethylated version of tamoxifen (see Section II). On the basis of this assumption, they suggested that steady state levels of this metabolite could be as high as 40 ng/ml; however, no data on serum levels of this metabolite were presented, so it is unclear if this compound is actually formed in patients on tamoxifen therapy. Metabolite B levels were not given in this report, as a result of technical problems in quantitating this metabolite in the presence of greater quantities of N-desmethyl-tamoxifen. If metabolite B was present in serum (as reported by Daniel et al. 1979, 1981), then its concentration was estimated to be < 11 ng/ml.

VI. Effect of Tamoxifen on the Metabolism of Other Drugs

Since tamoxifen is metabolized by microsomal enzymes *in vitro* to a number of metabolites, it might be expected that tamoxifen would inhibit the metabolism of other drugs by these same enzymes. This prediction has been shown to be true in several studies. Al-turk et al. (1981) have shown that the treatment of rats *in vivo* with tamoxifen reduced the levels of hepatic and intestinal aryl hydrocarbon hydroxylase (AHH) activity and 7-ethoxycoumarin-O-deethylase activity. Studies conducted *in vitro* (Al-turk and Stohs 1983) indicated that inhibition of rat liver AHH activity by tamoxifen was noncompetitive, whereas inhibition of intestinal AHH was competitive. Liver AHH activity was more sensitive to tamoxifen inhibition than was intestinal AHH activity; apparent K_i values for tamoxifen were 0.085 mM and 1.11 mM, respectively. Thus, inhibition of drug metabolizing enzymes by tamoxifen depended on the tissue examined as well as the concentration of tamoxifen used.

Ruenitz and Toledo (1980) demonstrated that tamoxifen (and enclomiphene) inhibited rabbit liver ethylmorphine-N-demethylase activity *in vitro* and, to a lesser extent, aniline hydroxylase activity. These triphenyl-ethylene derivatives also interfered with the binding of SKF-525A to liver microsomes; spectral and kinetic analysis suggested that both tamoxifen and enclomiphene were interacting directly with cytochrome P_{450}.

One problem in studying the effects of tamoxifen on other drug metabolism enzymes is that tamoxifen itself is metabolized *in vitro* (see above); therefore, it may not be easy to resolve whether it is tamoxifen itself or a metabolite that is having the observed effect. Meltzer et al. (1984) addressed this problem by testing the ability of several tamoxifen metabolites to function as drug metabolism inhibitors. Using rat liver microsomes, these workers found that tamoxifen, N-desmethyltamoxifen, and 4-hydroxytamoxifen were all inhibitors of a number of cytochrome P_{450} mixed-function oxidation reactions, and that the potency of these compounds was essentially equal. The inhibitory effect of tamoxifen and its metabolites was similar to those effects observed with SKF-525A, a classical inhibitor of cytochrome P_{450} function. This study, and the others mentioned above, indicate that tamoxifen may alter the metabolism of other drugs *in vivo* and vice versa. Given that many cancer patients routinely take a variety of medications, these potential drug interactions require further study. To date, only one such report has been published (Shah et al. 1982); tamoxifen was found to exacerbate the normally mild hepatotoxicity induced by chronic allopurinol treatment.

VII. Biological Properties of Tamoxifen Metabolites

There appear to be no published reports on the biological activity of tamoxifen metabolites A, C, and F, and so these compounds will not be discussed further.

Metabolite B (4-hydroxytamoxifen) is the major metabolite of tamoxifen in a number of species (see Section III) and has the same biological properties as tamoxifen in various bioassay systems. Like tamoxifen, 4-hydroxytamoxifen is a full estrogen agonist in the mouse uterus and a partial estrogen agonist/antagonist in the rat uterus (Jordan et al. 1978). Both compounds inhibit the growth of MCF-7 and T47D cells *in vitro* (Bates et al. 1982; Reddel et al. 1983; Tayor et al. 1984) and this inhibition is estrogen-reversible. Similarly, both compounds inhibit the induction of prolactin by estradiol in rat pituitary cells (Lieberman et al. 1983) and produce slight increases in progesterone receptor synthesis (Katzenellenbogen et al. 1984). In all of these studies, 4-hydroxytamoxifen was found to be more potent than tamoxifen; this presumably reflects the much higher relative binding affinity of 4-hydroxytamoxifen for estrogen receptor compared to tamoxifen (Jordan et al. 1977). However, Wakeling and Slater (1980) reported that the potencies of tamoxifen, 4-hydroxytamoxifen, and N-desmethyltamoxifen were equal in preventing egg implantation in rats. Allen et al. (1980) found that the p-methyl, p-fluoro, and p-chloro derivatives of tamoxifen were less potent uterotrophic compounds in rats than tamoxifen itself. Since these derivatives cannot undergo p-hydroxylation, these data suggest that at least part of the uterotrophic activity of tamoxifen in rats results from its conversion *in vivo* to 4-hydroxytamoxifen.

Metabolite D (3,4-dihydroxytamoxifen) has been shown to be an estrogen antagonist in the immature rat uterus (Jordan et al. 1977) and a partial estrogen agonist/antagonist in ovariectomized mice (Jordan et al. 1978). This compound, which has a high binding affinity for the estrogen receptor, was an antagonist of the induction of prolactin synthesis by estradiol in rat pituitary cells (Jordan et al. 1984).

Metabolite E is the only tamoxifen metabolite that is devoid of antiestrogenic activity. Jordan and Gosden (1982) reported that this metabolite was fully uterotrophic in rats, and we have found (Lyman and Jordan 1985) that this metabolite is also fully uterotrophic in ovariectomized mice. Metabolite E is an estrogen agonist in rat pituitary cells, since this compound induces prolactin synthesis (Jordan et al. 1984). This compound has a low relative binding affinity (RBA) for rat uterus estrogen receptors (Jordan and Gosden 1982).

Metabolite X (N-desmethyltamoxifen) has been shown by several groups to be a partial estrogen agonist/antagonist in immature rats (Jordan et al. 1983; Kemp et al. 1983); this compound also has a low binding affinity for estrogen receptors (Jordan et al. 1983), and it was less potent than tamoxifen in both studies. However, the potency of this compound to prevent egg implantation in rats was equal to tamoxifen (Wakeling and Slater 1980; Kemp et al. 1983). Metabolite X also inhibited the growth *in vitro* of MCF-7 cells (Bates et al. 1982; Reddel et al. 1983); this inhibition was reversible by estradiol, suggesting that this effect was estrogen receptor mediated.

Metabolite Y, like metabolite X, is a partial estrogen agonist/antagonist in the rat uterus (Jordan et al. 1983; Kemp et al. 1983) and also prevents egg implantation in the rat (Kemp et al. 1983). Metabolite Y was found to be a somewhat less potent estrogen antagonist than metabolite X in one study (Jordan et al. 1983), whereas it was slightly more potent in the other (Kemp et al.1983). The RBA of this compound was 0.5 for rat uterus estrogen receptor (Jordan et al. 1983).

Metabolite Z (N-didesmethyltamoxifen) has been shown to be antiuterotrophic, since it prevents egg implantation in rats (Kemp et al. 1983). This compound has yet to be tested in a uterine weight test for its uterotrophic and antiuterotrophic properties.

The only published report on the biological activity of tamoxifen-N-oxide (Bates et al. 1982) indicated that this compound had antiestrogenic effects against MCF-7 cells in culture.

VIII. Analytical Measurement of Tamoxifen and Its Metabolites

The first method for the analytical measurement of tamoxifen and its metabolites in humans was reported by Fromson et al. (1973b). These workers administered [14C]tamoxifen to female patients with either breast cancer or dysfunctional uterine bleeding, and at various times extracted the radioactivity from serum with methanol. The radioactive extracts were then analyzed by thin-layer chromatography on silica gel. Most of the radioactivity (28–47%) did not migrate from the point of application on the TLC plate; no attempts were made to identify or further analyze this material, which was probably sulfate and glucuronide conjugates of polar tamoxifen metabolites. The principal serum metabolite was reported to be metabolite B (4-hydroxytamoxifen); however, subsequent work (Adam et al. 1979) has shown that N-desmethyltamoxifen is actually the principal tamoxifen metabolite in female patients on tamoxifen therapy. The misidentification of metabolite B as the principal tamoxifen metabolite occurred because the TLC solvent system used by Fromson et al. (1973b) was not capable of separating this compound from N-desmethyltamoxifen. This work illustrates the dangers of identifying unknown materials based solely on their comigration with a synthetic standard in a single chromatography solvent system. Based on the specific activity of the [14C]tamoxifen used in this study, the limit of detection of tamoxifen metabolites was probably about 10 ng.

Analytical methods based on the use of radiolabeled drug to determine the levels of a drug and its metabolites are not generally useful for performing routine clinical assays. Therefore, Mendenhall et al. (1978) developed a new method for measuring the levels of tamoxifen and 4-hydroxytamoxifen in plasma based on the discovery by Mallory et al. (1964) that triphenylethylene compounds are converted by ultraviolet light into fluorescent phenanthrene derivatives (Fig. 11.2). Tamoxifen and 4-hydroxytamoxifen were extracted from plasma with diethyl ether, placed in a reaction vessel, and irradiated with UV light. The phenanthrene derivatives of these compounds were then separated by reversed-phase HPLC

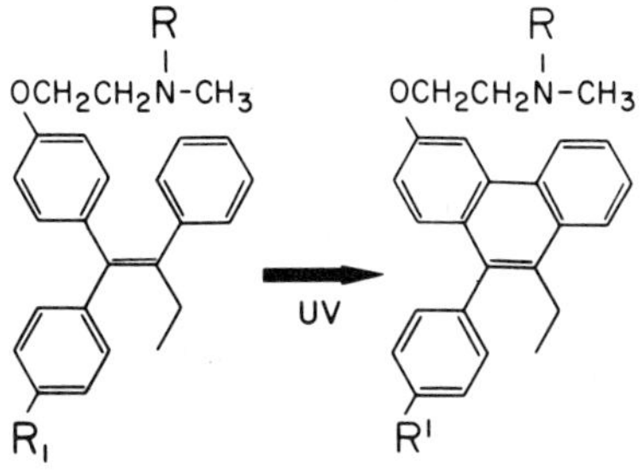

R   R
| |
OCH$_2$CH$_2$N-CH$_3$ OCH$_2$CH$_2$N-CH$_3$

UV →

R$_1$ R^1

                    R   R^1
Tamoxifen   CH$_3$ H
Desmethyltamoxifen   H   H
Monohydroxytamoxifen (Met B) CH$_3$ OH

Figure 11.2. Conversion of tamoxifen and several of its metabolites to fluorescent phenanthrene derivatives by UV light.

and quantitated with a fluorescence detector; the detection limit for both compounds was reported to be 1–2 ng/ml plasma. The authors in this study limited their analysis to tamoxifen and 4-hydroxytamoxifen and did not attempt to measure N-desmethyltamoxifen levels because, as explained above, 4-hydroxytamoxifen was thought (erroneously) to be the principal metabolite.

As a result of the problems caused by the misidentification of N-desmethyltamoxifen as 4-hydroxytamoxifen in the original paper of Fromson et al. (1973b), Daniel et al. (1979, 1981) developed an analytical GC-MS method for measuring tamoxifen and 4-hydroxytamoxifen levels in plasma. These compounds were extracted from plasma with diethyl ether, the extract was purified by ion-exchange chromatography, and after elution with methanol these compounds were separated and quantitated by GC-MS. The detection limit for these two compounds was reported as 1 ng/ml plasma; no efforts were made to quantitate any other metabolites. The high specificity of this method (determination of molecular weights by mass spectrometry) allowed these workers to confirm that N-desmethyltamoxifen, not 4-hydroxytamoxifen, was the major tamoxifen metabolite in female patients. This method has not been widely adapted because (1) the equipment required is expensive; (2) the method is slow, since tamoxifen and 4-hydroxytamoxifen are quantitated in separate chromatographic procedures; and (3) 4-hydroxytamoxifen must be derivatized before it can be injected into the GC-MS. It is for these reasons that most research groups have adapted the approach taken by Mendenhall et al. (1978) and have quantitated tamoxifen and its metabolites as their phenanthrene derivatives. The major disadvantage of these procedures is that they cannot be used to quantitate metabolites that are not converted to phenanthrene derivatives by UV light (e.g., metabolite A).

Adam et al. (1980a) developed a thin-layer densitometry method for measuring tamoxifen levels in serum. Tamoxifen and its metabolites were extracted from sera with hexane:amyl alcohol (197:3) and then separated by TLC on silica gel. After chromatography, the TLC plates were irradiated with UV light, then scanned with a densitometer to measure the fluorescence of these compounds *in situ*. Despite the fact that conversion of tamoxifen and its metabolites to phenanthrene derivatives was incomplete (because the UV light was unable to penetrate beyond the top layers of the silica gel), this method was reported to be as sensitive as the method of Mendenhall et al. (1978), with a detection limit of about 2 ng tamoxifen/ ml serum. Unlike previous methods, this densitometry assay allowed for the simultaneous quantitation of a number of tamoxifen metabolites. Few laboratories have thin-layer densitometers, however, and for this reason most workers have developed analytical methods to measure tamoxifen levels using HPLC.

Golander and Sternson (1980) modified the HPLC assay of Mendenhall et al. (1978) so that they could quantitate the levels of N-desmethyltamoxifen in plasma as well as tamoxifen and 4-hydroxytamoxifen. These workers had difficulty in resolving the phenanthrene derivatives of these three compounds by either normal or reversed-phase HPLC, and therefore they developed a paired-ion HPLC system. Tamoxifen and its metabolites were extracted from plasma with ether, the ether was removed by evaporation, and the compounds were then redissolved in a solvent mixture containing the ion-pairing agent sodium pentanesulfonate. This solution was then irradiated with UV light, and the pentanesulfonate-paired phenanthrene derivatives were separated by reversed-phase HPLC. Sensitivity of this technique was reported to be 0.1 ng/ml plasma for tamoxifen as well as for its metabolites.

Brown et al. (1983) developed an HPLC method that enabled them to quantitate metabolites E and Y, as well as tamoxifen, 4-hydroxytamoxifen, and N-desmethyltamoxifen. These workers improved the methodology by placing the UV light irradiation step on-line after the separation of these compounds by HPLC. This improvement eliminated most of the problems associated with the breakdown of unstable phenanthrene derivatives encountered by other groups. Serum was extracted with hexane:butanol (98:2), these solvents were then evaporated under nitrogen, and the extract was then redissolved in HPLC solvent. Following separation by HPLC, the compounds were irradiated with UV light and the fluorescence of the phenanthrene derivatives was quantitated with a fluorometer. This method is nearly as sensitive as that of other workers, with a detection limit of 2–5 ng tamoxifen or metabolite/ml serum, but its principal disadvantage is that three different HPLC separation systems requiring two different chromatography columns are needed to quantitate all five of the compounds listed above.

Camaggi et al. (1983) developed an approach similar to that of Brown et al. (1983) when they modified the procedure of Golander and Sternson (1980), because they also placed the photocyclization step on-line and post–HPLC column. Their method was to extract tamoxifen, N-desmethyltamoxifen, and 4-hydroxytamoxifen from plasma with methanol and then to purify this extract on a small reversed-phase cartridge. After elution from the cartridge with phosphoric acid, the compounds were separated by reversed-phase HPLC, converted to their phenanthrene derivatives, and quantitated. The limit of sensitivity of this method was given at 1 ng tamoxifen or metabolites/ml plasma. These authors did not attempt to quantitate tamoxifen metabolites E and Y.

IX. *Metabolism of Other Nonsteroidal Antiestrogens*

A. OVERVIEW

A large number of nonsteroidal antiestrogens have been synthesized and tested for their biological activity; however, the metabolism of only a small number of these compounds has been examined in any detail. A common finding in these studies was that the antiestrogens were metabolized to phenolic derivatives that have a much higher binding affinity for estrogen receptors than the parent compounds. These reactions are therefore analogous to the metabolic conversion of tamoxifen to 4-hydroxytamoxifen. Thus, Ruenitz et al. (1983a) found 4-hydroxyenclomiphene as a metabolite of enclomiphene in rat feces (Fig. 11.3), and Borgna et al. (1982) identified the 4-hydroxy derivative of LN 1643 in uterine nuclear fractions prepared from rats dosed with LN 1643 (Fig. 11.4). Similarly,

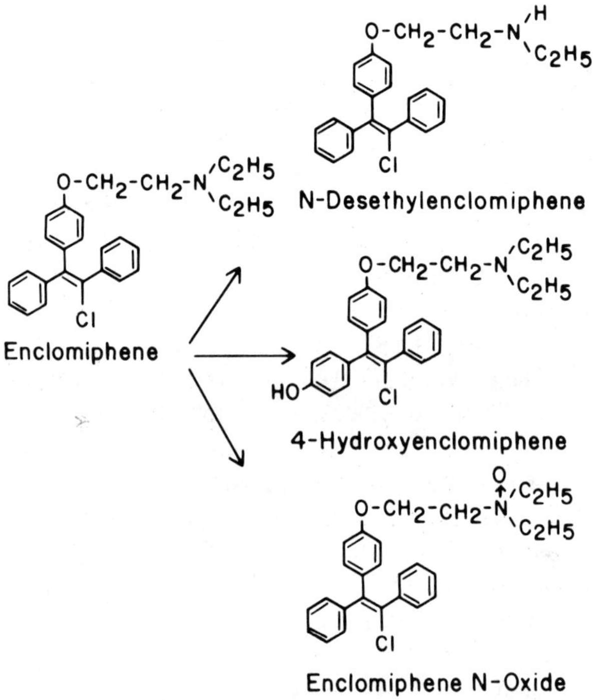

Figure 11.3. Structures of enclomiphene and its metabolites.

both nitromiphene (Fig. 11.5) (Katzenellenbogen et al. 1981) and U 23,469 (Fig. 11.4) (Tatee et al. 1979) were shown to be demethylated in the rat to their corresponding 4-hydroxy derivatives, and these metabolites were selectively accumulated in the uterus. These latter reactions are comparable to the demethylation of mestranol to ethinyl estradiol (Eisenfeld 1974). It should be noted that in most of these studies the workers looked for metabolites only in uterine nuclei; thus, their analytical methods are biased towards identifying those metabolites with a high affinity for the estrogen receptor. These studies should not be interpreted as indicating that these hydroxylated compounds are the sole metabolites formed. This having been said, the metabolism of these compounds will now be discussed in detail.

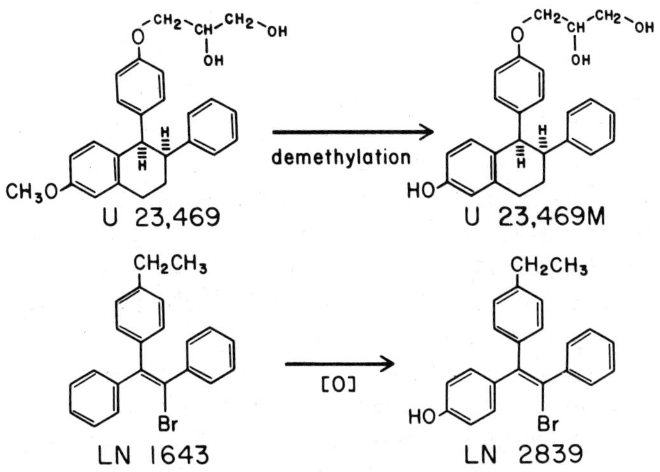

Figure 11.4. Metabolic activation of U 23,469 (by demethylation) and LN 1643 (by hydroxylation) to phenolic derivatives.

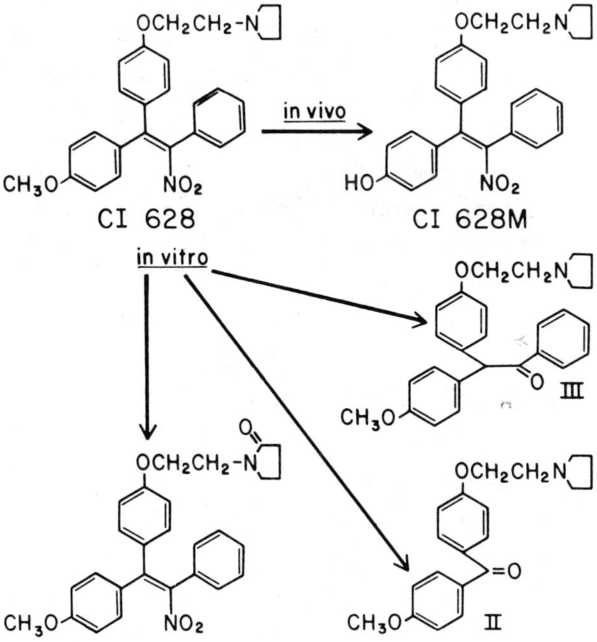

Figure 11.5. Metabolism of CI 628 (nitromiphene); II is the benzophenone derivative formed by ethylene bond cleavage, and III is the diarylacetophenone metabolite.

B. ENCLOMIPHENE

The metabolism of enclomiphene (Fig. 11.3) (the *trans* isomer of clomiphene) was studied by Ruenitz et al. (1983a) and Ruenitz (1981) both *in vitro* and *in vivo* in several species. In the presence of rabbit liver microsomes, enclomiphene was converted to 4-hydroxy and N-desmethyl derivatives; this is analogous to the conversion of tamoxifen to its 4-hydroxy and N-desmethyl derivatives (see Section II).

In contrast to these results, incubation of enclomiphene with rat liver microsomes resulted in the formation of three metabolites: the N-desethyl and 4-hydroxy metabolites, as well as enclomiphene N-oxide (Ruenitz et al. 1983a). Thus, it appears that rat microsomes can catalyze the formation of N-oxides of antiestrogens (e.g., tamoxifen [Foster et al. 1980], enclomiphene), whereas rabbit microsomes are unable to do so. Whether this finding is generally applicable to other compounds that form N-oxides remains to be seen.

Rats were also dosed orally with enclomiphene, and their urine and feces were collected for several days and then analyzed for the presence of enclomiphene metabolites. Neither enclomiphene nor any of its metabolites were found in urine, and the only compound identified in feces was 4-hydroxyenclomiphene. That more metabolites were not detected in feces is probably a reflection of the insensitivity of the detection techniques employed by these workers. Ruenitz et al. (1983a) did not use radiolabeled enclomiphene in these studies and therefore would not be expected to uncover as many metabolites as Fromson et al. (1973a) did in their studies with [^{14}C]tamoxifen.

C. NITROMIPHENE (CI 628)

Ruenitz and Toledo (1981) showed that incubation of nitromiphene with rat cecal contents resulted in the formation of two metabolites (Fig. 11.5); one was a benzophenone derivative formed by ethylene bond cleavage, and the other was an α,α-diarylacetophenone compound that was suggested to result from reduction of the nitro group of nitromiphene to an amino group, followed by enolization and hydrolysis to the ketone. Standards of these compounds were synthesized and shown to comigrate with these metabolites on thin-layer chromatography; the mass spectral characteristics of these standards were the same as the metabolites. Incubation of rat liver 9000 $\times$ g supernatant with nitromiphene resulted in the formation of two metabolites (Ruenitz and Bagley 1983). The major metabolite was not identified, although it was thought to be the O-demethylated derivative (see above); the minor metabolite was characterized by mass spectroscopy and identified as oxonitromiphene. This compound was presumably formed by N-methylene oxidation of the pyrrolidine ring, and it was suggested (Ruenitz et al. 1983b) that this reaction was analogous to the metabolism of nicotine to cotinine and the conversion of tremorine to oxotremorine. A limited study on the biological activity of these metabolites has been reported (Ruenitz et al. 1983b).

None of these types of metabolites has ever been identified *in vivo* in a metabolism study with any antiestrogen; therefore, these metabolites will probably receive little attention unless their formation *in vivo* can be demonstrated.

Katzenellenbogen et al. (1978) studied the metabolism of tritium-labeled nitromiphene (CI 628) in the rat. [³H]Nitromiphene was injected into rats and at appropriate times the animals were killed and their estrogen receptors were salt-extracted from uteri and purified on sucrose gradients. The fractions containing estrogen receptors were found to contain both a polar metabolite of nitromiphene and the parent compound; levels of the metabolite increased at later times, whereas levels of the parent compound decreased. This polar metabolite appeared to bind selectively to estrogen receptors because it was present only at very low levels in serum and in nuclear ethanol extracts. This metabolite was not identified in this paper; however, subsequent work (Katzenellenbogen et al. 1981) from this same group demonstrated that this metabolite was the O-demethylated derivative of nitromiphene (designated CI 628M). This metabolite was shown to comigrate with a synthetic standard in three different TLC solvent systems, and it could be converted back into nitromiphene by treatment with diazomethane (which methylates phenolic hydroxyl groups). However, it should be noted that the structure of this metabolite was not confirmed by mass spectrometry. The biological activity and potency of CI 628M in rats was found to be nearly identical to that of the parent compound (Hayes et al. 1981).

D. U 23,469

The metabolism of U 23,469 by both rat liver microsomes *in vitro* and by immature rats *in vivo* was studied by Tatee et al. (1979). This compound, like nitromiphene, was found to undergo O-demethylation of the methoxy group to form the phenolic derivative (Fig. 11.4). This metabolite was shown to accumulate over time in extracts of rat uterine nuclei, as was previously reported for the phenolic metabolite of nitromiphene (Katzenellenbogen et al. 1978). The metabolite of U 23,469 was also shown to comigrate with a synthetic standard. The biological properties of this polar metabolite (designated U 23,469M) were explored in a subsequent paper (Hayes et al. 1981) and shown to be nearly identical to the parent compound.

E. LN 1643

Borgna et al. (1982) studied the metabolism of the triphenylbromoethylene antiestrogen LN 1643 in immature female rats (Fig. 11.4). As with CI 628 and U 23,469, a polar metabolite of LN 1643 was selectively accumulated in uterine nuclear fractions containing estrogen receptors. This metabolite was shown to comigrate in several TLC solvent systems with LN 2839, which is a phenolic derivative of LN 1643. Thus, it appears that LN 1643 is converted *in vivo* into a hydroxylated metabolite in the same way that tamoxifen is converted to 4-hydroxytamoxifen (metabolite B). However, the metabolite that comigrated with LN 2839 was never characterized by any spectral techniques; therefore, identification of this metabolite as the 4-hydroxy derivative of LN 1643 must be considered tentative.

F. CHLOROTRIANISENE

Although chlorotrianisene is not an antiestrogen, its metabolism is similar to that of the compounds already described. This compound is an estrogenic triphenylethylene derivative that is used to suppress breast engorgement in nonnursing mothers and to treat estrogen deficiency and prostate cancer. Chlorotrianisene was incubated with rabbit liver microsomes (Ruenitz 1978) and then extracted with ethyl acetate; like nitromiphene and U 23,469, this compound was O-demethylated to yield a 4-hydroxy derivative designated as desmethyl chlorotrianisene (see above) (Fig. 11.6). In a subsequent study (Ruenitz and Toledo 1981), extracts of incubation mixtures containing rat liver microsomes and chlorotrianisene were found to contain three metabolites of the parent compound. Two of these metabolites were not present in sufficient quantities for isolation, whereas the third metabolite was shown by chromatographic and spectral techniques to be desmethylchlorotrianisene.

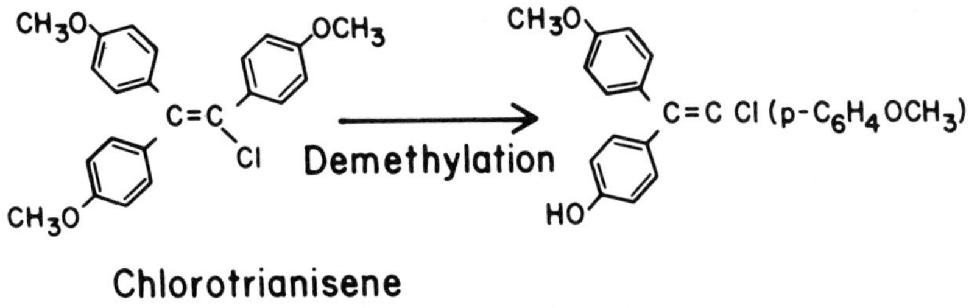

Chlorotrianisene

Figure 11.6. Demethylation of chlorotrianisene; the metabolite is a 1:1 mixture of *cis* and *trans* metabolites.

X. Discussion

Several conclusions about the metablism of nonsteroidal antiestrogens can be drawn from the data presented in this review. The overall biological effect of an antiestrogenic compound *in vivo* will be the sum of the effects of the parent compound as well as each of the metabolites. The contribution of each of these compounds will depend on both the tissue concentration of that compound and the binding affinity of the compound for estrogen receptors.

In general, it appears that most metabolites of the nonsteroidal antiestrogens have the same biological activities as the parent molecules. For example, tamoxifen has mixed agonistic/antagonistic properties in the rat uterus; similarly, metabolites B, D, X, Y, and Z of this compound also show mixed estrogenic and antiestrogenic effects in rat uterus. However, it should be noted that the biological potency of these metabolites and the maximum response (either estrogenic or antiestrogenic) that they elicit are different from tamoxifen and from each other. These differences probably result from a combination of three factors: (1) relative binding affinity of the molecules for estrogen receptors *in vivo;* (2) half-lives of the metabolites *in vivo;* and (3) capacity of the metabolites to undergo further metabolic changes that will in turn affect the first two factors mentioned above. For example, it seems probable that N-desmethyltamoxifen could be hydroxylated (like metabolite B) *in vivo,* and that metabolite B could also undergo N-demethylation. Although metabolites such as these have not yet been identified, it must be remembered that in studies with [^{14}C]tamoxifen, most of the radioactivity extracted from the bile and feces of many species did not comigrate on TLC with any known metabolite standards.

An exception to the general rule stated above is metabolite E of tamoxifen, which has been reported to have estrogenic but no antiestrogenic properties. Jordan and Gosden (1982) have argued that the side chain of antiestrogen molecules is required for antiestrogenic activity, and that removal of this portion of the molecule converts antiestrogens into estrogens. It is interesting to note that the only species from which metabolite E has been isolated is the dog (Fromson et al. 1973a), and tamoxifen has been reported to be estrogenic in this species (Furr et al. 1979).

A second general observation about the metabolism of antiestrogens is that these compounds are frequently converted into phenolic derivatives both *in vitro* and *in vivo*. These phenolic metabolites may be formed by either hydroxylation (tamoxifen, enclomiphene) or by demethylation (nitromiphene and U 23,469). The binding affinity of these metabolites for estrogen receptors is invariably much higher than that of the parent compound. The phenolic hydroxyl group in each of these molecules is thought to be functionally equivalent to the phenolic 3-hydroxyl group of estradiol. The biological activity of these phenolic metabolites is the same as that of the parent molecules; they are also more potent compounds, presumably as a result of the higher affinity of these compounds for estrogen receptors.

Studies on the metabolism of antiestrogens in humans have generally been restricted to identifying metabolites in serum (or plasma). A major question arises from these studies: are the compounds (parent drug and metabolites) found in serum the same ones that are present in other tissues (e.g., breast tumor, uterus) and at the same relative levels? Molecules will be retained or accumulated in a given tissue based on their binding affinities (both specific and nonspecific) for components of that tissue. Antiestrogen molecules in breast or uterus would be expected to bind (with high affinity) to estrogen receptors and to antiestrogen binding sites, a recently described binding species (Sutherland et al. 1980; Sudo et al. 1983) in these tissues. In serum, however, most of these molecules will be bound (with low affinity) to serum proteins (e.g., albumins). Thus, the distribution of metabolites measured in one tissue (serum) may not accurately reflect the distribution of these molecules in another tissue. Daniel et al. (1981), in the only study to address this issue, found that the concentrations of tamoxifen and its metabolites in plasma were not related to the levels present in breast tumor tissue. Retention of tamoxifen and its metabolites by breast tumor tissue may result from the presence of estrogen receptors in that tissue. Similarly, the levels of various metabolites in tissues with a high capacity to metabolize drugs (e.g., liver) would not be expected to be the same as found in a tissue with poor drug-metabolizing capacity (e.g., muscle). Measurement of serum levels of tamoxifen and its metabolites may correlate with relative levels of drug in other tissues, but it may not reflect the ratio of the parent drug to metabolites that will exist in various tissues. The relationship between serum levels of antiestrogen and the levels of these compounds (both parent drug and metabolite) in those tissues where one hopes to achieve a desired therapeutic effect requires further investigation.

Acknowledgments

Studies supported by grants R01-CA-32713, P01-CA-20432 and P30-CA-14520. Support from Stuart Pharmaceuticals, Wilmington, Delaware, and ICIplc Pharmaceuticals Division, England, is gratefully acknowledged.

References

Adam, H. K. 1981. A review of the pharmacokinetics and metabolism of "Nolvadex" (tamoxifen). In *Non-steroidal antioestrogens: molecular pharmacology and antitumour activity,* ed. R. L. Sutherland and V. C. Jordan, 59–74. Sydney: Academic Press.

Adam, H. K., E. J. Douglas, and J. V. Kemp. 1979. The metabolism of tamoxifen in humans. *Biochemical Pharmacology* 27:145–147.

Adam, H. K., M. A. Gay, and R. H. Moore. 1980a. Measurement of tamoxifen in serum by thin layer densitometry. *Journal of Endocrinology* 84:35–42.

Adam, H. K., J. S. Patterson, and J. V. Kemp. 1980b. Studies on the metabolism and pharmacokinetics of tamoxifen in normal volunteers. *Cancer Treatment Reports* 64:761–764.

Allen, K. E., E. R. Clark, and V. C. Jordan. 1980. Evidence for the metabolic activation of non-steroidal antioestrogens: a study of structure-activity relationships. *British Journal of Pharmacology* 71:83–91.

Al-turk, W. A., and S. J. Stohs. 1983. Kinetics of tamoxifen inhibition of aryl hydrocarbon hydroxylase activity of intestinal and hepatic microsomes from male rats. *Research Communications in Chemical Pathology and Pharmacology* 39:69–76.

Al-turk, W. A., S. J. Stohs, and E. B. Roche. 1981. Effect of tamoxifen treatment on liver, lung and intestinal mixed-function oxidases in male and female rats. *Drug Metabolism and Disposition* 9:327–330.

Bain, R. R., and V. C. Jordan. 1983. Identification of a new metabolite of tamoxifen in patient serum during breast cancer therapy. *Biochemical Pharmacology* 32:373–375.

Bates, D. J., A. B. Foster, L. J. Griggs, M. Jarman, G. Leclerq, and N. Devleeschouwer. 1982. Metabolism of tamoxifen by isolated rat hepatocytes: antiestrogenic activity of tamoxifen N-oxide. *Biochemical Pharmacology* 31:2823–2827.

Binart, N., M. G. Catelli, C. Geynet, V. Puri, R. Hähnel, J. Mester, J. and E. E. Baulieu.

1979. Monohydroxytamoxifen: an antiestrogen with high affinity for the chick oviduct oestrogen receptor. *Biochemical and Biophysical Research Communications*
91:812–818.

Borgna, J. L., and H. Rochefort. 1981. Hydroxylated metabolites of tamoxifen are formed
in vivo and bound to estrogen receptor in target tissues. *Journal of Biological Chemistry* 256:859–868.

Borgna, J. L., E. Coezy, and H. Rochefort. 1982. Mode of action of LN1643 (a triphenyl-
bromo-ethylene antiestrogen) probable mediation by the estrogen receptor and high
affinity metabolite. *Biochemical Pharmacology* 31:3187–3191.

Bowman, S. P., A. Leake, and I. D. Morris. 1982. Hypothalamic, pituitary and uterine
cytoplasmic and nuclear oestrogen receptors and their relationship to the serum concentration of tamoxifen and its metabolite, 4-hydroxytamoxifen, in the ovariectomized rat. *Journal of Endocrinology* 94:167–175.

Brown, R. R., R. Bain, and V. C. Jordan. 1983. Determination of tamoxifen and metabolites in human serum by high performance liquid chromatography with postcolumn
fluorescence activation. *Journal of Chromatography* 272:351–358.

Camaggi, C. M., E. Strocchi, N. Canova, and F. Pannuti. 1983. High performance liquid
chromatographic analysis of tamoxifen and major metabolites in human plasma.
Journal of Chromatography 275:436–442.

Daniel, C. P., S. J. Gaskell, H. Bishop, and R. I. Nicholson. 1979. Determination of tamoxifen and an hydroxylated metabolite in plasma from patients with advanced
breast cancer using gas chromatography mass spectrometry. *Journal of Endocrinology* 83:401–408.

Daniel, C. P., S. J. Gaskell, H. Bishop, C. Campbell, and R. I. Nicholson. 1981. Determination of tamoxifen and biologically active metabolites in human breast tumours
and plasma. *European Journal of Cancer and Clinical Oncology* 17:1183–1189.

Dorfman, R. I. (ed.). 1968. *Methods in hormone research*. New York: Academic Press.

Eisenfeld, A. 1974. Oral contraceptives: ethinyl estradiol binds with higher affinity than
mestranol to macromolecules from sites of contraceptive action. *Endocrinology*
94:803–807.

Foster, A. B., L. J. Griggs, M. Jarman, J. M. S. van Maanen, and H. R. Schulten. 1980.
Metabolism of tamoxifen by rat liver microsomes, formation of the N-oxide, a new
metabolite. *Biochemical Pharmacology* 29:1977–1979.

Fromson, J. M., and D. S. Sharp, 1974. The selective uptake of tamoxifen by human
uterine tissue. *Journal of Obstetrics and Gynaecology of the British Commonwealth*
81:321–323.

Fromson, J. M., S. Pearson, and S. Bramah. 1973a. The metabolism of tamoxifen (ICI
46,474). Part I. In laboratory animals. *Xenobiotica* 3:693–709.

Fromson, J. M., S. Pearson, and S. Bramah. 1973b. The metabolism of tamoxifen (ICI
46,474). Part II. In female patients. *Xenobiotica* 3:711–713.

Furr, B. J., J. S. Patterson, D. N. Richardson, S. R. Slater, and A. E. Wakeling. 1979.
Tamoxifen. In *Pharmacological and biochemical properties of drug substances*, vol.
2, ed. M. E. Goldberg, 355–399. Washington, D.C.: American Pharmaceutical Association.

Golander, Y., and L. A. Sternson, 1980. Paired ion chromatographic analysis of tamoxifen
and two major metabolites in plasma. *Journal of Chromatography* 181:41–49.

Hayes, J. A., E. A. Rorke, D. W. Robertson, B. S. Katzenellenbogen, and J. A. Katzenellenbogen. 1981. Biological potency and uterine estrogen receptor interactions of
the metabolites of the antiestrogens CI 628 and U 23,469. *Endocrinology* 108:164–
172.

Horwitz, K. B., Y. Koseki, and W. L. McGuire. 1978. Estrogen control of progesterone receptor in human breast cancer: role of estradiol and antiestrogen. *Endocrinology* 103:1742–1751.

Jordan, V. C., and B. Gosden. 1982. Importance of the alkyl aminoethoxy side chain for the estrogenic and antiestrogenic actions of tamoxifen and trioxifene in the immature rat uterus. *Molecular and Cellular Endocrinology* 27:291–306.

Jordan, V. C., M. M. Collins, L. Rowsby, and G. Prestwich. 1977. A monohydroxylated metabolite of tamoxifen with potent antioestrogenic activity. *Journal of Endocrinology* 75:305–316.

Jordan, V. C., C. J. Dix, K. E. Naylor, G. Prestwich, and L. Rowsby. 1978. Non-steroidal antiestrogens: their biological effects and potential mechanisms of action. *Journal of Toxicology and Environmental Health* 4:364–390.

Jordan, V. C., R. R. Bain, R. R. Brown, B. Gosden, and M. A. Santos. 1983. Determination and pharmacology of a new hydroxylated metabolite of tamoxifen observed in patient sera during therapy for advanced breast cancer. *Cancer Research* 43:1446–1450.

Jordan, V. C., M. E. Lieberman, E. Cormier, R. Koch, J. Bagley, and P. Ruenitz. 1984. Structural requirements for the pharmacological activity of nonsteroidal antiestrogens *in vitro*. *Molecular Pharmacology* 26:272–278.

Katzenellenbogen, B. S., J. A. Katzenellenbogen, E. R. Ferguson, and N. Krauthammer. 1978. Antiestrogen interaction with uterine estrogen receptors: studies with a radiolabelled antiestrogen (CI 628). *Journal of Biological Chemistry* 253:697–707.

Katzenellenbogen, B. S., H. S. Bhakoo, E. R. Ferguson, N. C. Lan, T. Tatee, T. S. Tsai, and J. A. Katzenellenbogen. 1979. Estrogen and antiestrogen action in reproductive tissues and tumors. *Recent Progress in Hormone Research* 35:259–300.

Katzenellenbogen, B. S., E. J. Pavlik, D. W. Robertson, and J. A. Katzenellenbogen. 1981. Interaction of a high affinity antiestrogen (α-[4-pyrrolidinoethoxy]phenyl-4-hydroxy-α'-nitrostilbene, CI-628M) with uterine estrogen receptors. *Journal of Biological Chemistry* 256:2908–2915.

Katzenellenbogen, B. S., M. J. Norman, R. L. Eckert, S. W. Peltz, and W. F. Mangel. 1984. Bioactivities, estrogen receptor interactions and plasminogen activator-inducing activities of tamoxifen and hydroxytamoxifen isomers in MCF-7 human breast cancer cells. *Cancer Research* 44:112–119.

Kemp, J. V., H. K. Adam, A. E. Wakeling, and R. Slater. 1983. Identification and biological activity of tamoxifen metabolites in human serum. *Biochemical Pharmacology* 32:2045–2052.

Lerner, L. J. 1964. Hormone antagonists: inhibitors of specific activities of estrogen and androgen. *Recent Progress in Hormone Research* 20:435–476.

Lieberman, M. E., J. Gorski, and V. C. Jordan. 1983. An estrogen receptor model to describe the regulation of prolactin synthesis by antiestrogens *in vitro*. *Journal of Biological Chemistry* 258:4741–4745.

Lyman, S. D., and V. C. Jordan. 1985. Metabolism of tamoxifen and its uterotrophic activity. *Biochemical Pharmacology* 34:2787–2794.

Mallory, F. B., C. S. Wood, and J. T. Gordon. 1964. Photochemistry of stilbenes, III: some aspects of photocylisation to phenanthrenes. *Journal of the American Chemical Society* 86:3094–3102.

Meltzer, N. M., P. Stang, L. A. Sternson, and A. E. Wade. 1984. Influence of tamoxifen and its N-desmethyl and 4-hydroxy metabolites on rat liver microsomal enzymes. *Biochemical Pharmacology* 33:115–123.

Mendenhall, D. W., H. Kobayashi, L. A. Shih, L. A. Sternson, T. Higuchi, and C. Fabian. 1978. Clinical analysis of tamoxifen, an antineoplastic agent, in plasma. *Clinical Chemistry* 24:1518–1524.

Patterson, J. S. 1981. "Nolvadex" (tamoxifen) as an anti-cancer agent in humans. In *Non-steroidal antioestrogens: molecular pharmacology and antitumour activity,* ed. R. L. Sutherland and V. C. Jordan, 453–472. Sydney: Academic Press.

Patterson, J. S., R. S. Settatree, H. K. Adam, and J. V. Kemp. 1980. Serum concentrations of tamoxifen and major metabolites during long term Nolvadex therapy, correlated with clinical response. In *Breast cancer: experimental and clinical aspects,* ed. H. T. Mouridsen, and T. Palshof, 89–92. Oxford: Pergamon Press.

Reddel, R. R., L. C. Murphy, and R. L. Sutherland. 1983. Effects of biologically active metabolites of tamoxifen on the proliferation kinetics of MCF-7 human breast cancer cells *in vitro. Cancer Research* 43:4618–4624.

Robertson, D. W., J. A. Katzenellenbogen, D. J. Long, E. A. Rorke, and B. S. Katzenellenbogen. 1982. Tamoxifen antiestrogens. A comparison of the activity, pharmacokinetics and metabolic activation of the *cis* and *trans* isomers of tamoxifen. *Journal of Steroid Biochemistry* 16:1–13.

Ruenitz, P. C. 1978. Rabbit hepatic microsomal O-demethylation of chlorotrianisene. *Drug Metabolism and Disposition* 6:631–636.

Ruenitz, P. C. 1981. Rabbit liver microsomal metabolism of enclomiphene. *Drug Metabolism and Disposition* 9:456–460.

Ruenitz, P. C., and J. R. Bagley. 1983. Formation of benzophenone and α,α-diarylacetophenone metabolites of the antiestrogen nitromiphene (CI 628) in the presence of rat cecal contents. *Life Sciences* 33:1051–1056.

Ruenitz, P. C., and M. M. Toledo. 1980. Inhibition of rabbit liver microsomal oxidative metabolism and substrate binding by tamoxifen and the geometric isomers of clomiphene. *Biochemical Pharmacology* 29:1583–1587.

Ruenitz, P. C., and M. M. Toledo. 1981. Chemical and biochemical characteristics of O-demethylation of chlorotrianisene in the rat. *Biochemical Pharmacology* 30:2203–2207.

Ruenitz, P. C., J. R. Bagley, and C. M. Mobler. 1983a. Metabolism of clomiphene in the rat: estrogen receptor affinity and estrogenic activity of clomiphene metabolites. *Biochemical Pharmacology* 32:2941–2947.

Ruenitz, P. C., J. R. Bagley, and C. M. Mobler. 1983b. Estrogen receptor binding and estrogenic/antiestrogenic effects of two new metabolites of nitromiphene, 2-[p-[nitro-1-(4-methoxyphenyl)-2-phenylvinyl]phenoxy]-N-ethylpyrrolidine. *Journal of Medicinal Chemistry* 26:1701–1705.

Shah, K. A., J. Levin, N. Rosen, E. Greenwald, and B. Zumoff. 1982. Allopurinol hepatotoxicity potentiated by tamoxifen. *New York State Journal of Medicine* 82:1745–1746.

Sudo, K., F. J. Monsma, Jr., and B. S. Katzenellenbogen. 1983. Antiestrogen binding sites distinct from the estrogen receptor: subcellular localization, ligand specificity and distribution in tissues of the rat. *Endocrinology* 112:425–434.

Sutherland, R. L., and V. C. Jordan. 1981. Modes of action of antioestrogens *in vivo* and *in vitro:* summary and future prospects. In *Non-steroidal antioestrogens: molecular pharmacology and antitumour activity,* ed. R. L. Sutherland and V. C. Jordan, 473–486. Sydney: Academic Press.

Sutherland, R. L., L. C. Murphy, M. S. Foo, M. D. Green, A. M. Whybourne, and Z. S. Krozowski. 1980. High affinity antioestrogen binding site distinct from the oestrogen receptor. *Nature* (London) 288:273–275.

Tatee, T., K. E. Carlson, J. A. Katzenellenbogen, D. W. Robertson, and B. S. Katzenellenbogen. 1979. Antiestrogens and antiestrogen metabolites: preparation of tritium-labelled U 23,469 and characterization and synthesis of a biologically important metabolite. *Journal of Medicinal Chemistry* 22:1509–1517.

Taylor, C. M., B. Blanchard, and D. T. Zava. 1984. Estrogen receptor-mediated and cytotoxic effects of the antiestrogens tamoxifen and 4-hydroxytamoxifen. *Cancer Research* 44:1409–1414.

Wakeling, A. E., and S. R. Slater. 1980. Estrogen-receptor binding and biologic activity of tamoxifen and its metabolites. *Cancer Treatment Reports* 64:741–744.

Wilking, N., L. E. Applegren, K. Carlström, A. Pousette, and N. O. Theve. 1982. The distribution and metabolism of ^{14}C-labelled tamoxifen in spayed female mice. *Acta Pharmacologica and Toxicologica* 50:161–168.

12

Inhibitors of the Aromatase Enzyme System: Basic and Clinical Studies with 4-Hydroxyandrostenedione

A. M. H. BRODIE, L. Y. WING,
M. DOWSETT, P. GOSS, AND R. C. COOMBES

I. INTRODUCTION   222
II. STUDIES ON AROMATASE INHIBITION BY 4-OHA *IN VITRO* AND *IN VIVO*   223
III. ANTITUMOR EFFECTS OF 4-OHA   226
IV. OTHER ACTIONS OF 4-OHA   228
V. TOXICOLOGY   228
VI. THE EFFECT OF 4-OHA TREATMENT ON POSTMENOPAUSAL BREAST CANCER PATIENTS   229
REFERENCES   233

I. *Introduction*

Breast carcinomas in animals and humans respond to hormone manipulations, and tumor regression is correlated with the concentration of estrogen and progesterone receptors in the tumor tissue (McGuire 1980). Estrogens are synthesized not only by the ovary but by extraovarian tissues. This peripheral production of estrogens increases after menopause (Longcope 1971; Helmsell et al. 1974). Breast tumors themselves have been found to synthesize estrogens (Miller and Forrest 1974; Tilson-Mallet et al. 1983) and metabolize estrone sulfate to estrone (Tseng et al. 1983). Estrogens from all of these sources may stimulate tumor growth. The traditional surgical procedures for hormone ablation—ovariectomy, adrenalectomy, and hypophysectomy—are therefore incomplete in removing estrogens. Furthermore, these procedures carry significant morbidity and mortality. Thus, estrogen antagonists which either block estrogen action or estrogen synthesis in all tissue sites could be more effective and safer methods than surgical ablation; the antiestrogen tamoxifen has already proved useful in this regard.

Our approach was to develop a selective inhibitor of estrogen synthesis with little intrinsic hormonal activity and low toxicity. Aromatase (estrogen synthetase) is an enzyme complex that comprises NADPH-cytochrome c reductase and cytochrome P_{450} components and that mediates the conversion of androgens to estrogens. Aromatization is unique in steroid biosynthesis, as it involves the loss of the C-19 methyl group on the androgen precursor and the elimination of the 1β and 2β hydrogens to form the aromatic A ring of the estrogens (Fig. 12.1). This is the last step in the biosynthesis of cholesterol to estrogens, and compounds interacting with aromatase should therefore be selective in preventing estrogen synthesis without interfering with the production of other steroid hormones, such as the adrenal corticoids.

In 1973, we reported the first of a number of steroidal compounds that we have identified as aromatase inhibitors (Schwarzel et al. 1973). Subsequently, 4-hydroxyandrostene-3,17-dione (4-OHA) was found to be the most potent compound (Brodie et al. 1976, 1977). Aminoglutethimide (AG) (Chakraborty et al. 1972) and testolactone were also shown to be inhibitors of aromatase (Siiteri and Thompson 1975). However, AG is a

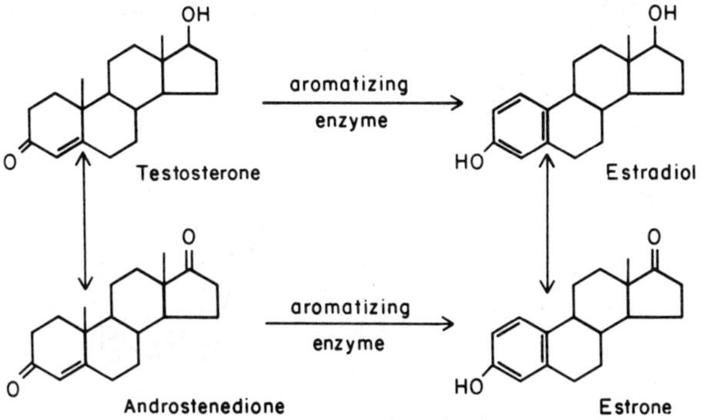

Figure 12.1. Aromatization of androgens to estrogens.

less specific inhibitor, as it binds competitively to the cytochrome P_{450} component of steroid hydroxylases including aromatase (Siiteri and Thompson 1975). As AG and testolactone had previously been approved for clinical use, it was possible to investigate them as aromatase inhibitors in the treatment of breast cancer (Barone et al. 1979; Santen et al. 1981; Santen and Brodie 1982). AG has been shown to lower estrogen levels and inhibit aromatase in animals (Wing et al. 1985) and in postmenopausal patients (Santen et al. 1980). This inhibitor is effective in the treatment of postmenopausal breast cancer patients, and recent studies indicate that it is effective in patients who have relapsed from tamoxifen treatment and in some tamoxifen-resistant patients (Santen and Brodie 1982). Thus, treatment with a compound which reduces estrogen synthesis may be of benefit in addition to the use of estrogen-blocking agents like tamoxifen. However, neither AG nor testolactone is sufficiently potent to inhibit the production of estrogens in premenopausal women (Santen et al. 1980).

II. *Studies on Aromatase Inhibition by 4-OHA* in Vitro *and* in Vivo

In our studies with 4-OHA carried out *in vitro* using human placental microsomes as a source of aromatase, this compound was found to be approximately 60 times more potent than AG in inhibiting the aromatization of androstenedione to estrogens (Fig. 12.2) (Johnston and Metcalf 1984; Wing et al. 1985). 4-OHA competes with androstenedione for aromatase, and we have demonstrated typical Line-Weaver Burke kinetics

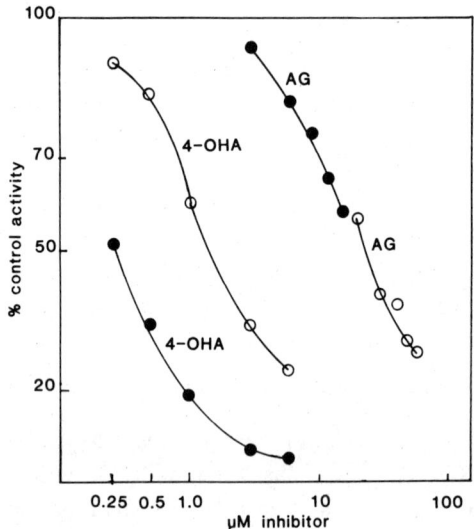

Figure 12.2. Inhibition of aromatization of androstenedione by 4-hydroxyandrostenedione and aminoglutethimide. Aromatization was determined from release of ^3H_2O from [1,2^{3}H]androstenedione (200,000 dpm/μM) incubated for 30 minutes with various concentrations of inhibitor, an oxygen-generating system, and microsomes from human placenta or pregnant mare's serum gonadotrophin (PMSG)-primed rat ovaries. (From Wing et al. [1985] with the permission of the editor.)

(Brodie et al. 1977) for this inhibitor. Unlike AG, which is solely a competitive inhibitor, 4-OHA also causes inactivation of the enzyme, which is evident when 4-OHA is preincubated with microsomes in the presence of NADPH, then removed and the enzyme activity estimated. 4-OHA appears to be converted by a catalytic process requiring NADPH to an intermediate which irreversibly binds to the aromatase and causes its inactivation (Brodie et al. 1981; Covey and Hood 1982). These reactions may be visualized by the following equation:

$$E + I \rightleftharpoons E - I \rightarrow EI$$

A number of enzyme inhibitors which act in this manner have been successfully developed as drugs in recent years (Sjoerdsma 1981); they have been called "suicide inhibitors" since the enzyme is inactivated by its own mechanism of action (Walsh 1982). Suicide inhibitors or K_{cat} inhibitors have advantages over competitive inhibitors because they bind to the active site of the enzyme and are therefore quite specific. Also, their inactivation of the enzyme should result in long-term effects *in vivo*, until new enzyme is formed.

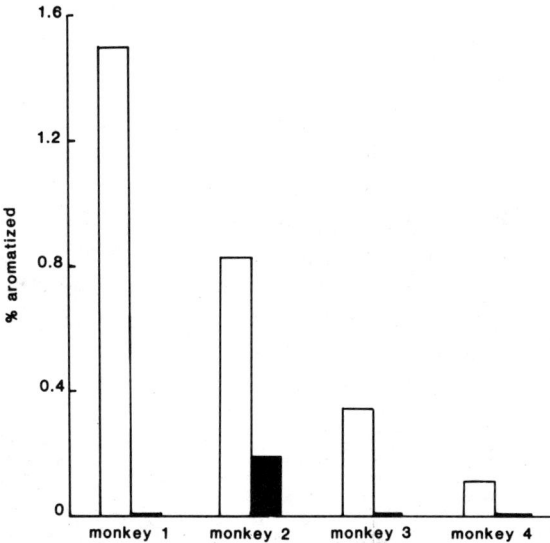

Figure 12.3. The effect of 4-OHA on peripheral aromatization. Male rhesus monkeys were infused with [7³H]androstenedione and the conversion to estradiol measured in plasma samples. Metabolic clearance rates of estrone were measured from [4-C¹⁴]estrone infused at the same time. The control infusion was carried out 1 week before 4-OHA treatment of monkeys 1 and 2 and 1 week after treatment of monkeys 3 and 4. A suspension of 4-OHA (50 mg/kg) was injected at 1700 hours the day before infusion of the radiolabeled steroid and at 1.5 hours (0830) before beginning the infusion. (From Brodie and Longcope 1980.)

Evidence that 4-OHA inhibits aromatase and blocks estrogen production *in vivo* has been demonstrated in animal models. Thus, in the normal-cycling rat, an injection of 4-OHA on proestrus caused marked inhibition of both ovarian estrogen secretion and aromatase activity 3 hours later (Brodie et al. 1981). In rats primed with pregnant mare's serum gonadotrophins to increase estrogen production and maintain a constant output, a subcutaneous injection of 4-OHA (50 mg/kg) suppressed ovarian aromatase and estrogen production for at least 72 hours (Brodie et al. 1981).

Peripheral aromatization was reduced to undetectable levels in three rhesus monkeys and to very low levels in the fourth monkey treated with 4-OHA (Fig. 12.3). Although the compound is cleared very rapidly from the blood (Brodie et al. 1982b), a lasting effect of the treatment was evident in these monkeys as well as in the rats described above. In the monkeys, peripheral aromatization had not returned to control levels when measured 7 days after treatment (Brodie and Longcope 1980). Whether this was due to inactivation of the enzyme, a depot effect of subcutaneous injections of 4-OHA suspension, or to both factors has not been determined. No specific effects of 4-OHA were observed on the metabolic clearance rates of androstenedione or estrone in the monkeys, indicating that aromatization was not affected by changes in clearance of the substrate or products of aromatization. The interconversion of androgens and of estrogens and the conversion of androstenedione to dihydrotestosterone (DHT) were unaffected by 4-OHA in the monkeys (Brodie and Longcope 1980). Some inhibition of androgen metabolism was observed *in vitro*. The enzymes, 5-α-reductase and 17 β-hydroxysteroid dehydrogenase, were inhibited by concentrations 5–100-fold greater than those required to inhibit aromatase (Brodie et al. 1982b).

III. Antitumor Effects of 4-OHA

Mammary tumors can be induced in the rat with carcinogens, dimethylbenz(a)anthracene (DMBA), or nitrosomethylurea. The growth of these tumors has been shown to be dependent on ovarian steroids. The tumors are measured with calipers and the tumor volume calculated. Because the tumors of each rat vary in size and number, the total tumor volume of the group is compared.

Several regimens of subcutaneous injections of 4-OHA suspension (50 mg/kg/day) have been evaluated in the DMBA model. Half the dose of 4-OHA administered twice a day for 4 weeks or during weeks 1 and 3 caused marked tumor regression in these rats to the same extent as ovariadrenalectomy. Approximately 90% of tumors are reduced to less than half their original volume and a large percentage of these completely eliminated (Brodie et al. 1977). After 4 weeks of treatment, ovarian estrogen secretion and aromatase activity are significantly reduced in the treated rats compared to control animals, suggesting that the antitumor effect of 4-OHA is due to reduced ovarian estrogen production (Brodie et al. 1982a) (Fig. 12.4). Furthermore, when physiological doses of estradiol are administered concomitantly with 4-OHA, tumor regression does not occur. Similar antitumor effects to the above were achieved with injections twice a day during the first 10 days. When this was followed with injections twice a week, tumor growth was suppressed for at least 5 months (Brodie et al. 1983).

Neither AG (50 mg/kg/day) (Wing et al. 1985) nor tamoxifen (20 µg/

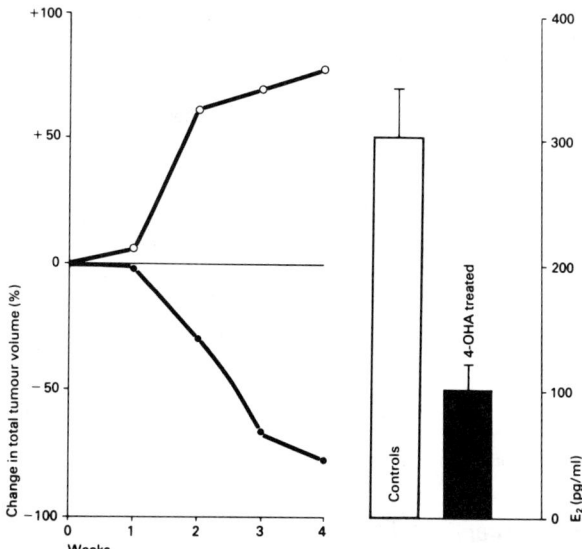

Figure 12.4. The effect of 4-OHA on DMBA-induced, hormone-dependent mammary tumors of the rat. Left panel: ●: percentage change in total volume of 13 tumors on six rats injected with 4-OHA (50 mg/kg/day) twice a day for 4 weeks; ○: tumors on five control rats injected twice a day with vehicle. Right panel: At the end of treatment, blood was collected from each rat by ovarian vein cannulation for estradiol (E_2) assay; controls were sampled during diestrus. (From Brodie et al. [1984] with the permission of the publishers.)

rat) (Brodie et al. 1983) treatment is as effective as 4-OHA treatment in causing tumor regression in the rat. Although some of the DMBA-induced tumors regressed with AG or tamoxifen, the proportion of tumors responding was less than with 4-OHA (Table 12.1). In addition, some tumor growth occurred. Although AG was highly effective in inhibiting ovarian aromatase and estrogen secretion in the rat during acute studies, after 4 weeks of treatment with AG, ovarian estrogen secretion was not significantly different from control values. This finding may be due to stimulation of ovarian aromatase by reflex increases in luteinizing hormone which occur in the rats after 4 weeks of AG treatment (Wing et al. 1985).

When 4-OHA was combined with the antiestrogen tamoxifen, tumor regression was not as great as with 4-OHA alone. Tamoxifen was also found to retard tumor regression following ovariectomy (Brodie et al. 1983). This effect may be due to its weak agonistic activity (Jordan 1984).

Table 12.1. The effect of 4-OHA, tamoxifen (TAM), and aminoglutethimide (AG) on
DMBA-induced mammary tumors in the rat[a]

Treatment	Number of rats	Number of tumors	Percent tumors regressing[b]
Control	7	24	34
Tamoxifen	5	17	42
4-OHA	5	16	94
4-OHA + TAM	5	14	78
Control	8	26	8
AG	8	23	43
4-OHA	10	22	94
4-OHA + AG	6	10	80

[a]Rats were treated for 4 weeks with subcutaneous injections of 4-OHA (50 mg/kg/day) and/
or AG twice daily and/or tamoxifen (1 mg/kg/day) once daily.
[b]Tumors regressing more than 50% of original volume.

IV. Other Actions of 4-OHA

4-OHA has little intrinsic hormonal activity; in bioassays the compound
was estimated to have $< 1\%$ the androgenic activity of testosterone (Brodie et al. 1977). 4-OHA does not bind to either estrogen or progesterone
receptors even at high concentrations. The effect of 4-OHA treatment on
estrogen, progesterone, and androgen receptors in long-term studies is
under investigation.

Unlike AG, 4-OHA does not cause a reflex increase in gonadotrophins. In ovariectomized rats treated for 4 weeks with gonadotrophin, levels are decreased, suggesting a direct action of the compound on pituitary
hormones (Brodie 1980). This effect appears to be due to the weak androgenic activity of 4-OHA or possibly a metabolite, since coadministration
with an antiandrogen, but not with an antiestrogen, could prevent suppression of gonadotrophins (Wing et al. 1985). Suppression of luteinizing hormone and follicle-stimulating hormone by 4-OHA treatment may contribute to maintaining low production of ovarian estrogens in chronically
treated rats.

V. Toxicology

Administered by intraperitoneal injection as a suspension in carboxymethyl cellulose, the acute LD_{50} of 4-OHA was 4.325 g/kg in mice
(Coombes et al. 1984), indicating that the compound has low toxicity.

VI. The Effect of 4-OHA Treatment on Postmenopausal Breast Cancer Patients

The above studies suggest that 4-OHA may reduce estrogen production from both ovarian and peripheral sources and thereby be effective in causing regression of hormone-dependent tumors in breast cancer patients.

The first clinical study with 4-OHA (Coombes et al. 1984), described below, was carried out in postmenopausal patients with advanced metastatic disease.

Eleven patients, aged 36–75 years, were treated with 4-OHA. All were either postmenopausal or ovariectomized and had histologically proven advanced progressive breast cancer with assessable tumors. None had received endocrine therapy or chemotherapy within 4 weeks of the start of treatment with 4-OHA. Four patients had estrogen receptor–positive tumors; the receptor content was unknown in the other cases. Patients were staged before treatment and every 8 weeks during treatment. Patients were examined each week and toxicity assessed using a standard questionnaire. The response of the disease was evaluated each week by standard criteria of the International Union Against Cancer.

4-OHA was synthesized in our laboratory by previously reported methods (Brodie et al. 1977) and purity checked as described (Coombes et al. 1984). The compound was ground to a fine powder and sonicated in 0.5% carboxymethyl cellulose in water. This suspension (500 mg 4-OHA) was injected intramuscularly once a week.

Blood samples were obtained for estradiol measurements from five patients every 2 hours for 12 hours on the day before and on the day of administration of 4-OHA and at 9 A.M. for 6 days thereafter to determine the acute effect of 4-OHA administration.

Estradiol concentrations were measured by radioimmunoassay after extraction of duplicate aliquots of serum with freshly purified ether. The assay sensitivity was 2.8 pmol/l and cross reaction with 4-OHA was $< 1 \times 10^{-6}$ % and with estrone was 0.03%. The within- and between-assay coefficients of variation were 10.4% and 12.8% respectively at a plasma concentration of 27 pmol/l. All samples from the same patient were assayed in the same batch.

The clinical results of 4-OHA treatment are shown in Table 12.2. In four patients, there was partial or complete response of soft tissue and bone metastases to 4-OHA treatment. In one patient the disease was stabilized. The disease progressed in the other six patients, three of whom

Table 12.2. Details of patients treated with 4-OHA

Patients	Age (yr)	Years since LMP	Estrogen receptor (fmol/mg)	Previous endocrine therapy and outcome	Dose of 4-OHA (mg)	Length of treatment (wk)	Sites of disease and response		Overall response	Duration response (wk)
Responders										
1	50	6	85	Oophorectomy — Unknown Tamoxifen — PD	500 weekly	> 10	Skin Bone	PR NC	PR	> 8
2	48	3	ND	Danazol — NC Oophorectomy — PR	500 weekly	> 16	Skin Nodes	PR CR	PR	16
3	41	2	ND	Oophorectomy — PR Buserelin — PD	500 weekly	> 12	Bone	PR	PR	> 6
4	60	18	ND	Tamoxifen — PR	500 weekly	> 20	Bone Nodes Skin	NC PR PR	PR	> 16

230

Nonresponders

5	75	25	80	None	PD	500 weekly	8	Skin	PD	PD	—
								Liver	PD		
6	52	4	ND	Tamoxifen	PD	500 biweekly	10	Bone	PD	PD	—
				Aminoglutethimide	PD			Liver	PD		
7	37	1	17	Oophorectomy	PD	500 weekly	> 12	Skin	NC	NC	> 12[a]
				Tamoxifen	PD			Lung	NC		
8	39	3	15	Oophorectomy	PD	500 biweekly	5	Bone	PD	PD	—
				Aminoglutethimide	PD			Skin	PD		
9	64	13	ND	Tamoxifen	PD	500 weekly	4	Skin	PD	PD	—
				Progesterone	PD			Breast	PD		
10	64	14	ND	Aminoglutethimide	PR	500 biweekly	3	Lung	PD	PD	—
				Progesterone	PD			Bone	PD		
11	40	7	0	Oophorectomy	NA	500 weekly	3	Lung	PD	PD	—
				Aminoglutethimide	PD						

From Coombes et al. 1984.

LMP = last menstrual period; PD = progressive disease; NC = no change; NA = not assessable; PR = partial response; CR = complete response; ND = not done.

[a] Duration of stabilization.

231

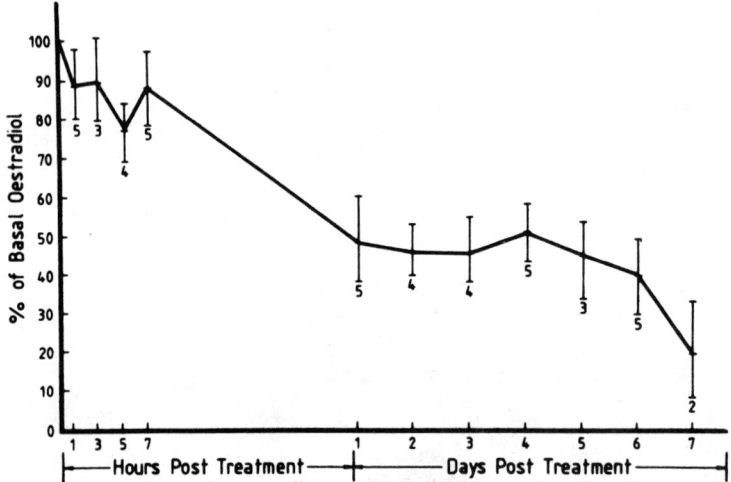

Figure 12.5. Effect of a single dose of 500 mg 4-OHA on plasma estradiol in five patients with breast cancer. The basal estradiol for each patient was calculated by averaging seven pretreatment values, and the posttreatment results were calculated as the percentage of that baseline. The mean of the percentage of baseline for the five patients is shown. Basal samples were obtained at four time points identical with those for the samples obtained 1 day post treatment. Results are as shown as mean ± SD. (From Coombes et al. 1984.)

had estrogen receptor–positive tumors. However, only one had responded to previous endocrine therapy.

The effect of a single dose of 4-OHA on plasma estradiol levels is shown in Figure 12.5. No significant change in level was noted during the first 7 hours after treatment, but after 24 hours significant suppression was evident. No further significant changes occurred during the ensuing 6 days. The mean ± SD levels of seven pretreatment samples from each of the five patients ranged from 12.5 ± 6.7 to 35.4 ± 3.7 pmol/l. The mean level of estradiol during days 1–6 after treatment was 46 ± 3% of the baseline level. It was not determined whether the apparent further suppression in two patients 7 days after injection is significant.

Side effects were evident in five patients. Three patients had pain at the site of injection, necessitating reduction in frequency of injections, and two patients experienced hot flashes. No other side effects were noted. Because of its low toxicity, 4-OHA may be effective as an adjuvant therapy. Improved formulation or route of administration may produce improved response rates.

Although the number of patients treated to date is small and the optimum dose and scheduling are not yet determined, the response to 4-OHA indicates that this aromatase inhibitor may be of significant benefit in advanced cases of breast cancer and after relapse from other agents such as tamoxifen.

References

Barone, R. M., I. M. Shamonki, P. K. Siiteri, and H. L. Judd. 1979. Inhibition of peripheral aromatizatioin of androstenedione to estrone in post-menopausal women with breast cancer using Δ^1-testolactone. *Journal of Clinical Endocrinology and Metabolism* 49:672–676.

Brodie, A. M. H. 1980. Inhibition of estrogen biosynthesis: an approach to treatment of estrogen-dependent cancer. In *Hormones and cancer. Progress in cancer research and therapy,* vol. 14, ed. S. Iacobelli, R. J. B. King, H. R. Lindner, and M. E. Lippman, 507–514. New York: Raven Press.

Brodie, A. M. H. 1982. Inhibition of estrogen biosynthesis and regression of mammary tumors by aromatase inhibitors. In *Hormones and cancer. Advances in experimental medicine and biology,* vol. 138, ed. W. W. Leavitt, 179–190. New York: Plenum Press.

Brodie A. M. H., and C. Longcope. 1980. Inhibition of peripheral aromatization by aromatase inhibitors, 4-hydroxy- and 4-acetoxyandrostenedione. *Endocrinology* 106: 19–21.

Brodie, A. M. H., W. C. Schwarzel, and H. J. Brodie. 1976. Studies on the mechanism of estrogen biosynthesis in the rat ovary. *Journal of Steroid Biochemistry* 7:787–793.

Brodie, A. M. H., W. C. Schwarzel, A. A. Shaikh, and H. J. Brodie. 1977. The effect of an aromatase inhibitor, 4-hydroxy-4-androstene-3,17-dione, on estrogen-dependent processes in reproduction and breast cancer. *Endocrinology* 100:1684–1695.

Brodie, A. M. H., W. M. Garrett, J. R. Hendrickson, C. H. Tsai-Morris, P. A. Marcotte, and C. H. Robinson. 1981. Inactivation of aromatase *in vitro* by 4-hydroxyandrostenedione and 4-acetoxyandrostenedione and sustained effects *in vivo. Steroids* 38:693–702.

Brodie, A. M. H., W. M. Garrett, J. R. Hendrickson, and C. H. Tsai-Morris. 1982a. Effects of 4-hydroxyandrostenedione and other compounds in the DMBA breast carcinoma model. *Cancer Research Supplement* 42:3360s–3364s.

Brodie, A. M. H., L. P. Romanoff, and K. I. H. Williams. 1982b. Metabolism of the aromatase inhibitor 4-hydroxyandrostenedione by male rhesus monkeys. *Journal of Steroid Biochemistry* 14:693–696.

Brodie, A. M. H., W. M. Garrett, J. R. Hendrickson, C. H. Tsai-Morris, and J. G. Williams. 1983. Aromatase inhibitors, their pharmacology and application. *Journal of Steroid Biochemistry* 19:53–58.

Brodie, A. M. H., W. M. Garrett, J. R. Hendrickson, C. H. Tsai-Morris, and L. C. Wing. 1984. Aromatase inhibition: a new perspective in the treatment of breast cancer. In *Aminoglutethimide as an aromatase inhibitor in the treatment of cancer,* ed. G. A. Nagel and R. J. Santen, 11–23. Vienna: Hans Huber.

Chakraborty, J., R. Hopkins, and D. V. Parke. 1972. Inhibition studies in the aromatization of androstenedione by human placental microsome preparations. *Biochemical Journal* 130:190.

Coombes, R. C., P. Goss, M. Dowsett, J. C. Gazet, and A. M. H. Brodie. 1984. 4-Hydroxyandrostenedione treatment of postmenopausal patients with advanced breast cancer. *Lancet* 2:1237–1240.

Covey, D. F., and W. F. Hood. 1982. Aromatase enzyme catalysis is involved in the potent inhibition of estrogen biosynthesis caused by 4-acetoxy- and 4-hydroxyandrostenedione. *Molecular Pharmacology* 21:173–180.

Helmsell, D. L., M. M. Grodin, P. F. Brenner, P. K. Siiteri, and P. D. MacDonald. 1974. Plasma precursors of estrogen. II. Correlation of the extent of conversion of plasma androstenedione to estrone with age. *Journal of Clinical Endocrinology and Metabolism* 38:476–479.

Johnston, J. O., and B. W. Metcalf. 1984. Aromatase: a target enzyme in breast cancer. In *Novel approaches to cancer chemotherapy,* ed. P. Sunkara, 307–328. New York: Academic Press.

Jordan, V. C. 1984. Biochemical pharmacology of antiestrogen action. *Pharmacological Reviews* 36:245–276.

Longcope, C. 1971. Metabolic clearance and blood production rates of estrogens in postmenopausal women. *American Journal of Obstetrics and Gynecology* 111:778–781.

McGuire, W. L. 1980. An update on estrogen and progesterone receptors in prognosis for primary and advanced breast cancer. In *Hormones and cancer. Progress in cancer research and therapy,* vol. 14, ed. S. Iacobelli, R. J. B. King, H. R. Lindner, and M. E. Lippman, 337–343. New York: Raven Press.

Miller, W. R., and A. P. M. Forrest. 1974. Oestradiol synthesis by a human breast carcinoma. *Lancet* 2:866–868.

Santen, R. J., and A. M. H. Brodie. 1982. Suppression of estrogen production as treatment of breast carcinoma: pharmacological and clinical studies with aromatase inhibitors. In *Clinics in oncology,* ed. B. J. A. Furr, 77–130. London: Saunders.

Santen, R. J., E. Samojlik, and S. A. Wells. 1980. Resistance of the ovary to blockade of aromatization with aminoglutethimide. *Journal of Clinical Endocrinology and Metabolism* 51:473–477.

Santen, R. J., T. J. Worgul, E. Samojlik, A. Interrante, A. E. Boucher, A. Lipton, H. A. Harvey, D. S. White, E. Smart, C. Cox, and S. A. Wells. 1981. Randomized trial comparing surgical adrenalectomy with aminoglutethimide plus hydrocortisone in women with advanced breast carcinoma. *New England Journal of Medicine* 305:545–551.

Schwarzel, W. C., W. Kruggel, and H. J. Brodie. 1973. Studies on the mechanism of estrogen biosynthesis. VII. The development of inhibitors of the enzyme system in human placenta. *Endocrinology* 92:866–880.

Segaloff, A., J. B. Weeth, K. K. Meyer, E. L. Rongone, and M. E. Cunningham. 1962. Hormonal therapy in cancer of the breast. XIX. Effect of oral administration of Δ^1-testololactone on clinical course and hormonal excretion. *Cancer* 15:633–640.

Siiteri, P. K., and E. A. Thompson. 1975. Studies on human placental aromatase. *Journal of Steroid Biochemistry* 6:317–322.

Sjoerdsma, A. 1981. Suicide inhibitors as potential drugs. *Clinical Pharmacology and Experimental Therapeutics* 30:3–22.

Tilson-Mallett, N., S. Santner, P. D. Feil, and R. J. Santen. 1983. Biological significance of aromatase activity in human breast tumors. *Journal of Clinical Endocrinology and Metabolism* 57:1125–1128.

Tseng, L., J. Mazella, L. Y. Lee, and M. L. Stone. 1983. Estrogen sulfatase and estrogen sulfatransferase in human primary mammary carcinoma. *Journal of Steroid Biochemistry* 19:1413–1417.

Walsh, C. 1982. Suicide substrates: mechanism-based enzyme inactivators. *Tetrahedron* 38:871–909.

Wing, L-Y, W. M. Garrett, and A. M. H. Brodie. 1985. The effects of aromatase inhibitors, aminoglutethimide and 4-hydroxyandrostenedione on cyclic rats with DMBA-induced mammary tumors. *Cancer Research* 45:2425–2428.

IV

Laboratory Models to Study Hormone-Dependent Breast Cancer

13

Estrogens Regulate Production of Specific Growth Factors in Hormone-Dependent Human Breast Cancer

Marc E. Lippman, Karen K. Huff,
Raimund Jakesz, Toby Hecht,
Attan Kasid, Susan Bates,
and Robert B. Dickson

I. Introduction 238
II. Estrogen-Induced Growth Factor Activities 240
    a. Identification of Insulin-like Growth Factor I 241
    b. Identification of Transforming Growth Factors 242
III. In Vivo Tests of Growth Factor Activities 243
IV. Future Prospects 244
    References 245

I. Introduction

Our laboratory has been interested in the mechanisms by which estrogens regulate the growth of human breast cancer. Many difficulties may complicate such studies in experimental animals or in humans. First, it is impossible to alter the activity of a single hormone *in vivo* without inducing a host of counterregulatory events which can alter the concentrations and activities of numerous other hormones and growth factors. Second, there can be no assurance that a response in the tumor is due to a direct effect on the malignant cells themselves as opposed to the immune system, supporting stroma, angiogenesis, or other factors. Using clonal lines of human breast cancer cells in long-term tissue culture, we succeeded in demonstrating direct proliferative responses to physiological doses of estrogen (Lippman et al. 1976a,b; Aitken and Lippman 1980) as well as in showing growth regulation by a variety of other trophic hormones, including insulin, glucocorticoids, iodothyronines, androgens, and retinoids. In addition, other groups have demonstrated receptors for or responses to prolactin, progestins, epidermal growth factor, vitamin D, and calcitonin (Lippman 1981). Following our initial observations of growth responses to estrogens, several groups reported marginal success or inability to induce direct estrogenic stimulation of growth (Edwards et al. 1980; Butler et al. 1981). Although the exact reasons for these discrepant results are unclear, several explanations, including clonal variation and culture conditions, are undoubtedly contributory. Nonetheless, more recently, many different groups (Weichselbaum et al. 1978; Barnes and Sato 1979; Chalbos et al. 1982; Leung et al. 1982; Darbre et al. 1983; Katzenellenbogen et al. 1983; Natoli et al. 1983; Page et al. 1983; Huseby et al. 1984) have all succeeded in verifying our finding by demonstrating primary mitogenic effects of physiological doses of estradiol on human breast cancer cells in continuous culture. Of course these direct effects of estrogens on purified cell culture systems *in vitro* do not exclude the possibility that more indirect effects (mediated, for example, by circulating estrogen-induced peptides produced by nonmammary cells) may play an important contributory role (Ikeda and Sirbasku 1984). Although isolated clonal lines of breast cancer have many advantages, they fail to take into account important potential tumor-host interactions. As a single hypothetical example, if estradiol could be replaced by some other cocktail of hormones for *in vitro* growth, but only estradiol was capable of inducing angiogenesis factors, then estradiol stimulation of *in vitro* growth might be variable and dependent on culture conditions, whereas it would be an absolute requirement for *in vivo* growth in athymic nude mice.

In previous work from our laboratory (Aitken and Lippman 1980, 1982; Lippman and Aitken 1980; Lippman et al. 1981; Cowan et al. 1982) we have shown that estrogens can directly regulate the activities of enzymes involved in nucleic acid synthesis. Using independent probes for *de novo*, salvage, and net DNA synthesis it was possible to demonstrate that the two pathways for pyrimidine biosynthesis were concurrently stimulated by estrogen and inhibited by antiestrogens. Specific enzyme activities—thymidine kinase, thymidylate synthetase, aspartate transcarbamylase, carbamyl phosphate synthetase, dihydroorotase uridine kinase, and dihydrofolate reductase—are all regulated by estrogen. Using a cDNA probe for thymidine kinase (Kasid and Lippman 1986), we have been able to show that estradiol regulates thymidine kinase mRNA activity, as would be predicted from enzyme activity studies (Bronzert et al. 1981). Similarly, we have shown that dihydrofolate reductase mRNA is also regulated by physiological doses of estradiol (Cowan et al. 1982; Levine et al. 1985). We are currently asking whether or not the control of mRNA concentration is at the transcriptional level.

None of these data however, either alone or in concert, necessarily implicates any of these inductions as growth regulatory. In fact, given the obvious necessity for complex interactions of cancer cells with the host in order to form a tumor, we wondered whether there might be important regulation by estrogens of substances secreted by breast cancer cells able to either stimulate cells in an autocrine fashion, other breast cancer cells, or surrounding nonmalignant cells. An additional reason for our interest in this phenomenon was the substantial difference between the action of estrogens on breast cancer cells *in vitro* and *in vivo*. As previously stated, *in vitro* conditions can be found in which estrogens can stimulate cell proliferation. However, extensive medium supplementation with nonsteroidal growth factors can replace any needed estrogen. On the other hand, several groups have found (Shafie 1980; Soule and McGrath 1980) and we have confirmed (Seibert et al. 1983) that estrogen supplementation is mandatory for tumorigenesis on MCF-7 human breast cancer cells in nude mice. McGrath and his colleagues further defined this system by showing that estrogens need not enter the systemic circulation in nude mice to have the effect; elevation of local estradiol concentration near the tumor was sufficient (Huseby et al. 1984). This did suggest that estrogens might be required to induce factors required by the tumor or host for tumorigenesis but also at least suggested that an endocrine (estromedin) pathway was unnecessary.

II. *Estrogen-Induced Growth Factor Activities*

Our attention to this possibility was stimulated most powerfully by an observation made with MCF-7 cells plated at various densities. We found that initial growth rate was directly proportional to number of cells plated (Jakesz et al. 1984). Doubling times varied from 44 hours to 20 hours for cells plated at the highest (subconfluent) densities. Although multiple interpretations of these data are possible, they are consistent with the production of auto- or paracrine-type growth factors by the MCF-7 cells. In preliminary experiments we found that conditioned medium (CM) harvested from MCF-7 cells was capable of stimulating thymidine incorporation and proliferation of other MCF-7 cells (Dickson et al. 1986a). This kind of result had also been obtained by Vignon and Rochefort and their colleagues (Vignon et al. 1983), who had noticed that MCF-7 cells grew faster with less frequent medium exchanges, compared to cells in which medium was changed every other day; they too had noted that CM was directly capable of stimulating other MCF-7 cells. In their preliminary work it had appeared that CM from estradiol-treated cells was more potent even after removal of the estradiol.

In previous work (Jakesz et al. 1984) we had also been able to show that partial synchrony of MCF-7 cells can be achieved by growth arrest which follows transfer to isoleucine-deficient medium for 24–30 hours. At this time, S fraction determined by flow cytometry is near zero, as is precursor incorporation into DNA, although viability remains close to 100% as assessed by trypan blue dye exclusion. If cells are now refed with fresh medium containing isoleucine, DNA synthesis resumes after a lag of about 24 hours. If instead the medium is supplemented with 1 nM estradiol, an accelerated and exaggerated growth response occurs, beginning at about 16 hours. Concentrated CM (even when completely devoid of estradiol as shown by both radioimmunoassay and radioreceptor assay) can exactly mimic this growth response to estradiol. The use of isoleucine deprivation (together with the serum-free system to be described) provides a convenient and sensitive assay for growth-promoting activity.

In order to study this matter further we felt that a defined medium system would substantially aid in both purification and assay of such activities. Previous work (Allegra and Lippman, 1978; Barnes and Sato 1979) was helpful in this regard. We found that MCF-7 cells could be propagated in improved minimal essential medium (IMEM) supplemented with fibronectin and transferrin (IMEM-SF). Thus MCF-7 cells could be plated in serum-containing medium, the medium removed, and exchanged for IMEM-SF with or without additional supplementation with estradiol. Following an additional 2 or 3 days in these media, the cells were replenished with fresh identical media, which after 2 days was collected and used as a starting material for assay of growth-promoting activities.

A. IDENTIFICATION OF INSULIN-LIKE GROWTH FACTOR I

The CM derived from MCF-7 cells grown in IMEM-SF with or without E_2 supplementation was harvested and filtered to remove cellular debris. Fibronectin and transferrin were removed by sequential gelatin sepharose chromatography and passage over an antitransferrin affinity column. This was followed by one of several different extraction procedures, including dialysis and concentration, acetic acid or acid ethanol extraction, and fractionation by Sephacryl S-200 or Biogel P60 chromatography.

Total concentrate and specific fractions of column eluates have been characterized by six distinct assay methodologies. These are radioimmunoassay for insulin-like growth factor I (somatomedin C), abbreviated IGF-I; epidermal growth factor (EGF) receptor reactive material measured by competition in a radioreceptor assay using A-431 cells as a source of receptor; transforming growth factor (TGF) activity assayed by measuring promotion of soft agar colony formation in normal rat kidney (NRK) cells; monoclonal antibody reactivity (described below); thymidine incorporation; and long-term growth-promoting activities. These six methodologies were applied to CM derived from MCF-7 cells which had or had not been stimulated with 1 nM estradiol. In addition, similar studies were performed using estrogen receptor–positive, estrogen-responsive ZR-75-1 cells and estrogen receptor–negative, estrogen-independent MDA-MB-231 and Hs578t human breast cancer cell lines.

All breast cell lines tested secrete IGF-I as assessed by specific radioimmunoassay (Huff et al. 1986). IGF-I activity from all breast cell lines gives a competition curve parallel to that of authentic IGF-I standard. Depending upon the extraction conditions employed, the IGF-I activity was eluted from chromatography columns at a higher apparent molecular weight than IGF-I standard, suggesting possible association with a binder. This contention is supported by the observation that when authentic ^{125}I-labeled IGF-I is incubated with MCF-7 CM, it shifts to a higher molecular weight form. With acid ethanol extraction, all of the IGF-I immunoassayable material co-elutes from Sephacryl S-200 with authentic IGF-I. Estradiol has minimal (less than 2-fold) and inconsistent effects on the quantity of IGF-I secreted by either MCF-7 cells or ZR-75-1 cells. Hs578t and MDA-MB-231 cells secrete up to 10 times more IGF-I activity than the former two cell lines, although estrogen has no effect on secretion. Cellular homogenates contain substantial amounts of IGF-I activity but whether this material is yet to be secreted, internalized previously secreted material, or subserves some other function is not yet known.

All of the four breast cancer cell lines respond to nanomolar concentrations of exogenously added authentic IGF-I. In cell lines secreting large amounts of IGF-I (MDA-MB-231 and Hs578t), the response is somewhat dampened and shifted to slightly higher concentrations (5 nM), possibly as a result of rapid accumulation of endogenous IGF-I–like material.

B. Identification of Transforming Growth Factors

Human breast cancer cell lines also secrete material able to compete with the binding of ^{125}I-labeled EGF to EGF receptor on A-431 epidermal carcinoma cell membrane (Dickson et al. 1986a; Salomon et al. 1984). When MCF-7 CM is chromatographed on Biogel P60 columns, a major 30 K peak of competitive activity is obtained. Total activity in CM from estradiol-treated cells is enhanced up to 5-fold, compared with cells not treated with estradiol. Authentic ^{125}I-labeled EGF does not elute on such columns in this position. Current work is addressing the question of the mechanism and function of induction of this growth factor. Authentic exogeneously supplied EGF is capable of stimulating growth of MCF-7 cells 2- to 3-fold in defined medium. We do not know at present whether any of the EGF receptor reactive material is responsible for autocrine growth promotion in these cells.

Transforming growth factors (TGFs) are a group of peptides capable of inducing the reversible acquisition of a malignant phenotype (as assessed by anchorage-independent growth in soft agar) of some nontransformed cells (DeLarco and Todaro 1978). Two classes of activities have been tentatively described (α and β). Others clearly exist. Both α and β TGF are acid- and heat-stable peptides which are sulfhydryl reagent sensitive. TGF-α-like peptides compete with EGF for receptor binding to

EGF receptor. They contain sequence homology with EGF but are not recognized by anti-EGF antibodies. Anti-EGF receptor antibodies, which block EGF binding, block TGF activity (Carpenter et al. 1983). TGF-α alone will not induce colonies of NRK cells in soft agar without concurrent administration of a source of TGF-β. TGF-β does not bind EGF receptor. By itself it induces small colonies or clusters of NRK cells in soft agar. Coincident addition of TGF-α and -β results in large colony formation. CM from all the breast cell lines tested contains TGF-α-like activity in that in the presence of a source of TGF-β, NRK colonies were induced. Preliminary evidence demonstrates that transforming activity corresponds to EGF receptor reactive material. In MCF-7 cells, although transforming activity is detectable in CM from cells not treated with estradiol, activity is induced by 48 hours of estrogen treatment (Dickson et al. 1986a). When eluted on gel exclusion columns, one major peak of transforming activity is obtained. The peak is 30 K in apparent molecular weight. Total induction of TGF activity is approximately 5-fold by estradiol. Addition of exogenous EGF to the MCF-7 cell CM results in some enhancement of NRK colony formation. This is consistent with production of some TGF-β activity as well. Further studies characterizing the nature and regulation of these activities are under way.

One of the difficulties in assessing growth-promoting activities in the CM of breast cancer cells is that it is not clear in any given case what should be used as an indicator cell. For example, for an autocrine growth factor a homologous cell is the appropriate choice (by definition), whereas for a paracrine factor the appropriate target cell is unknown. Thus far we have mostly assessed autocrine growth-promoting activities. Fractionation of CM activity on either Sephacryl S-200 or Biogel P60 columns reveals multiple peaks of autocrine growth-promoting activities when applied to other, growth-arrested MCF-7 cells. These individual peaks are induced 2- to 8-fold in CM prepared from estrogen-treated MCF-7 cells as compared to control cells. Several of these peaks do not correspond to previously described peaks of either IGF-I or EGF receptor reactive material. We are currently attempting further characterization of these activities.

III. In Vivo *Tests of Growth Factor Activities*

As previously stated, it is generally agreed that estrogen supplementation is an absolute requirement for the continued growth of MCF-7 cells in nude mice (Shafie 1980; Soule and McGrath 1980; Seibert et al. 1983). We asked whether CM, prepared from estrogen-treated MCF-7 cells (but from which all steroidal estrogens had been removed), could function in place of an estrogen pellet to support the growth of MCF-7 cells in nude mice. Concentrated CM from estradiol-treated cells was continuously injected subcutaneously by Alzet pump into nude mice bearing inocula of MCF-7 cells and results were compared to those obtained with animals bearing estradiol pellets or injected with control medium. Tumors were consistently seen in animals receiving CM from estradiol-treated MCF-7 cells or estrogen pellets; fewer tumors developed in animals treated with control medium. These data strongly suggest to us that a critical mechanism by which estrogens can induce tumors is through the induction of secreted factors, which critically regulate either tumor growth or necessary host responses (such as angiogenesis). These data are inconsistent with a critical role for estromedins as a necessary concomitant for tumorigenesis of MCF-7 cells, because substances produced by the tumor itself in response to estrogens are sufficient for partial tumorigenesis (Dickson et al. 1986b).

IV. Future Prospects

A variety of reasons suggest that the development of specific antibodies directed against breast cancer cell secreted (or shed) proteins might be of value. Not only would such antibodies aid in identifying and characterizing specific proteins, but they might be of value as immunodiagnostics or as therapeutic agents in their own right. Concentrated, acid-extracted, conditioned medium prepared as described above has been used as an immunogen to prepare monoclonal antibodies (MAB). Following primary immunization fusion and cloning, antibody-producing clones were initially screened by enzyme-linked immunoabsorbent assay (ELISA) for differential reactivity against secreted proteins as compared to fetal calf serum proteins. MABs were selected which reacted with cell-derived proteins but were unreactive with fetal calf serum. All of the MABs obtained also fail to react with normal human serum components. Most of the MABs thus far obtained reacted with CM concentrated from all breast cancer cell lines tested. In preliminary studies, one MAB, 1F-12, appears to react with CM concentrates from ZR-75-1 and MCF-7 when these cells are stimulated by estrogen, whereas control CM from these cells is not reactive. This same MAB reacts with CM from hormone-independent Hs578t and MDA-MB-231 in the absence of hormone stimulation. The identity and regulation of antigens recognized by these MABs is under study, as is the potential activity of these MABs, either alone or in concert, for interfering with breast cancer cell growth.

In summary, human breast cancer cells secrete a variety of potent growth-regulatory substances, at least some of which are regulated by estrogens. The data suggest that some of these hormone-regulated, secretory activities are required for *in vivo* tumor formation. The idea that a critical set of control elements which are required for tumor growth are externally secreted provides an attractive potential means of altering the malignant phenotype by immunological means, a strategy currently under active investigation.

References

Aitken, S. C., and M. E. Lippman. 1980. Hormonal regulation of DNA synthesis in human breast cancer cells. In *Control mechanisms in animal cells: specific growth factors,* ed. R. Jimenez de Asuya, P. Levi-Mortalcini, R. Shields, and S. Iacobelli, 133–156. New York: Raven Press.

Aitken, S. C., and M. E. Lippman. 1982. Hormonal regulation of net DNA synthesis in MCF-7 human breast cancer cells in tissue culture. *Cancer Research* 42:1727–1735.

Allegra, J. C., and M. E. Lippman. 1978. Growth of a human breast cancer cell line in serum-free hormone supplemented medium. *Cancer Research* 38:3823–3829.

Barnes, D., and G. Sato. 1979. Growth of a human mammary tumour cell line in a serum-free medium. *Nature* (London) 281:381–389.

Bronzert, D. A., M. E. Monaco, L. Pinkus, S. Aitken, and M. E. Lippman. 1981. Purification and properties of estrogen-responsive cytoplasmic thymidine kinase from human breast cancer. *Cancer Research* 41:604–610.

Butler, W. B., W. H. Kelsey, and N. Goran. 1981. Effects of serum and insulin in the sensitivity of the human breast cancer cell line MCF-7 to estrogen and antiestrogens. *Cancer Research* 41:82–88.

Carpenter, G., C. M. Stoscheck, Y. A. Preston, and J. DeLarco. 1983. Antibodies to the epidermal growth factor receptor block the biological activities of sarcoma growth factor. *Proceedings of the National Academy of Sciences* 80:5627–5630.

Chalbos, D., F. Vignon, I. Keydar, and H. Rochefort. 1982. Estrogens stimulate cell proliferation and induce secretory proteins in a human breast cancer cell line (T47D). *Journal of Clinical Endocrinology and Metabolism* 55:276–283.

Cowan, K., M. E. Goldsmith, R. M. Levine, S. C. Aitken, E. Douglass, N. Clendeninn, A. W. Nienhuis, and M. E. Lippman. 1982. Dihydrofolate reductase gene amplification and possible rearrangement in estrogen-responsive methotrexate resistant human breast cancer cell lines. *Journal of Biological Chemistry* 257:15079–15086.

Darbre, P., J. Yates, S. Curtis, and R. J. B. King. 1983. Effect of estradiol on human breast cancer cells in culture. *Cancer Research* 43:349–354.

DeLarco, J. E., and G. J. Todaro. 1978. Growth factors from murine sarcoma virus-transformed cells. *Proceedings of the National Academy of Sciences* 75:4001–4005.

Dickson, R. B., K. K. Huff, E. M. Spencer, and M. E. Lippman. 1986a. Induction of epidermal growth factor related polypeptides by 17β-estradiol in MCF-7 human breast cancer cells. *Endocrinology* 118:138–142.

Dickson, R. B., M. McManaway, and M. E. Lippman. 1986b. Estrogen-induced growth factors of breast cancer cells partially replace estrogen to promote tumor growth. *Science* (in press).

Edwards, D. P., S. R. Murphy, and W. L. McGuire. 1980. Effects of estrogen and antiestrogen on DNA polymerase in human breast cancer. *Cancer Research* 40:1722–1726.

Huff, K. K., D. K. Kaufman, E. M. Spencer, M. E. Lippman, and R. B. Dickson. 1986. Human breast cancer cells secrete an insulin-like growth factor I–related polypeptide. *Cancer Research* (in press).

Huseby, R. A., R. M. Maloney, and C. M. McGrath. 1984. Evidence for a direct growth-stimulating effect of estradiol on human MCF-7 cells *in vivo*. *Cancer Research* 44:2654–2659.

Ikeda, R., and D. A. Sirbasku. 1984. Purification and properties of a mammary-uterine-pituitary tumor cell growth factor from pregnant sheep uterus. *Journal of Biological Chemistry* 259:4049–4064.

Jakesz, R., C. A. Smith, S. Aitken, K. K. Huff, W. Schuette, S. Shackney, and M. E. Lippman. 1984. Influence of cell proliferation and cell cycles phase on expression of estrogen receptor in MCF-7 breast cancer cells. *Cancer Research* 44:619–625.

Kasid, A., N. Davidson, E. Gelmann, and M. E. Lippman. 1986. Transcriptional control of thymidine kinase gene expression by estrogen and antiestrogens in MCF-7 human breast cancer cells. *Journal of Biological Chemistry* 261:5562–5567.

Katzenellenbogen, B. S., M. J. Norman, R. L. Eckert, S. W. Peltz, and F. W. Mangel. 1983. Bioactivities, estrogen receptor interactions, and plasminogen activator-inducing activities of tamoxifen and hydroxytamoxifen isomers in MCF-7 human breast cancer cells. *Cancer Research* 44:112–119.

Leung, B. S., S. Querski, J. S. Leung. 1982. Response to estrogen by the human mammary carcinoma cell line CAMA-1. *Cancer Research* 42:5060–5066.

Levine, R. M., E. Rubalcaba, M. E. Lippman, M. E. Goldsmith, N. Clendeninn, and K. Cowan. 1985. Effects of estrogen and tamoxifen on the regulation of dihydrofolate reductase gene expression in a human breast cancer cell line. *Cancer Research* 45:1644–1650.

Lippman, M. E. 1981. Hormonal regulation of human breast cancer cells *in vitro*. In *Hormones and breast cancer*, ed. M. C. Pike, P. K. Siiteri, and C. W. Welsch, 171–184. New York: Cold Spring Harbor Laboratory.

Lippman, M. E., and S. C. Aitken. 1980. Estrogen and antiestrogen effects on thymidine utilization by MCF-7 human breast cancer cells in tissue culture. In *Hormones and cancer. Progress in cancer research and therapy*, vol. 14, ed. S. Iacobelli, R. J. B. King, H. R. Lindner, and M. E. Lippman, 3–19. New York: Raven Press.

Lippman, M. E., G. Bolan, and K. Huff. 1976a. The effects of estrogens and antiestrogens on hormone-responsive human breast cancer in long-term tissue culture. *Cancer Research* 36:4595–4601.

Lippman, M. E., G. Bolan, and K. Huff, 1976b. Interactions of antiestrogens with human breast cancer in long-term tissue culture. *Cancer Treatment Reports* 60:1421–1429.

Lippman, M. E., S. C. Aitken, and J. C. Allegra. 1981. Regulation of growth and DNA synthesis by oestrogens and antioestrogens in human breast cancer cell lines. In *Nonsteroidal antioestrogens: molecular pharmacology and antitumour activity, ed. R. L. Sutherland and V. C. Jordan, 365–396. Sydney: Academic Press.

Natoli, C., G. Sica, V. Natoli, V. Serra, and S. Iacobelli. 1983. Two new estrogen supersensitive variants of the MCF-7 human breast cancer cell line. *Breast Cancer Research and Treatment* 3:23–32.

Page, M., J. Field, N. Everett, and C. Green. 1983. Serum regulation of the estrogen responsiveness of the human breast cancer cell line MCF-7. *Cancer Research* 43:1244–1250.

Salomon, D. S., J. A. Zweibel, S. Mozeena, M. Bano, I. Losonczy, P. Fehnel, and W. R. Kidwell. 1984. Presence of transforming growth factors in human breast cancer cells. *Cancer Research* 44:4069–4077.

Seibert, K., S. M. Shafie, T. J. Triche, J. J. Whang-Peng, S. J. O'Brien, J. H. Toney, K. K. Huff, and M. E. Lippman. 1983. Clonal variation of MCF-7 breast cancer cells *in vitro* and in athymic nude mice. *Cancer Research* 43:2223–2239.

Shafie, S. M. 1980. Estrogen and growth of breast cancer: new evidence suggests indirect action. *Science* 209:701–702.

Soule, H. D., and C. M. McGrath. 1980. Estrogen responsive proliferation of clonal human breast carcinoma cells in athymic mice. *Cancer Letters* 10:177–189.

Vignon, F., D. Derocq, M. Chambon, and H. Rochefort. 1983. Endocrinologie: les protéines oestrogéno-induites sécrétées par les cellules mammaires cancéreuses humaines MCF-7 stimulent leur proliferation. *Compte rendu de l'Académie des sciences* 296:151–156.

Weichselbaum, R. R., S. Hellman, A. Piro, J. Nore, and J. B. Little. 1978. Proliferation kinetics of a human breast cancer line *in vitro* following treatment with 17 beta-estradiol and 1-beta-D-arabinofuranosylcytosine. *Cancer Research* 38:2339–2342.

14

Different Efficacy of Antiestrogens on Estrogen-Regulated Proteins in Human Breast Cancer Cell Lines

H. Rochefort, F. Vignon, S. Bardon, F. May, and B. Westley

I. Introduction 250
II. Regulation of the 52 K Protein by Antiestrogen in MCF-7 Cells 250
III. Inefficacy of Antiestrogen in Stimulating the Accumulation
    and Transcription of a Specific Estrogen-Regulated mRNA (pS2) 251
IV. Antiestrogen-Resistant Cell Lines and Autocrine Control of
    Cell Growth 255
V. Clinical Implications 259
VI. Conclusions 260
    References 261

I. Introduction

Nonsteroidal antiestrogens bind to the estrogen receptor (ER) and inhibit the proliferation of estrogen receptor–containing cells (Lippman et al. 1976; Rochefort et al. 1984a). The mechanism whereby antiestrogens control cell growth is not fully understood, although it appears that available estrogen receptor sites are required (Coezy et al. 1982; Bardon et al. 1984). The efficacy of antiestrogens in stimulating specific protein synthesis also appears to vary according to the species, since they have been described as full antagonists in chickens, full agonists in mice, and partial agonists/antagonists in rats and humans (Sutherland and Jordan 1981).

On the basis of the results we obtained in human breast cancer cell lines, we would like to emphasize in this review that the biological activity of antiestrogens also varies according to the nature of the specifically regulated proteins being measured. In the same species and in the same cells, antiestrogens can be full antagonists for some responses (such as the secreted 52 kilodalton protein) (Westley and Rochefort 1980) and pS2 mRNA (Masiakowsky et al. 1982) and partial agonists for others (such as the progesterone receptor) (Horwitz et al. 1978). We then describe a mechanism of antiestrogen resistance in cells containing biologically responsive estrogen receptors. Finally, we discuss the relationship between the regulation of a specific secreted protein of 52 kilodaltons and the regulation of cell proliferation. A complete description of the experimental procedure can be found in the quoted papers.

II. Regulation of the 52 K Protein by Antiestrogen in MCF-7 Cells

The production of the progesterone receptor, a classic estrogen-regulated protein, is known to be partly increased by tamoxifen and other nonsteroidal antiestrogens (Horwitz et al. 1978). We have confirmed this result in the MCF-7 cells that we use. This agonistic activity of tamoxifen contrasts with its marked inhibition of cell growth, suggesting that the assay of progesterone receptor sites may not be the best index of hormone responsiveness in breast cancer. It is obvious that for clinicians concerned with breast cancer therapy and monitoring, the proteins involved in the hormonal regulation of tumor growth are the most attractive.

In the past 5 years, we have extensively studied another estrogen-regulated protein which is secreted by hormone-dependent breast cancer cells in culture. This protein is defined by its molecular weight of 52 kilodaltons (52 K protein) in denaturing conditions (Westley and Rochefort 1980). The specificity, characteristics, and possible function of this protein have been discussed in several reviews (Rochefort et al. 1984b,c; Vignon et al. 1984a,b).

When measuring the 52 K protein by SDS-PAGE after ^{35}S methionine labeling of the secreted proteins, we found that its production in the medium was not stimulated by tamoxifen or 4-hydroxytamoxifen at any of the concentrations used (Westley and Rochefort 1980) (Figs. 14.1, 14.2) and for any period of stimulation. However, these antiestrogens prevented the induction of this protein by estradiol (Fig. 14.1). The 52 K protein has now also been characterized by its reactivity with specific monoclonal antibodies raised against it (Garcia et al. 1985), and it can be quantified using a double determinant, solid phase immunoradiometric assay. The same absence of 52 K protein stimulation by tamoxifen was observed using this radioimmunoassay (M. Garcia and D. Derocq, unpublished observations).

Since no cDNA probe corresponding to this estrogen-regulated protein is currently available, we have not been able to specify the mechanism by which estrogen and antiestrogen respectively increase and prevent the production of this protein released into the medium. By contrast, the 52 K protein appears to be useful both in the clinical monitoring of breast cancer and in studying the mechanism by which estrogens regulate cell proliferation.

III. Inefficacy of Antiestrogen in Stimulating the Accumulation and Transcription of a Specific Estrogen-Regulated mRNA (pS2)

The work described in this chapter was performed in collaboration with Pierre Chambon's laboratory, which kindly provided the pS2 cDNA probe. This probe allowing the titration of an estrogen-induced mRNA pS2 (Masiakowsky et al. 1982) was used in the Northern blot analysis of poly A+ RNA preparations of MCF-7 cells treated by tamoxifen, estra-

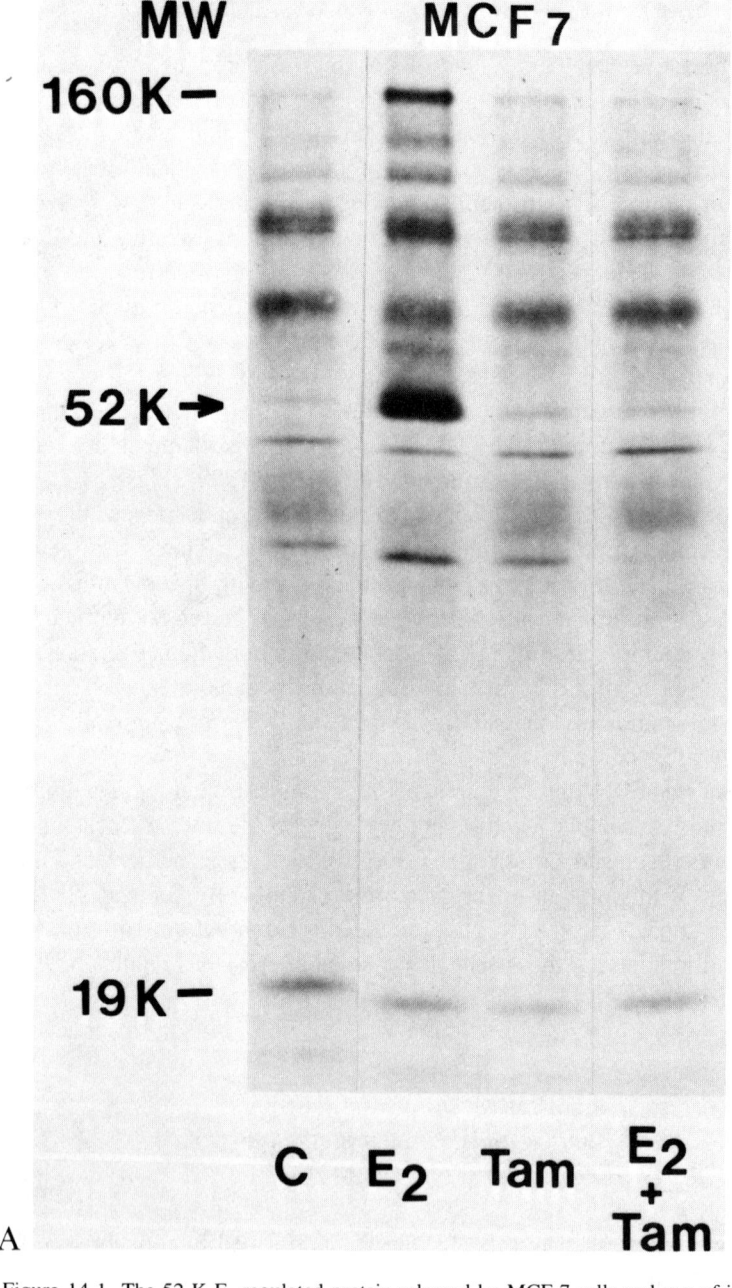

MW   MCF7

160K—

52K→

19K—

C   E₂   Tam   E₂ + Tam

A

Figure 14.1. The 52 K E_2-regulated protein released by MCF-7 cells and one of its antiestrogen-resistant variants, R27. (A) MCF-7 cells were grown in DMEM containing 10% FCS/DCC. They were then plated in 96-well microtiter plate and treated with either 1 nM E_2, 1 μM tamoxifen, E_2 + tamoxifen (1 nM + 1 μM), or with the solvent alone (control). After 2 days of treatment, the cells were labeled for 6 hours with ^{35}S-methionine. The labeled proteins of the medium were analyzed by SDS-polyacrylamide gel (15%) electro-

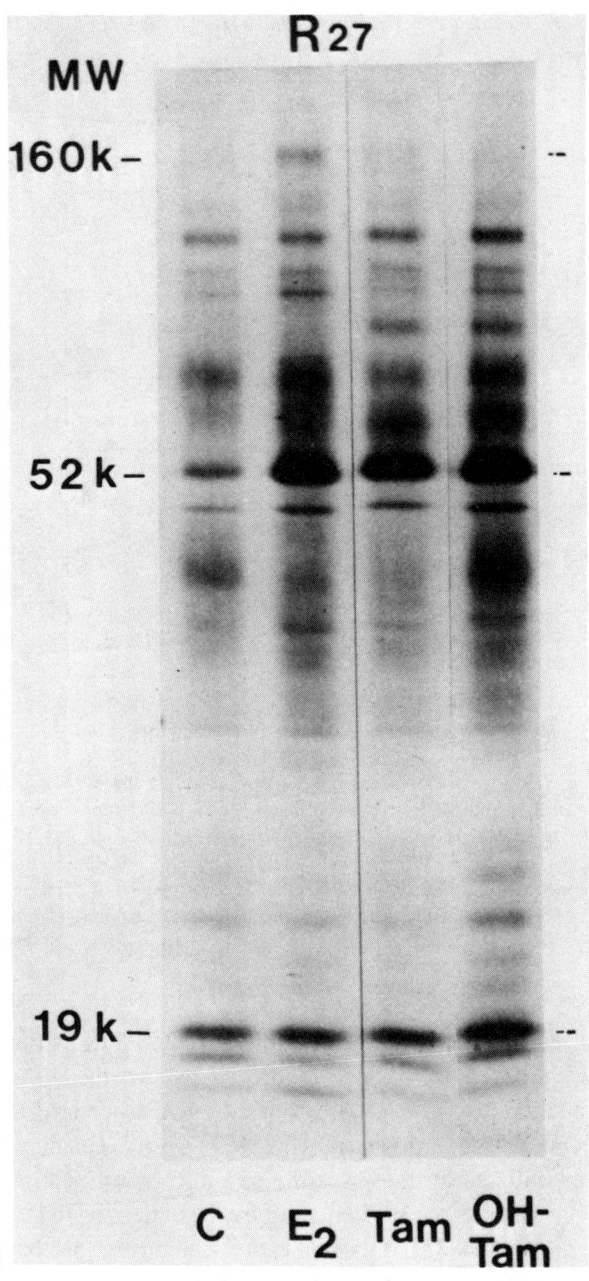

phoresis and processed for fluorography as described in Westley and Rochefort (1980). (B) Same protocol with the R27 cells. Concentrations of estradiol were 0.1 nM, 4-hydroxytamoxifen 1 nM, and tamoxifen 1 μM. The two major estradiol-regulated proteins of 52 and 160 kilodaltons are not induced by tamoxifen in MCF-7 cells (A), whereas only the 52 K protein is induced by tamoxifen and 4-hydroxytamoxifen in the R27 antiestrogen-resistant variant (B). (From Vignon et al. [1983] with the permission of the editor.)

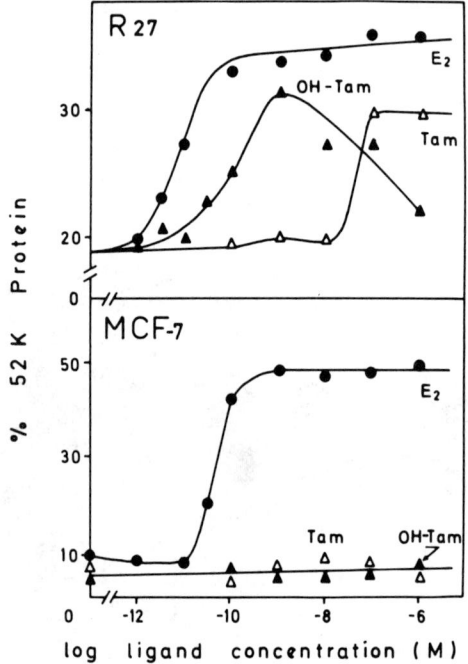

Figure 14.2. Dose-response curves for the production of the 52 K protein by E_2 and antiestrogens in R27 and MCF-7 cells. R27 and MCF-7 cells were exposed to increasing concentrations of E_2 (●) and antiestrogens (Tam, △; OH-Tam, ▲) and then labeled with ^{35}S-methionine. The secreted proteins were analyzed by SDS-PAGE. The films were developed and scanned using a Vernon densitometer. The absorbance of 52 K protein was then estimated as a percentage of the total absorbance of labeled proteins. (From Vignon et al. [1983] and Westley and Rochefort [1980] with the permission of the editors.)

diol, or untreated. The levels of pS2 mRNA could thus be quantified following these different treatments. Figure 14.3 shows the absence of a significant induction of pS2 mRNA by antiestrogen, whereas estradiol led to a 9-fold accumulation of this mRNA in MCF-7 cells. The number of RNA polymerases initiated to transcribe the pS2 mRNA was also increased by estradiol (Chambon et al. 1984) but not by the antiestrogen (Westley et al. 1984). To our knowledge, this is the first demonstration that tamoxifen has no agonistic activity on a specifically estrogen-regulated mRNA in humans. Since the induction of pS2 mRNA by estradiol is a direct transcriptional event (Brown et al. 1984), these results clearly demonstrate that the activation of the nuclear estrogen receptor–tamoxifen complex is unable to stimulate the transcription of pS2 mRNA.

Separate studies in our laboratory have shown several differences in the properties of the estrogen receptor, depending on whether it is bound to estradiol or to 4-hydroxytamoxifen. These relate to a decrease in the dissociation rate of the ligand from the hormone binding site (Rochefort and Borgna 1981), to the degree of interaction of ER with double-stranded DNA (Evans et al. 1982), and, as shown more recently, to the degree of interaction with monoclonal antibody to the calf nuclear ER (Borgna et al. 1984; Fauque et al. 1985). These results strongly suggest that ER activation is different following estrogen or antiestrogen binding. Since an additional blocking effect of antiestrogens has not been excluded, further studies are needed to relate these different conformations of the activated ER-ligand complex directly to the different capacities of these complexes for stimulating specific gene transcription.

IV. *Antiestrogen-Resistant Cell Lines and Autocrine Control of Cell Growth*

Five years ago we proposed the hypothesis that estrogens stimulate the growth of breast cancer cells via growth factors and/or mitogens, which are released into the culture medium (Rochefort et al. 1980). Since then, several experimental results have supported this hypothesis both in our laboratory and in others (Ikeda et al. 1984; Jakesz et al. 1984). Direct demonstrations of a mitogenic activity of estrogen-regulated secreted proteins (Vignon et al. 1983) and of an immunoaffinity-purified 52 K protein fraction (Vignon et al. 1986) have recently been obtained. Conversely, since tamoxifen decreases the production of secreted proteins, one can also hypothesize that one of the mechanisms by which this drug prevents cell growth is by decreasing the production of growth factor(s) (Rochefort et al. 1984c).

Results on antiestrogen-resistant cells were obtained with the collaboration of Marc Lippman, who kindly provided the R27 resistant clone (Nawata et al. 1981); of Francis Bayard, who gave us the RTx6 resistant clone; and of Pierre Chambon, who gave us the pS2 cDNA clone. These results provide additional support to our hypothesis that the 52 K protein is an estrogen-regulated glycoprotein acting as an autocrine mitogen (Vignon et al. 1984a; Westley et al. 1984). The two antiestrogen-resistant clones (R27 and RTx6) were selected for their ability to grow in the presence of 1 μM tamoxifen. Both clones contain estrogen receptors and respond to estradiol by increased progesterone receptor synthesis and in the

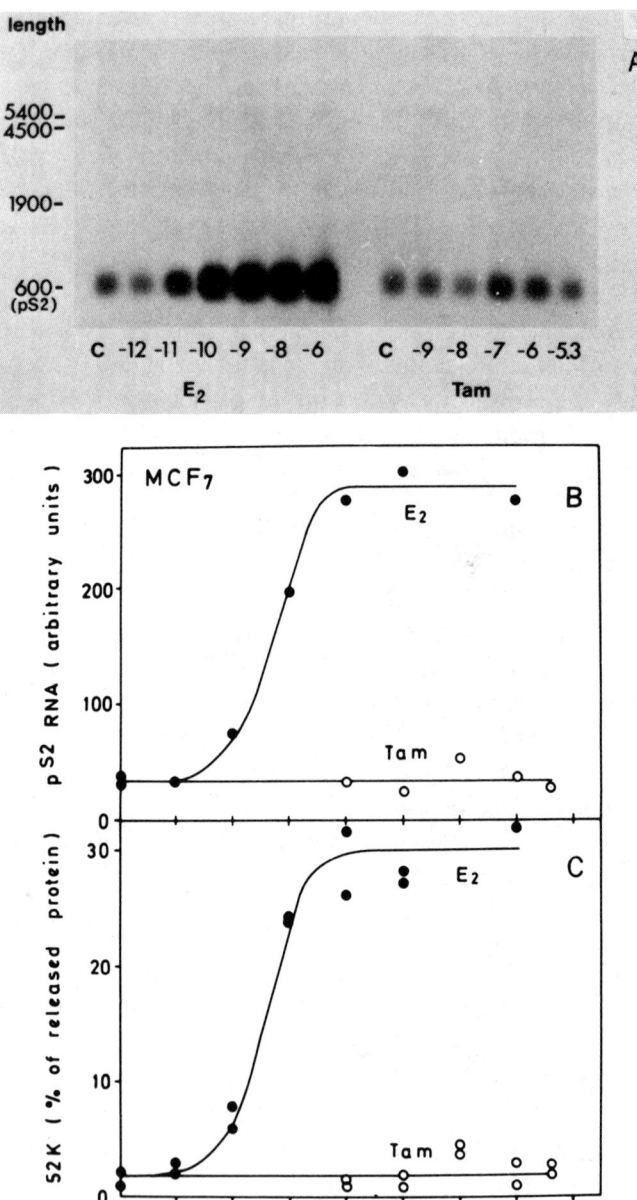

Figure 14.3. Effects of estradiol and tamoxifen on the levels of pS2 mRNA and 52 K protein in wild-type MCF-7 cells. MCF-7 cells were treated with various concentrations of

case of R27 by cell growth. However, contrary to the wild-type MCF-7 cells, they are able to grow with 1 μM tamoxifen. In these two resistant clones and in the antiestrogen-sensitive MCF-7 cells, we have quantified four estrogen-regulated parameters: the progesterone receptor sites, the pS2 mRNA, the secreted 52 K protein, and the secreted 160 K protein (Table 14.1). In all cells, tamoxifen increased the number of progesterone receptor sites, whereas it was ineffective with respect to the accumulation of pS2 mRNA in the cells and of the 160 K secreted protein in the medium (Figs. 14.3, 14.4). By contrast, a divergent effect of tamoxifen was observed in the case of the 52 K protein, since it was a full antiestrogen in the wild-type MCF-7 (Figs. 14.1, 14.2), whereas in the two antiestrogen-resistant clones, tamoxifen and 4-hydroxytamoxifen behaved as weak estrogens by inducing the 52 K protein. The activity of the two antiestrogens and of estradiol was correlated with the relative affinities of these three ligands for the ER (Fig. 14.4). Thus, tamoxifen acquired estrogenic activity in the regulation of the 52 K protein but not in the two other regulated events (pS2 and 160 K protein) (Table 14.1). The reason for this different efficacy of tamoxifen in the sensitive and resistant cell lines is unknown. It could be a discrete alteration of the estrogen receptor located on the acceptor domain but not on the estrogen binding domain. An alteration such as this could interfere with the recognition of the 52 K protein gene but not with that of other genes. It could also be the result of a modification in the localization, structure, or copy number of the gene coding the 52 K protein (Schimke 1984).

Regardless of the mechanism, these results support our hypothesis that the 52 K protein is an estrogen-induced mitogen. The 52 K protein is the only detectable estrogen-regulated protein modified when the pattern of ^{35}S methionine-labeled proteins is compared before and after tamoxifen treatment (Fig. 14.1B). It is therefore possible that MCF-7–resistant

---

estradiol (●) or tamoxifen (○) in T75 flasks (A and B) or 8 mm microwells (C). RNA was prepared from T75 flasks and assayed for pS2 mRNA by Northern blot. (A) Autoradiograph of the hybridization of ^{32}P-labeled pS2 ds-cDNA to 10 g of total RNA prepared from cells treated with the indicated concentrations of estradiol (E$_2$) or tamoxifen (Tam). (B) Relative amounts of pS2 mRNA measured by scanning the autoradiograph shown in panel A. Hybridization of the same filter with nick-translated 36B4 cDNA showed that the level of this RNA was the same in all RNA samples (not shown). (C) Amount of 52 K protein expressed as a percentage of total released proteins after scanning the fluorograph. Neither of the two estrogen-regulated responses was stimulated by tamoxifen. (From Westley et al. [1984] with the permission of the editor.)

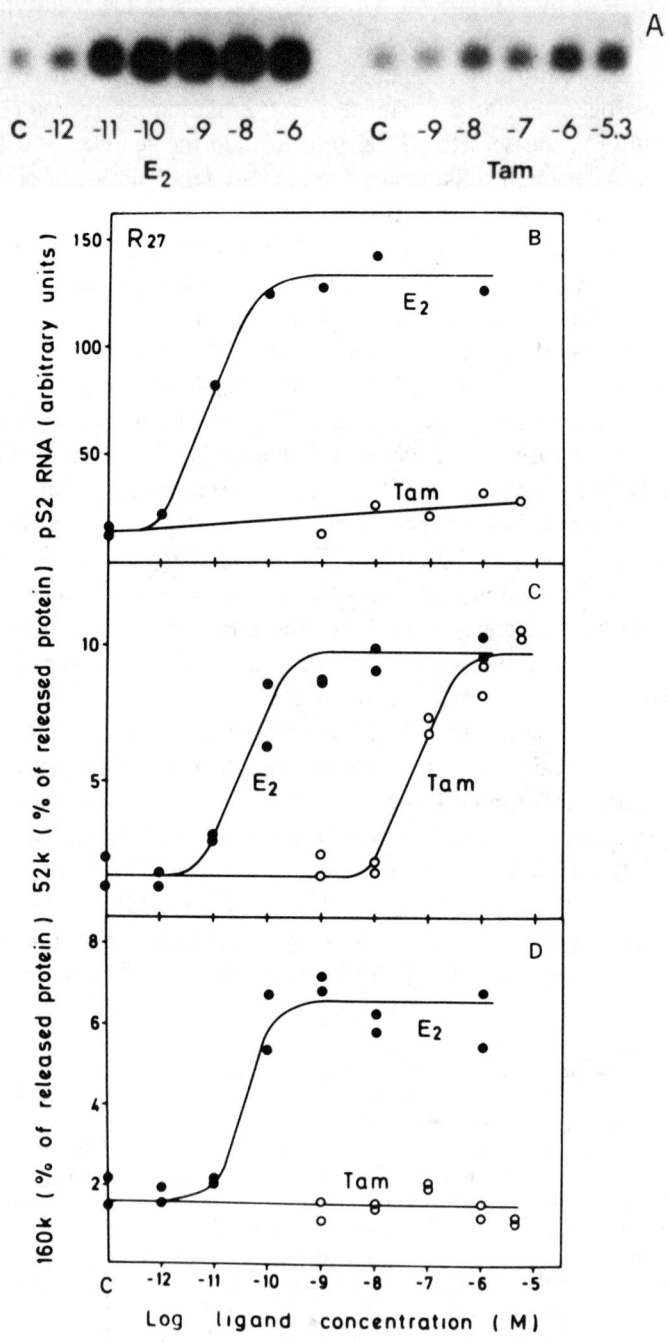

Table 14.1. Effect of tamoxifen on three estrogen receptor–positive cell lines, showing
that, in five estrogen-regulated responses in the antiestrogen-sensitive
(MCF-7) and resistant (R27 and RTx6) cell lines, only the 52 K secreted
protein behaves differently in the antiestrogen-resistant variants

	R_p	pS2 mRNA	160 K protein	52 K protein	Cell proliferation
MCF-7	+	−	−	−	Inhibition
R27 ⎱ RTx6 ⎰	+	−	−	+	Resistant

clones have been selected by their ability to produce autocrine growth factors under tamoxifen stimulation. If this is the case, tamoxifen may not only be inactive in these cells but may also be harmful by behaving as an estrogen for the production of growth factor. However, the mechanism of action of tamoxifen on cell growth may also involve additional mechanisms, as discussed previously (Rochefort et al. 1984a). For instance, an absence of antiestrogen binding sites has been proposed to explain the development of antiestrogen resistance (Faye et al. 1983). The presence of these specific antiestrogen binding sites in the R27 variant does not favor this hypothesis (Miller et al. 1984). We have also checked that tamoxifen was not metabolized differently (inactivated) in R27 cells compared to MCF-7 cells and that there was no defective entry of the drug into the resistant cells (Vignon et al. 1984b; J. L. Borgna, personal communication).

V. *Clinical Implications*

These results may have important clinical relevance, particularly for the monitoring of breast cancer patients treated by tamoxifen. Most of the metastatic ER-positive breast cancer patients with tumors who are treated

---

Figure 14.4. Effects of estradiol and tamoxifen on the induction of pS2 RNA, 52 K protein, and 160 K protein in R27 cells. R27 cells were treated with various concentrations of estradiol (●) or tamoxifen (○). pS2 mRNA levels (A) and (B), the amount of labeled 52 K (C), and 160 K (D) protein in the culture medium were determined as described in Section IV. Panel A shows an autoradiograph of the hybridization of ^{32}P-labeled pS2 ds-cDNA to the different RNA samples transferred to nitrocellulose; only the region containing pS2 RNA is shown. Only the 52 K protein is induced by tamoxifen. (From Westley et al. [1984] with the permission of the editor.)

by tamoxifen lose their responsiveness to antiestrogen therapy by developing antiestrogen resistance. A second-line endocrine therapy usually remains effective (Arafah and Pearson, Chapter 23 in this volume). It would be interesting to monitor the estrogen receptor and 52 K protein level in these patients in order to verify whether antiestrogen-resistant breast cancer R27 and RTx6 are frequently encountered in clinical practice. If this is the case, a test sensitive enough to detect antiestrogen-resistant cells at an early stage would be very useful for prognosis. In collaboration with clinical investigators, we are now carrying out studies based on the follow-up of patients treated by tamoxifen who have accessible tumoral tissue. The possible development of these antiestrogen-resistant clones during adjuvant treatment of breast cancer by tamoxifen is also being considered.

VI. Conclusions

In this short review we have discussed some aspects of the mechanism of action of the nonsteroidal antiestrogen tamoxifen, currently used in the treatment of breast cancer. The approach we used was to measure estrogen-specific responses in estrogen-responsive human breast cancer cell lines. In one response, the progesterone receptor is stimulated by tamoxifen, whereas in three other responses, the 52 K protein, 160 K protein, and pS2 mRNA, they are not induced by tamoxifen. Thus, tamoxifen behaves like a full estrogen antagonist in human MCF-7 cells if the last three responses are considered, whereas it behaves like a partial agonist/ antagonist with respect to the progesterone receptor response.

The work on pS2 mRNA transcription indicates, for the first time in humans, that tamoxifen is inactive in stimulating the transcription of estrogen-regulated responses. This was previously shown by Palmiter et al. (1977) on the ovalbumin gene in the chicken oviduct. The measurement of these estrogen-regulated responses in two antiestrogen-resistant variants of MCF-7 cells indicates that the 52 K protein is activated by tamoxifen. This provides a possible explanation for the mechanism of antiestrogen resistance in estrogen receptor–positive breast cancer, whereby the tamoxifen–estrogen receptor complex becomes active, like the estradiol–estrogen receptor complex, in stimulating the production of the 52 K protein, which acts as an estrogen-regulated autocrine mitogen.

Other studies based on the mitogenic activity of conditioned media (Vignon et al. 1983) and of purified 52 K protein (Vignon et al. 1986) strongly support this hypothesis.

Acknowledgments

This work was supported by the Institut National de la Santé et de la Recherche Médicale, the University of Montpellier, and the Fondation pour la Recherche Médicale Française; the paper was presented at the workshop on Estrogen and Antiestrogen Action in Madison, Wisconsin, June 26–29, 1984. We are grateful to Dr. Pierre Chambon (INSERM U 184, Faculté de Médecine, Institut de Chimie Biologique, 11 Rue Humann, 67085 Strasbourg, France) for the pS2 cDNA clone; Dr. Francis Bayard (INSERM U 168, Clinique Obstétricale, Hôpital de la Grave, 31052 Toulouse; France) for RTx6 cells; to the Michigan Cancer Foundation for MCF-7 cells; and to Dr. Marc Lippman (Medical Breast Cancer Section, Medicine Branch, National Institutes of Health (NIH), Bethesda, Maryland 20014) for R27 cells. We would also like to thank C. Prebois for technical assistance and M. Egea for preparing the manuscript.

References

Bardon, S., F. Vignon, D. Derocq, and H. Rochefort. 1984. The antiproliferative effect of tamoxifen in breast cancer cells: mediation by the estrogen receptor. *Molecular and Cellular Endocrinology* 35:2162–2168.

Borgna, J. L., J. Fauque, and H. Rochefort. 1984. A monoclonal antibody to the estrogen receptor discriminates between the inactive and activated estrogen and antiestrogen-receptor complexes. *Biochemistry* 23:2162–2168.

Brown, A. M. C., J. M. Jeltsch, M. Roberts, and P. Chambon. 1984. Activation of pS2 gene transcription is a primary response to estrogen in the human breast cancer cell line MCF-7. *Proceedings of the National Academy of Sciences* 81:6344–6348.

Chambon, P., A. Dierich, M. P. Gaub, S. Jakowlev, J. Jongstra, A. Krust, J. P. LePennec, P. Oudet, and T. Reudelhuber. 1984. Promoter elements of genes coding for proteins and modulation of transcription by estrogens and progesterone. In *The proceedings of the Laurentian Hormone Conference. Recent progress in hormone research*, vol. 40, ed. R. O. Greep, 1–40. New York: Academic Press.

Coezy, E., J. L. Borgna, and H. Rochefort. 1982. Tamoxifen and metabolites in MCF-7 cells: correlation between binding to estrogen receptor and inhibition of cell growth. *Cancer Research* 42:317–323.

Evans, E., P. P. Baskevitch, and H. Rochefort. 1982. Estrogen receptor DNA interaction: difference between activation by estrogen and antiestrogen. *European Journal of Biochemistry* 128:185–191.

Fauque, J., J. L. Borgna, and H. Rochefort. 1985. Activation of the estrogen receptor by estrogen and antiestrogen. Inhibition by a monoclonal antibody to the receptor. *Journal of Biological Chemistry* 260:15547–15553.

Faye, J. C., S. Jozan, G. Redeuilh, E. E. Baulieu, and F. Bayard. 1983. Physicochemical and genetic evidence for specific antiestrogen binding sites. *Proceedings of the National Academy of Sciences* 80:3158–3162.

Garcia, M., F. Capony, D. Derocq, D. Simon, B. Pau, and H. Rochefort. 1985. Monoclonal antibodies to the estrogen-regulated M_r 52,000 glycoprotein: characterization and immunodetection in MCF-7 cells. *Cancer Research* 45:709–716.

Horwitz, K. B., Y. Koseki, and W. L. McGuire. 1978. Estrogen control of progesterone receptor in human breast cancer: role of estradiol and antiestrogen. *Endocrinology* 103:1742–1751.

Ikeda, T., D. Danielpour, and D. A. Sirbasku. 1984. Isolation and properties of endocrine and autocrine type mammary tumor cell growth factors (estromedins). In *Hormones and cancer 2. Progress in cancer research and therapy,* vol. 31, ed. F. Bresciani, R. J. B. King, M. E. Lippman, M. Namer, and J. P. Raynaud, 171–186. New York: Raven Press.

Jakesz, R., C. A. Smith, K. Huff, S. Aitken, W. Schuette, S. Shackney, and M. E. Lippman. 1984. Influence of cell proliferation and cell cycle phase on expression of estrogen receptor in MCF-7 breast cancer cells. *Cancer Research* 44:619–625.

Lippman, M., G. Bolan, and K. Huff. 1976. The effects of estrogens and antiestrogens on hormone-responsive human breast cancer in long-term tissue culture. *Cancer Research* 36:4595–4601.

Masiakowski, P., R. Breathnach, J. Bloch, F. Gannon, A. Krust, and P. Chambon. 1982. Cloning of cDNA sequences of hormones-regulated genes from the MCF-7 human breast cancer cell line. *Nucleic Acids Research* 10:7895–7903.

Miller, M. A., M. E. Lippman, and B. S. Katzenellenbogen. 1984. Antiestrogen binding in antiestrogen growth-resistant estrogen-responsive clonal variants of MCF-7 human breast cancer cells. *Cancer Research* 44:5038–5045.

Nawata, H., D. Bronzert, and M. E. Lippman. 1981. Isolation and characterization of a tamoxifen-resistant cell line derived from MCF-7 human breast cancer cells. *Journal of Biological Chemistry* 256:5016–5021.

Palmiter, R. D., E. R. Mulvihill, G. S. McKnight, and A. W. Senear. 1977. Regulation of gene expression in the chick oviduct by steroid hormones. *Cold Spring Harbor Symposia on Quantitative Biology* 42:639–647.

Rochefort, H., and J. L. Borgna. 1981. Differences between the activation of the estrogen receptor by estrogen and by antiestrogen. *Nature* (London) 292:257–259.

Rochefort, H., E. Coezy, E. Joly, B. Westley, and F. Vignon. 1980. Hormonal control of breast cancer in cell culture. In *Hormones and cancer. Progress in cancer research and therapy,* vol. 14, ed. S. Iacobelli, R. J. B. King, H. R. Lindner, and M. E. Lippman, 21–29. New York: Raven Press.

Rochefort, H., S. Bardon, D. Chalbos, and F. Vignon. 1984a. Steroidal and nonsteroidal antiestrogen breast cancer cells in culture. *Journal of Steroid Biochemistry* 20:105–110.

Rochefort, H., F. Capony, M. Garcia, O. Massot, F. May, F. Veith, F. Vignon, and B. Westley. 1984b. The 52 K estrogen regulated protein secreted by human mammary cancer. In *Endocrinology,* ed. F. Labrie and L. Proulx, 443–446. *Proceedings of the Seventh International Congress of Endocrinology,* Excerpta Medica International Congress Series 655. Amsterdam: Elsevier.

Rochefort, H., D. Chalbos, F. Capony, M. Garcia, F. Veith, F. Vignon, and B. Westley. 1984c. Effect of estrogen in breast cancer cells in culture: released proteins and control of cell proliferation. In *Hormones and cancer. Progress in clinical and biological research,* vol. 142, ed. E. Gurpide, R. Calandra, C. Levy, and R. J. Soto, 37–51. New York: Alan R. Liss.

Schimke, R. T. 1984. Gene amplification in cultured animal cells. *Cell* 37:705–713.

Sutherland, R. L., and V. C. Jordan (eds.). 1981. *Non-steroidal antioestrogens: molecular pharmacology and antitumour activity.* Sydney: Academic Press.

Vignon, F., D. Derocq, M. Chambon, and H. Rochefort. 1983. Endocrinologie: les protéines oestrogéno-induites sécrétées par les cellules mammaires cancéreuses humaines MCF-7 stimulent leur proliferation. *Compte rendu de l'Académie des sciences* 296:151–156.

Vignon, F., F. Capony, D. Chalbos, M. Garcia, F. Veith, B. Westley, and H. Rochefort. 1984a. Estrogen regulated 52 K protein and control of cell proliferation of human breast cancer cells. In *Hormones and cancer 2. Progress in cancer research and therapy,* vol. 31, ed. F. Bresciani, R. J. B. King, M. E. Lippman, M. Namer, and J. P. Raynaud, 147–160. New York: Raven Press.

Vignon, F., M. E. Lippman, H. Nawata, D. Derocq, and H. Rochefort. 1984b. Induction of two estrogen-responsive proteins by antiestrogens in R27, a tamoxifen resistant clone of MCF-7 cells. *Cancer Research* 44:2084–2088.

Vignon, F., F. Capony, M. Chambon, G. Freiss, M. Garcia, and H. Rochefort. 1986. Autocrine growth stimulation of the MCF-7 breast cancer cells by the estrogen-regulated 52 K protein. *Endocrinology* 118:1537–1545.

Westley, B., and H. Rochefort. 1980. A secreted glycoprotein induced by estrogen in human breast cancer cell lines. *Cell* 20:352–362.

Westley, B., F. E. B. May, A. M. C. Brown, A. Krust, P. Chambon, M. E. Lippman, and H. Rochefort. 1984. Effects of antiestrogens on the estrogen regulated pS2 RNA, 52 kDa and 160 kDa proteins in MCF-7 cells and two tamoxifen resistant sublines. *Journal of Biological Chemistry* 259:10030–10035.

15

Effects of Antiestrogens on Cell Cycle Progression

ROBERT L. SUTHERLAND, ROGER R. REDDEL,
LEIGH C. MURPHY, AND IAN W. TAYLOR

I.	INTRODUCTION	266
II.	EFFECTS ON ASYNCHRONOUS CELLS	266
III.	EFFECTS ON SYNCHRONOUS CELLS	269
IV.	CELLULAR SELECTIVITY	271
V.	STRUCTURE-ACTIVITY RELATIONSHIPS	273
VI.	TAMOXIFEN STIMULATION	276
VII.	CONCLUSIONS	278
	REFERENCES	279

I. *Introduction*

ΓHE availability in recent years of several authentic human mammary carcinoma cell lines (Engel and Young 1978) has facilitated studies on the control of breast cancer cell proliferation by a number of natural and synthetic compounds. Since many human breast cancers show degrees of hormone dependence and hormone responsiveness *in vivo,* cell culture systems *in vitro* have helped to identify which hormones are involved in the control of replication of these cells.

Although it has long been appreciated that estrogens play an important role in the growth of human breast cancers, it was not until the mid-1970s that Lippman and his colleagues first demonstrated that estrogens had a direct effect on the growth of MCF-7 cells in culture (Lippman and Bolan 1975; Lippman et al. 1976).

After tamoxifen was successfully introduced for the treatment of advanced breast cancer, many researchers mounted laboratory studies to ascertain the molecular basis of the antitumor activity of this and other structurally related nonsteroidal antiestrogens. Cultures of human breast cancer cell lines have proven to be valuable experimental systems for such studies. In our laboratory we have used this model to investigate the cell cycle kinetic effects of antiestrogens, the cellular selectivity of responsiveness to these drugs, and the relationship between antiestrogen structure and antiproliferative activity. This chapter summarizes some of the studies that have emanated from this laboratory (Green et al. 1981; Sutherland and Taylor 1981; Murphy and Sutherland 1983, 1984; Reddel and Sutherland 1983, 1984; Reddel et al. 1983, 1984, 1985; Sutherland et al. 1983a, b,c,d, 1984; Taylor et al. 1983).

II. *Effects on Asynchronous Cells*

When estrogen receptor–positive (ER +) human breast cancer cell lines are treated with tamoxifen, their growth rate is affected in a time- and concentration-dependent manner (Fig. 15.1). In addition, the sensitivity of a particular cell line is markedly influenced by the *in vitro* culture conditions and the growth phase of the cells (Sutherland et al. 1983b; Reddel

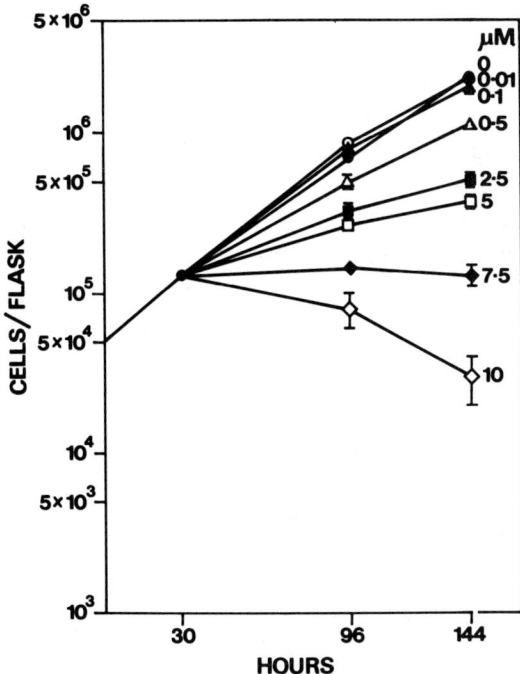

Figure 15.1. Effects of tamoxifen on the growth of MCF-7 cells. After 30 hours of exponential growth, cells were treated with various concentrations of tamoxifen. Drug-containing medium was replenished daily and cells were harvested and counted at 96 and 144 hours. Data points represent the mean ± SEM of triplicate flasks from two experiments (n = 6). (From Reddel et al. 1983.)

et al. 1984). When cells are cultured in medium supplemented with 5% fetal calf serum (FCS), concentrations of tamoxifen below 10 μM cause a dose-dependent inhibition of cell proliferation in the presence of a constant death rate, since in this dose range tamoxifen decreases growth rate but has no effect on clonogenic survival (Sutherland et al. 1983b).

Studies employing the technique of analytical DNA flow cytometry have illustrated that the tamoxifen-induced decrease in breast cancer cell proliferation rate is associated with an accumulation of cells in the G_0/G_1 phase of the cell cycle. This observation, first described by workers from this laboratory (Green et al. 1981; Sutherland and Taylor 1981; Sutherland et al. 1983a,b,d), was subsequently confirmed by others (Benz et al. 1983; Osborne et al. 1983, 1984; Lykkesfeldt et al. 1984). In an attempt to understand the kinetic basis of this G_0/G_1 accumulation further detailed experiments were carried out on the MCF-7 cell line. Studies employing stathmokinetic techniques revealed that this cell line contained two sub-populations of cells with markedly different G_1 transit times (Sutherland et al. 1983b). The "rapidly" cycling pool had a mean $t_{1/2}$ of efflux from G_1 phase of 2.3 hours, whereas in the "slowly" cycling pool the rate of efflux from G_1 was about 10-fold slower, i.e., $t_{1/2}$ of about 29 hours.

When MCF-7 cells were treated with increasing concentrations of tamoxifen, the rate of efflux of cells from the G_1 phase was reduced in a concentration-dependent fashion (Fig. 15.2). The predominant effect of tamoxifen appeared to be to shift cells from the "rapidly" cycling pool to the "slowly" cycling pool, with the net effect of increasing the mean cell cycle transit time mainly because of an increased G_1 phase duration (Sutherland et al. 1983b). It should be noted, however, that we currently have

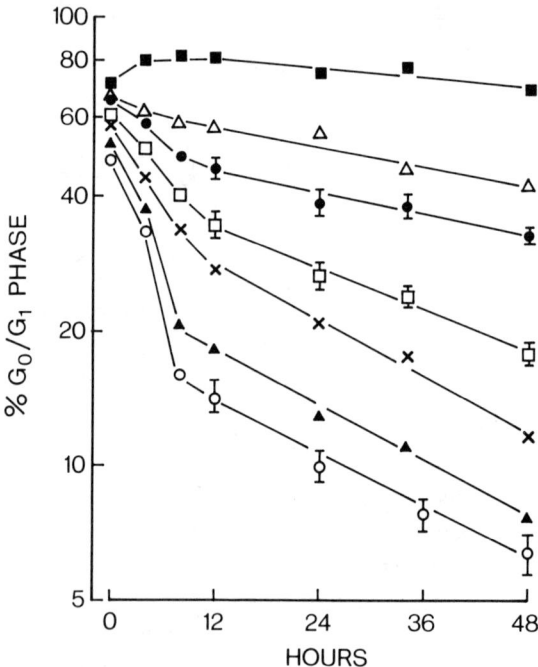

Figure 15.2. Effect of tamoxifen treatment on the rate of efflux of MCF-7 cells from the G_0/G_1 phase of the cell cycle. Exponentially growing cells were treated with tamoxifen for 42 hours and then ICRF 159 was added at zero time to block the re-entry of cell into G_1 phase. The proportion of the cell population remaining in G_0/G_1 phase was calculated from DNA histograms obtained by flow cytometry. Tamoxifen concentrations were: control (○), 100 (▲), 500 nM (x), 1 (□), 5 (●), 7.5 (△) and 10 μM (■). (From Sutherland et al. 1983.)

no information on the rate of passage of "slowly" cycling cells through S and G_2 + M phases of the cell cycle and the effects of tamoxifen on these parameters.

Together these data provide a rational kinetic explanation for the G_0/G_1 phase accumulation measured by DNA flow cytometry and the decreased growth rate observed after tamoxifen treatment of exponentially growing MCF-7 cells.

III. Effects on Synchronous Cells

Further studies, using MCF-7 cells synchronized by mitotic selection, confirmed the observations made with asynchronous populations (Taylor et al. 1983). As illustrated in Figure 15.3, those tamoxifen-treated cells that traversed the first cell cycle following mitotic selection did so at about the same rate as the untreated control population. These cells constituted the "rapidly" cycling pool. The major difference between the tamoxifen-treated and the untreated populations was not the rate at which cells traversed the cell cycle but the proportion of the total population that was able to do so. Such a result agrees with the previous suggestion, based on stathmokinetic studies of asynchronous populations, that the predominant effect of tamoxifen is to shift cells from a "rapidly" cycling to a "slowly" cycling pool. In the experiment presented in Figure 15.3, the cells in the "slowly" cycling pool are those cells remaining in G_1 phase when the proportion of cells in this phase reached its nadir at 12–16 hours, i.e., 18% for control cultures and approximately 40% for tamoxifen-treated cells.

Another series of experiments, which involved exposing synchronized cultures to 2-hour pulses of tamoxifen, illustrated that the effects of tamoxifen on cell cycle progression were confined predominantly to a 2–4-hour period in mid-G_1 phase (Taylor et al. 1983). These data added further support to the conclusion that tamoxifen is a cell cycle phase–specific growth-inhibitory agent in ER+ human breast cancer cells.

In addition to the growth-inhibitory effects discussed above, tamoxifen also demonstrated cytotoxicity when administered to MCF-7 cells at concentrations > 7.5 μM (Murphy and Sutherland 1983, 1985; Reddel et al. 1983, 1984, 1985; Sutherland et al. 1983a,b; Taylor et al. 1983). In all ER+ cell lines studied, this effect was accompanied by similar cell cycle kinetic changes, i.e., a further decrease in the percentage of S phase cells

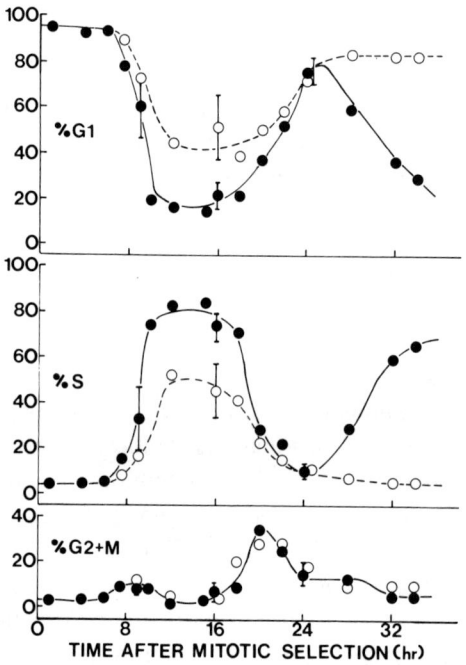

Figure 15.3. Effect of tamoxifen on the cell cycle distribution of MCF-7 cells with time after mitotic selection. Cells were synchronized by mitotic selection and then plated into flasks containing medium without drug (●) or medium containing 7.5 μM tamoxifen (○). Flasks were harvested at the times indicated and the cell cycle phase distribution calculated from DNA histograms obtained by flow cytometry. (From Taylor et al. 1983.)

and an increase in the proportion of G_1 phase cells (Reddel et al. 1985). Furthermore, studies with synchronized MCF-7 cells illustrated that, like the effect on cell cycle progression, the high-dose cytotoxic effect of tamoxifen was restricted to a specific period within the G_1 phase (Taylor et al. 1983).

Taken together, these cell cycle kinetic data, which are summarized schematically in Figure 15.4, illustrate that tamoxifen is a cell cycle phase–specific, growth-inhibitory, and cytotoxic agent acting at a very precise period in the G_1 phase of ER + human breast cancer cells. The apparent precision of the insult induced by tamoxifen, coupled with its reduced effect on cells outside the critical 2–4-hour period, suggests that tamoxifen controls some fundamental biochemical process critical in cell cycle regulation.

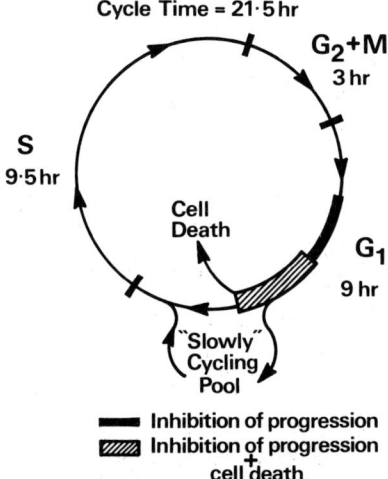

Figure 15.4. Schematic representation of the effects of tamoxifen on the cell cycle of MCF-7 cells. Cell cycle phase durations were determined from synchronized cell populations (Taylor et al. 1983). Tamoxifen acts predominantly during a specific time interval in mid-G$_1$ phase of the cell cycle. Lower concentrations of tamoxifen cause the cells to enter the "slowly" cycling pool, thus increasing their overall cell cycle transit time and decreasing the proliferation rate. Higher concentrations cause cells to embark upon a pathway that leads to cell death.

IV. Cellular Selectivity

It has been well documented that ER + human breast tumors have a considerably higher response rate to tamoxifen therapy than do estrogen receptor–negative (ER −) tumors (McGuire 1978). However, many ER + tumors fail to respond, whereas almost 10% of ER − tumors have been reported to show responsiveness (Seibert and Lippman 1982). To determine whether there are qualitative and/or quantitative differences in the response of human breast cancer cell lines to tamoxifen *in vitro*, we studied the effect of the drug on the proliferation kinetics of several ER + and ER − breast cancer cell lines. The concentrations of ER and antiestrogen binding sites (AEBS) were measured concurrently in an attempt to correlate these parameters with responsiveness (Reddel et al. 1985).

In ER + cell lines, a cell cycle phase–specific growth-inhibitory effect was seen with ID$_{20}$ values from < 0.1 to 1.0 μM (Fig. 15.5A). Within this group of cell lines, the degree of tamoxifen-induced inhibition of

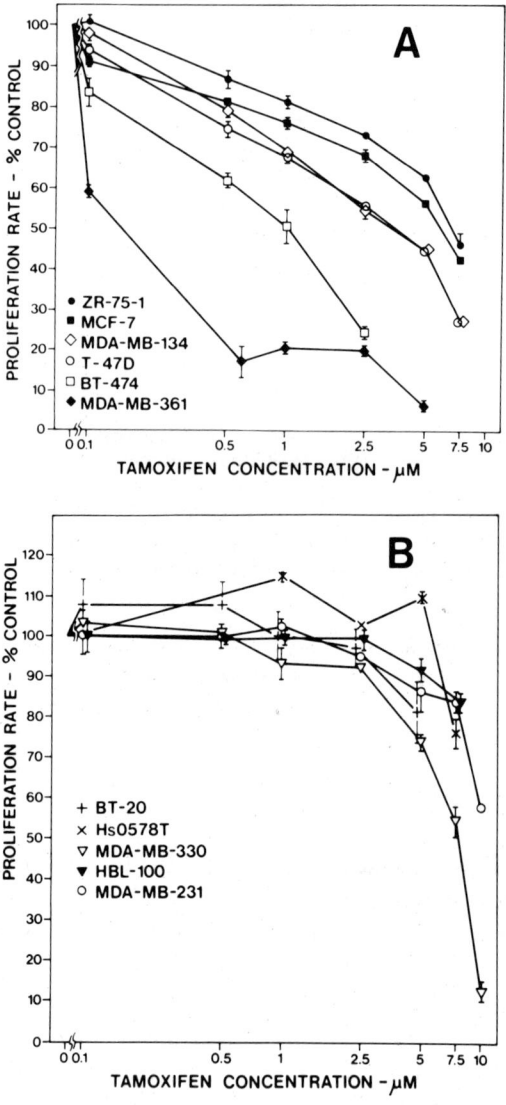

Figure 15.5. Effect of tamoxifen on the mean cellular proliferation rates of human breast cell lines. Cells were treated with various doses of tamoxifen, viable cell numbers were recorded after approximately four population doublings of control cultures, and the cell proliferation rate calculated. (A) ER+ lines; (B) ER− lines. Data points are the mean ± SEM for triplicate flasks. (From Reddel et al. 1985.)

growth correlated with the control population doubling time, but not with the ER or AEBS concentrations (Reddel et al. 1985). The changes in cell cycle kinetic parameters characteristic of all ER + lines were a decrease in the percentage of S phase cells and a corresponding increase in the percentage of G_0/G_1 phase cells (Fig. 15.6A).

In both ER + and ER − cell lines, 5–12.5 μM tamoxifen caused cytotoxicity and this was shown to be estrogen-irreversible. In ER + lines, grown in medium supplemented with 5–10% FCS, the cell cycle kinetic changes associated with cytotoxicity were similar to those accompanying growth inhibition (Reddel et al. 1983, 1984, 1985; Sutherland et al. 1983b), i.e., decreased proportions of S phase cells and G_0/G_1 phase accumulation. The cell cycle effects of tamoxifen in three ER − cell lines (Hs0578T, MDA-MB-231, MDA-MB-330) were increased proportions of S and G_2 + M phase cells with a decrease in the proportion of G_0/G_1 phase cells (Fig. 15.6B). These results implied that the mechanisms by which tamoxifen affects cell growth differ between ER + and these ER − breast cancer cells. However, in the ER − cell line BT-20, growth inhibition and cytotoxicity were associated with a slight decrease in the percentage of S phase cells (Fig. 15.6B), whereas in HBL-100 cells no changes in cell cycle kinetic parameters were observed (Fig. 15.6B). Thus, unlike the situation with ER + cell lines, tamoxifen-induced changes in cell cycle kinetics were not consistent within this group of ER − cell lines.

These results confirm that ER + breast cancer cells are more sensitive than ER − breast cancer cells to the growth-inhibitory effects of tamoxifen (5- to 75-fold in this study) and demonstrate that in all ER + cells, growth inhibition and cytotoxicity are accompanied by characteristic changes in cell cycle kinetic parameters. Different mechanisms are likely to be involved in tamoxifen action on ER − cells, with possible variation between different ER − lines as evidenced by the lack of uniform cell cycle changes within this group.

V. Structure-Activity Relationships

In an attempt to gain some insight into the role of ER in mediating the effects of antiestrogens on cell growth and cell cycle kinetics in ER + breast cancer, experiments were undertaken with a series of antiestrogens with differing affinities for ER. Since it had been previously demonstrated that the predominant effect of tamoxifen was to inhibit cell cyle progression in G_1 and thereby limit the proportion of cells entering S phase, it

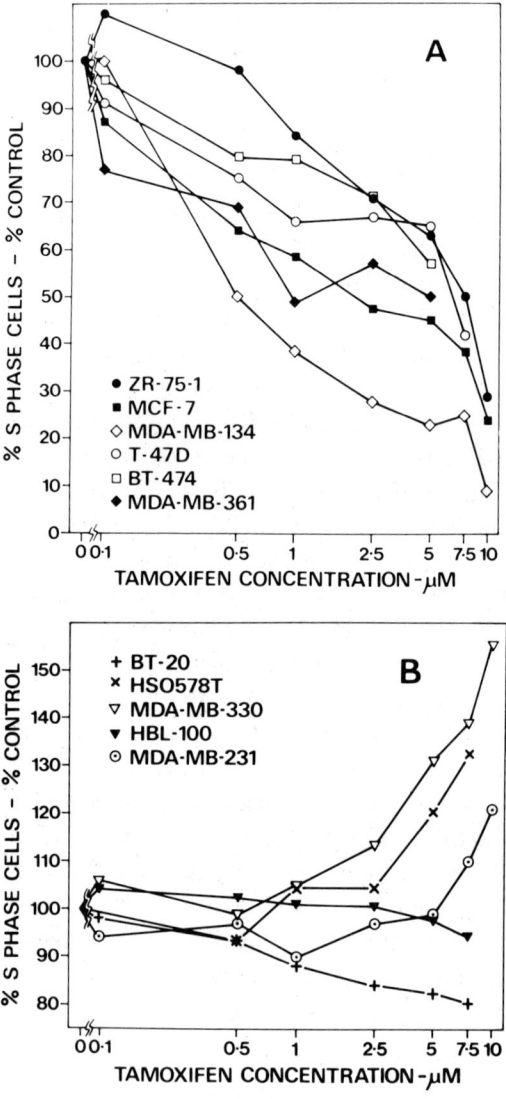

Figure 15.6. Effect of tamoxifen on the percentage of human breast cells in S phase of the cell cycle. Cells were treated as in Figure 15.5 and DNA histograms obtained by flow cytometry. Percentage of S phase cells was computed from these data and is expressed as a percentage of the value in control cultures. (A) ER + lines; (B) ER − lines. (From Reddel et al. 1985.)

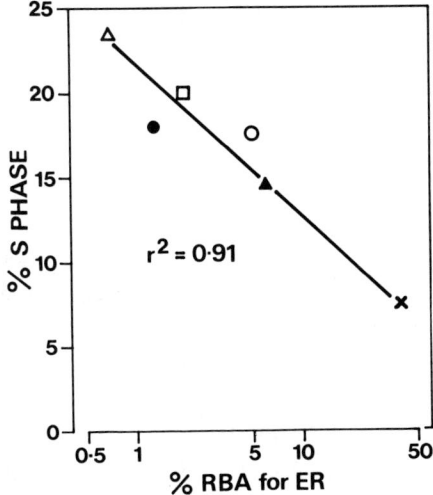

Figure 15.7. Relationship between the relative binding affinity of antiestrogens for the estrogen receptor and the percentage of cells in S phase of the cell cyle following antiestrogen treatment. Exponentially growing MCF-7 cells were exposed to 1 μM of the following antiestrogens for 6 days: tamoxifen (●), clomiphene (□), 6866 (▲), 9599 (△), 10222 (○), LY 117018 (x). Cells were harvested and the percentage of S phase cells calculated from DNA histograms obtained by flow cytometry. Relative binding affinities are from Murphy and Sutherland (1983).

was hypothesized that if this was an ER-mediated event one would find an inverse relationship between affinity for ER and the proportion of the total cell population in S phase; in other words, at a fixed concentration, ligands with high affinity for ER would be more effective at inhibiting cell cycle progression. When this hypothesis was tested by treating MCF-7 cells with six different antiestrogens having markedly different affinities for ER, and measuring the growth rate and percentage of S phase cells after 6 days, there was a highly significant negative correlation between affinity for ER and growth rate and between affinity for ER and percentage of S phase cells (Fig. 15.7). These data support the concept that estrogens and antiestrogens compete for a common event which regulates the rate of cell proliferation by controlling the rate at which cells leave G_1 phase.

Although this is an attractive hypothesis compatible with the current understanding of the effects of estrogens on cell growth and cell cycle kinetics (Sutherland et al. 1983c), it is complicated by two other observations made in this laboratory. First, we have previously shown that not all the effects of tamoxifen are reversed by simultaneous administration of estradiol to breast cancer cells (Murphy and Sutherland 1983, 1985; Reddel et al. 1983, 1984, 1985; Sutherland et al. 1983a,b), and second, we have demonstrated that antiestrogenic ligands with identical affinities for ER are not always equipotent in inhibiting breast cancer cell growth (Murphy and Sutherland 1983, 1985).

Although we have consistently demonstrated antiestrogen effects on breast cancer cell growth that are not reversed by estradiol, these effects occurred in the higher concentration range, i.e., > 5 μM tamoxifen. Since we know nothing of the mechanisms through which these effects are mediated, nor do we know what relationship concentrations of tamoxifen > 5 μM *in vitro* bear to the intratumor concentrations in patients receiving chronic tamoxifen therapy, the subject of the estrogen irreversibility will not be discussed further.

Two recent studies, in which the effects of various analogs of the antiestrogens clomiphene and tamoxifen on MCF-7 cell proliferation were investigated, revealed further interesting information on the relationship between structure and antiproliferative activity *in vitro* (Murphy and Sutherland 1983, 1985). In both studies we were able to identify analogs with similar or identical affinity for ER but markedly different affinities for the microsomal AEBS (Sutherland and Foo 1979; Sutherland and Murphy 1980; Sutherland et al. 1980; Murphy and Sutherland 1981; Watts et al. 1984). Interestingly, those ligands with enhanced affinity for AEBS were significantly more potent growth-inhibitory agents than their counterparts, with reduced (Murphy and Sutherland 1983) or no (Murphy and Sutherland 1985) affinity for this site. The simplest explanation for these results is that enhanced affinity for AEBS ensures a higher intracellular concentration of drug, which is then available for binding to ER, but other mechanisms may also be involved. These interesting and controversial observations require further investigation.

VI. *Tamoxifen Stimulation*

Nonsteroidal antiestrogens have long been known to be partial estrogen agonists/partial antagonists in a number of mammalian estrogen target tissues (Jordan 1976) and there have now been several reports of antiestrogens stimulating mammary tumor growth both in experimental animals (Gallez et al. 1973; Watson et al. 1981) and in humans (McIntosh and Thyme 1977; Legault-Poisson et al. 1979). It was therefore of considerable interest to test whether tamoxifen could stimulate cell proliferation *in vitro* and, if so, what cell cycle kinetic changes were associated with stimulation.

Since we had previously demonstrated a small but significant increase in the growth of T47D cells cultured in medium supplemented with 10% charcoal-stripped FCS (Reddel et al. 1984), we investigated the effects of various concentrations of tamoxifen and estradiol on this cell line when it was cultured in normal FCS or in FCS depleted of steroids by charcoal treatment (Reddel and Sutherland 1984). As can be seen from the data presented in Figure 15.8, both tamoxifen and estradiol were able to stimulate cell proliferation of T47D cells grown in steroid-depleted medium (Fig. 15.8A). Estradiol was consistently more potent, and both ligands had maximal effects at 10^{-9} M despite their different affinities for ER.

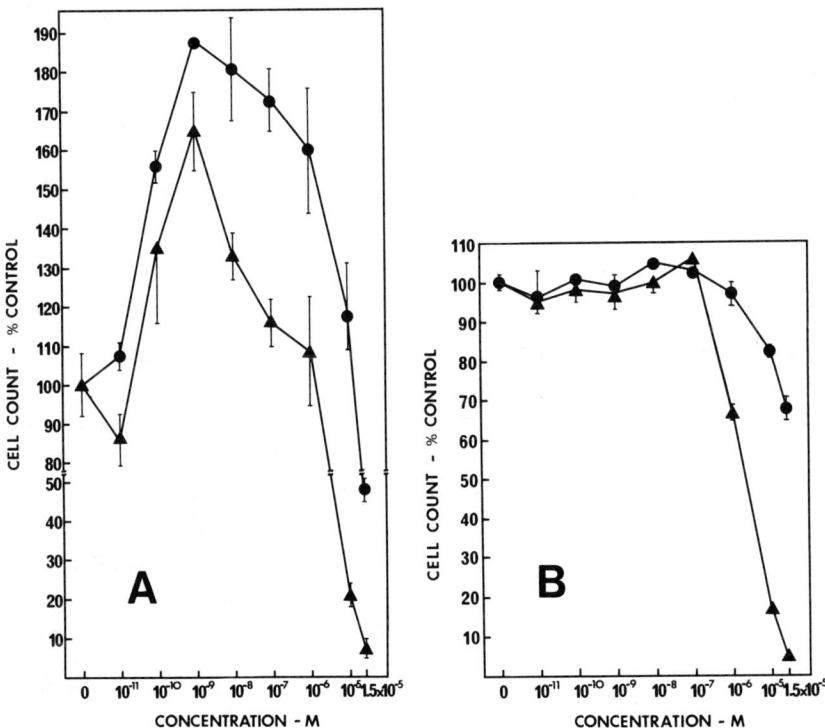

Figure 15.8. Effects of tamoxifen and estradiol on T47D cell proliferation. Cells were grown in medium supplemented with either 10% charcoal-treated fetal calf serum (A) or 10% normal fetal calf serum (B). After four population doublings of the control cultures, cells were harvested, counted, and expressed as a percentage of the numbers in untreated control cultures. Tamoxifen (▲), estradiol (●). (From Reddel and Sutherland 1984.)

This can probably be explained by the differential rates of metabolism of these compounds during the experimental period and differences in extracellular and intracellular binding. Both compounds were inhibitory at higher concentrations and thus showed bell-shaped dose-response curves typical of many estrogenic responses.

In contrast, cells grown in medium with untreated FCS were not stimulated by either estradiol or tamoxifen, but tamoxifen concentrations of 1 μM and greater caused a significant decline in cell numbers relative to control, as did 10 and 15 μM estradiol (Fig. 15.8B).

Cell cycle kinetic analysis of cells from these experiments yielded results which illustrated a correlation between growth rate and percentage of S phase cells; that is, when cell proliferation was stimulated by either ligand, the percentage of S phase cells was increased in proportion to the degree of growth stimulation. These data are tentatively interpreted as indicating that the increased cell proliferation rate induced by estradiol or tamoxifen is due mainly to a decrease in the G_1 transit time. Such a conclusion is in agreement with earlier studies in which the effects of estrogens on the cell cycle kinetics of epithelial cells in immature or castrated rodent reproductive tissues were investigated (Sutherland et al. 1983c).

VII. *Conclusions*

The data presented here are compatible with a model in which estrogens and antiestrogens, acting through the ER, compete for a common biochemical event in G_1 phase of the cell cycle, which controls the rate of cell cycle progression by determining the length of the G_1 phase and thus the overall cell cycle generation time. This simplistic model is in agreement with previously published data on cell cycle regulation by estrogens (Sutherland et al. 1983c). Such a model does not, however, explain why tamoxifen can be either an estrogen agonist or an estrogen antagonist, depending on the *in vitro* culture conditions, nor does it account for the estrogen-irreversible effects of tamoxifen or the enhanced antiproliferative effects of analogs with high affinity for AEBS. Further studies are being undertaken to develop a model of antiestrogen action that can account for all these effects.

References

Benz, C., E. Cadman, J. Gwin, T. Wu, J. Amara, A. Eisenfeld, and P. Dannies. 1983. Tamoxifen and 5-fluorouracil in breast cancer: cytotoxic synergism *in vitro*. *Cancer Research* 43:5298–5303.

Engel, L. W., and N. A. Young. 1978. Human breast carcinoma cells in continuous culture: a review. *Cancer Research* 38:4327–4339.

Gallez, G., J. C. Heuson, and C. Waelbroeck. 1973. Growth-stimulating effect of nafoxidine on rat mammary tumor after ovariectomy. *European Journal of Cancer* 9:699–700.

Green, M. D., A. M. Whybourne, I. W. Taylor, and R. L. Sutherland. 1981. Effects of antioestrogens on the growth and cell cycle kinetics of cultured human mammary carcinoma cells. In *Non-steroidal antioestrogens: molecular pharmacology and antitumour activity*, ed. R. L. Sutherland and V. C. Jordan, 397–412. Sydney: Academic Press.

Jordan, V. C. 1976. Antiestrogenic and antitumor properties of tamoxifen in laboratory animals. *Cancer Treatment Reports* 60:1409–1419.

Legault-Poisson, S., J. Jolivet, R. Poisson, M. Beretta-Piccoli, and P. R. Band. 1979. Tamoxifen-induced tumor stimulation and withdrawal response. *Cancer Treatment Reports* 63:1839–1841.

Lippman, M. E., and G. Bolan. 1975. Oestrogen-responsive human breast cancer in long term tissue culture. *Nature* (London) 256:592–593.

Lippman, M. E., G. Bolan, and K. Huff. 1976. The effects of estrogen and antiestrogen on hormone-responsive human breast cancer in long-term tissue culture. *Cancer Research* 36:4595–4601.

Lykkesfeldt, A. E., J. K. Larsen, I. J. Christensen, and P. Briand. 1984. Effects of the antioestrogen tamoxifen on the cell cycle kinetics of the human breast cancer cell line, MCF-7. *British Journal of Cancer* 49:717–722.

McGuire, W. L. 1978. Hormone receptors: their role in predicting prognosis and response to endocrine therapy. *Seminars in Oncology* 5:428–433.

McIntosh, I. H., and G. S. Thynne. 1977. Tumour stimulation by anti-oestrogens. *British Journal of Surgery* 64:900–901.

Murphy, L. C., and R. L. Sutherland. 1981. Modifications in the aminoether side chain of clomiphene influence affinity for a specific antiestrogen binding site in MCF-7 cell cytosol. *Biochemical and Biophysical Research Communications* 100:1353–1361.

Murphy, L. C., and R. L. Sutherland. 1983. Antitumor activity of clomiphene analogs *in vitro*: relationship to affinity for estrogen receptor and another high affinity antiestrogen binding site. *Journal of Clinical Endocrinology and Metabolism* 57:373–379.

Murphy, L. C., and R. L. Sutherland. 1985. Differential effects of tamoxifen and analogs with nonbasic sidechains on cell proliferation *in vitro*. *Endocrinology* 116:1071–1078.

Osborne, C. K., D. H. Boldt, G. M. Clark, and J. M. Trent. 1983. Effects of tamoxifen on human breast cancer cell cycle kinetics: accumulation of cells in early G_1 phase. *Cancer Research* 43:3583–3585.

Osborne, C. K., D. H. Boldt, and P. Estrada. 1984. Human breast cancer cell cycle synchronization by estrogens and antiestrogens in culture. *Cancer Research* 44:1433–1439.

Reddel, R. R., and R. L. Sutherland. 1983. N-desmethyltamoxifen inhibits growth of

MCF-7 human mammary carcinoma cells *in vitro*. *European Journal of Cancer and Clinical Oncology* 19:1179–1181.

Reddel, R. R., and R. L. Sutherland. 1984. Tamoxifen stimulation of human breast cancer cell proliferation *in vitro:* a possible model for tamoxifen tumour flare. *European Journal of Cancer and Clinical Oncology* 20:1419–1424.

Reddel, R. R., L. C. Murphy, and R. L. Sutherland. 1983. Effects of biologically active metabolites of tamoxifen on the proliferation kinetics of MCF-7 human breast cancer cells *in vitro*. *Cancer Research* 43:4618–4624.

Reddel, R. R., L. C. Murphy, and R. L. Sutherland. 1984. Factors affecting the sensitivity of T47D human breast cancer cells to tamoxifen. *Cancer Research* 44:2398–2404.

Reddel, R. R., L. C. Murphy, R. E. Hall, and R. L. Sutherland. 1985. Differential sensitivity of human cell lines to the growth inhibitory effects of tamoxifen. *Cancer Research* 45:1525–1531.

Seibert, K., and M. Lippman. 1982. Hormone receptors in breast cancer. *Clinics in Oncology* 1:735–794.

Sutherland, R. L., and M. S. Foo. 1979. Differential binding of antiestrogens by rat uterine and chick oviduct cytosol. *Biochemical and Biophysical Research Communications* 91:183–191.

Sutherland, R. L., and L. C. Murphy. 1980. The binding of tamoxifen to human mammary carcinoma cytosol. *European Journal of Cancer* 16:1141–1148.

Sutherland, R. L., and I. W. Taylor. 1981. Effect of tamoxifen on the cell cycle kinetics of cultured human mammary carcinoma cells. *Reviews on Endocrine-Related Cancer* Suppl. 8:17–25.

Sutherland, R. L., L. C. Murphy, M. S. Foo, M. D. Green, A. M. Whybourne, and Z. S. Krozowski. 1980. High-affinity anti-oestrogen binding site distinct from the oestrogen receptor. *Nature* (London) 288:273–275.

Sutherland, R. L., M. D. Green, R. E. Hall, R. R. Reddel, and I. W. Taylor. 1983a. Tamoxifen induces accumulation of MCF-7 human mammary carcinoma cells in the G_0/G_1 phase of the cell cycle. *European Journal of Cancer and Clinical Oncology* 19:615–621.

Sutherland, R. L., R. E. Hall, and I. W. Taylor. 1983b. Cell proliferation kinetics of MCF-7 human mammary carcinoma cells in culture and effects of tamoxifen on exponentially growing and plateau phase cells. *Cancer Research* 43:3998–4006.

Sutherland, R. L., R. R. Reddel, and M. D. Green. 1983c. Effects of oestrogens on cell proliferation and cell cycle kinetics: a hypothesis on the cell cycle effects of antioestrogens. *European Journal of Cancer and Clinical Oncology* 19:307–318.

Sutherland, R. L., R. R. Reddel, R. E. Hall, P. J. Hodson, and I. W. Taylor. 1983d. Effects of tamoxifen on the cell cycle kinetics of MCF-7 human mammary carcinoma cells in culture. *Rational basis for chemotherapy*, ed. B. A. Chabner, 177–193. *UCLA Symposia on Molecular and Cellular Biology*, vol. 4. New York: Alan R. Liss.

Sutherland, R. L., L. C. Murphy, R. E. Hall, R. R. Reddel, C. K. W. Watts, and I. W. Taylor. 1984. Effects of antioestrogens on human breast cancer cells *in vitro:* interaction with high affinity intracellular binding sites and effects on cell proliferation kinetics. *Hormones and cancer 2. Progress in cancer research and therapy*, vol. 31, ed. F. Bresciani, R. J. B. King, M. E. Lippman, M. Namer, and J. P. Raynaud, 193–212. New York: Raven Press.

Taylor, I. W., P. J. Hodson, M. D. Green, and R. L. Sutherland. 1983. Effects of tamoxifen on cell cycle progression of synchronous MCF-7 human mammary carcinoma cells. *Cancer Research* 43:4007–4011.

Watson, C. S., D. Medina, and J. H. Clark. 1981. Estrogenic effects of nafoxidine on ovarian-dependent and -independent mammary tumor lines in the mouse. *Endocrinology* 108:668–672.

Watts, C. K. W., L. C. Murphy, and R. L. Sutherland. 1984. Microsomal binding sites for nonsteroidal antiestrogens in MCF-7 human mammary carcinoma cells: demonstration of high affinity and narrow specificity for basic ether derivatives of triphenylethylene. *Journal of Biological Chemistry* 259:4223–4229.

16

Animal Models
to Study the Therapy of
Hormone-Dependent Breast Cancer

Marco M. Gottardis and V. Craig Jordan

I. Introduction   284
II. Historical Development of Carcinogen-Induced Models   284
III. Antitumor Actions of Antiestrogens in Carcinogen-Induced
     Models   287
IV. Mode of Action of Antiestrogens   289
    A. Inhibition of Estrogen Binding   290
    B. Inhibition of Ovarian Estrogen Synthesis   291
    C. Inhibition of Gonadotrophin Release   291
    D. Inhibition of Prolactin Secretion   291
V. Transplantation of Human Breast Tumors in Athymic Mice   292
VI. Conclusions   293
    References   295

I. Introduction

Beatson's (1896) early observation that women with late advanced breast cancer can have improvement of their disease by oophorectomy focused attention on the ovary as a source of factors which stimulate tumor growth. Lathrop and Loeb (1916) provided the first laboratory evidence for the decisive influence of estrogens on the development of mammary cancer in an inbred strain of mice. Ovariectomy of young female mice prevented the appearance of mammary cancer. Lacassagne (1932) followed up this observation by demonstrating that injections of folliculin (estrone) could induce mammary cancer in the males of a high-incidence strain of mice. Untreated males had a low incidence of mammary cancer, as did males of a low-incidence strain treated with folliculin.

Our understanding of the hormone dependency of breast cancer has increased dramatically in the past 30 years. In this chapter we will describe the evolution of interest in the study of hormone dependency in carcinogen-induced mammary cancer to the current attempts to study the action of hormones and antiestrogens on the growth of human breast cancer in athymic mice.

II. Historical Development of Carcinogen-Induced Models

Model development has focused on differential strain sensitivity to the carcinogens, sex differences, and the duration of the exposure to carcinogens. The compounds that induce mammary cancer in laboratory animals are shown in Figure 16.1.

2-Acetylaminofluorene (2AAF) was synthesized as a potential insecticide. The acute toxicity is very low, but there is a dramatic increase in toxicity if rats are fed continuously with food containing 0.25% 2AAF; all female rats died during the 100-day experiment (Wilson et al. 1941). Early toxicological studies showed carcinomas in various organs, and mammary tumors were noted but not confirmed (Wilson et al. 1941). Mammary tumor formation with 2AAF was subsequently found to be dependent upon the strain of rat (Bielschowsky 1944, 1946; Dunning et al. 1947); estradiol decreased, but progesterone dramatically increased, mammary tumor development (Cantarow et al. 1948).

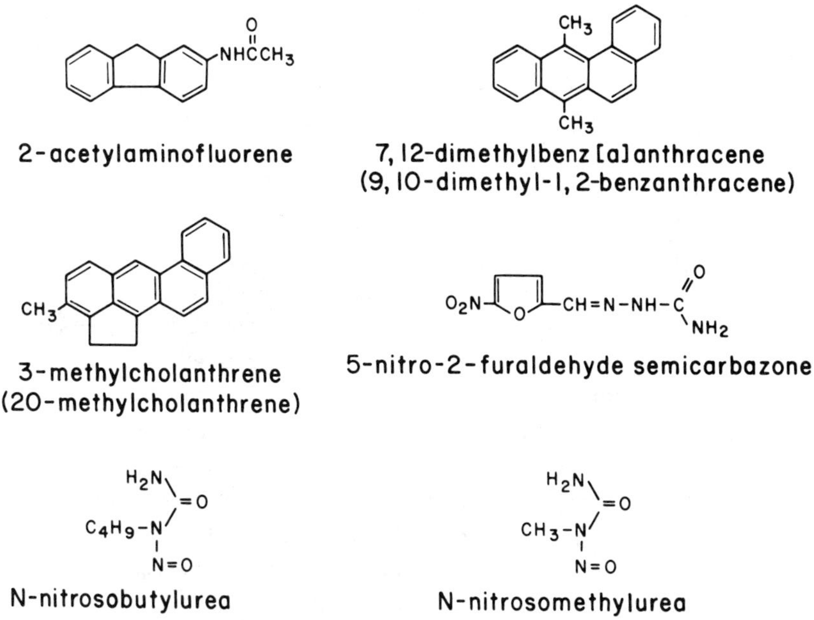

2-acetylaminofluorene

7,12-dimethylbenz[a]anthracene
(9,10-dimethyl-1,2-benzanthracene)

3-methylcholanthrene
(20-methylcholanthrene)

5-nitro-2-furaldehyde semicarbazone

N-nitrosobutylurea

N-nitrosomethylurea

Figure 16.1. Mammary carcinogens.

Polycyclic hydrocarbons are more potent mammary carcinogens than 2AAF. Shay et al. (1949) first described the formation of mammary tumors in Wistar rats following the repeated gastric instillation of 3-methylcholanthrene (3MC). The induction of mammary tumors is dependent upon (1) dosage, (2) the timing of administration of the carcinogen, and (3) a favorable hormonal environment (Shay et al. 1952; Huggins et al. 1959). Pregnancy increases the growth rate of tumors and regression occurs following parturition (Dao and Sutherland 1959).

The repeated intravenous injection of dimethylbenz[a]anthracene (DMBA) is extremely efficient at inducing mammary tumors (Geyer et al. 1951, 1953). However, a major advance was made by Huggins and co-workers (1961), who described mammary cancer models produced by a single feeding of carcinogens (3MC, 2AAF, and DMBA). The simplicity of the hormone-dependent DMBA-induced rat mammary carcinoma model was an exciting advance for the laboratory study of breast cancer. Nevertheless, the hormone dependency appears to be predominantly of pituitary origin. Although the mammary tumors regress in response to ovariectomy and regrow during estrogen administration, this does not occur if the animals are hypophysectomized (Sterental et al. 1963). These and other results indicate that DMBA-induced tumors are primarily dependent upon pituitary hormones (Meites 1972; Manni et al. 1977; Arafah et al. 1980b). DMBA-induced tumors contain estrogen receptors (King et al. 1965, 1966; Mobbs 1966; Vignon and Rochefort 1976; Asslin et al. 1977) but these probably do not mediate estrogen action directly; estrogen-stimulated prolactin release from the pituitary gland could account for the growth effects of estrogen in ovariectomized animals. Inhibition of prolactin release with dopamine agonists prevents the induction of tumors (Meites 1972; Chan and Cohen 1974; Quadri et al. 1974), and major tranquilizers, which increase prolactin secretion, can reverse the regression of tumors by antiestrogens (Manni et al. 1977). Nevertheless, increases in circulating prolactin alone are insufficient to cause tumor regrowth in ovariectomized rats. Ovarian transplants are necessary to stimulate the tumors to grow (Sinha et al. 1973).

With these reservations, carcinogen-induced mammary cancer models have been widely used to investigate potential agents for breast cancer therapy. Chemotherapy is effective in causing tumor regression (Griswold et al. 1966; Teller et al. 1966) but caution must be exercised in interpretating the results, because dietary restrictions retard tumor growth (Gropper and Shimkin 1967) and chemotherapy causes weight loss. Various approaches to an alteration of the hormonal milieu will result in the regression of DMBA-induced tumors. Inhibitors of steroidogenesis (Levin et al. 1976; Brodie et al. 1983), high-dose estrogen (Quadri et al. 1974), inhibitors of prolactin release (Quadri et al. 1974), androgen (Griswold and Green 1970), synthetic inhibitors of gonadotrophin release (Shay et al. 1964), or luteinizing hormone-releasing hormone (LH-RH) agonist (Nicholson and Maynard 1979) have all been reported to be effective agents for controlling tumor growth.

Additional laboratory models that might more closely represent human breast cancer have been sought. Exposing rats to the nitro compound 5-nitro-furaldehyde semicarbazone (Fig. 16.1) in their feed induces a small incidence of mammary tumors, but their hormone dependency has not been investigated (Erturk et al. 1970). In contrast, the continuous exposure of selected strains of rats to N-nitrosobutyl urea (Fig. 16.1) causes the induction of ovarian-dependent mammary tumors (Hosokawa et al. 1971; Takizawa and Yamasaki 1971). Consistent with the previous experiences with the polycyclic hydrocarbons, a precise protocol has been developed to produce tumors in all treated rats. Gullino and coworkers (1975) demonstrated that mammary tumors are induced by three intravenous injections of 5 mg N-nitrosomethyl urea (NMU) (Fig. 16.1) per 100 gm body weight 4 weeks apart, the first injection given when the rats are 50 days old. Another important observation was that, unlike all other carcinogen-induced models, NMU-induced mammary tumors metastasized. Unfortunately, this finding has not been confirmed (Rose et al. 1980; Williams et al. 1981).

Unlike the polycyclic hydrocarbons, NMU does not require metabolic activation to cause DNA alkylation. Indeed, a recent report (Sukumar et al. 1983) indicates that carcinogenesis with NMU involves the malignant activation of H-ras-1 locus by a single point mutation. This results in the encoding of a p21 protein with glutamic acid in place of glycine (the twelfth codon is GAA instead of GGA of the normal allele).

Mammary tumors induced by NMU have estrogen, progesterone, and prolactin receptors (Arafah et al. 1980a; Rose et al. 1980; Turcot-Lemay and Kelly 1980; Gandilhon et al. 1983) and the tumors regress in response to ovariectomy (Arafah et al. 1980a; Rose et al. 1980; Turcot-Lemay and Kelly 1981). However, the attractive feature of NMU-induced tumors is their partial direct dependence upon estrogen for homeostasis. If rats with NMU-induced tumors are hypophysectomized and then treated daily with estrogen, there is only a small decrease in tumor size (Arafah et al. 1982). Thus, the NMU-induced mammary tumor appears to be dependent upon both pituitary and ovarian hormones.

In conclusion, the evolution of carcinogen-induced models for the study of the hormone dependency of mammary cancer in the laboratory has been consistent. A single dose of a carcinogen is effective if administered at the optimal age or endocrine status in female rats. The models have been used extensively to study the pharmacology and antitumor properties of the nonsteroidal antiestrogens.

III. *Antitumor Actions of Antiestrogens in Carcinogen-Induced Models*

The coadministration of tamoxifen (Fig. 16.2) with DMBA prevents the initiation of mammary tumors in female rats (Jordan 1974, 1976). Different doses of tamoxifen, administered for a 4-week period, 4 weeks after DMBA administration, causes a dose-related decrease in the resulting number of mammary tumors. Although larger doses of tamoxifen cause a longer delay in the first appearance of tumors, eventually the tumor inci-

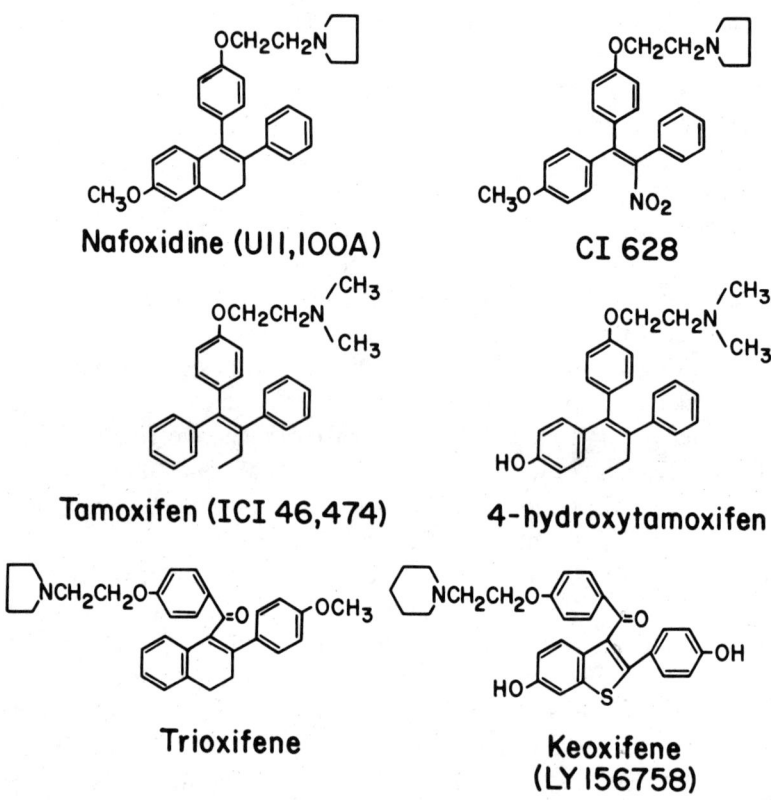

Figure 16.2. Nonsteroidal antiestrogens that have antitumor activity in carcinogen-induced rat mammary cancer.

dence is similar to controls (Jordan et al. 1979). Tamoxifen has a long biological half-life and it appears that the drug prevents tumor promotion as long as the compound is present. Thus, tamoxifen appears to be tumoristatic as well as tumoricidal in this model. This is exemplified by the finding (Jordan et al. 1980) that continuous daily treatment with tamoxifen starting 4 weeks after tumor initiation with DMBA maintains most animals in the tumor-free state.

These findings have been used to support the use of long-term tamoxifen treatment as an adjuvant to breast cancer therapy. The initial clinical findings are extremely encouraging (Tormey and Jordan 1984) and have been used to support the development of nationwide clinical trials through the Eastern Cooperative Oncology Group (EST 5181, EST 4181).

One of the aims of laboratory studies with antiestrogens has been to attempt to develop a compound with more potent, and perhaps more specific, antitumor actions. Tamoxifen is metabolized to 4-hydroxytamoxifen (Fig. 16.2), which is more potent as an antiestrogen than the parent compound (Jordan et al. 1977; Jordan et al. 1978; Dix and Jordan 1980a,b). However, 4-hydroxytamoxifen has not proved to be a more effective antitumor agent than tamoxifen in the DMBA-induced rat mammary carcinoma model (Jordan and Allen 1980).

A whole range of different antiestrogens has been shown to be effective at causing the regression of established DMBA-induced tumors. Nafoxidine (Terenius 1971), CI 628 (DeSombre and Arbogast 1974), and tamoxifen (Nicholson and Golder 1975; Jordan and Dowse 1976; Jordan and Jaspan 1976; Jordan and Koerner 1976) (Fig. 16.2) all have equivalent antitumor activity, but the polyphenolic compound keoxifene is less active (Clemens et al. 1983) and, indeed, appears to promote tumor growth at higher doses (Wakeling and Valacaccia 1983). This finding, like the observation with 4-hydroxytamoxifen in the DMBA model, is rather perplexing because the phenolic antiestrogens are potent antiestrogens with binding affinities for the estrogen receptor equivalent to that of estradiol.

Although most of the published reports of antiestrogens used as antitumor agents have focused upon the DMBA-induced rat mammary carcinoma model, several studies have been undertaken in the NMU-induced model. Tamoxifen appears to be the most effective compound, both in causing the regression of established NMU-induced tumors (Turcot-Lemay and Kelly 1980; Rose et al. 1981) and "adjuvant" models (Wilson et al. 1982; Jordan et al. 1984). Trioxifene (Jordan and Gosden 1982) and keoxifene (Black et al. 1983) (Fig. 16.2) are both more potent antiestrogens in immature rat uterine weight tests but are less active antitumor agents than tamoxifen in the NMU model (Rose et al. 1981; Jordan and Gottardis 1984). Clearly, these inconsistencies require resolution in the future.

IV. *Mode of Action of Antiestrogens*

There are many mechanisms by which antiestrogens could provoke tumor regression (these are illustrated in Figure 16.3). In general, antiestrogens could either affect the direct action of estrogen and prolactin or modify the hormonal environment in which the tumor cells are growing.

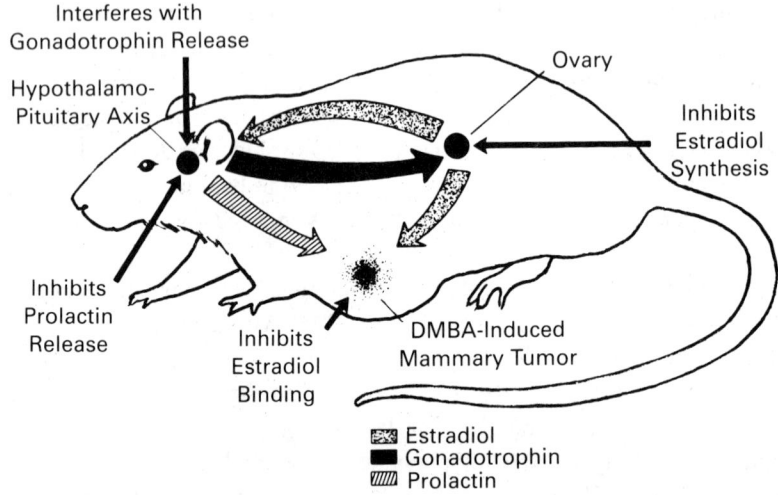

Figure 16.3. Potential sites of action of nonsteroidal antiestrogens.

The major sites that may be involved in the mode of action of antiestrogens are (1) inhibition of estrogen binding in the tumor, (2) inhibition of ovarian estrogen synthesis, (3) inhibition of gonadotrophin release, and (4) inhibition of prolactin secretion.

A. INHIBITION OF ESTROGEN BINDING

Tamoxifen inhibits the binding of [³H]estradiol in DMBA-induced tumor tissue whether this is determined *in vivo* (Jordan and Dowse 1976) or *in vitro* (Nicholson and Golder 1975; Jordan and Jaspan 1976). At the subcellular level, tamoxifen inhibits the binding of [³H]estradiol to the 8S estrogen receptor protein derived from DMBA-induced tumors (Jordan and Dowse 1976).

The estrogen receptor system in DMBA-induced tumors has been studied extensively (King et al. 1965, 1966; Mobbs 1966). Tamoxifen, like estradiol, will cause the location of estrogen receptors in the nuclear compartment, but unlike estradiol, tamoxifen seems unable to maintain a rise in tumor RNA polymerase (Nicholson et al. 1977). If tamoxifen has an antitumor action via this sequence of events, then a decrease in the protein synthetic capacity of the cells may be an important first step in tumor regression.

The significance of estrogen receptors in the tumors is poorly understood, but it is possible that they are indicators of hormone dependency. Low levels of estrogen receptors indicate that the tumors will not respond to tamoxifen therapy (Jordan and Jaspan 1976).

B. INHIBITION OF OVARIAN ESTROGEN SYNTHESIS

An inhibition of estrogen synthesis and the resulting reduction in circulating levels of estrogen would facilitate the competitive blockade of estrogen receptors by tamoxifen in estrogen target tissues. The short-term administration of tamoxifen reduced the level of circulating estradiol in the rat (Watson et al. 1975) by inhibiting synthesis of estradiol in the ovary (Watson and Alam 1976; Watson and Howson 1977). There is very little information about the long-term effects of tamoxifen on ovarian function in rats with DMBA-induced mammary tumors. The few reports suggest that antiestrogens can lower circulating estrogen concentrations (Nicholson and Golder 1975; Jordan and Koerner 1976). It is clear, though, that any fluctuation in the cyclical synthesis of estrogen will have a profound effect on the regulation of both gonadotrophin and prolactin secretion.

C. INHIBITION OF GONADOTROPHIN RELEASE

Evidence from studies in rats and hamsters suggests that antiestrogens can inhibit the positive feedback effects of estrogens on the ovulatory release of luteinizing hormone (Labhsetwar 1970).

D. INHIBITION OF PROLACTIN SECRETION

Nonsteroidal antiestrogens inhibit estrogen-stimulated increases in plasma prolactin (Heuson et al. 1971; Jordan et al. 1975), but this inhibition is incomplete (Jordan and Koerner 1976). Unlike estrogen, tamoxifen and 4-hydroxytamoxifen do not stimulate large rises in circulating prolactin in ovariectomized rats. Results in the intact rat have been confusing. Antiestrogens inhibit (or delay) the surge of prolactin at proestrus (Jordan et al. 1975) but studies in rats with DMBA-induced tumors have failed to show a uniform decrease in the concentrations of circulating prolactin (Nicholson and Golder 1975; Jordan and Koerner 1976). It is interesting to note, however, that tamoxifen-induced regression of tumors can be reversed by perphenazine, a stimulant of prolactin release (Manni et al. 1977).

V. Transplantation of Human Breast Tumors in Athymic Mice

The study of human breast cancer cells *in vitro* has provided valuable information about the biochemical pharmacology of antiestrogens (Jordan 1984). However, the information that can be obtained about the pharmacology and antitumor actions of tamoxifen is limited *in vitro* because during therapy the drug is metabolized to a variety of compounds that interact with the tumor in different ways. Furthermore, the bioavailability of the drug to the tumor may be limited *in vivo*. Thus, the direct effect of antiestrogens can be studied precisely using cell culture systems but the drug and hormone interactions encountered *in vivo* are difficult to duplicate.

The description of the immune-deficient athymic mouse (Pantelouris 1968) and its development for the heterotransplantation and growth of human cancer cells (Rygaard and Poulsen 1969) provided an important research model to study the pharmacology of antitumor agents *in vivo*. Giovenella and coworkers (1974) showed that human tumors grown in athymic mice maintained their pathological morphology and breast tumors could be transplanted and used for chemotherapy studies (Giovenella et al. 1978). However, since one-third of breast tumors are hormone dependent, one goal of research has been to establish a hormone-dependent human breast tumor model to study endocrine therapies.

MCF-7 breast cancer cells (Soule et al. 1973) contain hormone receptors (Brooks et al. 1973; Horwitz et al. 1975) and can be inoculated into athymic mice to produce tumors (Soule and McGrath 1980). However, solid tumors develop only if animals are supplemented with estrogen, because athymic animals have a hypothalamo-pituitary lesion (Weinstein 1978), resulting in very low circulating levels of estradiol (Soule and McGrath 1980). Estrogen supplementation is sufficient to cause tumor growth and the ovaries do not appear to be necessary (Shafie and Grantham 1981) for the development of MCF-7 cells as solid tumors. However, progesterone can act synergistically with estrogen to stimulate MCF-7 solid tumor growth (Soule and McGrath 1980). Unlike the hormone-dependent MCF-7 cells, the hormone-independent breast cancer cell line MDA-MB-231 will grow in athymic mice without hormone supplementation (Siebert et al. 1983; Osborne et al. 1985).

Several investigators have described experiments to determine the hormonal modulation of MCF-7 tumor growth in athymic mice (Shafie 1980; Kubota et al. 1983; Huseby et al. 1984), but there is a paucity of studies

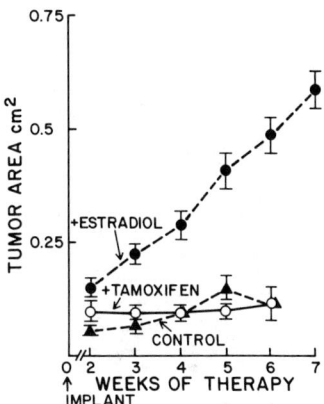

Figure 16.4. The growth of tumors in athymic mice inoculated with 10^7 human breast cancer cells (MCF-7). Mice were implanted with pellets containing a sustained-release preparation of estradiol (1.7 mg), or tamoxifen (5 mg), or placebo (cholesterol pellet control). Tumor areas were measured weekly. Six mice per group with inoculations in the left and right axillary mammary fat pads.

to describe the pharmacology of nonsteroidal antiestrogens. Shafie and Grantham (1981) have demonstrated, however, that unlike estradiol, tamoxifen does not support the growth of breast tumors. This report on the regression of MCF-7 breast tumors *in vivo* by tamoxifen contrasts with the recent report that tamoxifen causes the partial growth of human endometrial cells in athymic mice (Satyaswaroop et al. 1984).

Osborne and coworkers (1985) have recently shown that tamoxifen is unable to cause the growth of MCF-7 cells in athymic mice. This is illustrated in Figure 16.4, showing that estradiol causes the growth of MCF-7 into solid tumors, whereas neither placebo nor tamoxifen causes tumor growth. The treatment of animals with tamoxifen does not destroy the breast cancer cells, as subsequent administration of estradiol can cause tumor growth (Fig. 16.5). These observations strongly support the long-term adjuvant therapy of breast cancer with tamoxifen (Tormey and Jordan 1984).

VI. Conclusions

In the past 30 years researchers have developed several laboratory models to study the hormone dependency of breast cancer. The current interest in the growth of human breast cancer cell lines in athymic mice has provided

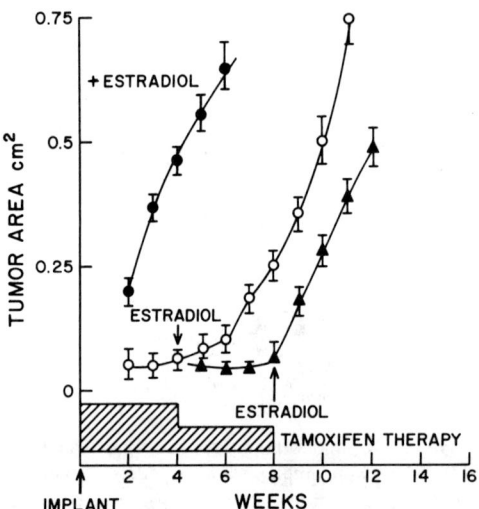

Figure 16.5. The growth of implanted MCF-7 derived breast tumors in athymic mice. Mice were implanted with either estradiol pellets (1.7 mg) or tamoxifen pellets (5 mg). The tamoxifen pellets were removed at weeks 4 and 8 and replaced with estradiol pellets. Tumor areas were measured weekly. Six mice per group with tumor implants on each side of the axillary mammary fat pads.

an additional dimension to focus upon human disease. However, this change in focus has come about in part because of the dependency of carcinogen-induced models upon pituitary hormones and the general belief that human breast cancer is dependent upon estrogen. Leung and Shiu (1981) recently demonstrated that the T47D breast cancer cell line, which has a high level of progesterone receptors but almost undetectable levels of estrogen receptor (Horwitz et al. 1982), will grow in response to estrogen in athymic mice. However, the hormone dependency of these cells is perhaps more complex, as the cotransplantation of GH_3 rat pituitary cells provides the optimal environment for T47D tumor growth (Leung and Shiu 1981). It is therefore very important to study the hormone dependency of a broad range of breast cancer cell lines and then transplanted cells from primary cultures. In this way realistic models can be established to test novel therapeutic agents before clinical trials are initiated.

Acknowledgments

Studies supported by P01-CA-20432.

References

Arafah, B. M., P. M. Gullino, A. Manni, and O. H. Pearson. 1980a. Effect of ovariectomy on hormone receptors and growth of N-nitrosomethylurea–induced mammary tumors in the rat. *Cancer Research* 40:4628–4630.

Arafah, B. M., A. Manni, and O. H. Pearson. 1980b. Effect of hypophysectomy and hormone replacement on hormone receptor levels and the growth of 7,12-dimethylbenz(a)anthracene–induced mammary tumors in the rat. *Endocrinology* 107:1364–1369.

Arafah, B. M., H. M. Finegan, J. Roe, A. Manni, and O. H. Pearson. 1982. Hormone dependency in N-nitrosomethylurea–induced rat mammary tumors. *Endocrinology* 111:584–588.

Asselin, J., P. A. Kelly, M. G. Caron, and F. Labrie. 1977. Control of hormone receptor levels and growth of 7,12-dimethylbenz(a)anthracene–induced mammary tumors by estrogens, progesterone and prolactin. *Endocrinology* 101:666–671.

Beatson, G. T. 1896. On the treatment of inoperable cases of carcinoma of the mamma: suggestions for a new method of treatment with illustrative cases. *Lancet* 2:104–107, 162–167.

Bielschowsky, F. 1944. Distant tumours produced by 2-amino- and 2-acetyl-aminofluorene. *British Journal of Experimental Pathology* 25:1–4.

Bielschowsky, F. 1946. Comparison of the tumours produced by 2-acetaminofluorene in Piebald and Wistar rats. *British Journal of Experimental Pathology* 27:135–139.

Black, L. J., C. D. Jones, and J. F. Falcone. 1983. Antagonism of estrogen action with a new benzothiophene-derived antiestrogen. *Life Sciences* 32:1031–1036.

Brodie, A. M. H., W. M. Garrett, J. R. Hendrickson, C. H. Tsai-Morris, and J. G. Williams. 1983. Aromatase inhibitors, their pharmacology and application. *Journal of Steroid Biochemistry* 19:53–58.

Brooks, S. C., E. R. Locke, and H. D. Soule. 1973. Estrogen receptor in a human cell line (MCF-7) from breast carcinoma. *Journal of Biological Chemistry* 248:6251–6253.

Cantarow, A., J. Stasney, and K. E. Paschkis. 1948. The influence of sex hormones on mammary tumors induced by 2-acetaminofluorene. *Cancer Research* 8:412–417.

Chan, P. C., and L. A. Cohen. 1974. Effect of dietary fat, antiestrogen and antiprolactin on the development of mammary tumors in rats. *Journal of the National Cancer Institute* 52:25–30.

Clemens, J. A., D. R. Bennett, L. J. Black, and C. D. Jones. 1983. Effect of a new antiestrogen, keoxifene (LY 156758) on growth of carcinogen-induced mammary tumors and on LH and prolactin levels. *Life Sciences* 32:2869–2875.

Dao, T. L., and H. Sutherland. 1959. Mammary carcinogenesis by 3-methyl-cholanthrene. 1. Hormonal aspects in tumor induction and growth. *Journal of the National Cancer Institute* 23:567–585.

DeSombre, E. R., and L. Y. Arbogast. 1974. Effect of the antiestrogen CI628 on the growth of rat mammary tumors. *Cancer Research* 34:1971–1976.

Dix, C. J., and V. C. Jordan. 1980a. Subcellular effects of monohydroxytamoxifen in the rat uterus: steroid receptors and mitosis. *Journal of Endocrinology* 85:393–403.

Dix, C. J., and V. C. Jordan. 1980b. Modulation of rat uterine steroid hormone receptors and estrogen and antiestrogen. *Endocrinology* 107:2011–2020.

Dunning, E. F., M. R. Curtis, and M. E. Madsen. 1947. The induction of neoplasms in five strains of rats with acetylaminofluorene. *Cancer Research* 7:134–140.

Erturk, E., J. E. Morris, S. M. Cohen, J. M. Price, and G. T. Bryan. 1970. Transplantable rat mammary tumors induced by 5-nitro-2-furaldehyde semicarbazone and by formic acid 2-[4-5-nitro-2-furyl)-2(thiazolyl]-hydrazide. *Cancer Research* 30:1409–1412.

Gandilhon, P., R. Malancon, F. Gandilhon, J. Djane, and P. A. Kelley. 1983. Prolactin receptors in N-nitroso-N-methylurea–induced rat mammary tumors: relationship to tumor age and down-regulation in short-term explant culture. *Anticancer Research* 3:203–206.

Geyer, R. P., V. R. Bleisch, J. E. Bryant, A. N. Robbins, I. M. Saslow, and F. J. Stare. 1951. Tumor production in rats injected intravenously with oil emulsions containing 9,10-dimethyl-1,2-benzanthracene. *Cancer Research* 112:474–478.

Geyer, R. P., J. E. Bryant, V. R. Bleisch, E. M. Peirce, and F. J. Stare. 1953. Effect of dose and hormones on tumor production in rats given emulsified 9,10-dimethyl-2, 2-benzanthracene intravenously. *Cancer Research* 13:503–506.

Giovenella, B. C., J. S. Stehlin, and L. J. Williams. 1974. Heterotransplantation of human malignant tumors in "nude" thymusless mice. *Journal of the National Cancer Institute* 52:921–927.

Giovenella, B. C., J. S. Stehlin, L. J. Williams, S. Lee, and R. Shepard. 1978. Heterotransplantation of human cancers into "nude" mice: a model system for human cancer therapy. *Cancer* 42:2269–2281.

Griswold, D. P., and C. H. Green. 1970. Observations on the hormone sensitivity of 7,12-dimethylbenz(a)anthracene–induced mammary tumors in the Sprague-Dawley rat. *Cancer Research* 30:819–826.

Griswold, D. P., H. E. Skipper, W. R. Laster, W. S. Wilcox, and F. M. Schabel. 1966. Induced mammary carcinoma in the female rat as a drug evaluation system. *Cancer Research* 26:2169–2180.

Gropper, L., and M. B. Skimkin. 1967. Combination therapy of 3-methyl-cholanthrene–induced mammary carcinomas in rats: effect of chemotherapy, ovariectomy and food restriction. *Cancer Research* 27:26–32.

Gullino, P. M., H. M. Pettigrew, and F. H. Granthram. 1975. N-nitrosomethyl-urea as mammary gland carcinogen in rats. *Journal of the National Cancer Institute* 54:401–414.

Heuson, J. C., C. Waelbrock, and N. Legros. 1971. Inhibition of DMBA-induced mammary carcinogensis in the rat by 2 Br-α-ergocryptine (CB154) an inhibitor of prolactin secretion, and by nafoxidine (U-11,100A) an estrogen antagonist. *Gynecologic Investigation* 2:130–137.

Horwitz, K. B., M. E. Costlow, and W. L. McGuire. 1975. MCF-7—a human breast cancer cell line with estrogen, androgen, progesterone and glucocorticoid receptors. *Steroids* 26:785–795.

Horwitz, K. B., M. B. Mockus, and B. A. Lessey. 1982. Variant T47D human breast cancer cells with high progesterone receptor levels despite estrogen and antiestrogen resistance. *Cell* 28:633–642.

Hosokawa, M., E. Gotahda, and H. Kobayashi. 1971. Leukemia and mammary tumor in rats administered N-nitrosobutylurea. *Gann* 62:557–559.

Huggins, C., G. Briziarelli, and H. Sutton. 1959. Rapid induction of mammary carcinoma in the rat and the influence of hormones on the tumors. *Journal of Experimental Medicine* 109:25–41.

Huggins, C., L. C. Grand, and F. B. Brillantes. 1961. Mammary cancer induced by a single feeding of polynuclear hydrocarbons and its suppression. *Nature* (London) 189:204–207.

Huseby, R. A., T. M. Maloney, and C. M. McGrath. 1984. Evidence for a direct growth stimulating effect of estradiol on human MCF-7 cells *in vivo*. *Cancer Research* 44:2654–2659.

Jordan, V. C. 1974. Antitumour activity of the antioestrogen ICI46,474 (tamoxifen) in the dimethylbenzanthracene (DMBA)-induced rat mammary carcinoma model. *Journal of Steroid Biochemistry* 5:354.

Jordan, V. C. 1976. Effect of tamoxifen (ICI46,474) on initiation and growth of DMBA-induced rat mammary carcinomata. *European Journal of Cancer* 12:419–424.

Jordan, V. C. 1984. Biochemical pharmacology of antiestrogen action. *Pharmacological Reviews* 36:245–276.

Jordan, V. C., and K. E. Allen. 1980. Evaluation of the antitumour activity of the non-steroidal antioestrogen monohydroxytamoxifen in the DMBA-induced rat mammary carcinoma model. *European Journal of Cancer* 16:239–251.

Jordan, V. C., and L. J. Dowse. 1976. Tamoxifen as an antitumour agent: effect on oestrogen binding. *Journal of Endocrinology* 68:297–303.

Jordan, V. C., and B. Gosden. 1982. Importance of the alkylaminoethoxy side chain for the estrogenic and antiestrogenic actions of tamoxifen and trioxifene in the immature rat uterus. *Molecular and Cellular Endocrinology* 27:291–306.

Jordan, V. C., and M. M. Gottardis. 1984. A comparative study of antiestrogens LY156758 and tamoxifen on N-nitrosomethylurea–induced rat mammary carcinomas: a potential model for adjuvant therapy. *Journal of Steroid Biochemistry* 20:1631.

Jordan, V. C., and T. Jaspan. 1976. Tamoxifen as an antitumour agent: oestrogen binding as a predictive test for tumour response. *Journal of Endocrinology* 68:453–460.

Jordan, V. C., and S. Koerner. 1976. Tamoxifen as an antitumour agent: role of oestradiol and prolactin. *Journal of Endocrinology* 68:305–311.

Jordan, V. C., S. Koerner, and C. Robison. 1975. Inhibition of oestrogen-stimulated prolactin release by antioestrogens. *Journal of Endocrinology* 65:151–152.

Jordan, V. C., M. M. Collins, L. Rowsby, and G. Prestwich. 1977. A monohydroxylated metabolite of tamoxifen with potent antioestrogenic activity. *Journal of Endocrinology* 75:305–316.

Jordan, V. C., L. Rowsby, C. J. Dix, and G. Prestwich. 1978. Dose-related effect of non-steroidal antioestrogens and non-steroidal oestrogens on the measurement of cytoplasmic oestrogen receptors in the rat and mouse uterus. *Journal of Endocrinology* 78:71–81.

Jordan, V. C., C. J. Dix, and K. E. Allen. 1979. The effectiveness of long-term tamoxifen treatment in a laboratory model for adjuvant hormone therapy of breast cancer. In *Adjuvant therapy of cancer II*, ed. S. E. Jones and S. E. Salmon, 19–26. New York: Grune and Stratton.

Jordan, V. C., K. E. Allen, and C. J. Dix. 1980. Pharmacology of tamoxifen in laboratory animals. *Cancer Treatment Reports* 64:745–759.

Jordan, V. C., D. Mirecki, and M. M. Gottardis. 1984. Continuous tamoxifen therapy prevents the appearance of mammary tumors in a laboratory model of adjuvant therapy. In *Adjuvant therapy of cancer IV*, ed. S. E. Jones and S. E. Salmon, 27–33. New York: Grune and Stratton.

King, R. J. B., D. M. Cowan, and D. R. Inman. 1965. The uptake of [6,7-³H]oestradiol by dimethylbenzanthracene-induced rat mammary tumours. *Journal of Endocrinology* 32:83–90.

King, R. J. B., J. Gordon, D. M. Cowan, and D. R. Inman. 1966. The intranuclear localisation of [6,7-³H]oestradiol-17β in dimethylbenzanthracene-induced rat mammary adenocarcinoma and other tissues. *Journal of Endocrinology* 36:139–150.

Kubota, T., H. Kubouchi, and K. Jin-ichi. 1983. Human breast carcinoma (MCF-7) serially transplanted into nude mice. *Japanese Journal of Surgery* 13:381–384.

Labhsetwar, A. P. 1970. Role of estrogen in ovulation: a study using the estrogen antagonist ICI46,474. *Endocrinology* 87:542–551.

Lacassagne, A. 1932. Apparition de cancers de la mamelle chez le souris mâle, sourmise à des injections de folliculine. *Compte rendu de l'Académie des sciences* 195:630.

Lathrop, A. E. C., and L. Loeb. 1916. Further investigations on the origin of tumors in mice. III. On the part played by internal secretion in the spontaneous development of tumors. *Journal of Cancer Research* 1:1–19.

Leung, C. K. H., and R. P. C. Shiu. 1981. Required presence of both estrogen and pituitary factors for the growth of human breast cancer cells in athymic nude mice. *Cancer Research* 41:546–551.

Levin, J. M., A. S. Goldman, F. E. Rosato, and E. E. Rosato. 1976. Therapy of dimethylbenzanthracene-induced mammary carcinomas in the rat by selective inhibition of steroidogenesis. *Cancer* 38:56–61.

Manni, A., T. E. Trujillo, and O. H. Pearson. 1977. Predominant role of prolactin in stimulating the growth of 7,12-dimethylbenz(a)-anthracene-induced rat mammary tumors. *Cancer Research* 37:1216–1219.

Meites, J. 1972. Relation of prolactin and estrogen to mammary tumorigenesis in the rat. *Journal of the National Cancer Institute* 48:1217–1224.

Mobbs, B. J. 1966. The uptake of tritiated oestradiol by dimethylbenzanthracene-induced mammary tumours of the rat. *Journal of Endocrinology* 36:409–414.

Nicholson, R. I., and M. P. Golder. 1975. The effect of synthetic antioestrogens on the growth and biochemistry of rat mammary tumours. *European Journal of Cancer* 11:571–579.

Nicholson, R. I., and P. V. Maynard. 1979. Antitumour activity of ICI118,630, a potent luteinizing hormone-releasing hormone agonist. *British Journal of Cancer* 39:268–273.

Nicholson, R. I., P. Davis, and S. Griffiths. 1977. Early increases in ribonucleic acid polymerase activities of dimethylbenzanthracene-induced mammary tumour nuclei in response to oestradiol-17β and tamoxifen. *Journal of Endocrinology* 73:135–142.

Osborne, C. K., K. Hobbs, and G. M. Clark. 1985. Effect of estrogens and antiestrogens on growth of human breast cancer cells in athymic nude mice. *Cancer Research* 45:584–590.

Pantelouris, E. M. 1968. Absence of thymus in a mouse mutant. *Nature* (London) 217:370–371.

Quadri, S. K., G. S. Kledzik, and J. Meites. 1974. Enhanced regression of DMBA-induced mammary cancer in rats by combination of ergocornine with ovariectomy or high doses of estrogen. *Cancer Research* 34:499–501.

Rose, D. P., B. Pruitt, P. Stauber, E. Ertürk, and G. T. Bryan. 1980. Influence of dosage schedule on the biological characteristics of N-nitrosomethylurea–induced rat mammary tumors. *Cancer Research* 40:235–239.

Rose, D. P., A. H. Fischer, and V. C. Jordan. 1981. Activity of the antioestrogen trioxifene against N-nitrosomethylurea–induced rat mammary carcinoma. *European Journal of Cancer and Clinical Oncology* 17:893–898.

Rygaard, J., and C. O. Poulsen. 1969. Heterotransplantation of a human malignant tumour to "nude mice." *Acta Pathologica et Microbiologica Scandinavica* 77:758–760.

Satyaswaroop, P. B., R. J. Zaino, and R. Mortel. 1984. Estrogen-like effects of tamoxifen on human endometrial carcinoma transplanted into nude mice. *Cancer Research* 44:4006–4010.

Shafie, S. M. 1980. Estrogen and the growth of breast cancer: new evidence suggests indirect action. *Science* 209:701–702.

Shafie, S. M., and F. H. Grantham. 1981. Role of hormones in the growth and regression of human breast cancer cells (MCF-7) transplanted into athymic mice. *Journal of the National Cancer Institute* 67:51–56.

Shay, H., E. A. Aegerter, M. Gruenstein, and S. A. Komarov. 1949. Development of adenocarcinoma of the breast in the Wistar rat following the gastric instillation of methylcholanthrene. *Journal of the National Cancer Institute* 10:255–266.

Shay, H., C. Harris, and M. Gruenstein. 1952. Influence of sex hormones on the incidence and form of tumors produced in male or female rats by gastric instillation of methylcholanthrene. *Journal of the National Cancer Institute* 13:307–331.

Shay, H., M. Gruenstein, and M. B. Shimkin. 1964. Inhibition of mammary cancer in the rats by a dithiocarbamoyl hydrazine (ICI33,828). *Cancer Research* 24:998–1001.

Siebert, K., S. Shafie, T. Triche, J. Wing-Peng, S. O'Brien, J. Tovey, K. Huff, and M. Lippman. 1983. Clonal variation of MCF-7 cells *in vitro* and in athymic animals. *Cancer Research* 43:2223–2239.

Sinha, D., D. Cooper, and T. L. Dao. 1973. The nature of estrogen and prolactin effect on mammary tumorigenesis. *Cancer Research* 33:411–414.

Soule, H. D., and C. M. McGrath. 1980. Estrogen responsive proliferation of clonal human breast carcinoma cells in athymic mice. *Cancer Letters* 10:177–189.

Soule, H. D., J. Vasquez, A. Long, S. Albert, and M. J. Brennan. 1973. Human cell line from pleural effusion derived from breast carcinoma. *Journal of the National Cancer Institute* 51:1409–1413.

Sterental, A., J. M. Dominguez, C. Weissman, and O. H. Pearson. 1963. Pituitary role in the estrogen dependency of experimental mammary cancer. *Cancer Research* 23:481–484.

Sukumar, S., V. Notario, D. Martin-Zanca, and M. Barbacid. 1983. Induction of mammary carcinomas in rats by nitroso-methylurea involves malignant activation of H-ras-1 locus by single point mutations. *Nature* (London) 306:658–661.

Takizawa, S., and T. Yanasoki. 1971. Role of ovarian hormones in mammary tumorigenesis by a continuous oral administration of N-nitrosobutylurea in Wistar/Furth rats. *Gann* 62:485–493.

Teller, M. N., C. C. Stock, G. Stohr, P. C. Merker, R. J. Kaufman, G. C. Escher, and M. Bowie. 1966. Biologic characteristics and chemotherapy of 7,12-dimethyl-benz(a)anthracene–induced tumors in rats. *Cancer Research* 26:245–252.

Terenius, L. 1971. Antioestrogens and breast cancer. *European Journal of Cancer* 7:57–64.

Tormey, D. C., and V. C. Jordan. 1984. Long-term tamoxifen adjuvant therapy in node positive breast cancer—a metabolic and pilot clinical study. *Breast Cancer Research and Treatment* 4:297–302.

Turcot-Lemay, L., and P. A. Kelly. 1980. Characterization of estradiol, progesterone, and prolactin receptors in nitrosomethylurea-induced mammary tumors and effect of antiestrogen treatment on the development and growth of these tumors. *Cancer Research* 40:4628–4630.

Turcot-Lemay, L., and P. A. Kelly. 1981. Response to ovariectomy of N-methyl-N-nitrosourea–induced mammary tumors in the rat. *Journal of the National Cancer Institute* 66:97–102.

Vignon, F., and H. Rochefort. 1976. Regulation of estrogen receptors in ovarian-dependent rat mammary tumors. 1. Effect of castration and prolactin. *Endocrinology* 98:722–729.

Wakeling, A. F., and B. Valacaccia. 1983. Antioestrogenic and antitumour activities of a series of non-steroidal antioestrogens. *Journal of Endocrinology* 99:455–464.

Watson, J., and M. Alam. 1976. Oestrogen synthesis during delayed implantation in the rat. *Contraception* 13:101–107.

Watson, J., and J. W. H. Howson. 1977. Inhibition by tamoxifen of the stimulatory action of FSH on oestradiol-17β biosynthesis by rat ovaries *in vitro. Journal of Reproduction and Fertility* 49:375–380.

Watson, J., F. B. Anderson, M. Alam, J. E. O'Grady, and P. J. Heald. 1975. Plasma hormones and pituitary luteinizing hormone in the rat during the early stages of pregnancy and after post-coital treatment with tamoxifen (ICI46,474). *Journal of Endocrinology* 65:7–17.

Weinstein, Y. 1978. Impairment of the hypothalamo-pituitary-ovarian axis of the athymic "nude" mouse. *Mechanisms of Ageing and Development* 8:63–68.

Williams, J. C., B. Gusterson, S. J. Humphrey, P. Managhar, R. C. Coombes, P. Rudland, and A. M. Neville. 1981. N-methyl-N-nitrosourea–induced rat mammary tumors. Hormone responsiveness but lack of spontaneous metastases. *Journal of the National Cancer Institute* 66:147–152.

Wilson, A. J., F. Tehrani, and M. Baum. 1982. Adjvuant tamoxifen therapy for early breast cancer: an experimental study with reference to oestrogen and progesterone receptors. *British Journal of Surgery* 69:121–125.

Wilson, R. H., F. DeEds, and A. J. Cox. 1941. The toxicity and carcinogenic activity of 2-acetaminofluorene. *Cancer Research* 1:595–608.

V

Hormone Receptors:
Clinical
Applications

17

Estrogen Receptor Studies: Laboratory Investigations and Clinical Applications

EUGENE R. DESOMBRE, WILLIAM J. KING,
GEOFFREY L. GREENE, SUSAN M. THORPE,
CARSTEN ROSE, AND ELWOOD V. JENSEN

I. INTRODUCTION 304
II. HISTORICAL EVIDENCE FOR THE HORMONE DEPENDENCY OF BREAST
   CANCER 304
III. INTERACTION OF ESTROGENS WITH NORMAL AND NEOPLASTIC TISSUES 305
   A. ESTROGEN RECEPTORS IN NORMAL TISSUES 307
   B. ESTROGEN RECEPTORS IN BREAST CANCER 308
IV. ANTIBODIES TO THE ESTROGEN RECEPTOR PROTEIN 312
   A. LIMITATIONS OF CURRENT RECEPTOR ASSAYS 312
   B. ANTIBODY-BASED ASSAYS FOR ESTROGEN RECEPTOR 312
   C. CLINICAL UTILITY OF ESTROGEN RECEPTOR IMMUNOCHEMICAL
      ASSAYS 313
   REFERENCES 320

303

I. Introduction

T HE application of new knowledge in basic science to the diagnosis and treatment of breast cancer is a classic example of how clinical medicine can benefit from advances in the basic sciences. In this chapter we present some of these relationships, originating from the study of the interaction of radioactive estrogens with normal and neoplastic tissues and extracts and also from the more recent application to breast cancer tissues of immunochemical studies of the estrogen receptor using monoclonal antibodies to the receptor protein. Even though we do not yet understand the molecular details of estrogen action at the gene level, nor do we fully appreciate the intricacy of hormonal control of breast cancer growth at either the cellular or tissue level, nonetheless the studies of steroid receptors in breast cancer have had a clear impact on breast cancer diagnosis and treatment today.

II. Historical Evidence for the Hormone Dependency of Breast Cancer

The application of endocrine methods for the control of breast cancer predated the field of endocrinology and in fact the identification of the hormones whose concentration the treatments affect. The use of surgical oophorectomy by Beatson in 1896, effecting remission of metastatic breast cancer in several premenopausal women, led to what is probably the first endocrine trial for breast cancer (Boyd 1900). The results of this early study of the use of bilateral oophorectomy for advanced breast cancer indicated, interestingly enough, that about 30% of the 54 premenopausal breast cancer patients benefitted from such endocrine-ablative therapy, a response rate not significantly different than is found today. Since breast cancer most frequently affects postmenopausal patients, the major stimulus to renewed interest in endocrine therapy for breast cancer followed the important reports of remissions of advanced breast cancer in postmenopausal women following adrenalectomy (Huggins and Bergenstal 1952) and hypophysectomy (Luft and Olivecrona 1953; Pearson et al. 1956). Modulation of the hormonal milieu of the patient by endocrine-additive therapy was also found to be effective using androgens (Nathanson 1952), large doses of estrogen (Haddow et al. 1944), as well as more recently the use of antiestrogens (Cole et al. 1971; Ward 1973). The results of these and many other endocrine-therapy studies for breast cancer have clearly shown that, for those patients who respond, endocrine therapy provides the best treatment. These recent studies have also confirmed that only 25–30% of nonselected metastatic breast cancer patients respond to the various types of endocrine therapy. The ability to identify those patients who are most likely to respond to such endocrine therapies followed basic studies of the endocrine nature of breast cancer and led to methods which have proved to be of considerable diagnostic and therapeutic utility.

III. Interaction of Estrogens with Normal and Neoplastic Tissues

The large body of current knowledge about steroid hormone mechanism of action has been derived almost entirely from studies in which a radio-labeled steroid hormone has been used as the marker to elucidate the details of the interaction of the hormone with responsive cells. Following the preparation of tritiated estrogens of sufficiently high specific activity to study at the dilute, physiological concentrations found *in vivo*, reports of studies using hexestrol (Glascock and Hoekstra 1959) and estradiol (Jensen and Jacobson 1960) demonstrated that certain tissues of the reproductive tract, such as the uterus, vagina, and anterior pituitary, contained a characteristic estrogen-binding capacity; these target tissues for the hormone were found to take up and retain physiological amounts of the tritiated estrogens against a concentration gradient with the blood. An important characteristic of this process was that the administered estradiol was taken up and retained by the target tissues without change despite the considerable metabolism in the animal, reflected in the mixture of tritiated metabolites in the blood (Jensen and Jacobson 1962).

Following the recognition of the specific uptake of tritiated estrogens by target tissues *in vivo*, it was found that a similar interaction of estradiol with target tissues could be demonstrated with physiological solutions of tritiated estradiol *in vitro* (Jungblut et al. 1965; Terenius 1966). Furthermore, the specific inhibition of the uptake of tritiated estradiol *in vivo* or *in vitro* by certain triphenylethylene antagonists such as Upjohn U 11,100 (Nafoxidine) and Parke Davis CI 628 (Jensen et al. 1972) paralleled the

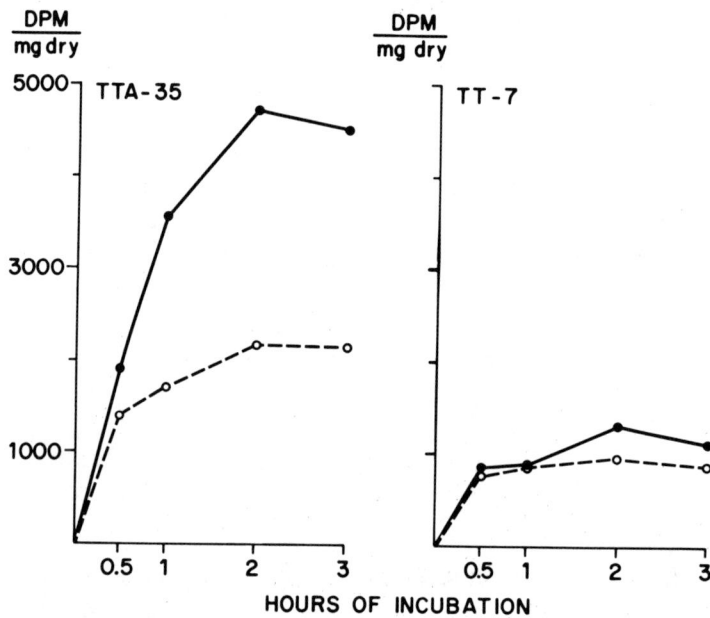

Figure 17.1. Stadie-Riggs slices of freshly excised DMBA-induced rat mammary tumors, either hormone-dependent (*left*) or hormone-independent (*right*), were incubated in Krebs-Ringer Henseleit buffer at 37°C with 0.1 nM 6,7 [³H]estradiol alone (solid lines) or in the presence of 10 μM U 11,100A. At the various time points five replicate tumor slices were removed, rinsed, dried, and oxidized to obtain tritiated water, which was counted in a scintillation counter.

antiuterotrophic effect of such compounds. Indeed, investigations with the DMBA-induced rat mammary carcinoma (Fig. 17.1), where thin slices of tumors were incubated with tritiated estradiol *in vitro*, gave the first evidence that the interaction of tritiated estradiol with slices of breast cancers, in the presence or absence of competitive binding inhibitors, could provide a useful technique to differentiate hormone-dependent and hormone-independent lesions (Jensen et al. 1967). Therefore, with the collaboration of several surgeons at the University of Chicago, initial studies of the interaction of tritiated estradiol with excised human breast cancer tissue *in vitro* were carried out to correlate with patient responses to endocrine-ablative therapy (Jensen et al. 1971). Although such *in vitro* uptake procedures suffered from several significant limitations, especially the requirement for at least a gram of fresh tissue, the early results clearly indicated that the patients whose tumors showed substantial, antiestrogen-

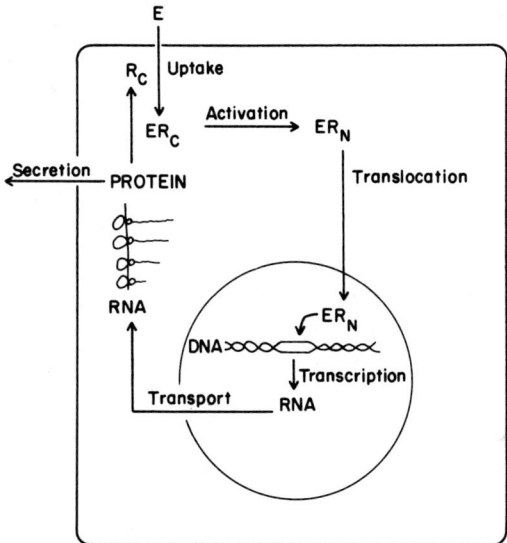

Figure 17.2. Interaction pathway for estrogen with a target cell.

inhibitable uptake of tritiated estradiol were the patients who subsequently responded to endocrine therapies.

A. ESTROGEN RECEPTORS IN NORMAL TISSUES

Numerous laboratories throughout the world have contributed to the rapid expansion of knowledge concerning the molecular details of the interaction of estrogen with its target cells. These studies have led to a generally accepted interaction pathway based on biochemical studies (Fig. 17.2). Most of the estrogen taken up by target tissues *in vivo,* or at physiological temperatures *in vitro,* was associated with the cell nuclei, but smaller amounts were found in low salt extracts and were believed to be extranuclear (Jensen et al. 1968). Following the introduction by Toft and Gorski (1966) of sedimentation analysis to characterize steroid receptors, it was found that upon homogenization of the uterus of untreated immature rats with hypotonic/EDTA buffer, almost all of the tissue content of the receptor protein was obtained in a high-speed supernatant, a so-called cytosolic fraction. When cytosolic estrogen receptor was incubated with estrogen it was found to give rise to a temperature-dependent change (Gorski et al. 1968; Jensen et al. 1968), which could be recognized by a change in the sedimentation character of the complex, changing from 4S to 5S in 0.4 M KCl. This transformed estrogen receptor complex was indistinguishable from the receptor complex extracted by KCl from nuclei of uteri of estrogen-treated immature rats. Hence, the general interaction pathway for estrogen and its target cell (Fig. 17.2) evolved, in which the steroid entered the cell, probably by passive diffusion, and rapidly bound to its receptor protein, which was believed to be present in excess amounts as free receptor in the extranuclear region of the cell. The association of estrogen with its receptor protein led to an activation, possibly involving a dimerization (Notides et al. 1975) to a form believed to translocate to the nucleus and associate with a putative nuclear acceptor. This association of estrogen receptor complex with acceptor or DNA is believed to lead to the subsequent initiation of new nucleic acid synthesis leading to new protein, growth, and the cellular responses that are characteristic of the response of the tissue to estrogen. As described subsequently, the evidence from recent immunohistochemical studies of estrogen receptor indicates that the native estrogen receptor probably resides predominantly in the nucleus, even before estrogen enters the cell. Despite this change in the apparent localization of the native receptor within the cells, the steroid-dependent activation of the receptor protein as a prerequisite for the tight association of the receptor complex with the chromatin and DNA remains as the key process preceding the estrogen-dependent regulation of cellular function.

B. ESTROGEN RECEPTORS IN BREAST CANCER

Following the recognition that the basis for the specific uptake of radioactive estradiol in hormone-responsive cancers was the specific cellular receptor protein, assays for the actual receptor proteins themselves were carried out on breast cancer tissue. Our results (Jensen et al. 1971) indicated that patients whose breast cancers lacked estrogen receptors seldom responded to endocrine therapy, whereas most, but not all, patients with receptor-containing lesions benefitted from such treatment. These findings were soon confirmed and extended by others (Maass et al. 1972; Engelsman et al. 1973; Leung et al. 1973; Savlov et al. 1974), and it was soon generally recognized that the estrogen receptor status of human breast cancer tissue was an important indicator for proper treatment (McGuire et al. 1975).

As receptor assays were refined and became more sensitive, investi-

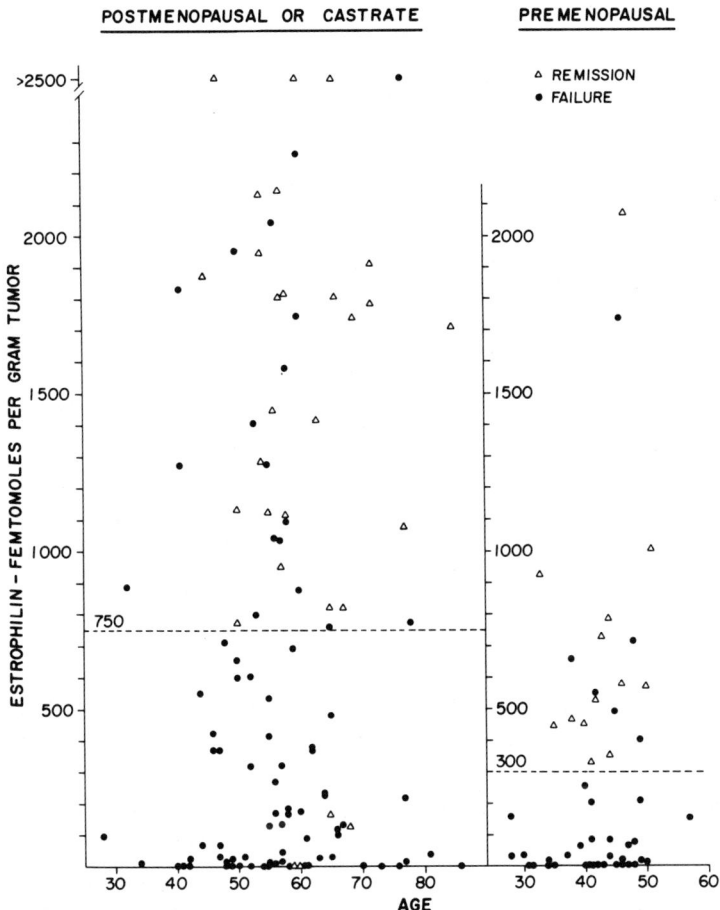

Figure 17.3. Correlation of breast cancer cytosol estrogen receptor content with response to endocrine therapy for 160 patients with metastatic breast cancer. Assays were carried out using the subsaturating sedimentation analysis method (Jensen et al. 1976). (From De-Sombre et al. 1978.)

gators found that a greater proportion of breast cancers contained detectable amounts of estrogen receptor (Leclercq et al. 1975). Since only 25–30% of unselected breast cancer patients were found to respond to endocrine therapies, this increased sensitivity in the assay actually reduced the ability of the assay to predict endocrine responses. One solution to this problem was not only to consider the presence of estrogen receptor in the lesion, but to assess the possible significance of the concentration of receptor. As shown in Figure 17.3, based on sedimentation analyses at sub-

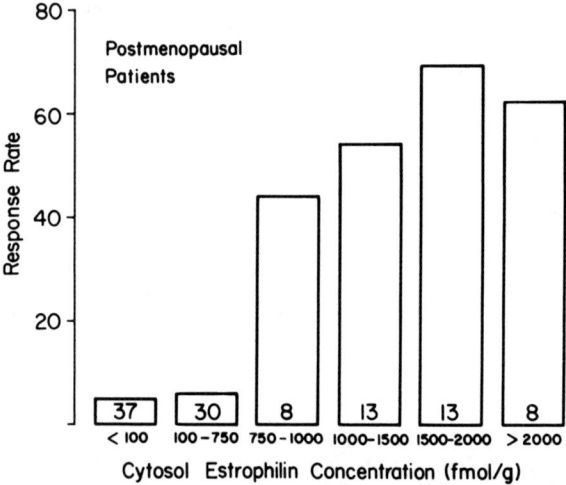

Figure 17.4. Relation of response rate of postmenopausal breast cancer patients to endocrine therapy to the tumor cytosol estrogen receptor concentration. The number in each bar designates the number of patients in the group, and the range of receptor values is given under each bar (ER assay by sedimentation analysis at subsaturating estradiol concentration, Jensen et al. [1976]). (From DeSombre et al. 1978.)

saturating concentrations of estrogen, those patients whose lesions contained a low concentration of estrogen receptor, as well as those with no receptor at all, seldom responded to endocrine therapy (DeSombre et al. 1978). Although some patients with cancers found to contain high concentrations of estrogen receptor nonetheless do not benefit from endocrine therapies, most of such treatment failures occurred in patients whose cancers had only low-to-moderate receptor content. When patient response rates were related directly to tumor estrogen receptor content for lesions of the postmenopausal patients (Fig. 17.4), the low response rate for patients whose tumors have low estrogen receptor content was evident. Thus, rather than characterizing breast cancers as receptor-positive or negative, it seemed to be more appropriate to indicate whether the lesions were receptor rich or poor, with the classification based upon clinical response rate (Jensen et al. 1976). Furthermore, as seen in Figure 17.4, there appeared to be an increasing response rate with increasing receptor content of the tumor (DeSombre and Jensen 1980). This relationship has been observed by others as well (Dao and Nemoto 1980; Lippman and Allegra 1980; Osborne et al. 1980; Paridaens et al. 1980). Using such a quantitative cutoff for estrogen receptor (as indicated by the dashed lines

Table 17.1. Objective remissions to endocrine ablation[a]

| | Tumor classification | |
Treatment	Receptor-rich	Receptor-poor
Adrenalectomy	4/6	0/20
Adrenalectomy + oophorectomy	14/19	1/17
Hypophysectomy	2/4	0/9
Oophorectomy	9/12	1/30
Total (n = 117)	29/41 (71%)	2/76 (3%)

[a]Objective remissions/total cases.

in Fig. 17.3), one finds improved predictability of endocrine responses (Table 17.1). In this series of 117 patients treated by endocrine-ablative surgery, 71% of those classified as having estrogen receptor–rich cancers responded to one of the various endocrine-ablative procedures. Even though the receptor-poor category contains lesions which have identifiable, albeit low, concentrations of estrogen receptor as well as the receptor-negative lesions, only a very low response rate, 3%, was observed. The overall accuracy of prediction of response in these patients approaches 90% (29 plus 74 of 117 equals 88%) with the overall response rate (29 plus 2 divided by 117 equals 26.5%) similar to that observed in unselected populations of breast cancer patients. Nonetheless, as is evident from Table 17.1 as well as Figures 17.3 and 17.4, some patients whose breast cancers contain even high concentrations of estrogen receptor do not respond to endocrine therapy. Knowledge of the progestin receptor content of breast cancer has also been found to improve the predictability of endocrine response in the patient. Results presented at the Consensus Meeting on Steroid Receptors in Breast Cancer in 1979 (DeSombre et al. 1979), which consisted of clinical correlations of responses to endocrine therapy with the estrogen and progestin receptor status of the cancers, from 10 institutions, and which included more than 500 patient trials, showed that 78% of patients whose lesions contained both estrogen and progestin receptor had objective responses to endocrine therapy, but 33% responded when only one of the two receptors was present (DeSombre 1982). Although conventional steroid-binding assays for estrogen and progestin receptor are indeed useful in predicting breast cancer response to endocrine therapies and also in providing prognostic information (see review in DeSombre 1982), there is room for improvement of the accuracy of response prediction and there is a critical need for more insight into the nature of hormone-regulated processes in normal and neoplastic cells.

IV. *Antibodies to the Estrogen Receptor Protein*

A. LIMITATIONS OF CURRENT RECEPTOR ASSAYS

Despite the considerable clinical utility of steroid-binding assays for estrogen and progestin receptor, such assays suffer from distinct limitations. As has been well documented, especially in cancer tissue, the binding of the steroid to its receptor protein can be very labile, and often the reproducibility of steroid-binding assay results among several laboratories is less than optimal. Futhermore, in recent years there has been increased recognition of the importance of obtaining pathological confirmation of the nature of the tissue being assayed for receptor by having pathological assessment of the tissue adjacent to that taken for the assay, but the actual composition of various benign and metastatic, as well as connective tissue and stromal, components within the actual lesion being assayed cannot be assessed, since the tissue is homogenized. Perhaps the quantity of receptor reflects the proportion of cancer cells within the tissue, but it is also possible that there is heterogeneity in the expression of estrogen receptor, reflecting also a heterogeneity in the hormone dependency of the various cancer cells of the lesion. Such information obviously cannot be obtained from the conventional steroid-binding assays.

B. ANTIBODY-BASED ASSAYS FOR ESTROGEN RECEPTOR

With the availability of monoclonal antibodies to the estrogen receptor from human breast cancer cells (Greene et al. 1980; Jensen et al. 1982; Greene 1984), it became possible to develop assays for the estrogen receptor protein itself, independent of steroid binding. In separate studies the antibodies have been found to react with both the estrogen receptor complex and the naked receptor protein (Greene 1984), thereby allowing detection of receptor complexed to endogenous estrogen (which is difficult to assay by exchange assays using steroid-binding procedures), as well as the uncomplexed receptor. These antibodies have therefore been used to develop both immunoradiometric and immunocolorimetric assays for estrogen receptor (Greene and Jensen 1982).

A number of the monoclonal antibodies have been studied as reagents for immunohistochemical detection of receptor in normal and neoplastic tissues (King and Greene 1984; Press et al. 1985). The results have shown an essentially exclusive nuclear localization of estrogen receptor by immunohistochemical staining. Indeed, the possibility that the estrogen receptor may be a nuclear protein, even in the absence of hormone, was also suggested previously by others (Siiteri et al. 1973; Martin and Sheridan 1982). This conclusion that the receptor is in the nucleus even in the absence of estrogen is also consistent with the recent report by Welshons et al. (1984), who found that cytochalasin-induced enucleation of GH_3 pituitary cells leads to the partition of the estrogen receptor almost exclusively with the nucleoplasts, although the cytoplasts retain most of the total cellular protein.

Although under certain conditions it is possible to carry out estrogen receptor–immunocytochemical assays (ER-ICA) in paraffin blocks of fixed tissues, we have found that the epitopes of most, if not all, of the antibodies are highly sensitive to fixation procedures and the most dependable results with normal or neoplastic tissues are obtained with brief fixation of frozen sections of tissue. Several studies of fixation conditions (Press and Greene 1984; King et al. 1985) have indicated that using short fixation times (less than 10 minutes) with ethanol, buffered formalin, or acetone all give acceptable immunocytochemical results. The most sensitive method results from short fixation with picric acid:paraformaldehyde (Stefanini et al. 1967) or periodic acid:lysine:paraformaldehyde (McLean and Nakane 1974). As has been presented in detail elsewhere (King and Greene 1984; King et al. 1985) and can be seen in Figure 17.5, the positive staining in cell nuclei of breast cancer sections incubated with monoclonal antibody to estrogen receptor is specific. Sequential sections of the same tumor incubated with control rat IgG (since the monoclonal antibodies are rat IgG) show no such staining. Furthermore, if the antibody is first exposed to a sufficient concentration of crude or purified estrogen receptor, the nuclear staining is prevented (King and Greene 1984).

C. CLINICAL UTILITY OF ESTROGEN RECEPTOR IMMUNOCHEMICAL ASSAYS

In a study comparing immunocytochemical and steroid-binding assays for estrogen receptor in human breast cancers, we found a clear relationship between steroid-binding assays for estrogen receptor and ER-ICA nuclear staining of the same cancers (King et al. 1985). In this study ER-

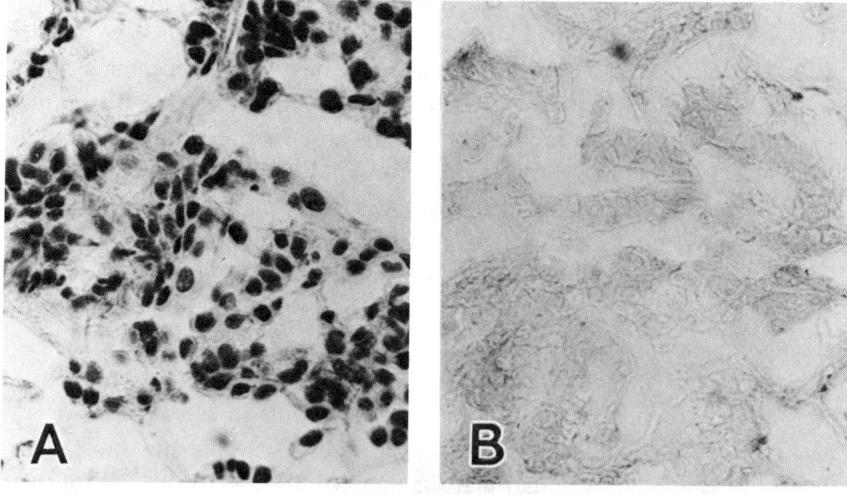

Figure 17.5. Immunocytochemical staining of an ER-rich breast cancer. Adjacent 8 μm frozen sections of the cancer were fixed in ethanol and stained using the immunoperoxidase technique with 10 μg/ml of anti-ER antibody H226 (A) or normal rat IgG (B), followed by goat antirat IgG and rat peroxidase, antiperoxidase complex. After washing with PBS, the sections were incubated with chromagen (1.7 mM diaminobenzadine and 0.06% hydrogen peroxide in PBS) for staining. (From King et al. 1985.)

ICA results were designated positive in all cases in which any specific nuclear staining was found, independent of its intensity or distribution. As shown in Figure 17.6, all those premenopausal or postmenopausal patients whose lesions would be considered receptor-rich according to criteria discussed earlier were found to contain ER-ICA–positive cells. In addition, some tumors found to be receptor-poor, but having measurable receptor, were also found to contain specific nuclear staining for receptor. In a group of 38 of these ER-ICA–positive tumors, staining intensity and distribution were evaluated for comparison with quantitative receptor values. Staining intensity showed a weak correlation with receptor content alone ($R = 0.382$, $p < 0.05$), but the proportion of stained epithelial cells showed a stronger correlation ($R = 0.565$, $p < 0.01$) (King et al. 1985). An important feature of this relationship, however, was the consistently high proportion of ER-ICA–positive tumor cells in ER-rich lesions. However, tumors with low cytosolic estrogen receptor by steroid-binding assays showed a range in heterogeneity of nuclear staining. Thus, classification of a lesion as ER-poor may arise from either a lack of tumor cells

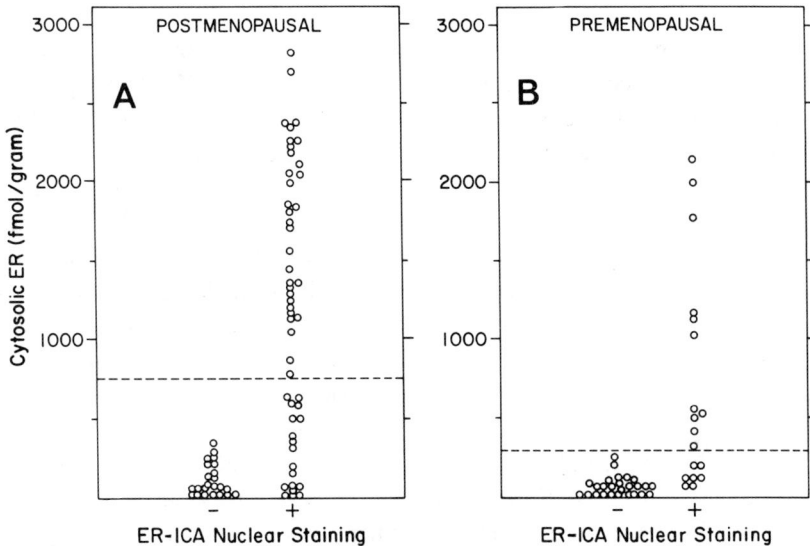

Figure 17.6. Comparison of immunocytochemical and sucrose density gradient assays for ER in breast cancers from postmenopausal (A) and premenopausal (B) patients. Frozen sections of the cancers were briefly fixed in ethanol, incubated with anti-ER antibody H226Sp2, and stained as described in Figure 17.5. Cytosolic ER was determined on another portion of each cancer by sucrose gradient assay (Jensen et al. 1976). The cancers were classified as ER-ICA–positive if they showed any specific nuclear staining regardless of the staining intensity or distribution.

in the lesion, even if the tumor cells are largely ER-positive, or in the case of highly cellular cancers, from a low percentage of ER-positive cells.

A recent collaborative study has as one of its goals to assess the clinical usefulness of ER-ICA in breast cancers. The patients are high-risk, postmenopausal, stage II breast cancer patients entered into randomized adjuvant therapy trials conducted by the Danish Breast Cancer Group. In this study we wished to confirm and possibly refine the correlation of ER-ICA features with quantitative estrogen receptor assays, which in this case were performed by more standard steroid-binding methods; dextran-coated charcoal (DCC) titration assays with Scatchard plots according to the EORTC protocol (EORTC Breast Cancer Cooperative Group 1980). However, we also wished to determine whether there might be any relationship between any ER-ICA features and the disease-free interval or survival of the patients. Patients were treated by total mastectomy and partial axillary dissection, following which most were randomized to receive radiotherapy to the mastectomy area and the supraclavicular and axillary lymph nodes at a dose equivalent to 1335 rets (rad). They were randomized to receive either no drug treatment or tamoxifen, 10 mg three times daily for 48 weeks (see Rose et al. 1985). A small number of patients entered into a subsequent protocol which randomized patients among rad + TAM, TAM alone, or TAM + CMF (cyclophosphamide, methotrexate, and 5-flourouracil). At the time of ER analysis by DCC, a central portion of the tumor tissue was removed, placed in a cryotube, and kept frozen at −70°C until the time of ER-ICA analysis. In this study frozen sections of the cancers were fixed for 5 minutes at room temperature with picric acid:paraformaldehyde, but other aspects of the immunocytochemical procedure of the coded biopsies was performed essentially the same as in the earlier study (King et al. 1985).

As noted above, in this study cancers were assayed by steroid-binding methods as well as ER-ICA evaluation. Unlike the previous study (King et al. 1985), however, an overall judgment was made as to whether the sample was to be designated ER-ICA–positive or –negative to reflect the predominant nature of the tumor, that is, combining qualitatively the intensity of staining and staining distribution. Correlation with steroid-binding assays showed that all but two of the lesions found to be estrogen receptor–negative by steroid-binding assays were also judged ER-ICA–negative. However, the ER-ICA–negative lesions also included some cancers with up to 50 fmols ER/mg cytosol protein. In this study both the staining intensity and the percentage of ER-ICA positive cells correlated strongly with the quantitative estrogen receptor assay. The intensity of ER-ICA staining was coded as 0 or 1, 2, or 3 +, corresponding to increasing intensity of staining. As shown in Table 17.2, greater staining intensity

Table 17.2. Correlation of ER-ICA staining intensity and ER-DCC[a]

ER-ICA staining intensity	Number of samples	Median ER-DCC (fmol/mg protein)
0	26	< 10
1	11	20
2	56	150
3	21	600

[a] Samples of breast cancers from the Danish Breast Cancer Group high-risk adjuvant therapy protocol study.

corresponded in a direct way to more receptor as determined by DCC assay.

Regression analysis of the features of ER-ICA as predictors of the quantity of estrogen receptor indicated a strong relationship between ER-ICA and the quantitative ER value (Fig. 17.7). These results suggest that by combining the ER-ICA staining intensity and features representing the

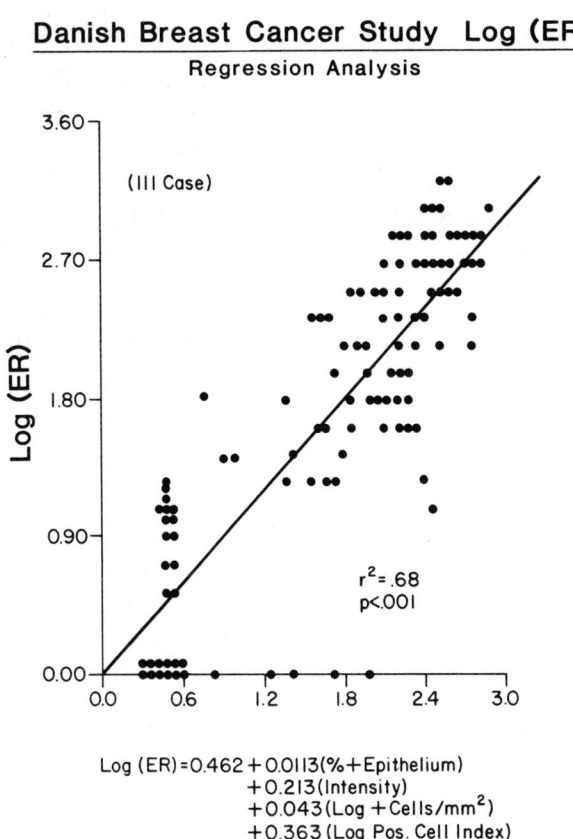

Danish Breast Cancer Study Log (ER)
Regression Analysis

$$Log (ER) = 0.462 + 0.0113(\% + Epithelium)$$
$$+ 0.213(Intensity)$$
$$+ 0.043(Log + Cells/mm^2)$$
$$+ 0.363 (Log\ Pos.\ Cell\ Index)$$

Figure 17.7. Regression analysis of the best linear fit of ER-ICA parameters to predict the log of the ER-DCC value. The positive cells/mm^2 of cross section was determined with the aid of an ocular grid, scanning the entire tissue section. The positive cell index was based on three randomly chosen fields (at 100×) for each section by recording the frequency with which an ER-ICA–stained cell coincided with any of the 99 intersections on the 1 mm^2 ocular grid. The major contributions to the correlation are derived from the percentage of positive epithelium and intensity results, with the other two parameters, also reflecting the tissue distribution, making only minor additions to the overall correlation.

distribution of stained cells one can obtain a reasonably accurate prediction of the quantity of estrogen receptor which would be obtained by conventional steroid-binding assays. The statistically significant relationship between the quantity of "cytosolic" estrogen receptor, by steroid-binding assays, and the intensity and distribution or heterogeneity of *nuclear* immunohistochemical staining for ER also provides strong support for the conclusion that ER-ICA and ER-DCC are measuring the same receptor, or at least that what ER-ICA is showing is directly related to the amount of ER found by steroid-binding assays of low salt extracts of the tumor.

Initial evaluation of recurrence and survival statistics for these patients suggests that ER-ICA parameters are of prognostic usefulness as well. As shown in Figure 17.8, there is a statistically significant difference in disease-free interval of patients whose lesions were judged to be ER-ICA–positive compared with those to be judged to be ER-ICA–negative. Analyses at this time suggest that this prognostic usefulness of ER-ICA is in-

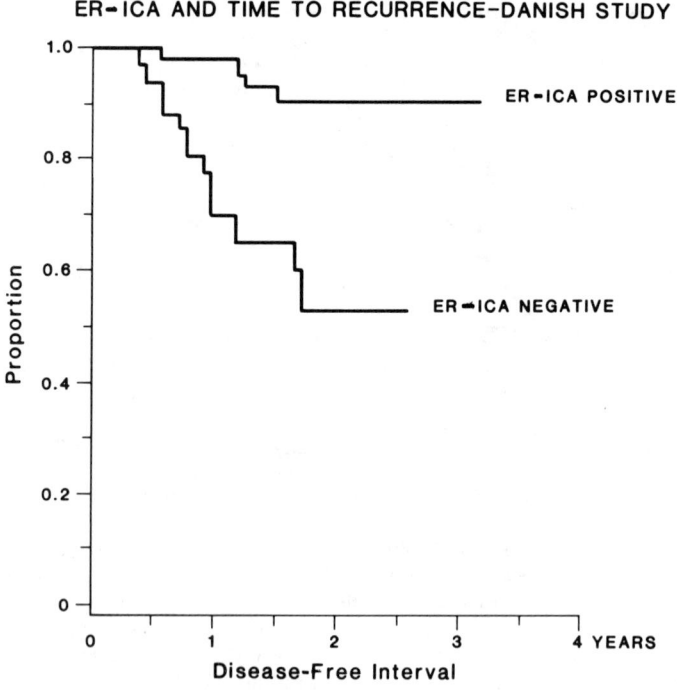

Figure 17.8. Proportional hazard regression analysis of ER-ICA status with the time to recurrence for the breast cancer patients.

dependent of the lymph node status and serves to further stratify patient prognosis for recurrence and survival based on lymph node status alone (DeSombre et al. 1986). Similarly, statistically significant differences between ER-ICA–positive and –negative lesions have been found with regard to patient survival. It appears that these prognostic differences relate both to ER-ICA staining intensity and heterogeneity within the lesion. It is probable that some of these differences are related to the improved prognosis, if not survival, of the patients treated with tamoxifen in the adjuvant setting, but the trends of the data at present suggest that responses to tamoxifen are only a part of the basis for these differences. Earlier studies with this patient population indicated that overall there was no statistically significant difference in disease-free interval related to tamoxifen treatment (Rose et al. 1985), but the analysis of specific subgroups indicated that patients whose ER content was greater than 100 fmols/mg cytosol protein appeared to benefit from treatment with antiestrogen in the adjuvant setting. Interestingly, initial results from evaluation of ER-ICA status, treatment protocol, and disease-free interval indicate that, although not statistically different at the present time, the proportional hazard curves for ER-ICA–positive patients treated with radiation alone as well as with radiation plus tamoxifen show prolonged disease-free intervals compared to patients with ER-ICA–negative lesions treated by both of these adjuvant treatments.

Although there are too few data presently available to know whether immunocytochemical evaluation of estrogen receptor in breast cancer can more readily predict which patients will respond to endocrine therapies, the intensity and distribution of ER-ICA–stained cells within breast cancers are clearly of considerable value. Certainly the ability to identify whether the receptor is present in the invasive lesion or associated with benign or hyperplastic elements of the specimen will be of considerable value. Early indications from the Danish study suggest that there is significantly better prognosis for patients whose lesions are ER-ICA–positive. Continued follow-up with this patient group as well as future studies should help assess the actual clinical usefulness of such measurements.

In our experience thus far, it is clear there are certain areas for which immunocytochemical assays for ER are particularly attractive. These include lesions too small for conventional steroid-binding assays and the evaluation of ER in needle aspiration biopsies. The identification of the cellular origin of the ER-positive conventional assay can be reassuring, since we now have several examples of ER-positive lesions where the stained cells were in the noninvasive, hyperplastic or *in situ* lesions within a sample also containing a nonstaining invasive breast cancer. Although the extent of the role of such immunocytochemical assays has yet to be established, it is clear that the new reagents provide information not available by conventional assays. One may also expect that with the availability of these new immunochemical tools to study the basis of the biochemical dependence of normal and neoplastic tissues upon estrogen as mediated by its receptor, we may thereby obtain knowledge to provide new and better methods for the diagnosis and treatment of breast cancer.

Acknowledgments

These investigations were supported by grants from the National Cancer Institute (CA-02897, CA-14599, CA-27476), the American Cancer Society, the UICC Technology Transfer Fellowship Program (to W.J.K.), Abbott Laboratories, the Women's Board of the University of Chicago Cancer Research Foundation, and the Danish Cancer Society.

References

Beatson, G. T. 1896. On the treatment of inoperable cases of carcinoma of the mamma: suggestions for a new method of treatment with illustrative cases. *Lancet* 2:104–107.

Boyd, S. 1900. On oophorectomy in cancer of the breast. *British Medical Journal* 2:1161–1167.

Cole, M. P., C. T. A. Jones, and I. D. H. Todd. 1971. A new antioestrogenic agent in late breast cancer. *British Journal of Cancer* 25:270–275.

Dao, T. L., and T. Nemoto. 1980. Steroid receptors and response to endocrine ablations in women with metastatic cancer of the breast. *Cancer* 46:2779–2782.

DeSombre, E. R. 1982. Breast cancer: hormone receptors, prognosis and therapy. *Clinics in Oncology* 1:191–213.

DeSombre, E. R., and E. V. Jensen. 1980. Estrophilin assays in breast cancer: quantitative features and application to the mastectomy specimen. *Cancer* 46:2783–2788.

DeSombre, E. R., G. L. Greene, and E. V. Jensen. 1978. Estrophilin and endocrine responsiveness of breast cancer. In *Hormones, receptors, and breast cancer. Progress in cancer research and therapy,* vol. 10, ed. W. L. McGuire, 1–14. New York: Raven Press.

DeSombre, E. R., P. P. Carbone, E. V. Jensen, W. L. McGuire, S. A. Wells, J. L. Wittliff, and M. B. Lipsett. 1979. Special report: steroid receptors in breast cancer. *New England Journal of Medicine* 301:1011–1012.

DeSombre, E. R., S. M. Thorpe, C. Rose, R. M. Blough, K. W. Andersen, B. B. Rasmussen, and W. J. King. 1986. Prognostic usefulness of estrogen receptor immunocytochemical assays (ER-ICA) for human breast cancer. *Cancer Research* (in press).

Engelsman, E., J. P. Persijn, C. B. Korsten, and F. J. Cleton. 1973. Oestrogen receptors in human breast cancer tissue and response to endocrine therapy. *British Medical Journal* 2:750–752.

EORTC Breast Cancer Cooperative Group. 1980. Revision of standards for the assessment of hormone receptor in human breast cancer. Report of the second EORTC workshop. *European Journal of Cancer* 16:1513–1515.

Glascock, R. F., and W. G. Hoekstra. 1959. Selective accumulation of tritium-labeled hexoestrol by the reproductive organs of immature female goats and sheep. *Biochemical Journal* 72:673–682.

Gorski, J., D. Toft, G. Shyamala, D. Smith, and A. Notides. 1968. Hormone receptors: studies on the interaction of estrogen with the uterus. *Recent Progress in Hormone Research* 24:45–80.

Greene, G. L. 1984. Application of immunochemical techniques to the analysis of estrogen receptor structure and function. In *Biochemical actions of hormones,* vol. 11, ed. G. Litwack, 207–239. New York: Academic Press.

Greene, G. L. and E. V. Jensen. 1982. Monoclonal antibodies as probes for estrogen receptor detection and characterization. *Journal of Steroid Biochemistry* 16:353–359.

Greene, G. L., C. Nolan, J. P. Engler, and E. V. Jensen. 1980. Monoclonal antibodies to human estrogen receptor. *Proceedings of the National Academy of Sciences* 77: 5115–5119.

Haddow, A., J. M. Watkinson, and E. Patterson. 1944. Influence of synthetic estrogens upon advanced malignant disease. *British Medical Journal* 2:393–398.

Huggins, C., and D. M. Bergenstal. 1952. Inhibition of human mammary and prostatic cancers by adrenalectomy. *Cancer Research* 12:134–141.

Jensen, E. V., and H. I. Jacobson. 1960. Fate of steroid estrogens in target tissues. In *Biological activities of steroids in relation to cancer,* ed. G. Pincus and E. P. Vollmer, 161–174. New York: Academic Press.

Jensen, E. V., and H. I. Jacobson. 1962. Basic guides to the mechanism of estrogen action. *Recent Progress in Hormone Research* 18:387–414.

Jensen, E. V., E. R. DeSombre, and P. W. Jungblut. 1967. Estrogen receptors in hormone-responsive tissues and tumors. In *Endogenous factors influencing host-tumor balance,* ed. R. W. Wissler, T. L. Dao, and S. Wood, Jr., 15–30. Chicago: University of Chicago Press.

Jensen, E. V., T. Suzuki, T. Kawashima, W. E. Stumpf, P. W. Jungblut, and E. R. DeSombre. 1968. A two-step mechanism for the interaction of estradiol with rat uterus. *Proceedings of the National Academy of Sciences* 59:632–638.

Jensen, E. V., G. E. Block, S. Smith, K. Kyser, and E. R. DeSombre. 1971. Estrogen receptors and breast cancer response to adrenalectomy. In *Prediction of response in cancer therapy,* ed T. C. Hall, 55–70. Cancer Institute Monograph 34. Bethesda, Md.

Jensen, E. V., H. I. Jacobson, S. Smith, P. W. Jungblut, and E. R. DeSombre. 1972. The use of estrogen antagonists in hormone receptor studies. *Gynecologic Investigation* 3:108–122.

Jensen, E. V., S. Smith, and E. R. DeSombre. 1976. Hormone dependency in breast cancer. *Journal of Steroid Biochemistry* 7:905–962.

Jensen, E. V., G. L. Greene, L. E. Closs, E. R. DeSombre, and M. Nadji. 1982. Receptors reconsidered: a 20-year perspective. *Recent Progress in Hormone Research* 38:1–40.

Jungblut, P. W., R. I. Morrow, G. L. Reeder, and E. V. Jensen. 1965. *Forty-Seventh Meeting of The Endocrine Society,* New York. Abstract, p. 56.

King, W. J., and G. L. Greene. 1984. Monoclonal antibodies localize oestrogen receptor in the nuclei of target cells. *Nature* (London) 307:745–747.

King, W. J., E. R. DeSombre, E. V. Jensen, and G. L. Greene. 1985. Comparison of immunocytochemical and steroid binding assays for estrogen receptor in human breast tumors. *Cancer Research* 45:293–304.

Leclercq, G., J. C. Heuson, M. C. Deboel, and W. H. Mattheiem. 1975. Oestrogen receptors in breast cancer: a changing concept. *British Medical Journal* 1:185–189.

Leung, B. S., W. S. Fletcher, T. D. Lindell, D. C. Wood, and W. W. Krippaehne. 1973. Predictability of response to endocrine ablation in advanced breast carcinoma. *Archives of Surgery* 106:515–519.

Lippman, M. E., and J. C. Allegra. 1980. Quantitative estrogen receptor analyses: the response to endocrine and cytotoxic chemotherapy in human breast cancer and the disease free interval. *Cancer* 46:2829–2834.

Luft, R., and H. Olivecrona. 1953. Experiences with hypophysectomy in man. *Journal of Neurosurgery* 10:301–316.

Maass, H., B. Engel, H. Hohmeister, F. Lehmann, and G. Trams. 1972. Estrogen receptors in human breast cancer tissue. *American Journal of Obstetrics and Gynecology* 113:377–382.

Martin, P. M., and P. J. Sheridan. 1982. Toward a new model for the mechanism of action of steroids. *Journal of Steroid Biochemistry* 16:215–229.

McGuire, W. L., P. P. Carbone, and E. P. Vollmer (eds.). 1975. *Estrogen receptors in human breast cancer.* New York: Raven Press.

McLean, I. W., and P. K. Nakane. 1974. Periodate-lysine-paraformaldehyde fixative. A new fixative for immunoelectron microscopy. *Journal of Histochemistry and Cytochemistry* 22:1077–1083.

Nathanson, I. T. 1952. Clinical investigative experience with steroid hormones in breast cancer. *Cancer* 5:754–762.

Notides, A., D. E. Hamilton, and H. E. Auer. 1975. A kinetic analysis of the estrogen receptor transformation. *Journal of Biological Chemistry* 250:3945–3950.

Osborne, C. K., M. G. Yochmowitz, W. A. Knight, III, and W. L. McGuire. 1980. The value of estrogen and progesterone receptors in the treatment of breast cancer. *Cancer* 46:2884–2888.

Paridaens, R., R. J. Sylvester, E. Ferrazzi, N. Legros, G. Leclercq, and J. C. Heuson. 1980. Clinical significance of the quantitative assessment of estrogen receptors in advanced breast cancer. *Cancer* 46:2889–2895.

Pearson, O. H., B. S. Ray, and C. C. Harrold. 1956. Hypophysectomy in treatment of advanced cancer. *Journal of the American Medical Association* 161:17–21.

Press, M. F., and G. L. Greene. 1984. An immunocytochemical method for demonstrating estrogen receptor in human uterus using monoclonal antibodies to human estrophilin. *Laboratory Investigation* 50:480–486.

Rose, C., S. M. Thorpe, K. W. Andersen, B. V. Pedersen, H. T. Mouridsen, M. Beichert-Toft, and B. B. Rasmussen. 1985. Beneficial effect of adjuvant tamoxifen therapy in primary breast cancer patients with high oestrogen receptor values. *Lancet* 1:16–19.

Savlov, E. D., J. L. Wittliff, R. Hilf, and T. C. Hall. 1974. Correlations of certain biochemical properties of breast cancer and response to therapy: a preliminary report. *Cancer* 33:303–309.

Siiteri, P. K., B. E. Schwarz, I. Moriyama, R. Ashby, D. Linkie, and P. C. MacDonald. 1973. Estrogen binding in the rat and human. In *Receptors for reproductive hormones. Advances in Experimental Medicine and Biology,* vol. 36, ed. B. W. O' Malley and A. R. Means, 97–112. New York: Plenum Press.

Stefanini, M., C. DeMartino, and L. Zamboni. 1967. Fixation of ejaculated spermatozoa for electron microscopy. *Nature* (London) 216:173–174.

Terenius, L. 1966. Specific uptake of oestrogens by the mouse uterus *in vitro*. *Acta Endocrinologica* 53:611–618.

Toft, D., and J. Gorski. 1966. A receptor molecule for estrogens: isolation from the rat uterus and preliminary characterization. *Proceedings of the National Academy of Sciences* 55:1574–1581.

Ward, H. W. C. 1973. Anti-oestrogen therapy for breast cancer: a trial of tamoxifen at two dose levels. *British Medical Journal* 1:13–14.

Welshons, W. V., M. E. Lieberman, and J. Gorski. 1984. Nuclear localization of unoccupied oestrogen receptors: cytochalasin enucleation of GH_3 cells. *Nature* (London) 307:747–749.

18

Estrogen Receptor Determinations: Studies in Relation to Rapidly Progressive Carcinoma of the Breast

K. Griffiths, R. I. Nicholson, R. W. Blamey, and C. W. Elston

I. Introduction 326
II. Patients and Clinical Study 327
III. Methodology: Receptor Analysis 327
IV. Disease Recurrence and Prognostic Index 328
V. Survival after Recurrence 333
   A. Response to Therapy 333
   B. Site of Recurrence and Response 335
   C. Tumor Growth Rate 336
References 338

325

I. *Introduction*

A MOST interesting and well-established feature of breast cancer is that, generally, the condition can be considered to encompass two types of disease. Certain tumors are hormone-responsive and will regress after endocrine therapy, ablative or additive. In such patients, therefore, representing approximately 30% of women with advanced metastatic cancer, endocrine therapy offers a reasonable and important means of palliating the disease. In contrast, other tumors are hormone-independent and conventional endocrine treatment provides no substantial benefit in the management of patients with this form of breast cancer. Estrogens are involved in the regulation of gene expression and cell proliferation in the hormone-responsive breast cancer, their biological effects being mediated through a specific estrogen receptor (ER) protein (Jensen and DeSombre 1973), and although certain clinical features have been found useful in predicting the response to endocrine therapy, in recent years it has become clear that the determination of the ER concentration of the tumor offers a more valuable, objective predictive factor. Clinical studies have shown that the presence of the estrogen receptor protein in secondary breast cancer is associated with a 50–60% objective response rate to endocrine therapy (McGuire et al. 1975) and during the past few years, routine ER analysis has been used to preselect patients likely to benefit from this treatment.

It is equally clear, however, that although estrogen dependence or independence represent two biological variants of breast cancer, clinical experience shows that the disease presents with a variable range of malignancy, degree of differentiation, rates of growth, and invasiveness. Of particular interest must therefore be the relationship among these various clinical and biological features of breast cancer, the estrogen receptor status of the tumor, and the natural history of the disease. This communication deals with the monitoring of breast cancer progression in a series of patients studied from clinical presentation and treatment to recurrence and secondary therapy, relating various clinical and biological features of the disease to survival.

II. Patients and Clinical Study

Over the past decade, the Breast Cancer Research Laboratory (Head, R.I.N.) of the Tenovus Institute for Cancer Research (Director, K.G.) has been responsible for the measurement of the ER content of over 10,000 breast cancer specimens. This analysis was undertaken in association with various clinical research studies (Bishop et al. 1979; Croton et al. 1981; Nicholson et al. 1981; Blamey et al. 1983; Griffiths et al. 1983; Nicholson et al. 1984a) and as a routine service for the management of patients with breast cancer in the various hospitals in Wales.

A considerable amount of information has been generated from this analytical program, but the investigations associated with one particular center, the Breast Clinic, City Hospital, Nottingham, have provided invaluable data for the study of the natural history of the disease in relation to various biological and clinical characteristics (Blamey et al. 1983).

The women in this study form part of a consecutive series of patients with operable primary breast cancer, under the care of one surgeon (R.W.B.), whose tumors had been typed and graded according to their degree of malignancy (consultant pathologist, C.W.E.).

This Nottingham-Tenovus research program was initiated in 1973 with preliminary reports (Griffiths et al. 1978; Maynard et al. 1978a,b) describing the study. Patients underwent a single or subcutaneous mastectomy and in the majority of women, further treatment was withheld until symptomatic advanced disease had developed (Blamey et al. 1980). On recurrence, endocrine therapy was initiated, premenopausal women undergoing bilateral oophorectomy and postmenopausal patients receiving the antiestrogen tamoxifen (Campbell et al. 1981b). Radiotherapy was administered to patients with secondary disease where appropriate.

Response to therapy was externally assessed according to the criteria of the UICC (Hayward et al. 1977) but with a mandatory response period of 6 months (British Breast Group 1974).

III. Methodology: Receptor Analysis

The procedure for ER determination has been described previously (Nicholson et al. 1981, 1984a). Simply, tumor tissue was rapidly frozen after removal and stored in liquid nitrogen before transportation in dry ice to Cardiff, where ER status was determined within 2–3 weeks. ER levels were measured using a saturation analysis technique incubating high-speed supernatant with 10 concentrations of [³H]estradiol-17β ranging from 200–5000 pmol/l for 16 hours at 4°C. The inefficiency of separating free from bound label, and nonspecific binding were also estimated, computation of values being based on the method of least squares using a Newton-Raphson iterative technique (Feldman 1972).

Throughout the period of study, these laboratories have been particularly concerned with the problems of quality control of the procedures for determining ER status (Wilson et al. 1981). Tumor sampling at surgery (Mumford et al. 1983) and the storage of tissue specimens prior to analysis require care and a responsible pathology laboratory. Computation of assay data is important to determine the minimum detectable level that can be distinguished from zero with given probability, which is dependent on assay precision. The errors concerned in the analytical procedure and in the computation of results have been thoroughly investigated (Wilson et al. 1981; Richards et al. 1983; Nicholson et al. 1984a) in these laboratories, studies which clearly have directed attention to the inherent errors in the methodology and the care required in the quality-assessment program.

IV. Disease Recurrence and Prognostic Index

The basis of the Tenovus-Nottingham study was the development of a better understanding of the natural history of breast cancer and the identification of biological and clinical characteristics that influence prognosis. Clearly, improvements in therapy can only be derived from a greater ability to predict the behavior of *individual* tumors, and it should be accepted that no single therapeutic regimen is appropriate for all patients. In this study, therefore, patient follow-up after mastectomy was carried out at regular intervals and patients *did not* receive systemic adjuvant therapy, treatment being witheld until the disease recurred.

It is now well established that approximately 60% of breast tumors contain measurable amounts of estrogen receptor (McGuire et al. 1975). In accord with the accumulated data of many studies (Consensus Meeting 1980), the early results from this investigation indicated that there was no correlation between ER status and tumor size or disease stage (Maynard et al. 1978a). It is also now accepted that the ER status reflects the degree of tumor differentiation (Maynard et al. 1978b), the majority of undifferentiated grade III cancers being ER-negative. It is noteworthy, however,

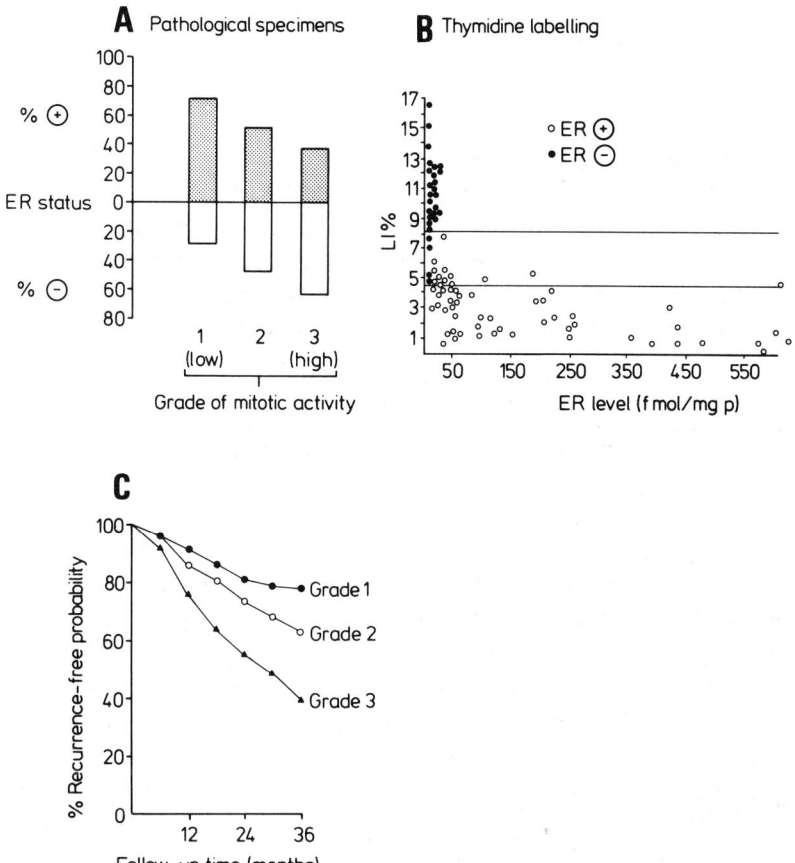

Figure 18.1. Relationship between estrogen receptor status and (A) mitotic index of tissue specimens and (B) thymidine-labeling index; (C) relationship between the grade of mitotic activity observed for histological sections of the tumor and disease recurrence.

that three parameters are used for this semiquantitative assessment of the degree of differentiation, essentially, nuclear pleomorphism, the presence of tubular structures, and mitotic rate; and it is the mitotic rate which shows the most significant relationship with ER status (Fig. 18.1A). Tumors with low mitotic activity are more often (71%) ER-positive, with higher levels of receptor, whereas the intermediary group and those with a high mitotic index have a greater proportion of ER-negative tumors (52% and 36% are ER-positive, respectively). Only 16% of postmenopausal, ER-negative tumors were seen to have a low mitotic activity. Equally,

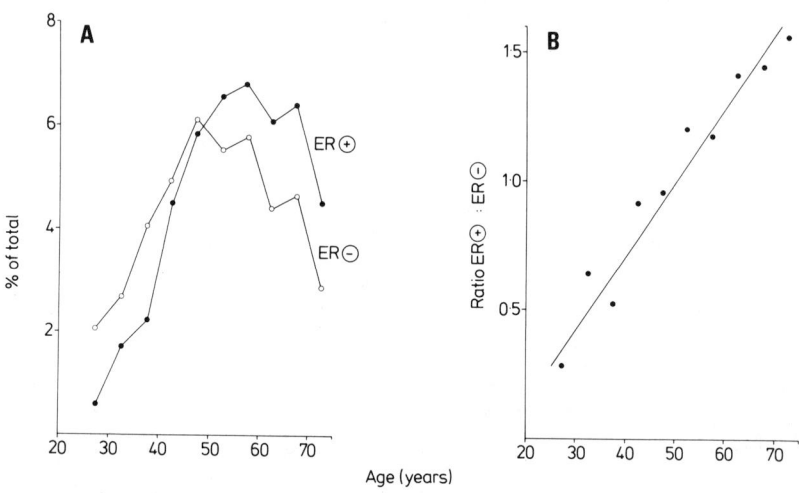

Figure 18.2. Relationship between ER status of primary tumor and the age of patients at mastectomy. The data are derived from 2000 patients.

the thymidine-labeling index, as might be expected, related to ER status (Fig. 18.1B) and the rate of mitotic activity correlates well with disease recurrence (Fig. 18.1C) as does tumor grade (Griffiths et al. 1983).

Receptor status in relation to age at presentation with breast cancer and to recurrence and survival is of particular interest. Breast cancer is comparatively rare in young women, but the incidence rises steeply during middle age and in women over 55 years of age represents the major form of cancer (Logan 1975). Data on the ER status of primary tumors in relation to the age distribution shows that less than 50% are ER-positive in women between the ages of 25 and 40 years. The figure rises to 58% in women who present with breast cancer between the ages of 41 and 50 years, and to 65% in patients older than 50 (51–60 years). This relationship is illustrated in Figure 18.2.

Although earlier reports (Knight et al. 1977; Griffiths et al. 1978; Maynard et al. 1978a) suggested that patients with ER-negative tumors recurred earlier and that this advantage for patients with tumors with measurable amounts of receptor was also seen in relation to survival (Bishop et al. 1979), longer-term follow-up at 7 years indicates that these differences are small (Fig. 18.3). Certainly ER status alone cannot be considered a good prognostic factor, although the measurement of the amount of receptor does appear to contribute significantly to prognosis in the pres-

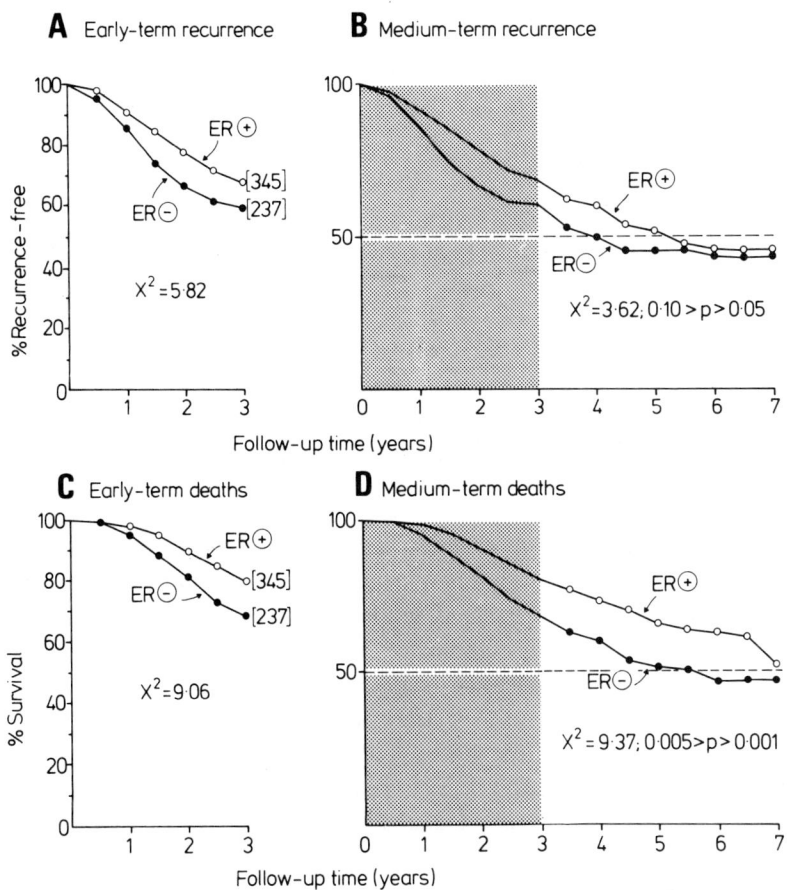

Figure 18.3. ER status and prognosis.

ence of therapy (Fig. 18.4). Some evidence has been presented earlier (Nicholson et al. 1981; Griffiths et al. 1983) to show that prognosis can be better predicted if stage and grade are assessed in relation to ER status. The risk category of an *individual* patient must be seen to be important in determining the appropriate treatment regimen, particularly when adjuvant therapy is to be considered. More important, possibly, may be the decision that immediate adjuvant therapy is *not* appropriate.

Development of procedures to stratify patients into controlled clinical trials on the basis of good, objective prognostic indices is of paramount importance and, as part of the Tenovus-Nottingham program, multivariate

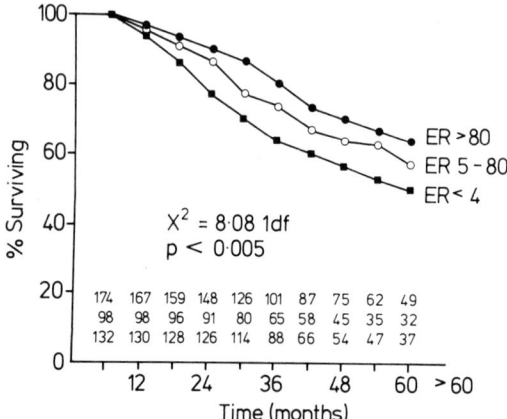

Figure 18.4. Relationship between survival of patients and the amount of estrogen receptor in the primary tumor.

analysis has been used to establish a prognostic index (Haybittle et al. 1982; Blamey et al. 1983). The independent contribution of the various factors such as tumor size, stage, grade, ER status, age, menopausal status, and other factors, was evaluated in relation to subsequent survival, with the statistical procedure (Cox 1972) estimating the independent contribution of each factor to the hazard function, or risk of dying. Tumor size, stage, and either ER status or grade were found significant, the contribution being measured by a coefficient. Using the various coefficients, a prognostic index (PI) was calculated for each patient, for example:

PI = 0.76 (lymph node stage) + 0.82 (grade) + 0.17 (tumor size)

The use of the index was found to offer better discrimination between patients than using staging alone. Patients with a PI of 2.8 or less were found to have an excellent prognosis, with a survival curve similar to that of the age-matched normal female population (Fig. 18.5). Patients with indices greater than 4.4 have a very bad prognosis, with more than 90% dead within 5 years.

The reliable histopathological evaluation of tumor grade has been a particular feature of the Nottingham-Tenovus study, which became clear with the early observation (Maynard et al. 1978b) that there was a significant correlation between tumor grade and ER status. Consequently, ER status can be substituted for grade (ER being coded as follows: negative = 0, positive = 1). Therefore, the prognostic index can be derived from the equation:

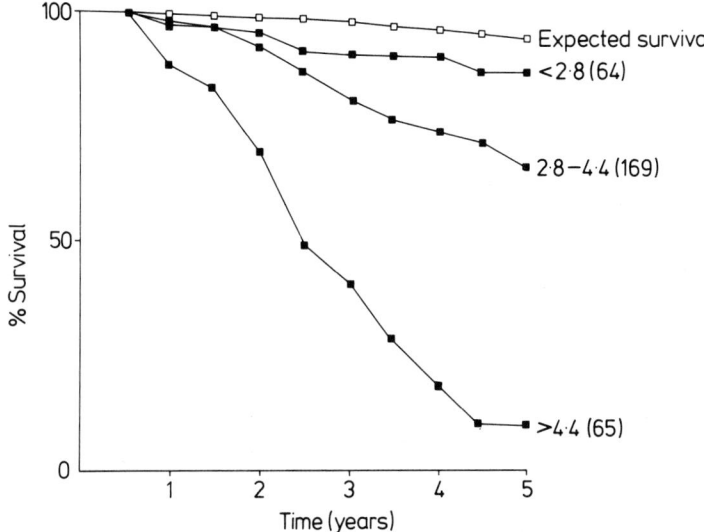

Figure 18.5. Survival of patients according to their prognostic index shown against the expected survival of an age-matched population free of breast cancer (□).

$$PI = 0.18 \text{ (size)} + 0.68 \text{ (stage)} - 0.52 \text{ (ER)}$$

The principal advantage of ER status over histological grade is that the former is a more reliable indicator of response to endocrine therapy than the latter and, in general, offers a more objective form of analysis. The current investigations on the use of preparations of labeled antibodies against the receptor will soon offer new and interesting data that should be of particular prognostic value.

V. Survival after Recurrence

A. RESPONSE TO THERAPY

For the larger proportion of patients, the prognosis after the first major recurrence is poor, with only 50% surviving beyond 12 months, and 20% until the end of the second year. All patients with a prolonged survival of greater than 5 years had an ER-positive tumor and responded to endocrine therapy. Figure 18.6A shows patient survival after recurrence (first 101 patients to recur in this study) and following endocrine therapy. Of the patients studied, 23% responded to endocrine therapy and all but one had an ER-positive tumor. Only one person with a "reported" ER-negative

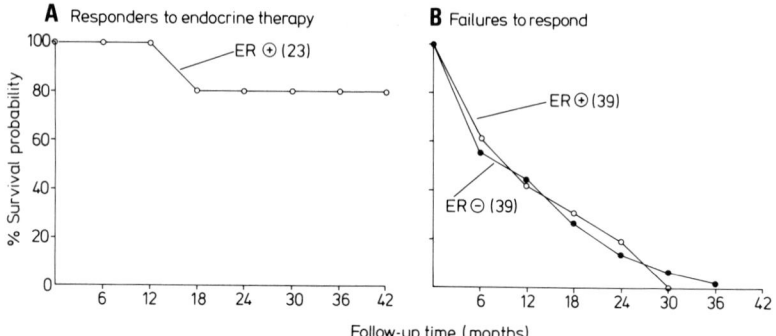

Figure 18.6. Patient survival after disease recurrence: (A) responses to endocrine therapy; (B) patients who failed to respond.

tumor responded. A large proportion (77%) failed to respond, of whom 39/78 had ER-positive tumors (Fig. 18.6B). As previously reported (Campbell et al. 1981b; Nicholson et al. 1984a), the responders were those patients whose tumors had the higher levels of estrogen receptor. Of those patients who failed to respond to endocrine therapy, those with ER-positive tumors fared just as badly as those in whom the tumor was shown to be ER-negative (Fig. 18.6B). When the patients who failed endocrine therapy were studied, age at recurrence appeared to have little or no effect in relation to survival after recurrence (Fig. 18.7).

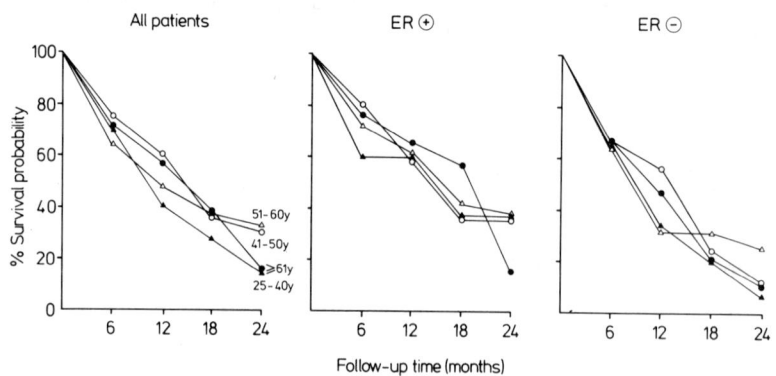

Figure 18.7. Relationship between patient survival after disease recurrence and the age of the patient at recurrence.

B. SITE OF RECURRENCE AND RESPONSE

It has been recognized for some time that the anatomical site of distant metastases offers a guide to the clinician, not only with regard to response to endocrine therapy (Baum 1980) but also to survival (Papaioannou et al. 1967; Cutler et al. 1969). Patients with skeletal metastases respond much better to endocrine therapy than those with visceral secondaries, whose prognosis is much less favorable. Although generally the overall incidence of distant metastases is unrelated to ER status of the primary tumor, the site of the metastatic spread is related (Campbell et al. 1981a; Nicholson et al. 1981). Patients with ER-positive primary tumors tended to develop bone metastases, whereas the ER-negative tumor disseminated to the viscera. However, of the patients with either visceral or bone metastases, those with ER-positive primary tumors tended to fare a little better than those with ER-negative disease (Fig. 18.8).

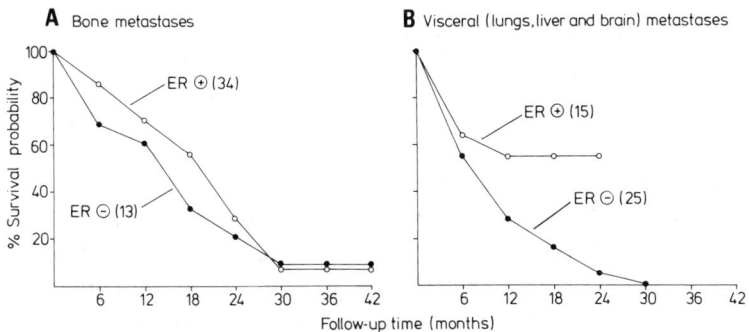

Figure 18.8. Relationship betwen patient survival after recurrence and receptor status of those with (A) bone metastases and (B) visceral metastatic deposits.

It is interesting that the response rate is similar for all patients with ER-positive tumors, regardless of whether they have skeletal or visceral metastatic spread (Fig. 18.9). The difference essentially between the groups is that there are more patients with ER-positive tumors who appear with skeletal metastases (Fig. 18.8). Again, regardless of whether a patient had visceral metastases or secondaries in bone, if the tumor is ER-positive and the patient responds to endocrine therapy, the responders subsequently do well. The failures, patients with either ER-positive or ER-negative tumors, fare badly and generally are dead within 3 years (Fig. 18.9).

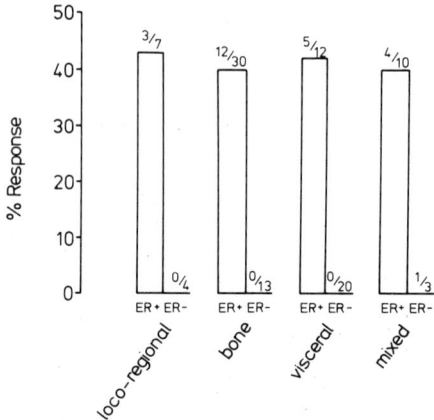

Figure 18.9. Response of patients to endocrine therapy in relation to site of metastatic deposit.

C. TUMOR GROWTH RATE

It would probably be expected that the mitotic rate of the primary tumor and the related disease-free interval are factors that would be seen to relate to survival after recurrence. Patients with tumors showing a low mitotic index and with a long disease-free interval (DFI) have a much more favorable prognosis than those with a high index and short DFI (Nicholson et al. 1984b). ER-negative tumors are generally associated with poor prognosis (Fig. 18.10), even in women with a DFI greater than 2 years. Conversely, 10/11 women with ER-positive tumors had a DFI longer than 4 years (Fig. 18.11). Such tumors were more frequently found in older women, the postmenopausal group of patients having a greater proportion of ER-positive tumors with low mitotic index. Patients with ER-positive primary tumors and a short DFI, or with high mitotic index, die after recurrence, at a rate similar to patients with ER-negative tumors.

Figure 18.12 shows the relationship between ER status, response of the secondary disease to endocrine therapy, and duration of the disease-free interval. Clearly patients with ER-positive tumors which respond to endocrine therapy are drawn from a group of women with slower recurring, and by inference, slower growing, disease. Patients with ER-positive or -negative primary tumors who subsequently fail to respond to endocrine therapy have relatively short disease-free intervals.

Overall, a patient's prognosis after mastectomy is dependent on a com-

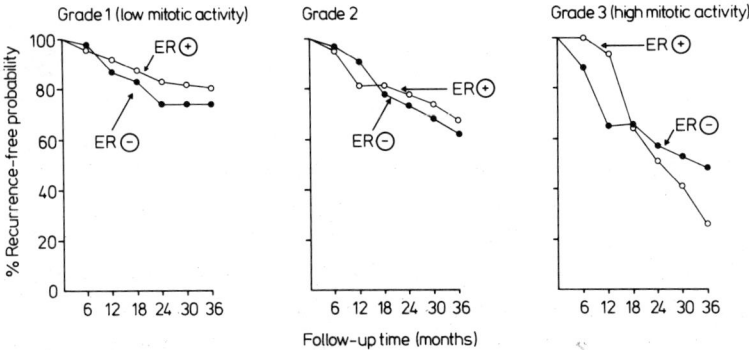

Figure 18.10. Relationship between disease-free interval and mitotic activity of the primary tumor.

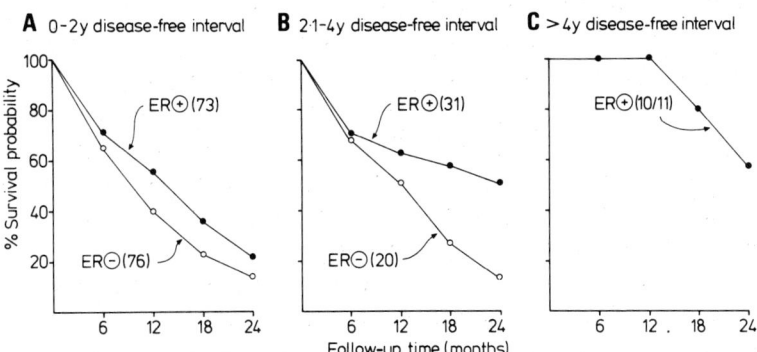

Figure 18.11. Survival of patients after recurrence in relation to disease-free interval and ER status.

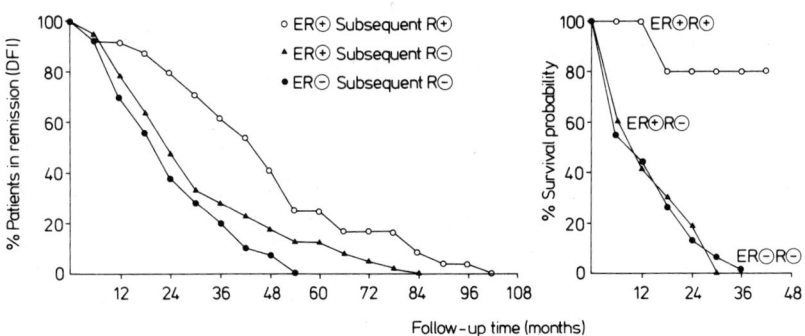

Figure 18.12. Relationship between ER status, duration of disease-free interval, and response of the secondary disease to endocrine therapy (R + represents responder, R − a nonresponder). The data are also shown in relation to survival after recurrence.

337

posite of all the various clinical and biological features described. The Nottingham-Tenovus study was aimed at increasing our understanding of the biological nature of breast cancer and the factors that influence its development. It was hoped that such knowledge would be of value in future adjuvant-controlled clinical trials when prognosis and biological responsiveness to subsequent endocrine therapy could be accurately predicted and patients could be effectively stratified on the basis of data relating to certain facets of tumor behavior.

In general, the presence of estrogen receptor in a primary breast tumor is often associated with well-differentiated tissue of low mitotic activity, tumors which have retained hormone sensitivity. Higher levels of the receptor are generally seen in the tumors from postmenopausal women. Conversely, patients with ER-negative tumors are more likely to present earlier with their disease. These tumors are generally hormone insensitive and have high mitotic rates.

On recurrence, prognosis is poor for all women with ER-negative tumors, no patients being alive after 3 years in the Nottingham-Tenovus series, despite an initial response to cytotoxic therapy. The prognosis for patients with ER-positive tumors on recurrence is also poor. Only 15% survived 5 years, and the patients who survived this longer period were those with ER-positive tumors with a low mitotic rate, who had an extended DFI and generally responded to endocrine therapy. It is clear that in terms of survival, the present regimens for the treatment and management of breast cancer are not particularly successful and after an early recurrence of the disease, such forms of therapy make little impression on the progress of the cancer. Obviously much remains to be done!

References

Baum, M. 1980. The management of advanced breast cancer. *British Journal of Hospital Medicine* 23:32–38.

Bishop, H. M., R. W. Blamey, C. W. Elston, J. L. Haybittle, R. I. Nicholson, and K. Griffiths. 1979. Relationship of oestrogen-receptor status to survival in breast cancer. *Lancet* 2:283–284.

Blamey, R. W., H. M. Bishop, J. R. S. Blake, P. J. Doyle, C. W. Elston, J. L. Haybittle, R. I. Nicholson, and K. Griffiths. 1980. Relationship between primary breast tumour receptor status and patient survival. *Cancer* 46:2765–2769.

Blamey, R. W., C. W. Elston, J. L. Haybittle, and K. Griffiths. 1983. Prognosis in breast cancer: the Nottingham-Tenovus trial. *Commentaries on Research in Breast Disease* 3:93–112.

British Breast Group. 1974. Assessment of response to treatment in advanced breast cancer. *Lancet* 2:38–39.

Campbell, F. C., R. W. Blamey, P. J. Doyle, H. M. Bishop, R. I. Nicholson, and K. Griffiths. 1981a. Oestrogen receptor status, histological grade and patterns of metastasis of breast cancer. *British Journal of Cancer* 44:456–459.

Campbell, F. C., R. W. Blamey, C. W. Elston, A. H. Morris, R. I. Nicholson, and K. Griffiths. 1981b. Quantitative oestradiol receptor values in primary breast cancer and response of metastases to endocrine therapy. *Lancet* 2:1317–1319.

Consensus Meeting on steroid receptors in breast cancer, National Institutes of Health, Bethesda, Md., U.S.A. 1980. *Cancer* 46: (no. 12).

Cox, D. R. 1972. Regression models and life-tables. *Journal of the Royal Statistics Society* 34:187–194.

Croton, R., T. Cooke, W. D. George, R. I. Nicholson, and K. Griffiths. 1981. Oestrogen receptors and survival in early breast cancer. *British Medical Journal* 283:1289–1291.

Cutler, S. J., A. J. Asire, and S. G. Taylor. 1969. Classification of patients with disseminated cancer of the breast. *Cancer* 24:861–869.

Feldman, H. 1972. Mathematical theory of complex ligand-binding systems at equilibrium: some methods for parameter fitting. *Analytical Biochemistry* 48:317–338.

Griffiths, K., P. V. Maynard, D. W. Wilson, and P. Davies. 1978. Endocrine aspects of primary breast cancer. In *Reviews on endocrine related cancer* Suppl., ed. M. Mayer, S. Saez, and B. A. Stoll, 221–236. Macclesfield: I.C.I.

Griffiths, K., R. I. Nicholson, B. Joyce, M. Morton, C. Campbell, and R. W. Blamey. 1983. Steroid receptor analysis and the clinical management of breast cancer. In *Recent clinical developments in gynecologic oncology. Progress in cancer research and therapy*, vol. 24, ed. C. P. Morrow et al., 107–121. New York: Raven Press.

Haybittle, J. L., R. W. Blamey, C. W. Elston, J. Johnson, P. J. Doyle, F. C. Campbell, R. I. Nicholson, and K. Griffiths. 1982. A prognostic index in primary breast cancer. *British Journal of Cancer* 45:361–366.

Hayward, J. L., R. D. Rubens, P. P. Carbone, J. -C. Heuson, S. Kumaoka, and A. Segaloff. 1977. Assessment of response to therapy in advanced breast cancer. *British Journal of Cancer* 35:292–298.

Jensen, E. V., and E. R. DeSombre. 1973. Estrogen-receptor interaction. *Science* 182:126–134.

Knight, W. A., R. B. Livingston, E. J. Gregory, and W. L. McGuire. 1977. Estrogen receptor as an independent prognosis factor in early recurrence in breast cancer. *Cancer Research* 37:4669–4671.

Logan, W. P. D. 1975. *World Health Organization Statistics Report* 28:232.

Maynard, P. V., R. W. Blamey, C. W. Elston, J. L. Haybittle, and K. Griffiths. 1978a. Oestrogen receptor assay in primary breast cancer and early recurrence of the disease. *Cancer Research* 38:4292–4295.

Maynard, P. V., C. I. Davies, R. W. Blamey, C. W. Elston, J. Johnson, and K. Griffiths. 1978b. Relationship between oestrogen receptor content and histological grade in human primary breast tumours. *British Journal of Cancer* 38:745–748.

McGuire, W. L., P. P. Carbone, and E. P. Vollmer, (eds.). 1975. *Estrogen receptors in human breast cancer.* New York: Raven Press.

Mumford, C. J., C. W. Elston, F. C. Campbell, R. W. Blamey, J. Johnson, R. I. Nicholson, and K. Griffiths. 1983. Tumor epithelial cellularity and quantitative oestrogen receptor concentrations in primary breast cancer. *British Journal of Cancer* 47:549–552.

Nicholson, R. I., F. C. Campbell, R. W. Blamey, C. W. Elston, D. George, and K. Griffiths. 1981. Steroid receptors in early breast cancer: value in prognosis. *Journal of Steroid Biochemistry* 15:193–199.

Nicholson, R. I., F. C. Campbell, R. W. Blamey, C. W. Elston, J. L. Haybittle, D. W. Wilson, and K. Griffiths. 1984a. Steroid receptors and primary breast cancer: their prognostic value. In *Regulation of target cell responsiveness,* vol. 2, ed. K. W. McKerns, A. Aakvaag, and V. Hansson, 257–282. New York: Plenum Press.

Nicholson, R. I., D. W. Wilson, G. Richards, K. Griffiths, M. Williams, C. W. Elston, and R. W. Blamey. 1984b. Biological and clinical aspects of oestrogen receptor measurements in rapidly progressing breast cancer. In *Proceedings of the IUPHAR Ninth International Congress of Pharmacology,* vol. 3, ed. W. Paton, J. Mitchell, and P. Turner, 75–79. London: Macmillan Press Ltd.

Papaioannou, A. N., F. J. Tany, and M. Volk. 1967. Fate of patients with recurrent carcinoma of the breast. *Cancer* 20:371–376.

Richards, G., D. W. Wilson, and K. Griffiths. 1983. Computer-aided assessment of receptor status in human breast cancer. *Computers and Biomedical Research,* 16:483–498.

Wilson, D. W., S. J. Gaskell, and K. W. Kemp, (eds.). 1981. *Quality control in clinical endocrinology. Proceedings of the Eighth Tenovus Workshop.* Cardiff: Alpha Omega Publishers.

19

*Progesterone Receptor
Determinations:
A Refinement of Predictive Tests
for Hormone Dependency of
Breast Cancer*

C. F. LeMaistre and W. L. McGuire

I. Introduction 342
II. Estrogen Receptors in Breast Cancer 342
III. Progesterone Receptor as a Prognostic Factor in Early Breast Cancer 344
    a. Estrogen Receptor and Disease-Free Interval 344
    b. Progesterone Receptor and Disease-Free Interval 344
IV. Progesterone Receptor in Advanced Breast Cancer 347
V. Consistency of Progesterone Receptor Assays 348
    a. Simultaneous Assays 349
    b. Sequential Assays 349
VI. Conclusion 351
    References 351

"In short, I believe that the major diseases of human beings
have become approachable biologic puzzles, ultimately solvable."
Lewis Thomas

I. *Introduction*

$\mathbf{T}$HE role of the female reproductive organs in the genesis of breast cancer has long been highlighted. Bernardo Ramazzini (1713) commented on the "mysterious sympathy" that exists between the female genital organs and the breast over two centuries ago. More than a century elapsed before this observation was exploited and tumor regression was achieved through endocrine manipulation (Schinzinger 1889; Beatson 1896). In this century, surgical ablative procedures were systematically exploited, but the results of prophylactic ablative measures were disappointing, leading to their application in advanced disease (Taylor 1939; Huggins and Dao 1954; Horsley and Horsley 1962; Kennedy et al. 1964; Nissen-Meyer 1964; Huggins and Bergenstal 1981). Less than a third of patients were found to respond to surgical endocrine ablation, prompting a search for the characteristics of breast malignancies that define hormone sensitivity.

A greater understanding of the biochemical mechanism of steroid hormone action in breast cancer has developed over the last 20 years, allowing the clinician to more accurately assess prognosis and predict response to endocrine therapies. The initial observations that radiolabeled estrogens localized in estrogen-responsive tissues in animals (Glascock and Hoekstra 1959; Jensen and Jacobson 1960) was followed by the realization that labeled estrogens were concentrated in metastasis of patients who had responded to adrenalectomy (Folca et al. 1961). A plausible explanation for these observations was forwarded upon the discovery that a protein present in the cytoplasm, the estrogen receptor, was responsible for the specific binding of estrogen by both normal target tissues and breast cancer (Jensen et al. 1967). This discovery caused Jensen and coworkers to venture that by using this estrogen receptor, "it should be possible to predict in advance which (tumors) will respond . . ."

II. *Estrogen Receptors in Breast Cancer*

Jensen's speculation about the utility of the estrogen receptor in predicting response to hormonal therapy in breast cancer proved correct. This hypothesis was confirmed by cumulative data from a number of investigators at an international meeting in 1974 (McGuire et al. 1975). No matter which assay was used, patients with tumors lacking estrogen receptor rarely responded to endocrine manipulation. Thus patients with estrogen receptor–negative tumors have been spared the morbidity of ablative surgery and the long delays in waiting for a response to hormonal therapy.

For patients whose tumors contain estrogen receptor, there is a 50–60% chance of objective response with endocrine therapies. When compared to clinical criteria used to select patients for endocrine therapy, the estrogen receptor is clearly superior. However, the high rate of treatment failure in the estrogen receptor–positive group represented a challenge to better understand mechanisms of hormone action at a cellular level so that additional markers of hormone sensitivity could be identified. As will be discussed, the progesterone receptor is such a marker.

In vitro systems utilizing cell lines established from human breast cancers have provided some definition of the mechanism of action of steroid hormones. Care must be taken in the use of such a cell line as a model, as certain minimal criteria must be met to confirm mammary origin. The MCF-7 cell line is among the best characterized in terms of karyology, protein phenotyping, and differentiated function (Soule et al. 1973; Russo et al. 1976). Further, it contains receptors for a number of steroid hormones (Horwitz et al. 1975a). To be sure, the direct application of information learned in *in vitro* systems to the clinic is fraught with hazard (Lippman 1981). Nevertheless, using such models we have gained new insights into hormone dependency.

The mechanism by which gene activity is induced by a steroid hormone is not well defined. The cell membrane is freely traversed by steroids. In the case of estradiol, the hormone is rapidly bound by an high affinity estrogen receptor in the target cell cytoplasm. In MCF-7 cells the estrogen–estrogen receptor complex is translocated to the nucleus within minutes (Horwitz and McGuire 1980). Rapid processing of the receptor complex then occurs such that by 3–5 hours, 70% of the nuclear estrogen receptor is lost from the cells. Although the way in which the hormone complex interacts with DNA at a molecular level is not clear, the results of this interaction impact on the production of a multitude of proteins and on cell growth.

Of all the estrogen-regulated proteins, the progesterone receptor has stimulated the most interest. Horwitz and McGuire (1978) have clearly demonstrated the induction of progesterone receptor by estrogen in human breast cancer *in vitro*. Since the binding of estrogen by the estrogen receptor is only the initial step in a complex biochemical pathway, it is possible that lesions might exist in later steps, rendering an ER-positive tumor unresponsive to endocrine manipulation. The fact that 30–40% of estrogen receptor–positive tumors will not respond to endocrine therapy caused Horwitz et al. (1975b) to postulate that a product of hormone action such as progesterone receptor would be a better marker of hormone dependence.

III. Progesterone Receptor as a Prognostic Factor in Early Breast Cancer

A. Estrogen Receptor and Disease-Free Interval

The estrogen receptor is a useful tool to predict disease-free interval after mastectomy. Knight et al. (1977) were the first to show that patients whose tumors contained estrogen receptor recurred less frequently than those whose tumors did not contain estrogen receptor. This finding was independent of the size of the primary tumor, the number of involved lymph nodes, menopausal status, or duration of adjuvant therapy. Those patients whose tumors involved axillary lymph nodes and did not contain estrogen receptor represent a subgroup at especially high risk, as half of this subgroup recurred within 18 months of surgery. Subsequent studies have confirmed these observations (Rich et al. 1978; Allegra and Lippman 1980; Furmanski et al. 1980; Hartveit et al. 1980; Leake et al. 1981). As one might expect, the differences observed in disease-free interval based on the estrogen receptor also translate into differences in survival (Bishop et al. 1979; Hahnel et al. 1979; Kinne et al. 1981; Samaan et al. 1981; Stewart et al. 1981).

B. Progesterone Receptor and Disease-Free Interval

If the estrogen receptor is an effective marker for predicting disease-free interval, it is possible that an end product of estrogen action such as the progesterone receptor may be an even better predictor of time to recurrence for patients with primary breast cancer. We recently examined this question in a randomized adjuvant therapy protocol that was conducted in Cleveland, Ohio (Clark et al. 1983). All patients had a radical or modified radical mastectomy and documented stage II breast cancer. Patients were stratified according to the estrogen receptor status of their tumors and the number of involved lymph nodes. Within each stratum,

Table 19.1. Univariate disease-free-survival analyses in stage II
breast cancer

Prognostic factor	*p*-Value
Number of positive nodes	< 0.0001
Size of primary tumor	0.0062
Log (ER + 0.5)	0.0008
Log (PgR + 0.5)	< 0.0001
Menopausal status	0.4592
Treatment	0.5696

patients were randomly assigned to one of three treatment combinations: cyclophosphamide, methotrexate, and flourouracil (CMF); CMF plus tamoxifen; or CMF plus tamoxifen plus bacille Calmette-Guerin vaccine.

Table 19.1 shows the results of the disease-free-survival analysis for the patients with progesterone receptor measurements when the prognostic factors are considered one at a time. The number of positive axillary nodes and the size of the primary tumor were both negatively correlated with time to recurrence. On the other hand, both estrogen receptors and progesterone receptors were positively correlated with time to recurrence, whether expressed as qualitative or quantitative factors. There were no overall significant differences in disease-free survival based on menopausal status or treatment regimen.

The finding that the qualitative expression of progesterone receptor content is highly correlated with disease-free survival indicated that patients with high levels of progesterone receptor in their tumors should have longer time to recurrence. As shown in Table 19.2, patients with low receptor levels had a significantly shorter disease-free survival than did patients with moderate levels; patients with high receptor levels fared better than those with moderate levels.

Table 19.2. Progesterone receptor and disease-free survival

Femtomoles of PgR/mg cytosol protein	Number of patients	Percentage with disease-free survival for	
		18 months	36 months
< 5	41	68	50
5–49	68	88	65
≥ 50	80	100	90

The patients were divided into three groups to examine the association between receptors: (1) estrogen receptor–positive/progesterone receptor–positive (ER + /PgR +), (2) estrogen receptor–positive/progesterone receptor–negative (ER + /PgR −), and (3) estrogen receptor–negative/progesterone receptor–negative (ER − /PgR −). Disease-free survival was significantly better for the group of patients whose tumors contained progesterone receptor than for the other two groups. However, the disease-free survival of the ER + /PgR − group was only marginally better than that of the ER − /PgR − group.

One problem with using two or more variables to create subgroups in this fashion is that the sample sizes become small. Moreover, the interactions between variables cannot be examined. To overcome these problems a multivariate model was used which simultaneously incorporated several prognostic variables and their interactions. Table 19.3 shows the results of this analysis. Consistent with the univariate analysis, the number of positive nodes and the level of progesterone receptor were significant prognostic factors ($p < 0.0001$), whereas the size of the primary tumor was only of borderline significance ($p = 0.11$).

The surprising result in this analysis was the lack of significance of the ER level, either as a single variable or as an interaction with any other variables. No matter what combinations of variables were examined, as long as both receptor levels were considered simultaneously, estrogen receptor content never enhanced the prediction of recurrence. On the other hand, progesterone receptor status and the number of positive nodes always remained significant prognostic factors, suggesting that the additional knowledge of the progesterone receptor level will help predict disease-free survival, even if estrogen receptor is known.

Table 19.3. Multivariate disease-free-survival analyses in stage II
        breast cancer

Prognostic factor	p-Value	Rank
Number of positive nodes	< 0.0001	1
Size of primary tumor	0.07	3
Log (ER + 0.5)	0.07	
Log (PgR + 0.5)	0.004	2
Menopausal status	0.77	
Treatment	0.24	

IV. *Progesterone Receptor in Advanced Breast Cancer*

As an end product of hormone action, and therefore a marker of an intact receptor pathway, the progesterone receptor might also be expected to effectively predict endocrine responsiveness of breast cancer. Retrospective examination of data pooled from a number of different centers appears to support this concept (Table 19.4).

Central to this hypothesis is that tumors lacking both estrogen receptor and progesterone receptor should not respond to endocrine manipulations, whereas tumors containing both receptors should have the highest response rate. As predicted, the least frequent response rate is found in the tumors lacking both receptors (9%) and the highest response rate is found among tumors containing both receptors (73%). These observations are consistent with the concept that progesterone receptor may be a good marker for endocrine dependence.

The fact that progesterone receptors are found in estrogen receptor–negative tumors is a consistent finding, though usually accounting for only 3–5% of tumors (McGuire and Horwitz 1978; Bloom et al. 1980; Young et al. 1980; Maas and Jonat 1985). This discordance has evoked a number of technical as well as nonmethodological explanations and it is possible that inadequacy of assay techniques might account for a portion of this group (Zava et al. 1977; Panko and MacLeod 1978; Edwards et al. 1979). Sarrif and Durant (1981) reported evidence that some apparently estrogen receptor–negative/progesterone receptor–positive $(ER-/PgR+)$ tumors do, in fact, contain estrogen receptor. In any event, 59% of these tumors regress with endocrine therapy.

There is a 35% response rate to endocrine therapy among those tumors that are $ER+/PgR-$. According to the hypothesis, these tumors should not regress with endocrine therapy. Again, methodological problems may

Table 19.4. Response to endocrine therapy

	Number of patients	Objective response (%)
$ER-/PgR-$	285	9
$ER-/PgR+$	29	59
$ER+/PgR-$	368	35
$ER+/PgR+$	434	73

Data from McGuire et al. 1975; Leake et al. 1981.

account for some of these cases, or perhaps the synthesis of progesterone receptor may not be a sufficient marker of endocrine control in all cases.

Although these data are generally supportive of the progesterone receptor as a marker of hormone sensitivity in breast cancer, interpretation of retrospective, pooled data must be done cautiously. The receptor assays were done in many different laboratories utilizing several different methods. Criteria for patient selection were not uniform and a variety of endocrine therapies were employed. Finally, the criteria for response can vary from center to center.

A number of groups have initiated prospective clinical trials designed to study the relationship between progesterone receptor and response to endocrine therapy in metastatic breast cancer. While these trials will be evaluable in the near future, there is at least one prospective trial that supports these retrospective data. Cavalli et al. (1984) have demonstrated that the response rate to high-dose medroxyprogesterone acetate is 73% for patients whose tumors contain progesterone receptor and 10% for those that do not. Future studies will accurately define the value of the progesterone receptor in predicting responsiveness in advanced breast cancer.

V. Consistency of Progesterone Receptor Assays

We have suggested that the knowledge of the progesterone receptor content of a tumor allows an improved ability to predict response to endocrine therapy and that it is predictive of disease-free interval and survival. Because of the chronic nature of breast cancer, in which a typical case is fraught with recurrences, we can expect an increasing dependence on hormone receptor assays in treatment planning. Obviously, the clinician must know if each recurrence need be biopsied to evaluate hormone receptor status in order to optimize treatment planning. Further, a better understanding of the impact of time, therapy, and other factors on receptor status must be reached.

In an attempt to gain insight into some of these issues, we retrospectively evaluated a large series of patients on whom multiple simultaneous or sequential biopsies were assayed for progesterone receptor (Gross et al. 1984). From more than 5500 specimens analyzed in San Antonio since 1975, we identified 280 patients in whom multiple breast cancer biopsies were assayed for progesterone receptor. The samples were considered simultaneous if the specimens were obtained less than 14 days apart without intervening therapy. The samples were considered sequential if the interval between biopsies was greater than 6 weeks. In this analysis a value of greater than 10 fmol/mg cytosol protein was considered positive, a value less than 5 fmol/mg cytosol protein was considered negative, and values between 5 and 10 fmol/mg cytosol protein were considered intermediate.

A. SIMULTANEOUS ASSAYS

Multiple biopsy specimens from 109 patients fulfilled the criteria for simultaneous assays and were analyzed for progesterone receptor concordance. As can be seen in Table 19.5, 14% were found to have major discordance and 18% were found to have a minor discordance. The discordance observed for simultaneous progesterone receptor assays may be a result of several factors. As has been demonstrated for estrogen receptor (Van Netten et al. 1982; Hull et al. 1983), it seems evident that an ade-

Table 19.5. Simultaneous assays for progesterone receptor (%; N = 109)

Concordance rate	68
Major discordance rate	14
Minor discordance rate	18

quate tumor sample is necessary to perform an accurate assay. Variability inherent in the sucrose density gradient technique for measurement of the receptor may also be an explanation for at least part of the observed discordance. Finally, heterogeneity within the tumor may contribute to discordant assay results (Kiang and Kennedy 1977; Brennan et al. 1979). Our major discordance rate of 14% of simultaneous progesterone receptor assays is considerably higher than the 3% reported for estrogen receptor (Hull 1983). Nevertheless, this serves as a useful baseline for evaluation of progesterone receptor discordance between sequential biopsies.

B. SEQUENTIAL ASSAYS

The content of progesterone receptor was studied in 174 sequential pairs of assays. Of the 106 patients whose initial biopsy was negative, 9% were found to have major discordance. However, among those patients whose initial biopsy was positive for progesterone receptor, there was a striking major discordance of 44% (see Table 19.6).

Table 19.6. Sequential assays for progesterone receptor (%; N = 174)

		Discordance	
First specimen	Concordance	Minor	Major
PgR −	89	3	8
PgR +	49	8	44

A univariate analysis was performed to identify factors that could influence progesterone receptor status. Tumor size, the number of axillary nodes, and menopausal status were not associated with the impressive discordance in receptor-positive patients. The time interval between biopsies was also examined to evaluate the potential presence of a biological "drift" (time-dependent change) on tumor receptor status. Whether patients' tumors were initially progesterone receptor positive or negative, the median interval between biopsies was not significantly different for concordant versus discordant results. This suggests that a longer time interval cannot be implicated in the evolution of tumors from positive to negative. In fact, there was a tendency to shorter time to second biopsy in the major discordance groups, suggesting a possible relationship between discordance and aggressiveness.

It is reasonable to expect intervening therapy to have a significant impact on the receptor content of tumors. Whereas the analysis of progesterone receptor–negative patients revealed little discordance whether or not there was intervening therapy, this was not the case for the progesterone receptor–positive patients. Those patients who were progesterone receptor–positive and received no intervening therapy or chemotherapy alone demonstrated a major discordance of 21%. However, a remarkable 56% of the patients who received internal endocrine therapy showed apparent loss of progesterone receptor. These findings were consistent for both adjuvant and therapeutic intervening therapy. In fact, a multivariate analysis of possible factors contributing to discordance in progesterone receptor patients (menopausal status, nodal status, tumor size, and intervening therapy) demonstrated intervening endocrine therapy to be the only variable of significance.

The central issue pertaining to this loss of progesterone receptor is whether it has clinical or biological significance. To examine this, patients were divided into three groups: (1) those initially PgR − who remained so; (2) those initially PgR + who remained so; (3) those initially PgR +

who experienced loss of PgR. As expected, the worst survival was seen in the group of patients who were consistently progesterone receptor–negative. Of great interest, however, was the finding that patients who were initially positive, but who lost their receptor between biopsies, had a significantly poorer survival than did those who remained positive. The estimated median survival times were 36, 76, and 51 months, respectively, in the three groups. Based on these findings, it would appear that a tumor which loses progesterone receptor is, in fact experiencing an ominous evolution to a more aggressive cancer. Further, in patients whose tumors initially contain progesterone receptor, reassessment of tumor receptor content upon disease recurrence seems indicated for optimal treatment planning.

VI. *Conclusion*

Remarkable progress has been made over the last decade in our understanding of hormone-dependent breast cancer. There can be no question that the identification of the estrogen receptor has allowed us an improved ability to determine both prognosis and potential for response to endocrine manipulation. The progesterone receptor now appears to surpass the estrogen receptor in both these determinations, allowing the clinician an intelligent framework upon which therapy for the individual patient can be more closely constructed. This particular "biologic puzzle" is far from being solved, however, and it is only with a more basic understanding of the disease that we can more accurately diagnose, assess, and design individual treatment for patients with breast cancer.

References

Allegra, J. C., and M. E. Lippman. 1980. Estrogen receptor status and the disease free interval in breast cancer. In *Endocrine treatment of breast cancer. Recent results in cancer research,* vol. 71, ed. B. Henningsen, F. Linder, and C. Steichele, 20–25. Berlin: Springer-Verlag.

Beatson, G. T. 1896. On the treatment of inoperable cases of carcinoma of the mamma: suggestions for a new method of treatment, with illustrative cases. *Lancet* 2:104–107, 162–165.

Bishop, H. M., R. W. Blamey, C. W. Elston, J. L. Haybittle, R. I. Nicholson, and K. Griffiths. 1979. Relationship of oestrogen-receptor status to survival in breast cancer. *Lancet* 2:283–284.

Bloom, W. D., E. H. Tobin, B. Schreibman, and G. A. Degenshein. 1980. The role of progesterone receptors in the management of advanced breast cancer. *Cancer* (Philadelphia) 45:2992–2997.

Brennan, M. J., W. L. Donegan, and D. E. Appleby. 1979. The variability of estrogen receptors in metastatic breast cancer. *American Journal of Surgery* 137:260–263.

Cavalli, F., A. Goldhirsch, F. Jungi, G. Martz, B. Mermillad, and P. Alberto, for the Swiss Group for Clinical Cancer Research. 1984. *Journal. of Clinical Oncology* 2:414–419.

Clark, G. M., W. L. McGuire, C. A. Hubay, O. H. Pearson, and J. S. Marshall. 1983. Progesterone receptors as a prognostic factor in stage II breast cancer. *New England Journal of Medicine* 309:1343–1347.

Edwards, D. P., G. C. Chamness, and W. L. McGuire. 1979. Estrogen and progesterone receptor proteins in breast cancer. *Biochimica et Biophysica Acta* 560:457–486.

Folca, P. J., R. F. Glascock, and W. T. Irvin. 1961. Studies with tritium-labelled hexoestrol in advanced breast cancer. *Lancet* 2:796–798.

Furmanski, P., D. E. Saunders, S. C. Brooks, M. A. Rich, and the Breast Cancer Prognostic Study Clinical and Pathology Associates. 1980. The prognostic value of estrogen receptor determinations in patients with primary breast cancer. *Cancer* (Philadelphia) 46:2794–2796.

Glascock, R. F., and W. G. Hoekstra. 1959. Selective accumulation of tritium labelled hexoestrol by the reproductive organs of immature female goats and sheep. *Biochemical Journal* 72:673–682.

Gross, G. E., G. M. Clark, G. L. Chamness, and W. L. McGuire. 1984. Multiple progesterone receptor assays in human breast cancer. *Cancer Research* 44:836–840.

Hahnel, R., T. Woodings, and A. B. Vivian. 1979. Prognostic value of estrogen receptors in primary breast cancer. *Cancer* (Philadelphia) 44:671–675.

Hartveit, F., H. Maartman-Moe, K. F. Stou, M. Tangen, and T. Thorenson. 1980. Early recurrence in oestrogen receptor negative breast carcinomas. *Acta Chirurgica Scandinavica* 146:93–95.

Horsley, J. S., III, and G. W. Horsley. 1962. Twenty years of experience with prophylactic bilateral oopherectomy in the treatment of carcinoma of the breast. *Annals of Surgery* 155:935–942.

Horwitz, K. B., and W. L. McGuire. 1978. Estrogen control of progesterone receptor in human breast cancer: correlation with nuclear processing of estrogen receptor. *Journal of Biological Chemistry* 253:2223–2228.

Horwitz, K. B., and W. L. McGuire. 1980. Studies on mechanisms of estrogen and antiestrogen action in human breast cancer. In *Endocrine treatment of breast cancer. Recent results in cancer research,* vol. 71, ed. B. Henningsen, F. Linder, and C. Steichele, 45–58. Berlin: Springer-Verlag.

Horwitz, K. B., M. E. Costlow, and W. L. McGuire. 1975a. MCF-7: A human breast cancer cell line with estrogen, androgen, progesterone and glucocorticoid receptor. *Steroids* 26:785–795.

Horwitz, K. B., W. L. McGuire, O. Pearson, and A. Segaloff. 1975b. Predicting response to endocrine therapy in human breast cancer: a hypothesis. *Science* 189:726–727.

Huggins, C., and D. M. Bergenstal. 1951. Inhibition of human mammary and prostatic cancer by adrenalectomy. *Cancer Research* 12:134–141.

Huggins, C., and T. L. Dao. 1954. Characteristics of adrenal dependent mammary cancer. *Annals of Surgery* 12:497–501.

Hull, D. F., III, G. M. Clark, C. K. Osborne, G. C. Chamness, and W. A. Knight, III. 1983. Multiple estrogen receptor assays in human breast cancer. *Cancer Research* 43:413–416.

Jensen, E. V., and H. I. Jacobson. 1960. Fate of steroid estrogens in target tissues. In *Biological activities of steroids in relation to cancer*, ed. G. Pincus and E. P. Vollmer, 191. New York: Academic Press.

Jensen, E. V., E. R. DeSombre, and P. W. Jungblut. 1967. Estrogen receptors in hormone-responsive tissues and tumors. In *Endogenous factors influencing host-tumor balance*, ed. R. W. Wissler, T. L. Dao, and S. Wood, Jr., 15–68. Chicago: University of Chicago Press.

Kennedy, B. J., P. W. Mielke, and T. E. Fortuny. 1964. Therapeutic castration versus prophylactic castration in breast cancer. *Surgery, Gynecology, and Obstetrics* 118:524–540.

Kiang, D. T., and B. J. Kennedy. 1977. Factors affecting estrogen receptors in breast cancer. *Cancer* (Philadelphia) 40:1571–1576.

Kinne, D. W., R. Ashikari, S. Butler, C. Menendez-Botet, P. R. Rosen, and M. Schwartz. 1981. Estrogen receptor protein in breast cancer as a predictor of recurrence. *Cancer* (Philadelphia) 47:2364–2367.

Knight, W. A., III, R. B. Livingston, E. J. Gregory, and W. L. McGuire. 1977. Estrogen receptor is an independent prognostic factor for early recurrence in breast cancer. *Cancer Research* 37:4669–4671.

Leake, R. E., L. Laing, C. McArdle, and D. C. Smith. 1981. Soluble and nuclear oestrogen receptor status in human breast cancer in relation to prognosis. *British Journal of Cancer* 43:67–71.

Lippman, M. E. 1981. Hormonal regulation of human breast cancer cells *in vitro*. In *Hormones and Breast Cancer*, ed. M. C. Pike, P. K. Siiteri, and C. W. Welsch, 171–184. New York: Cold Spring Harbor Laboratory.

Maass, H., and W. Jonat. 1983. Steroid receptors as a guide for therapy of primary and metastatic breast cancer. *Journal of Steroid Biochemistry* 19:833–837.

McGuire, W. L., and G. M. Clark. 1983. The prognostic role of progesterone receptors in human breast cancer. *Seminars in Oncology* 10:2–5.

McGuire, W. L., and K. B. Horwitz. 1978. Progesterone receptors in breast cancer. In *Hormones, receptors, and breast cancer. Progress in cancer research and therapy*, vol. 10, ed. W. L. McGuire, 31–42. New York: Raven Press.

McGuire, W. L., P. P. Carbone, M. E. Sears, and G. C. Escher. 1975. Estrogen receptors in human breast cancer: an overview. In *Estrogen receptors in human breast cancer*, ed. W. L. McGuire, P. P. Carbone, and E. P. Vollmer, 1–7. New York: Raven Press.

Nissen-Meyer, R. 1964. Prophylactic endocrine treatment in carcinomas of the breast. *Clinical Radiology* 15:152–160.

Panko, W. B., and R. M. McLeod. 1978. Uncharged nuclear receptors for estrogen in breast. *Cancer Research* 38:1948–1951.

Ramazzini, B. 1713. *Diseases of workers*, 167–202. Trans. W. C. Wright, 1964. New York: Hafner.

Rich, M. A., P. Furmanski, S. C. Brooks, and the Breast Cancer Prognostic Surgery and Pathology Associates. 1978. Prognostic value of estrogen receptor determination in patients with breast cancer. *Cancer Research* 38:4296–4298.

Russo, J., H. D. Soule, C. McGrath, and M. A. Rich. 1976. Re-expression of the original tumor pattern by a human breast carcinoma cell line (MCF7) in sponge culture. *Journal of the National Cancer Institute* 56:279–283.

Samaan, W. A., A. N. Buzdar, K. A. Aldinger, P. N. Schultz, K. P. Yong, M. M. Romsdahl, and R. Martin. 1981. Estrogen receptor: a prognostic factor in breast cancer. *Cancer* (Philadelphia) 47:554–560.

Sarrif, A. M., and J. R. Durant. 1981. Evidence that estrogen-receptor-negative, progesterone-receptor-positive breast and ovarian carcinomas contain estrogen receptor. *Cancer* (Philadelphia) 48:1216–1220.

Schinzinger, A. 1889. Über Carcinoma Mammae. *Verhandlungen der Gesellschaft fuer Orthopaedische Chirurgie* 18:28.

Soule, H. D., J. Vasquez, A. Long, S. Albert, and M. Brennan. 1973. Human cell line from a pleural effusion derived from a breast carcinoma. *Journal of the National Cancer Institute* 51:1409–1413.

Stewart, J. F., R. J. B. King, S. A. Sexton, R. R. Millis, R. D. Ruben, and J. L. Hayward. 1981. Oestrogen receptors, sites of metastatic disease and survival in recurrent breast cancer. *European Journal of Cancer* 17:449–453.

Taylor, G. W. 1939. Ovarian sterilization for breast cancer. *Surgery, Gynecology, and Obstetrics* 68:452.

Van Netten, J. P., F. T. Algard, P. Coy, J. J. Carlyle, M. L. Brudgen, I. C. R. Thorton, and M. P. To. 1982. ER assay on breast cancer microsamples. *Cancer* (Philadelphia) 79:2383–2388.

Young, P. C. M., C. E. Ehrlich, and L. H. Einhorn. 1980. Relationship between steroid receptors and response to endocrine therapy and cytotoxic chemotherapy in metastatic breast cancer. *Cancer* (Philadelphia) 46:2961–2963.

Zava, D. T., G. C. Chamness, K. B. Horwitz, and W. L. McGuire. 1977. Biologically active estrogen receptor in the absence of estrogen. *Science* 196:663–664.

VI

Antibodies to
Steroid Hormone
Receptors

20

Antibodies to Estrogen Receptor: New Probes for the Analysis of Receptor Structure and Function

GEOFFREY L. GREENE, WILLIAM J. KING,
MICHAEL F. PRESS, AND ELWOOD V. JENSEN

I. INTRODUCTION   358
II. PURIFICATION OF MAMMALIAN ESTROGEN RECEPTORS   360
III. ANTIBODIES TO THE ESTROGEN RECEPTOR PROTEIN   362
    A. POLYCLONAL ANTIBODIES   362
    B. MONOCLONAL ANTIBODIES   363
IV. IMMUNOCHEMICAL ANALYSIS OF RECEPTOR STRUCTURE AND FUNCTION   365
    REFERENCES   371

357

I. Introduction

CONSIDERABLE effort has been devoted to the elucidation of the molecular mechanisms by which steroid hormones regulate gene expression, growth, and function in hormone-responsive cells. Virtually everything that is known about steroid receptors and their postulated role as transcriptional modulators has come from the use of radiolabeled hormones (Jensen and Jacobson 1962) and analogs to detect, quantify, and characterize these intracellular proteins, primarily in reproductive tissues. The model of hormone action (Gorski et al. 1968; Jensen et al. 1968) that has emerged from numerous studies of steroid-receptor interactions has several important features. Among these is that the steroid, upon entering a responsive cell, associates with a specific extranuclear receptor protein and induces its conversion to a form that has increased affinity for chromatin and DNA. This steroid-dependent process is accompanied by translocation of the hormone receptor complex to the nucleus, where it interacts with the genome and stimulates the production or accumulation of specific RNAs. The net result is the production of intracellular and secreted proteins that are involved in the regulation of growth and/or function of the initial target tissue or other tissues (Beato 1980). Despite considerable effort by many investigators, most of the processes involved in steroid uptake and binding to appropriate receptor proteins, as well as virtually all of the cellular interactions of steroid receptor complexes, including activation, binding to chromatin, synthesis and degradation of receptor, and the events involved in transcriptional modulation, remain obscure and controversial. Also unclear is the intracellular location of the "extranuclear" unoccupied receptor found in the cytosol of tissue homogenates. Recent biochemical (Welshons et al. 1984) and immunocytochemical data (King and Greene 1984; Press and Greene 1984; Press et al. 1985) suggest that the majority of functional estrogen receptor may reside in the nucleus regardless of hormone status and that binding of hormone to receptor leads to a tighter association of steroid receptor complex with nuclear components. The nature of this association is not known, although a number of nuclear acceptor sites have been proposed, including specific DNA sequences (Compton et al. 1983; Payvar et al. 1983; Cato et al. 1984; Jost et al. 1985), ribonucleoprotein (Ling and Liao 1974), basic nonhistone proteins (Puca et al. 1974), the nuclear matrix (Barrack and Coffey 1980; Barrack 1983), and acidic nonhistone protein/DNA complexes (Spelsberg et al. 1983). The biological significance of these results has not been established and, as yet, no one has been able to reconstitute all of the cellular components required for steroid hormone response in any cell-free system.

It is clear that a means of locating, measuring, and purifying steroid receptors that does not depend on the binding of radiolabeled hormone would complement and extend our knowledge of receptor-mediated events. The recent availability of specific polyclonal and monoclonal antibodies to various steroid receptors has led to new approaches to the study of the structure, composition, and dynamics of steroid receptors. As independent probes for the receptor molecule, these antibodies are being used to detect, measure, and purify receptor in tissue extracts, to determine the distribution and intracellular location of receptors in various responsive tissues, as well as to map the hormone- and DNA-binding domains of the receptor and to study the structural changes that accompany the binding of steroids to their receptors.

This chapter summarizes the results of our efforts to purify and characterize calf and human estrogen receptors as well as to prepare specific polyclonal and monoclonal antibodies to these proteins. As a consequence of their high specificity and affinity for receptor, the resulting antibodies have proved to be valuable probes for analyzing receptor structure and function. Monoclonal antibodies have been particularly useful for purifying receptor from various sources, mapping functional domains on the receptor molecule, comparing receptors from various sources, and for determining the distribution and intracellular location of estrogen receptor (ER) in reproductive tissues and cancers in the presence and absence of hormone or antagonist. One of the more significant and unexpected observations to emerge from our immunocytochemical analyses of ER in various estrogen-sensitive tissues was the exclusively nuclear localization of specific immunoperoxidase staining for receptor in all stained cells, suggesting that the native, unoccupied receptor that is present in low salt cytosols may actually reside inside the nuclear compartment in the intact cell. The application of the estrogen receptor immunocytochemical assay (ER-ICA) to the assessment of prognosis and hormone responsiveness in breast cancer is particularly promising. In addition, a quantitative sandwich immunoassay for ER in tissue or tumor extracts has also been developed and tested on a number of breast tumor cytosols. The clinical utility of receptor immunoassays, especially ER-ICA, is discussed by DeSombre et al. in Chapter 17 of this volume.

II. Purification of Mammalian Estrogen Receptors

All of our early polyclonal (Greene et al. 1977, 1979) and monoclonal (Greene et al. 1980a) antibodies were prepared by immunization of animals with nuclear [^{3}H]estradiol receptor complex (E*R$_n$) obtained from calf uteri after *in vitro* translocation of cytosolic receptor with [^{3}H]estradiol. Purification of this complex was achieved by a sequence of extraction of E*R$_n$ from nuclear pellets with 400 mM KCl, followed by ammonium sulfate precipitation, gel filtration, and polyacrylamide gel electrophoresis (Greene et al. 1979). A 12,000-fold purification of receptor afforded a 1% yield of E*R$_n$ that was essentially pure and that contained one molecule of [^{3}H]estradiol per protein molecule of M$_r$ 68,000. Immunizations were carried out with receptor that was about 20% pure.

As part of our more recent efforts to isolate estrogen receptor in a pure form for detailed analysis of amino acid composition and sequence as well as physiochemical properties, we have developed a two-step affinity chromatography procedure for the purification of unoccupied cytosolic ER (Greene 1984). The use of steroid affinity chromatography for the purification of receptors has generally been limited by the resistance of the bound receptor to elution under conditions compatible with its stability as well as by cleavage of ester and amide groups in the spacer arms that link steroids to the supporting matrix. For estrogen receptors, the elution problem was solved by including chaotropic salts such as sodium thiocyanate (Greene et al. 1980b) with dimethylformamide (Musto et al. 1977) in the eluting medium with estradiol to facilitate release of the receptor protein. A stable steroid affinity adsorbent was prepared by linking estradiol to Sepharose 6B via a thioether bridge in the 17α position of the steroid (Greene et al. 1980b). As a result, we have established a purification scheme that is simple and reproducible, and that affords a good yield of highly purified receptor as the steroid receptor complex (E*R$_c$) (Greene et al. 1980b; Greene 1984). Following the examples of Puca (Molinari et al. 1977) and Bresciani (Sica and Bresciani 1979), who used heparin-Sepharose to improve their purification of calf uterine estrogen receptor, we included heparin-Sepharose in our protocol.

The cytosolic forms of estrogen receptor from calf uterus and from

Table 20.1. Purification of MCF-7 estrogen receptor

Step	Protein (mg)	Total receptor[a] (nmol)	Specific activity (pmol/mg)	Yield (%)	Purity[b] (%)	Purification factor
1. Cytosol	3979	5.61	1.41	100	—	1
2. Affinity eluate	N.D.	4.58	N.D.	82	—	—
3. G25 eluate	26.6	4.03	152	72	1	108
4. Heparin-Sepharose eluate	0.26	2.33	9058	42	> 59	6424

From Greene 1983.
[a]Determined by specific binding to controlled-pore glass beads.
[b]Assuming one E* bound to a protein of M_r 65,000 (determined by SDS-gel electrophoresis).

MCF-7 human breast cancer cells are now routinely purified to virtual homogeneity by the above protocol. A typical purification sequence is summarized in Table 20.1 for MCF-7 receptor. The overall recovery of receptor as E^*R_c is 30–45% and the purity ranges from 60% to greater than 90% of the specific radioactivity expected for one molecule of [^{3}H]estradiol bound to a 4S monomer of M_r 65,000. We have isolated as much as 5 nmol (315 μg) of receptor in a single experiment. Recent modifications of the protocol include omission of the gel filtration step prior to heparin-Sepharose chromatography and replacement of the original di-n-propyl thioether bridge in the steroid resin with a 1,4-bis(2,3-epoxypropoxy)butyl thioether spacer. The latter estradiol resin affords more highly purified receptor (300- to 1000-fold), indicating that less nonspecific adsorption of proteins to the adsorbent occurs when the steroid is linked through the longer diglycidyl ether bridge.

The highly purified MCF-7 E*R has properties that are similar to, if not the same as, the activated steroid receptor complex found in high salt nuclear extracts of MCF-7 cells. Thus, the purified cytosol E*R binds DNA and sediments as a 5.3S species in sucrose gradients containing 400 mM KCl. In addition, an apparent molecular weight of 140,000, calculated from a Stokes radius of 5.74 Å and the 5.3S sedimentation coefficient, is consistent with the formation of a homodimer of two 65 K (4S) monomers. Chemical crosslinking experiments and dense amino acid labeling of unpurified nuclear MCF-7 ER also indicate that activated E*R is a homodimer (Miller et al. 1985). Interestingly, the purified E*R has lost its ability to form an 8–9S complex in low salt gradients and sediments as a 5.9S species in 10 mM KCl, indicating that the factors, or factor, responsible for the formation of these larger complexes in cytosols are removed during purification. In fact, if purified receptor is added to receptor-depleted MCF-7 cytosol, a 7–8S complex is observed in 10 mM KCl. When highly purified receptor is analyzed by SDS-gel electrophoresis under reducing conditions, one major silver-stained band, M_r 65,000, is seen. The same band can be visualized by autoradiography if E* is exchanged with [^{3}H]tamoxifen aziridine, a specific covalent tag for estrogen receptor (Katzenellenbogen et al. 1983).

III. Antibodies to the Estrogen Receptor Protein

A. POLYCLONAL ANTIBODIES

The production of antibodies to steroid receptors has been hampered by difficulties in obtaining enough highly purified receptor for immunizations. Estrogen receptor in particular has proven difficult to purify because of receptor instability, proteolysis, and its low concentration in the cell. The availability in our laboratory of partially purified nuclear estradiol receptor complex (E*R_n) from calf uterus led to the preparation of the first well-characterized antibodies to a steroid receptor protein (Greene et al. 1977). Rabbits, a goat, and rats (Greene et al. 1979) immunized with E*R_n that was about 10–20% pure produced antibodies that recognized the cytosol and nuclear forms of ER from all tested mammalian and non-mammalian tissues, as well as some antibodies that were species specific. In all cases these antibodies have been specific for estrogen receptors, showing no tendency to react with androgen or progesterone receptors, free estradiol, or other steroid-binding proteins present in tissue extracts or serum. Since the generation of well-defined ER antibodies was first reported by this laboratory (Greene et al. 1977), polyclonal antibodies have been raised against partially purified preparations of glucocortoid receptors (Govindan 1979; Eisen 1980; Okret et al. 1981), calf and human uterine estrogen receptor (Radanyi et al. 1979; Coffer et al., 1980), and PgR isolated from rabbit and guinea pig uterus (Logeat et al. 1981; Feil 1983), as well as chick oviduct (Renoir et al. 1982). In general, these antibodies recognize corresponding receptors from other species. However, all antibodies directed against steroid-binding subunits appear to be hormone specific.

For virtually all of the experiments involving polyclonal antibodies, [^{3}H]estradiol (E*) has served as a marker for estrogen receptor, either before or after interaction of the receptor with antibody. This interaction does not cause the release of significant amounts of E* from E*R nor does it prevent the binding of hormone to uncomplexed receptor. However, our goat antibody to calf nuclear ER does cause a decrease in the affinity and number of binding sites for E* when antibody is associated with calf or MCF-7 cytosol ER (Greene et al. 1979). Interestingly, the same two binding parameters for [³H]monohydroxytamoxifen are unaffected, whereas the binding of nonsteroidal diethylstilbestrol to MCF-7 ER is so perturbed by goat antibody that it was not possible to quantify the affinity or number of sites (Tate et al. 1984). These results suggest that there are significant differences in the binding of estrogens and antiestrogens to cytosol ER, possibly indicating different ligand-receptor conformations, which are affected by the binding of one or more antibodies to sites near the hormone-binding region. Although it seems likely that these ligands all bind to the same site on ER, an allosteric model would also be consistent with the observed antibody effects.

B. Monoclonal Antibodies

Polyclonal ER antibodies have been of limited use for many receptor studies, especially in human reproductive tissues and cancers, because of a lack of cross reactivity, monospecificity, and supply. Also, it has been difficult to obtain enough highly purified ER for immunizations. For these reasons, we turned to the hybridoma technique developed by Kohler and Milstein (1976) to prepare monoclonal antibodies to the calf and human estrogen receptors.

The first monoclonal antibodies to mammalian estrogen receptors were prepared in our laboratory by polyethylene glycol–mediated fusion of splenic lymphocytes from male Lewis rats, immunized with partially purified nuclear E*R from calf uterus, with mouse myeloma cells (P3-X63-Ag8, P3-NSI/1-Ag4-1, and Sp2/0-Ag14) (Greene et al. 1980a). Rat antibodies were detected in hybridoma culture medium by double antibody precipitation of crude nuclear E*R from calf uterus. Both IgM- and IgG2a-secreting hybridomas were obtained. Like the polyclonal rat antiserum, all of the monoclonal antibodies recognized 4S cytosol E*R and 5S nuclear E*R from calf uterus. However, in contrast to monoclonal IgG, which showed comparable affinity for the cytosol and nuclear forms of calf E*R, the IgMs reacted preferentially with the nuclear form. The reasons for this distinction are not clear. All of these monoclonal antibodies were specific for calf estrogen receptor, as were the polyclonal antibodies

364 VI. Antibodies to Steroid Hormone Receptors

present in the serum of the immunized rat. These antibodies recognized occupied as well as unoccupied receptors and did not interfere with the binding of steroid to receptor. All of the data accumulated thus far indicate that the 10 monoclonal antibodies (IgM and IgG) recognize either the same epitope or mutually exclusive epitopes on the calf receptor.

Although the monoclonal antibodies prepared against calf ER have proven useful for the characterization and purification of cytosol and nuclear forms of calf ER, they are limited by their specificity and recognition of only one region of the receptor molecule. Because of our interest in being able to study estrogen receptors in other species, particularly in human reproductive tract and breast cancer, all subsequent efforts have been directed toward preparing monoclonal antibodies against human ER. With the successful partial purification of cytosol estrogen receptor obtained from MCF-7 human breast cancer cells, we began, in 1979, to immunize male Lewis rats with E^*R_c, eluted from the estradiol affinity resin, that was about 5–10% pure. Fusion of splenic lymphocytes from immunized animals with two different mouse myeloma lines (P3-X63-Ag8 and Sp2/0-Ag14) yielded three cloned hybridomas, each of which secretes a unique idiotype of antibody that recognizes a distinct region of the ER molecule (Table 20.2, D series). Subsequent fusions, carried out both in our own laboratory (Greene et al. 1984) and at Abbott Laboratories (Miller et al. 1982), have produced a total of 13 monoclonal antibodies (Miller et al. 1982; Greene et al. 1984) all of which (with one possible exception) recognize distinct regions of the receptor molecule (Table 20.2). These antibodies have high affinity ($K_d = 10^{-9}–10^{-10}$ M) for both steroid-occupied and unoccupied estrogen receptor and recognize nuclear as well as cytosol forms of the receptor molecule. Although they vary in their cross reactivity with estrogen receptors from various animal species, each antibody appears to be completely specific for the 65 kilodalton steroid-binding subunit of the estrogen receptor complex, as judged by extensive sucrose gradient and immunoblot analyses of cytosol and nuclear extracts from a variety of tissues and cell lines. Cross reactivity patterns (Table 20.1) indicate both sequence homology and heterogeneity among mammalian and nonmammalian estrophilins. Some determinants (e.g., H222 and H226) are common to all tested estrogen receptors, including those from hen oviduct, whereas others (e.g., D547 and D58) are present only in mammalian receptors, and one (D75) appears to be restricted to primate estrophilin.

Table 20.2. Cross reactivity of monoclonal antibodies to human estrophilin

			Receptor source				
	Breast cancer		Uterus				Oviduct
Antibody[a]	MCF-7	Human	Human	Monkey	Calf	Rat	Hen
Rat serum	+	+	+	+	+	+	+
D58P3μ	+	+	+	+	+	+	−
D75P3γ	+	+	+	+	−	−	−
D547Spγ	+	+	+	+	+	+	−
F88Spγ	+	+	+		+	+	+
F344Spμ	+		+		+	+	+
G5Spγ	+	+	+		+		−
G13Spγ	+						
H23Spγ	+	+	+	+		+	+
H142Spγ	+	+	+	+		+	+
H165Spγ	+	+	+	+		+	+
H221Spγ	+	+	+	+	+	+	+
H222Spγ	+	+	+	+	+	+	+
H226Spγ	+	+	+	+	+	+	+

From Greene et al. 1984.
[a]IgM antibodies indicated by μ and IgG by γ. P3 and Sp indicate hybridomas derived from P3-X63-Ag8 and Sp2/0-Ag14 mouse myeloma cells, respectively.

IV. Immunochemical Analysis of Receptor Structure and Function

Two of the more important uses of the antibodies listed in Table 20.2 have been the immunochemical purification of estrogen receptor from different sources and the mapping of functional domains of the receptor. MCF-7 cytosol estrogen receptor has been purified to near homogeneity in a single step by chromatography on an immunoadsorbent consisting of D547 IgG conjugated to Sepharose 4B (Greene 1984). Intact estradiol-receptor complex (E*R) can be eluted in good yield with a buffer containing sodium thiocyanate and dimethylformamide, similar to the conditions used for the elution of receptor from the estradiol affinity adsorbent. The E*R obtained by this procedure appears to be identical to receptor purified by the method outlined in Table 20.1. Immunopurification with D547 and H222 adsorbents is also being used to isolate occupied and unoccupied forms of estrophilin from mRNA translation mixtures, nuclear matrix preparations, and extracts of various reproductive tissues and cell lines.

In ongoing studies to map the location of various determinants in relation to each other and to the steroid- and DNA-binding domains, the relative positions of nine unique determinants have been determined by density gradient analysis of antibody-E*R interaction after limited proteolysis of MCF-7 cytosol E*R with trypsin, chymotrypsin, or papain (Fig. 20.1). As shown in Figure 20.1, determinants for three of the monoclonal rat antibodies are susceptible to selective cleavage by one or more of the enzymes tested. Six other antibodies are capable of binding the 2.6S steroid-binding fragment remaining after cleavage with trypsin. When tested for their ability to associate with ϕX174 double-stranded DNA in sucrose density gradients, none of the E*R fragments was able to bind DNA, whereas the intact 5S nuclear receptor cosedimented with the DNA. Preliminary results indicate that when nuclear E*R is cleaved with papain, a non-steroid-binding portion of the receptor retains its ability to recognize DNA, as shown by the formation of an immune complex consisting of ^{35}S-H226 IgG, ϕX174 DNA, and cleaved receptor. Although the H226 and H222 determinants appear to be well separated from each other on the polypeptide chain, the corresponding antibodies can not bind additively, suggesting that these regions of the receptor are spatially proximal to each other. Interestingly, the determinants that are most well conserved across all tested species (Table 20.2) are located either near the steroid-binding domain (H23, H142, H165, H221, H222) or the DNA-binding domain (H226).

A clinically important application of ER monoclonal antibodies has been the development of quantitative and cytochemical immunoassays for estrogen receptor in breast cancers. These assays are being used to assess the prognosis and probable response to endocrine therapy of estrogen-dependent reproductive cancers. Three antibodies (D547, D75, H222) were used to devise simple immunoradiometric (Greene and Jensen 1982) and immunocolorimetric (Nolan et al. 1984) sandwich assays for ER. When tumor cytosols from 82 human breast cancers were analyzed for receptor content by both methods, a linear correlation of results with sucrose gradient and dextran-coated charcoal analyses (with [^{3}H]estradiol) was obtained (Fig. 20.2). The enzyme immunoassay (ER-EIA), which is now available as a commercial kit, is simple and rapid, and does not depend on the binding of hormone to receptor.

The major disadvantage of all quantitative receptor assays performed

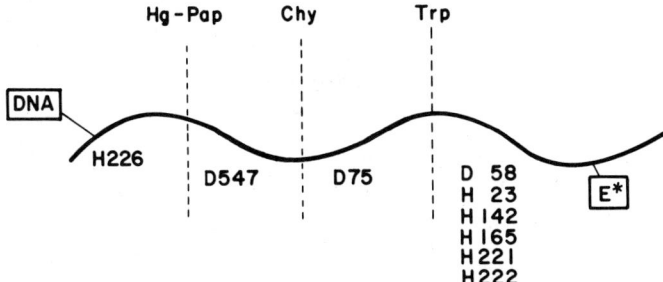

Figure 20.1. Map of antigenic determinants in relation to steroid-binding and DNA-binding domains of the MCF-7 cytosol estrogen receptor. Dashed lines indicate sites of cleavage for listed enzymes. Postulated recognition sites for nine antibodies are shown. (From Sobel 1982).

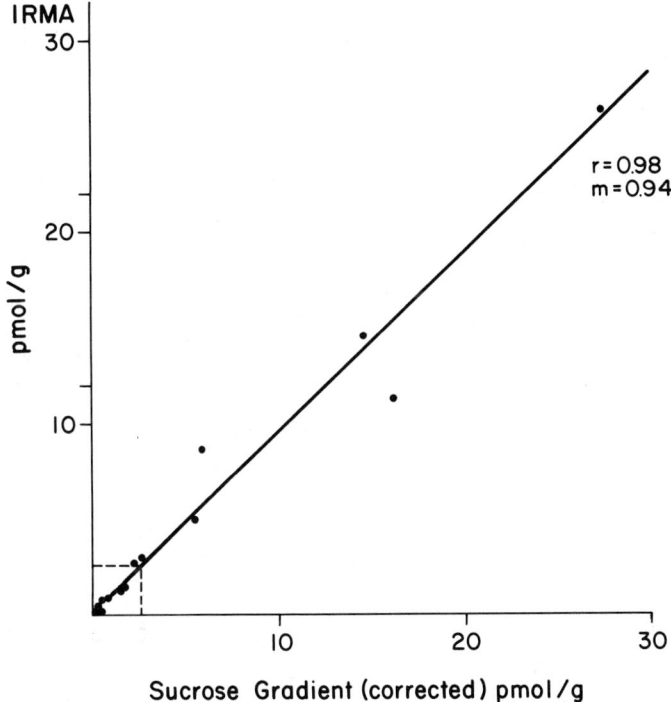

Sucrose Gradient (corrected) pmol/g

Figure 20.2. The estrogen receptor contents of 18 human breast cancer cytosols as determined by the immunoradiometric assay (IRMA) technique, compared with the results obtained by sucrose gradient ultracentrifugation. In the latter procedure, a subsaturating dose (0.5 nM) of [³H]estradiol was used and the results were corrected to total receptor binding capacity. (From Greene and Jensen 1982.)

in tissue extracts is their inability to provide information about receptor distribution in both normal and neoplastic cells. As part of our ongoing effort to determine the location and dynamics of the estrogen receptor protein in target tissues in the presence and absence of estrogens and antiestrogens, we have developed an immunocytochemical assay (ER-ICA) for visualizing receptor directly in tissues and cells. Five monoclonal antibodies (D547, D58, D75, H222, H226) have been used individually to localize estrophilin by an indirect human uterus, rabbit uterus (Fig. 20.3), and in other mammalian reproductive tissues, as well as in fixed MCF-7 cell cultures (King and Greene 1984; Press and Greene 1984; King et al. 1985). Specific immunoperoxidase staining for receptor in estrogen-sensitive tissues is confined to the nucleus of all stained cells, regardless of hormone status. Staining is absent in nontarget tissues, such as colon epithelium, and in receptor-negative breast cancers; in addition, it can be abolished by the addition of highly purified receptor to primary antibody (Fig. 20.3E). Heterogeneous staining has been observed in MCF-7 cells as well as in receptor-poor and receptor-rich breast cancers, possibly reflecting either variations in cell cycle or the presence of estrogen-sensitive and -insensitive cells. Little or no cytoplasmic staining for estrophilin has been observed in any of the tissues or tumor cells examined thus far, including those deprived of exogenous estrogens. In a study of 117 human breast cancers by the ER-ICA method, the presence or absence of nuclear staining was significantly associated with the concentration of cytosolic estrogen receptor determined by steroid-binding assay. Staining intensity, epithelial cellularity, and the proportion of tumor cells stained also correlated significantly with receptor concentration (King et al. 1985).

In view of the exclusively nuclear localization of specific immunoperoxidase staining for receptor in all estrogen-sensitive tissues and cells studied thus far, it appears that both cytosol and nuclear forms of the receptor may reside in the nuclear compartment in the presence and absence of steroid. We have seen little or no increase in nuclear staining intensity in MCF-7 cells and in uteri from immature rabbits or from postmenopausal women following short-term exposure of cells or tissue to estradiol. A notable exception is the increase in nuclear staining intensity observed by McClellan et al. (1984) in monkey endometrium following *in vitro* exposure to 100 nm estradiol. These observations are consistent with the hypothesis that unoccupied estrophilin recovered in the low salt cytosol fraction of a tissue homogenate represents receptor that is loosely as-

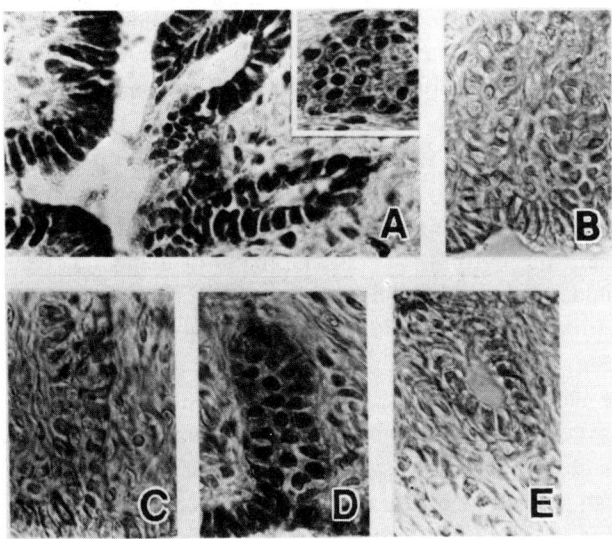

Figure 20.3. Immunocytochemical localization of estrogen receptor in a rabbit uterus taken from an animal that was ovariectomized 8 days prior to killing. Uteri from similarly treated rabbits contained 3.15 ± 0.85 pmol cytosol ER per mg of DNA ($n = 3$) and 0.16 ± 0.01 pmol of salt-extractable (0.4 M KCl) ER per mg of DNA, as measured by exchange assay with [^{3}H]estradiol. The insert in the upper right corner of panel A represents rabbit myometrium. Frozen sections (8 μm) fixed with picric acid–paraformaldehyde were incubated successively with primary antibody, goat antibody to rat IgG, and rat peroxidase-antiperoxidase complex (PAP) for 30 minutes each in a humidified chamber. Bound antibodies were visualized by treatment with diaminobenzidine. Sections A–E were treated identically, except for the first incubation, which consisted of either (A) 2μg/ml (13 pmol/ml) of H226 IgG in PBS; (B) 2 μg/ml of purified normal rat IgG; (C) 2μg/ml of H226 in MCF-7 cytosol (20 pmol ER per ml); (D) 2μg/ml of H226 in receptor-depleted (by adsorption to estradiol-Sepharose) MCF-7 cytosol; or (E) 2 μg/ml of H226 in receptor-depleted MCF-7 cytosol supplemented with 20 pmol/ml of highly purified estrophilin. (From King and Greene 1984.)

sociated with nuclear components and that binding of estradiol to receptor leads to a tighter association, a phenomenon previously interpreted as indicating translocation of the receptor from the cytoplasm to the nucleus. Several lines of evidence support this hypothesis, including the observation by Welshons et al. (1984) that cytochalasin-induced enucleation of rat pituitary (GH$_3$) cells leads to partitioning of unoccupied ER almost exclusively into the nucleoplast fraction. At least two forms of steroid receptor complex appear to be tightly bound to chromatin. One of these forms can be extracted with salt (0.4 M KCl) and one is resistant to salt extraction and may be associated with transcriptionally active DNA on the nuclear matrix (Alexander et al. 1985). Both forms are recognized by one or more of our monoclonal antibodies and both migrate as M_r 65,000 proteins in reducing SDS gels. We are currently trying to identify specific chromatin binding sites for ER, as a function of occupancy by estrogens and estrogen antagonists, by immunoelectron microscopy. Preliminary results (Press et al. 1985) indicate that unoccupied ER is localized in the euchromatin, but not in the heterochromatin or nucleoli of epithelial and stromal nuclei of human endometrium and MCF-7 cells.

The availability of specific, high affinity monoclonal antibody probes for estrogen receptor has clearly led to the development of new and complementary methods for analyzing receptor structure and function in hormone-responsive cells. Not only have these antibodies facilitated the purification and comparison of cytosol and nuclear forms of ER from various mammalian and nonmammalian sources, but they have also permitted the development of steroid-independent immunoassays for ER in tissues and their extracts. A particularly promising application for the immunocytochemical assay is the ultrastructural localization of ER in target cells during various stages of the cell cycle and as a function of hormone agonistic/antagonistic action. Future applications also include a more detailed analysis of receptor-chromatin interactions as well as the structural changes that accompany ligand-binding, activation, and DNA-binding. In addition, several antibodies are being used to screen an MCF-7 cDNA library for expressed immunoreactive human estrogen receptor. The availability of cloned gene sequences for ER will allow us to study the regulation of ER gene expression, as well as to determine the complete amino acid sequence of receptor and to obtain large quantities of receptor for structural studies and for a more detailed analysis of the physical and chemical properties of the steroid- and DNA-binding domains of ER. A combination of biochemical, immunochemical, and recombinant DNA techniques should provide new and valuable information about how steroid receptors regulate gene expression.

Acknowledgments

These investigations were supported by grants from the National Cancer Institute (CA-02897), the American Cancer Society (BC-86), Abbott Laboratories, and the Women's Board of the Cancer Research Foundation.

References

Alexander, R. B., G. L. Greene, and E. R. Barrack. 1985. Estrogen receptors in the liver nuclear matrix: direct demonstration using monoclonal anti-receptor antibody. *Endocrinology*. Submitted for publication.

Barrack, E. R. 1983. The nuclear matrix of the prostate contains acceptor sites for androgen receptors. *Endocrinology* 113:430–432.

Barrack, E. R., and D. S. Coffey. 1980. The specific binding of estrogens and androgens to the nuclear matrix of sex hormone responsive tissues. *Journal of Biological Chemistry* 255:7265–7275.

Beato, M. 1980. In *Steroid-induced uterine proteins*, ed. M. Beato, Amsterdam: Elsevier.

Cato, A. C. B., S. Geisse, M. Wenz, H. M. Westphal, and M. Beato. 1984. The nucleotide sequences recognized by the glucocorticoid receptor in the rabbit uteroglobin gene region are located far upstream from the initiation of transcription. *EMBO Journal* 3:2771–2778.

Coffer, A. I., R. J. B. King, and A. J. Brockas. 1980. Antibodies to human myometrial oestrogen receptor. *Biochemistry International* 1:126–132.

Compton, J. G., W. T. Schrader, and B. W. O'Malley. 1983. DNA sequence preference of the progesterone receptor. *Proceedings of the National Academy of Sciences* 80:16–20.

Eisen, H. J. 1980. An antiserum to the rat liver glucocorticoid receptor. *Proceedings of the National Academy of Sciences* 77:3893–3897.

Feil, P. D. 1983. Characterization of guinea pig anti-progestin receptor antiserum. *Endocrinology* 112:396–398.

Gorski, J., D. Toft, S. Shyamala, D. Smith, and A. Notides. 1968. Hormone receptors: studies on the interaction of estrogen with the uterus. *Recent Progress in Hormone Research* 24:45–80.

Govindan, M. V. 1979. Purification of glucocorticoid receptors from rat liver cytosol. Preparation of antibodies against the major receptor proteins and application of immunological techniques to study activation and translocation. *Journal of Steroid Biochemistry* 11:323–332.

Greene, G. L. 1983. Immunochemical studies of estrogen receptor. In *Gene regulation by steroid hormones II*, ed. A. K. Roy and J. H. Clark, 191–200. New York: Springer-Verlag.

Greene, G. L. 1984. Application of immunochemical techniques to the analysis of estrogen receptor structure and function. In *Biochemical actions of hormones*, vol. 11, ed. G. Litwack, 207–239. New York: Academic Press.

Greene, G. L., and E. V. Jensen. 1982. Monoclonal antibodies as probes for estrogen receptor detection and characterization. *Journal of Steroid Biochemistry* 16:353–359.

Greene, G. L., L. E. Closs, H. Fleming, E. R. DeSombre, and E. V. Jensen. 1977. Antibodies to estrogen receptor: immunochemical similarity of estrophilin from various mammalian species. *Proceedings of the National Academy of Sciences* 74:3681–3685.

Greene, G. L., L. E. Closs, E. R. DeSombre, and E. V. Jensen. 1979. Antibodies to estrophilin: comparison between rabbit and goat antisera. *Journal of Steroid Biochemistry* 11:333–341.

Greene, G. L., F. W. Fitch, and E. V. Jensen. 1980a. Monoclonal antibodies to estrophilin: probes for the study of estrogen receptors. *Proceedings of the National Academy of Sciences* 77:157–161.

Greene, G. L., C. Nolan, P. Engler, and E. V. Jensen. 1980b. Monoclonal antibodies to human estrogen receptor. *Proceedings of the National Academy of Sciences* 77:5115–5119.

Greene, G. L., N. B. Sobel, W. J. King, and E. V. Jensen. 1984. Immunochemical studies of estrogen receptors. *Journal of Steroid Biochemistry* 20:51–56.

Jensen, E. V., and H. I. Jacobson. 1962. Basic guides to the mechanism of estrogen action. *Recent Progress in Hormone Research* 18:387–414.

Jensen, E. V., T. Suzuki, T. Kawashima, W. E. Stumpf, P. W. Jungblut, and E. R. De-Sombre. 1968. A two-step mechanism for the interaction of estradiol with rat uterus. *Proceedings of the National Academy of Sciences* 59:632–638.

Jost, J. P., M. Geiser, and M. Seldran. 1985. Specific modulation of the transcription of cloned avian vitellogenin II gene by estradiol-receptor complex in vitro. *Proceedings of the National Academy of Sciences* 82:988–991.

Katzenellenbogen, J. A., K. E. Carlson, D. F. Heiman, D. W. Robertson, L. L. Weill, and B. S. Katzenellenbogen. 1983. Efficient and highly selective covalent labeling of the estrogen receptor with [^{3}H]tamoxifen aziridine. *Journal of Biological Chemistry* 258:3487–3495.

King, W. J., and G. L. Greene. 1984. Monoclonal antibodies localize oestrogen receptor in the nuclei of target cells. *Nature* (London) 307:745–747.

King, W. J., E. R. DeSombre, E. V. Jensen, and G. L. Greene. 1985. Comparison of immunocytochemical and steroid binding assays for estrogen receptor in human breast tumors. *Cancer Research* 45:293–304.

Kohler, G., and C. Milstein. 1976. Derivation of specific antibody-producing tissue culture and tumor lines by cell fusion. *European Journal of Immunology* 6:511–519.

Ling, T., and S. Liao. 1974. Association of the uterine 17β-estradiol-receptor complex with ribonucleoprotein in vitro and in vivo. *Journal of Biological Chemistry* 249:4671–4678.

Logeat, T., M. T. V. Mai, and E. Milgrom. 1981. Antibodies to rabbit progesterone receptor: crossreaction with human receptor. *Proceedings of the National Academy of Sciences* 78:1426–1430.

McClellan, M. C., N. B. West, D. E. Tacha, G. L. Greene, and R. M. Brenner. 1984. Immunocytochemical localization of estrogen receptors in the Macaque reproductive tract with monoclonal antiestrophilins. *Endocrinology* 114:2002–2014.

Miller, L. S., I. I. E. Tribby, M. R. Miles, J. T. Tomita, and C. Nolan. 1982. Hybridomas producing monoclonal antibodies to human estrogen receptor. *Federation Proceedings of the American Societies for Experimental Biology* 41:520.

Miller, M. A., A. Mullick, G. L. Greene, and B. S. Katzenellenbogen. 1985. Characterization of the subunit nature of nuclear estrogen receptors by chemical cross-linking and dense amino acid labeling. *Endocrinology* 117:515–522.

Molinari, A. M., N. Medici, B. Moncharmont, and G. A. Puca. 1977. Estradiol receptor of calf uterus: interaction with heparin-agarose and purification. *Proceedings of the National Academy of Sciences* 74:4886–4890.

Musto, N. A., G. L. Gunsalus, M. Miljkovic, and C. W. Bardin. 1977. A novel affinity column for isolation of androgen binding protein from rat epididymus. *Endocrine Research Communications* 4:147–157.

Nolan, C., L. W. Przywara, L. S. Miller, V. Susuikis, and J. Tomita. 1984. A sensitive solid-phase enzyme immunoassay for human estrogen receptor. In *Current controversies in breast cancer*, ed. F. C. Ames, G. R. Blumenschein, and E. D. Montague, 433–441. Austin: University of Texas Press.

Okret, S., J. Carlstedt-Duke, O. Wrange, K. Carlstrom, and J. A. Gustafsson. 1981. Characterization of an antiserum against the glucocorticoid receptor. *Biochimica et Biophysica Acta* 677:205–219.

Payvar, F., D. DeFranco, G. L. Firestone, G. Edgar, O. Wrange, S. Okret, J. A. Gustafsson, and K. R. Yamamoto. 1983. Sequence specific binding of glucocorticoid receptor to MTV DNA at sites within and upstream of the transcribed region. *Cell* 35:381–392.

Press, M. F., and G. L. Greene. 1984. An immunocytochemical method for demonstrating estrogen receptor in human uterus using monoclonal antibodies to human estrophilin. *Laboratory Investigation* 50:480–486.

Press, M. F., N. A. Nousek-Goebl, and G. L. Greene. 1985. Immunoelectron microscopic localization of estrogen receptor with monoclonal estrophilin antibodies. *Journal of Histochemistry and Cytochemistry* 33:915–924.

Puca, G. A., V. Sica, and E. Nola. 1974. Identification of a high affinity nuclear acceptor site for estrogen receptor of calf uterus. *Proceedings of the National Academy of Sciences* 71:979–983.

Radanyi, C., G. Redeuilh, E. Eigenmann, M. C. Lebeau, N. Massol, C. Secco, E. E. Baulieu, and H. Richard-Foy. 1979. Production et détection d'anticorps antirécepteur de l'oestradiol d'utérus de veau. Interaction avec le récepteur d'oviducte de poule. *Comptes Rendus Hebdomadaires des Séances de l'Académie des Sciences, Série D* 288:255–258.

Renoir, J. M., C. Radanyi, C. R. Yang, and E. E. Baulieu. 1982. Antibodies against progesterone receptor from chick oviduct cross-reactivity with mammalian progesterone receptors. *European Journal of Biochemistry* 127:81–86.

Sica, V., and F. Bresciani. 1979. Estrogen-binding proteins of calf uterus. Purification to homogeneity of receptor from cytosol by affinity chromatography. *Biochemistry* 18:2369–2378.

Sobel, N. 1982. Immunochemical characterization of estrogen binding fragments of the estrogen receptor protein from MCF-7 human breast cancer cells. Ph.D. dissertation, University of Chicago, Chicago, IL.

Spelsberg, T. C., B. A. Littlefield, R. Seelke, G. Martin-Dani, H. Toyoda, P. Boyd-Leinen, C. Thrall, and O. L. Kon. 1983. Role of specific chromosomal proteins and DNA sequences in the nuclear binding sites for steroid receptors. *Recent Progress in Hormone Research* 39:463–517.

Tate, A. C., G. L. Greene, E. R. DeSombre, E. V. Jensen, and V. C. Jordan. 1984. Differences between estrogen– and antiestrogen–estrogen receptor complexes from human breast tumors identified with an antibody raised against the estrogen receptor. *Cancer Research* 44:1012–1018.

Welshons, W. V., M. E. Lieberman, and J. Gorski. 1984. Nuclear localization of unoccupied oestrogen receptors: cytochalasin enucleation of GH_3 cells. *Nature* (London) 307:747–749.

21

The Generation of Antibodies
Against Partially Purified
Estradiol Receptor from
Human Myometrium

R. J. B. KING AND A. I. COFFER

I. INTRODUCTION   376
II. ANTIBODY PRODUCTION   377
   A. ANTIGEN   377
   B. POLYCLONAL ANTIBODIES   377
   C. MONOCLONAL ANTIBODIES   378
III. CHARACTERIZATION OF THE D5 ANTIGEN   379
IV. ASSAY OF P29   383
   A. IMMUNOASSAY   383
   B. IMMUNOHISTOCHEMICAL STUDIES   386
   C. COMPARISON OF IRMA AND HISTOCHEMISTRY   390
V. CONCLUSIONS   392
   REFERENCES   392

375

I. Introduction

The use of tritiated steroids to monitor the intracellular components of the estrogen receptor machinery has been extremely useful but has severe limitations. These became apparent at an early stage when autoradiography was used to determine the intracellular distribution of binding sites. Because of their lability and high solubility in aqueous media, the question of nuclear ys cytoplasmic sites could not be resolved (Stumpf and Sar 1976; Clark and Peck 1979; Sheridan et al. 1979). This problem has been compounded by the use of fluorescent ligands or labeled antibodies to the ligand, which have engendered often acrimonious debate as to what binding sites are being assayed by these techniques (McCarty et al. 1981; Pertschuk et al. 1981; Lee 1984). Likewise, it was soon discovered that binding sites were lost after cellular uptake of steroid. Extensive studies indicated that this "processing" of receptor was an important adjunct of hormone action (Horwitz and McGuire 1978), but this view has now been questioned; by changing the labeling methods, the number of binding sites remains constant (Jakesz et al. 1983). A third example of the limitations inherent in the use of labeled steroids is the question of the structure of the classic 8S receptor; is it composed of similar or dissimilar subunits (King and Mainwaring 1974b; Notides et al. 1975; Sherman 1984)?

In the same vein, are the estrogen receptors in one target cell different from those in another? These and other questions exist because of two features of the ligand receptor complex. First, the interaction is not a covalent one, which imposes technical limitations on our methodologies and, second, if the ligand binding site is either occupied with endogenous ligand, lost, or not present in each component of the receptor, the properties of that component cannot be monitored. The first problem can be, and is being, overcome by affinity labeling techniques (Katzenellenbogen, Chapter 5 in this volume). The second difficulty requires a method of detecting the protein moieties of the receptor; antibodies are the obvious candidate.

Several groups adopted this approach with, until recently, only limited success. Several polyclonal sera were raised, which produced some interesting results but which did not have the hoped-for impact on receptor information (reviewed in Coffer et al. 1985a). Monoclonal antibodies have, however, been more productive both in terms of clarifying established problems and in generating surprises. The present chapter will use our experiences to illustrate these points.

II. Antibody Production

A. ANTIGEN

Our prime interest concerns hormone action in humans and we therefore wished to ensure that any receptor antibodies reacted with human antigens. This dictated the choice of human source material. Other groups were using cultured human breast cancer cell lines as a source of receptor and, given the theoretical possibility that receptors from neoplastic cells might be different from those from nonmalignant sources, we opted for nonmalignant tissue. Myometrium, obtained at hysterectomy for various benign conditions, was the only practical choice, given the quantities of material required. Myometrium contains high levels of a serine-protease that cleaves the DNA-binding part of the receptor from the estradiol-binding region (Gregory and Notides 1982). This has the disadvantage of producing a degraded receptor but has the advantage that this 4S product does not aggregate, which simplifies purification. The antigen was purified by ammonium sulfate precipitation and affinity chromatography on an estradiol hemisuccinate-sepharose column. The immunogen was about 5% pure as judged from [^{3}H]estradiol binding, and the latter component had an isoelectric point of 6.15 and a molecular weight of 36 kilodaltons; after electrofocusing, the molecular weight decreased to 30 K (Coffer et al. 1976).

B. POLYCLONAL ANTIBODIES

The polyclonal antibodies were raised in sheep by an initial injection of 20 µg soluble estradiol receptor (ER), boosted at monthly intervals by further 20 µg injections. Two of the three animals produced antibodies capable of reacting with cytosol 8S ER from human, rat, and calf tissues as judged by sucrose gradient analysis. They did not react with androgen receptor (AR) or progesterone receptor (PgR), sex hormone–binding globulin (SHBG), or α-fetoprotein (Table 21.1) but, more significantly, no consistent reaction could be obtained with rat nuclear receptor, calcium-stabilized 4.6S or 4S, trypsin-treated rat uterine ER (Coffer and King

Table 21.1. Antibody specificity as judged by reaction with labeled estradiol-ER complex

	Polyclonal	Monoclonal	
	G3	D5	C3
ER (human)			
Cytosol	+	−	−
"Activated" cytosol[a]	+	+	+
Nuclear	−	−	+
ER cytosol (rat, calf)	+	−	+
Nuclear (rat)	−		
Cytosol (chick)	−	−	+
PgR, AR, SHBG, α-fetoprotein	−	−	−

[a] See Table 21.2.

1981). The antigenic determinants were lost on conversion of the rat 8S complex to smaller forms, and at the time we interpreted this as being due to loss of determinants from the estradiol-binding unit. Given the properties of the monoclonal antibodies (see below), that interpretation may need revising.

Further analysis indicated that the antisera contained other major species of antibody that were unrelated to ER and that were difficult to remove by adsorption methods. Hence, they were unsuitable for many of the experiments we wished to perform, and monoclonal antibodies would be more useful.

C. Monoclonal Antibodies

Mice were immunized with 5 injections, each of 1–3 μg of affinity-purified ER, after which the spleen cells were fused with mouse myeloma cells. Hybridoma supernatants were screened by double antibody precipitation of $[^{125}I]E_2$-ER complex from human myometrium that had been partially purified by ammonium sulfate precipitation. The choice of this method was dictated by experiments carried out with the polyclonal antibody G3. Double antibody precipitation experiments with G3 indicated that no precipitation of $[^{125}I]E_2$-ER occurred from cytosols, but it did if the receptor was first fractionated with ammonium sulfate. No explanation for this observation was available at the time.

Two monoclonal antibodies were produced, the specificities of which are summarized in Table 21.1. Thus far we have worked mainly with D5, which is specific for the human antigen.

Table 21.2. Immunoprecipitation of cytosol [^{125}I]estradiol-ER by D5: effect of labeling conditions

	Polyclonal	Monoclonal	
	G3	D5	C3
4°C	−	−	−
30°C	+	+	+
KCNS	Not tested	+	+
pH 6	Not tested	+	+
Ammonium sulfate 4°C	+	+	+
Molybdate 4°C	Not tested	−	+
Molybdate 30°C	Not tested	+	+

III. Characterization of the D5 Antigen

The specificity studies (Table 21.1) were all carried out with ammonium sulfate-treated samples. Clearly, D5 is capable of reacting with the E_2 binding unit under activating conditions as well as by immunoaffinity chromatography on protein A (Coffer et al. 1985a), but we have been unable to precipitate bound hormone from untreated cytosols. Likewise, no sedimentation changes in the presence of antibody have been detected on sucrose gradients. Although double antibody precipitation of bound estradiol from cytosols is ineffective, an interaction can be generated by carrying out the estradiol-labeling step at elevated temperatures, low pH, high salt, or in the presence of potassium thiocyanate; molybdate inhibits this effect (Table 21.2). It is noteworthy that, with the possible exception of thiocyanate, all these conditions also "activate" receptor for nuclear retention. Furthermore, molybdate has an inhibitory effect on both properties. It is, however, unlikely that epitope exposure on the estradiol-binding unit as a result of activation is a valid explanation, because D5 will not react with nuclear receptor either by double antibody precipitation or immunoradiometric assay (IRMA), and the antigen has a cytoplasmic location (see below).

To add to the confusion, the D5 antigen can be separated from the estradiol binding unit by either isoelectric focusing (Fig. 21.1A) or sucrose gradient analysis (Fig. 21.1B) and has a molecular weight of 29 K (p29) under reducing conditions (Fig. 21.2), as compared to the 60–70 K value reported for the E_2 binding unit (Redeuilh et al. 1980; Miller et al., Chapter 8 in this volume; Greene et al., Chapter 20 in this volume). The

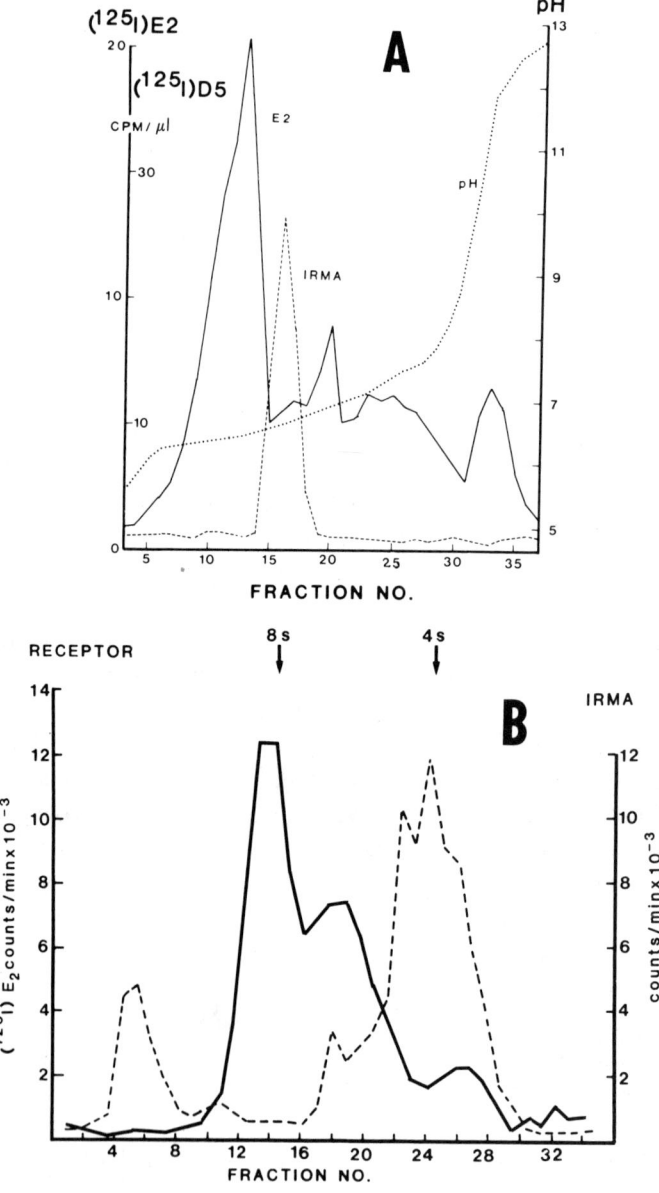

Figure 21.1. (A) Isoelectric focusing profile of estradiol-binding proteins and p29 in breast tumor cytosol. (B) Sucrose gradient analysis of estradiol receptor and p29 in cytosol from MCF-7 cells. The receptor counts have been corrected for nonspecific binding.

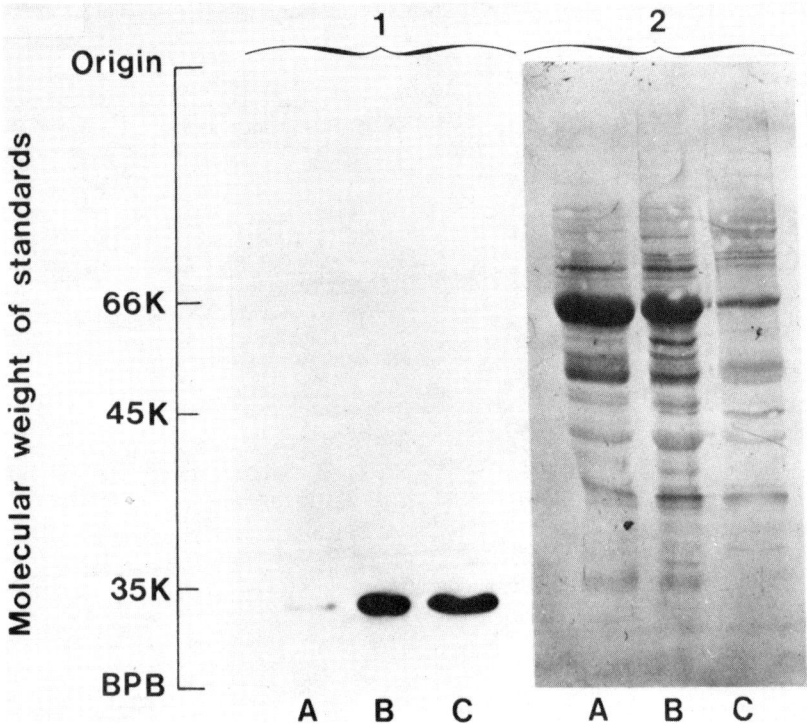

Figure 21.2. Comparison of immunoblotting (1) and Coomassie blue staining (2) of breast tumor cytosols. (A) ER-poor (< 5 fmol/mg protein); (B) and (C) ER-rich (> 20 fmol/mg protein); (B) cytosol; (C) ammonium sulfate fractions; BPB: bromophenol blue marker position.

simplest explanation for all these data would be that the antibody has been raised against an impurity which artifactually reacts with the receptor; there are many examples of such interactions of dubious physiological significance (King and Mainwaring 1974a; Puca et al. 1983). This possibility cannot be ruled out but is very unlikely because of the close qualitative and quantitative relationship between ER and the D5 antigen. We have developed both an IRMA and histochemical assay for p29 and compared the data so obtained with the [³H]estradiol binding assay. At a qualitative level, a 100% correlation exists among the three methods, regardless of whether the source material is normal or neoplastic, solid tissue or cultured cell line (Table 21.3). This statement does of course apply only

Table 21.3. Comparison of the specificity of immunoassays with [³H]estradiol binding
assay[a]

	Assay		
Sample	[³H]Estradiol	IRMA	Histochemistry
Solid tumors			
Breast	$\begin{cases} + \\ - \end{cases}$	+ −	+ −
Endometrium	$\begin{cases} + \\ - \end{cases}$	+ −	+ −
Ovary	−	−	−
Leiomyoma	+	+	+
Tumor cell lines			
Endometrium: HEC1A	−	−	−
Breast			
ZR-75	+	+	+
MCF-7	+	+	+
Epidermoid: trachea: HEP11	+	+	+
Epidermoid: vulva: A-431	−	−	−
Neuroblastoma: NB100	−	−	−
Leisch Nyan fibroblasts: LN75 (not tumor)	−	−	−
Normal tissues			
Endometrium	+	+	+
Myometrium	+	+	+
Fallopian tube	+	+	+
Biological fluids			
Pleural effusion (cells removed)	−	−	N.A.
Serum	−	−	N.A.

N.A. = not applicable.
[a]All samples were of human origin.

to human material; species such as rat, calf, and chick have estradiol receptors which do not react with D5 either by immunoprecipitation (Table 21.1) or IRMA. These qualitative results are further substantiated by the quantitative data on breast tumors (Fig. 21.3). This highly significant correlation between ER and p29 is discussed in more detail in Section IV.

Our conclusion is that a relationship exists between p29 and ER but we do not understand its basis. Activation exposes an epitope on either ER or p29 that allows an interaction to occur, the physiological significance of which remains in doubt, as p29 is not detectable in nuclear receptor. We considered the possibility that p29 was a component of the 8S receptor in which the epitope was masked in the native state, but p29 was not detectable even under denaturing conditions. Other possibilities, such as p29 being a product of processing or activation, have not yet been studied; it does not, however, appear to be a glycoprotein.

Two other examples have been described of monoclonal antibodies raised against steroid receptors reacting with antigens that do not bind steroid. Our antibody differs in some important respects from these. Thus, one monoclonal antibody raised against chick oviduct progesterone receptor recognises a 90 K protein that is common to androgen, estrogen, glucocorticoid, and progesterone receptors (Baulieu et al. 1983; Joab et al. 1984). However, it has been suggested that this 90 K protein has nothing to do with the receptor machinery (Birnbaumer et al. 1984); our antibody is specific for the estradiol receptor. Other monoclonal antibodies raised against highly purified 108 K B subunit of chick oviduct progesterone receptor recognizes a 108 K protein that has many similarities to the progesterone-binding B subunit of the receptor, except that it does not bind hormone (Edwards et al. 1984; Edwards et al., Chapter 22 in this volume). In contrast to our D5 antibody, the B subunit antibody will react on sucrose gradients with the 8S forms of progesterone, estradiol, androgen, and glucocorticoid receptor (Edwards et al., Chapter 22 in this volume).

In the absence of highly purified ER and p29, we cannot say if the two proteins have similarities analogous to those seen with progesterone receptor.

IV. *Assay of p29*

A. IMMUNOASSAY

Such an assay was desirable both for the work described above on the characterization of p29 and for clinical use with breast and endometrial cancer patients. The assay that we have developed gives a clear distinction between ER-rich and ER-poor endometrial tumors (Coffer et al. 1985b), but as yet, no further work has been done with these samples. We have mainly worked with breast tumors and, unless stated otherwise, all the following experiments were performed with this material.

We have developed two types of solid-phase assay, both based on the adsorption of antigen to plastic wells followed by reaction with labeled D5. The antibody is labeled either with [^{125}I] (IRMA) or peroxidase (enzyme-linked immunoabsorbent assay, ELISA). Both assays are effective

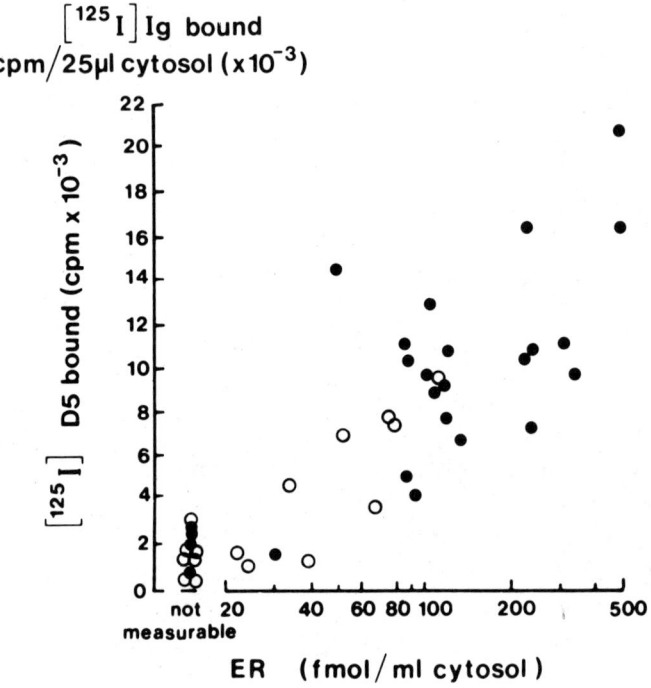

$\left[^{125}I\right]$ Ig bound
cpm/25µl cytosol $(\times 10^{-3})$

Figure 21.3. Correlation of ER (by [³H]estradiol-binding assay) with p29 (by IRMA) in individual breast tumors. Correlation coefficient $r = 0.758, p < 0.001.$ ○ ≤ 50 years old; ● > 50 years old.

but this chapter will deal only with IRMA. In contrast to the double antibody precipitation data (see above), IRMA with [¹²⁵I]D5 as the detecting reagent worked well with unactivated cytosols, and this method has therefore been used. In testing the effect of coating the wells with different proteins, we made the surprising observation that bovine serum albumin (BSA) markedly increased the final signal. This was specific in that it did not occur with other proteins such as ovalbumin and gamma globulin and only increased [¹²⁵I]D5 binding with ER-positive cytosols; addition of BSA to the cytosol prior to contact with coated wells had no effect (Coffer et al. 1985b). We assume that the BSA is altering the surface properties of the plastic in some unknown way. In more recent studies with a different plastic, BSA coating is not required for efficient antigen adsorption. Coating the plates with polyclonal antibody G3 or monoclonal C3 instead of BSA also enhanced subsequent [¹²⁵I]D5 binding as anticipated, and coating with D5 was inhibitory. As neither G3 nor C3 was as effective as BSA,

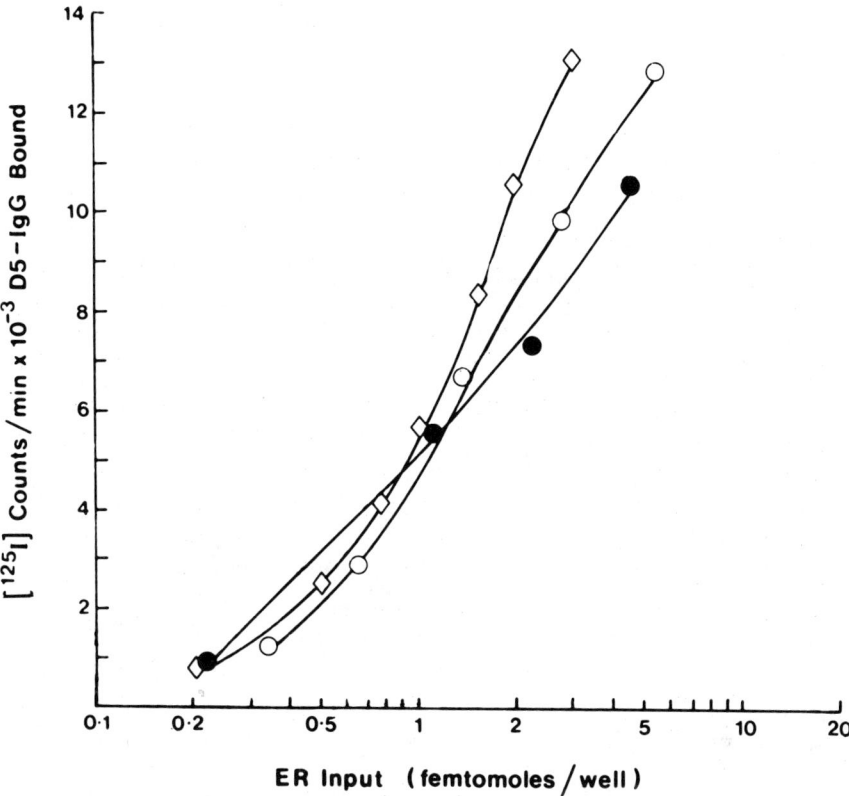

Figure 21.4. Dose response (ER and IRMA) for three breast tumor cytosols.

the latter reagent was chosen as the coating agent. Full details of the assay procedure are given elsewhere (Coffer et al. 1985b) but, in essence, it involves a 1-hour reaction at room temperature of cytosol with the BSA-coated wells, washing, a 2-hour incubation at room temperature with [^{125}I]D5, further washing, and counting. Good dose-response curves can be constructed with receptor concentrations in the clinically useful range (Fig. 21.4).

We have completed a pilot study in which breast tumor ER, measured with the routine, single concentration [^{3}H]estradiol $\pm$ diethylstilbestrol assay used in this institute, was compared with p29 quantitated by IRMA (Fig. 21.3). No example of an ER-negative tumor giving a significant IRMA response has yet been found, whereas a highly significant correlation between the two parameters was obtained. It is interesting that the younger women give lower values than the older women. Given the well-documented relationship of ER content and age (Braunsberg et al. 1974), we interpret the present observation as increasing the probability of a direct relationship between ER and p29.

The tissue specificity of the assay has been described above.

B. IMMUNOHISTOCHEMICAL STUDIES

1. General Experiments

A method for the localization of receptors to specific cell types within one tissue and to loci within one cell type has long been desired. Autoradiography has been useful for the localization of ^{3}H steroids but the long exposure times and potential artifacts have limited interpretation of these data (Stumpf and Sar 1976; Sheridan et al. 1979; Buell and Tremblay 1983). Immunohistochemical methods should circumvent these problems and indeed are doing so (King and Greene 1984; McClellan et al. 1984). We have found the indirect immunoperoxidase method useful at both a qualitative and semiquantitative level (King et al. 1985). Unfortunately, formalin fixation destroys most of the epitope, but ethanol or methacarn followed by routine wax embedding gives reproducibly positive results. All the data presented here were obtained after ethanol fixation, although now we use methacarn because it gives better tissue preservation and is easier to section than ethanol-fixed material.

Staining is specific in that omission of D5 or its replacement with monoclonal IgGs against progesterone or HLA-dr gave no color; monoclonal antibodies against human milk fat globule antigen gave a staining pattern different from that seen with D5. No staining was seen with human kidney (normal and neoplastic) ureter, parathyroid gland, skeletal (rectus) muscle, adenocarcinoma of the colon, DX3, SK23, and A32 SP human melanoma cell lines. Additional negative cells are listed in Table 21.3. Positive results were obtained with human ectocervical and vaginal squamous epithelia, skin epidermis, endocervical rest cells, but not with the glandular epithelium plus the positive cells listed in Table 21.3. In the fallopian tube, both the ciliated and secretory cells reacted, although stronger staining was seen with the ciliated cells. In all cases of positive reaction, the staining has been cytoplasmic. This agrees with the biochemical data indicating no reaction with putative nuclear antigen, and it reinforces the difference between D5 and the monoclonal antibodies described by Greene et al. (King and Greene 1984; DeSombre et al., Chapter 17 in this volume; Greene et al., Chapter 20 in this volume).

2. Human Breast Tumors

Of the positive tumors, about 85% showed relatively homogeneous staining (Fig. 21.5A), whereas the others showed marked heterogeneity of the two general types. Tumors could either be all positive with some cells exhibiting more intense staining (Fig. 21.5B), or the section could be predominantly negative intermingled with either single positive cells or clumps (Fig. 21.5C). The significance of this heterogeneity remains to be determined. In some cases, large areas of cells were all positive and adjacent large areas negative, which could be explained by clonal selection of negative cells. In other examples, the positive and negative cells were randomly intermingled. The clinical significance of these different staining patterns is unknown, although it may have prognostic significance. One could speculate that an ER-positive tumor with a heterogeneous staining pattern of the type shown in Figure 21.5B might respond better to combined endocrine and chemotherapy than to endocrine therapy alone. Likewise, the staining pattern of a tumor after relapse from a first round of hormone therapy might indicate whether a second round of hormone treatment or chemotherapy or a combination of both would be the most beneficial. Points such as this could not be answered by the biochemical assays, and they illustrate the clinical potential of the histochemical method.

Interesting as the heterogeneity is for biological reasons, it presents problems in quantitating the histochemical results and relating them to the biochemical assay of ER by conventional [^{3}H]estradiol-binding methods. In a pilot study we have compared the histochemical data with cytosol ER determined by the routine, single concentration [^{3}H]estradiol assay we use for clinical purposes (King et al. 1985). Quantitation of staining was attempted by assessing the proportion of tumor cells in a section (scale 0–6) and the proportion of those tumor cells that were positive, together with the staining intensity of those cells (scale 0–6). A simple multiple of these two results has been defined as the staining index. With this method we find a highly significant ($p < 0.001$) correlation between [^{3}H]E$_2$-ER and p29 staining with individual tumors. Interestingly, the one high-staining, ER-negative sample was ER-negative/PgR-positive. The data comparing ER with the staining index are shown in Figure 21.6. We have no explanation for the plateau in staining seen with the very high ER samples (> 200 fmol/mg protein). The ligand-binding assays were carried out on areas remote from those used for histochemistry. Given the heterogeneity of breast tumors, some discordance of results would be anticipated under

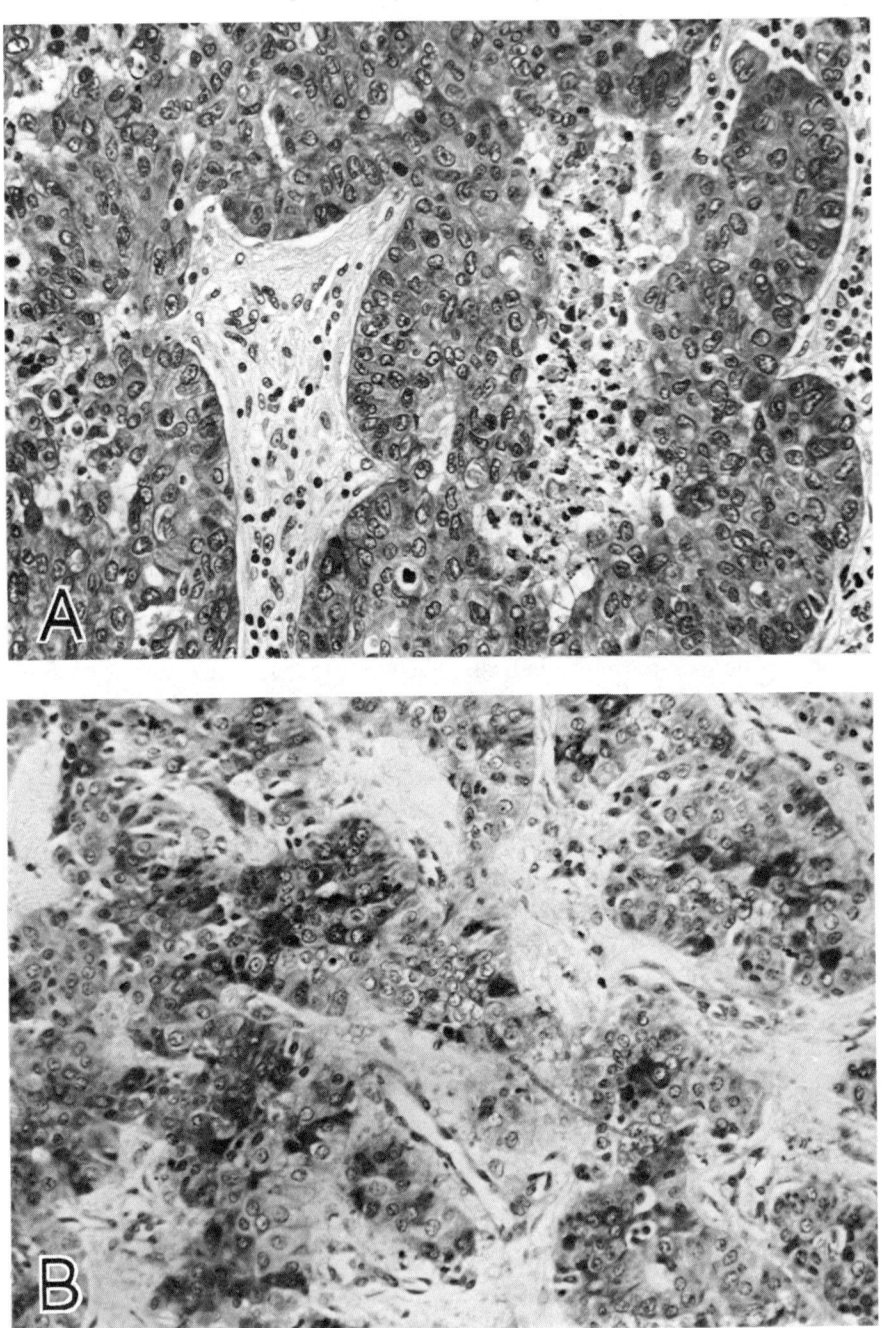

Figure 21.5. Histochemical localization of p29 in breast tumors (A–C) and normal breast epithelium (D). (A) Homogeneous pattern; (B) heterogeneous pattern in which all tumor cells are positive; (C) heterogeneous pattern in which some cells are negative; and (D)

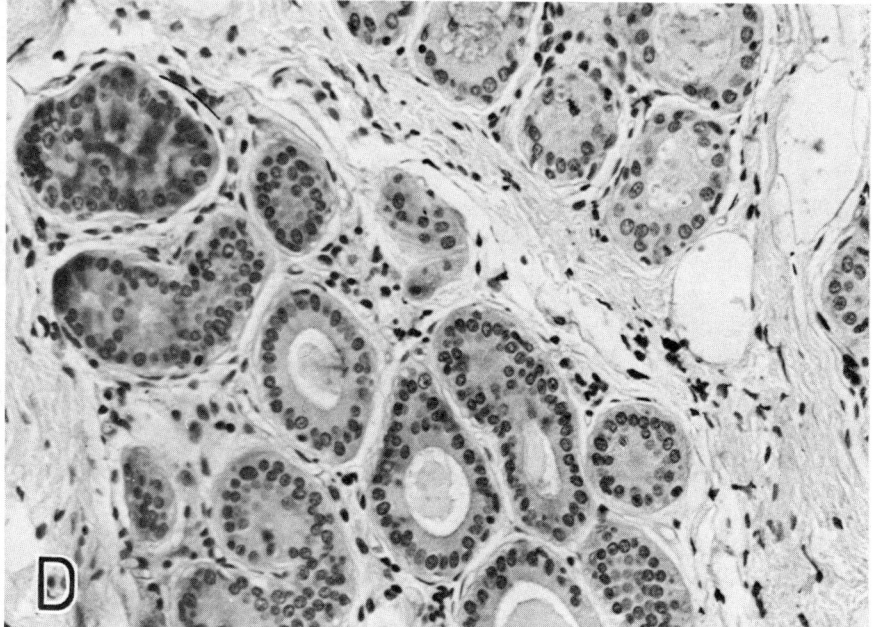

normal alveoli from an area of breast adjacent to a tumor. Some alveoli positive; others negative.

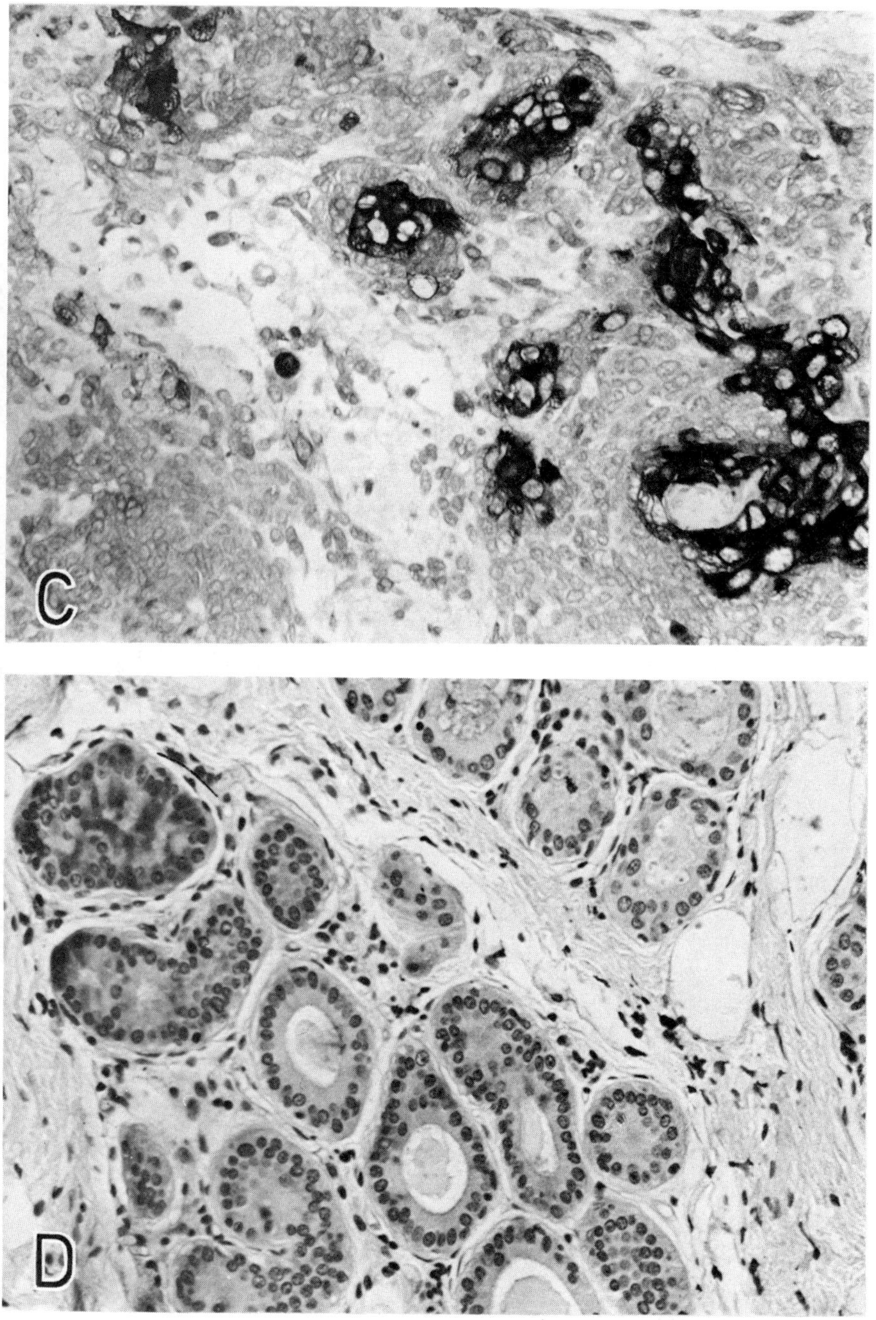

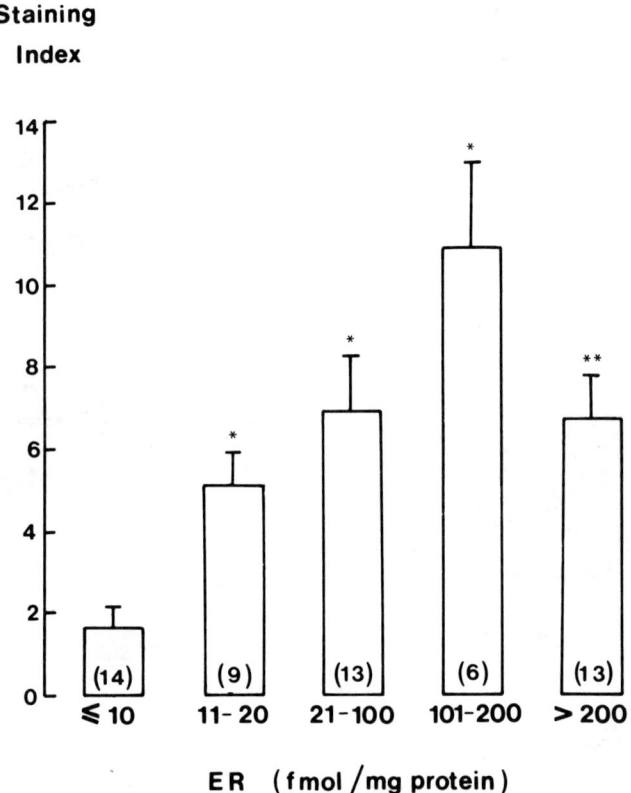

Figure 21.6. Comparison of histochemical staining index and ER content of breast tumors. Mean ± SEM. The number of samples is given in parentheses. Significantly different to ≤ 10 fmol/mg protein value: * $p < 0.01$; ** $p < 0.001$.

these conditions, and we currently feel that the results are encouraging but that some anomalies occur, in that occasional low-staining samples have high ER and vice versa (Table 21.4).

Normal mammary epithelium in areas adjacent to tumor rarely stains as strongly as the tumor cells but heterogeneity of staining occurs with alveoli in the same section showing either positive or negative reaction (Fig. 21.5D).

C. COMPARISON OF IRMA AND HISTOCHEMISTRY

Both assays measure an antigen that is related to ER and not PgR (Fig. 21.7). This indicates that p29 is not simply a product of estrogen action.

Table 21.4. Comparison of histochemical assay and IRMA of p29 in human breast tumors

	IRMA[a]		Histochemistry[a]	
ER status				
< 10 fmol/mg protein	0/11	(0)	2/14	(14)
10–19	2/6	(33)	6/8	(75)
≥ 20	31/32	(97)	28/33	(85)
Age				
< 50 years	5/16	(31)	3/10	(30)
≥ 50 years	25/28	(89)	33/45	(73)
Histology				
Lobular	4/4	(100)	5/5	(100)
Ductal				
Grade 2	13/15	(87)	13/15	(87)
Grade 3	7/13	(54)	8/18	(44)

[a]Number of tumors of high value versus total number; percentage in parentheses. High value defined as: IRMA > 3,000 dpm [^{125}I]D5 bound; histochemistry staining index > 3.

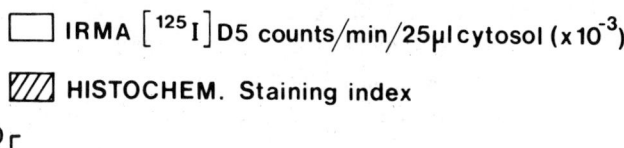

☐ IRMA [^{125}I] D5 counts/min/25 μl cytosol (x 10^{-3})

▨ HISTOCHEM. Staining index

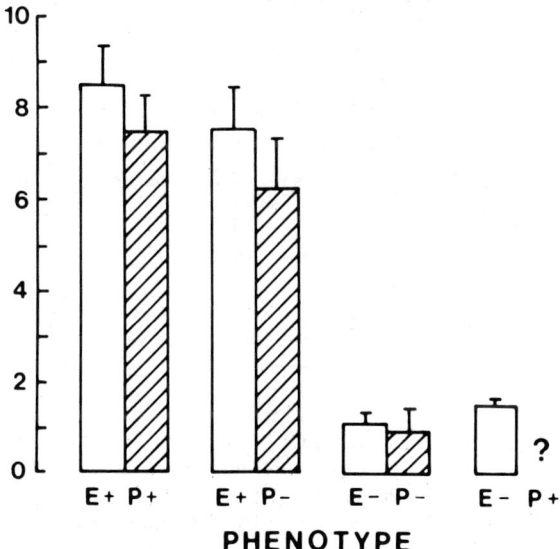

PHENOTYPE

+ { IRMA > 30 fmol/ml cytosol (2-3 mg P/ml)
{ HISTOCHEM. > 10 fmol/mgP

Figure 21.7. Relationship of IRMA and histochemical assays for p29 to ER and PgR phenotype of human breast tumors. (?) only two samples analyzed, one high, the other low.

Both assays indicate a qualitative and quantitative relationship to ER (Table 21.4), although the histochemical method produces occasional positive staining in ER-negative tumors. Whether this is due to errors in the biochemical or histochemical assay remains to be ascertained.

Both assays also point to the lower activity in tumors from young women (Table 21.4), an observation that has also been made for ER content.

V. Conclusions

The monoclonal antibodies we have produced do not behave in the anticipated manner. The 29 K antigen recognized by antibody D5 is clearly distinct from, but closely related to, ER. The nature of this relationship is under investigation, but both IRMA and histochemistry suggest that clinically useful information will be obtained with both types of assay. Furthermore, the histochemical assay may provide information as to the proportion of hormone-responsive and unresponsive cells in a tumor that cannot be obtained by the [^{3}H]estradiol-binding assay.

Acknowledgments

We thank the members of the Breast Unit, Guy's Hospital, and the Department of Obstetrics and Gynaecology, St. Thomas Hospital, for providing the clinical samples used in this work. Thanks are also due to Amersham International for their help in most of these studies and to Sarah Murdoch, who assayed the breast tumor receptors.

References

Baulieu, E.-E., N. Binart, T. Buchou, M. G. Catelli, T. Garcia, J.-M. Gasc, A. Groyer, I. Joab, B. Moncharmont, C. Radanyi, M. Renoir, P. Tuohimaa, and J. Mester. 1983. Biochemical and immunological studies of the chick oviduct cytosol progesterone receptor. In *Steroid hormone receptors: structure and function, Nobel symposium no. 57*, ed. J. Å. Gustafsson and H. Eriksson, 45–72. Amsterdam: Elsevier.

Birnbaumer, M., R. C. Bell, W. T. Schrader, and B. W. O'Malley. 1984. The putative molybdate-stabilized progesterone receptor subunit is not a steroid-binding protein. *Journal of Biological Chemistry* 259:1091–1098.

Braunsberg, H., V. H. T. James, C. W. Jamieson, S. Desai, A. E. Carter, and M. Hulbert. 1974. Effect of age and menopausal status on estimates of oestrogen binding by human malignant breast tumours. *British Medical Journal* 4:745–747.

Buell, R. H., and G. Tremblay. 1983. The localization of ³H-estradiol in estrogen receptor-positive human mammary carcinoma as visualized by thaw-mount autoradiography. *Cancer* 51:1625–1630.

Clark, J. H., and E. J. Peck, Jr. 1979. Cellular compartment and translocation of receptor steroid complex. In *Female sex steroids: receptors and function,* 37–45. *Monographs on endocrinology,* vol. 14. Berlin: Springer-Verlag.

Coffer, A. I., and R. J. B. King. 1981. Antibodies to estradiol receptor from human myometrium. *Journal of Steroid Biochemistry* 14:1229–1235.

Coffer, A. I., P. J. D. Milton, J. Pryse-Davies, and R. J. B. King. 1976. Purification of oestradiol receptor from human uterus by affinity chromatography. *Molecular and Cellular Endocrinology* 6:231–246.

Coffer, A. I., K. M. Lewis, A. J. Brockas, and R. J. B. King. 1985a. Monoclonal antibodies against a component related to soluble estrogen receptor. *Cancer Research* 45:3686–3693.

Coffer, A. I., G. H. Spiller, K. M. Lewis, and R. J. B. King. 1985b. Immunoradiometric studies with monoclonal antibody against a component related to human estrogen receptor. *Cancer Research* 45:3694–3698.

Edwards, D. P., N. L. Weigel, W. T. Schrader, and B. W. O'Malley, 1984. Structural analysis of chicken oviduct progesterone receptor using monoclonal antibodies to the subunit B protein. *Biochemistry* 23:4427–4435.

Gregory, M. R., and A. C. Notides. 1982. Characterization of two uterine proteases and their actions on the estrogen receptor. *Biochemistry* 21:6452–6457.

Horwitz, K. B., and W. L. McGuire. 1978. Antiestrogens: mechanism of action and effects in breast cancer. In *Breast cancer: advances in research and treatment.* Vol. 2: *Experimental biology,* ed. W. L. McGuire, 155–204. New York: Plenum Press.

Jakesz, R., A. Kasid, and M. E. Lippman. 1983. Continuous estrogen exposure in the rat does not induce loss of uterine estrogen receptor. *Journal of Biological Chemistry* 258:11798–11806.

Joab, I., C. Radanyi, M. Renoir, T. Buchou, M.-G. Catelli, N. Binart, J. Mester, and E.-E. Baulieu. 1984. Common non-hormone binding component in non-transformed chick oviduct receptors of four steroid hormones. *Nature* (London) 308:850–853.

King, R. J. B., and W. I. P. Mainwaring. 1974a. Properties: interaction with polycations. In *Steroid-cell interactions,* 206–207. London: Butterworths.

King, R. J. B., and W. I. P. Mainwaring. 1974b. Interrelationship of the different receptors. In *Steroid-cell interactions,* 212–214. London: Butterworths.

King, R. J. B., A. I. Coffer, J. Gilbert, K. Lewis, R. Nash, R. Millis, S. Raju, and R. W. Taylor. 1985. Histochemical studies with a monoclonal antibody raised against a partially purified soluble estradiol receptor preparation from human myometrium. *Cancer Research* 45:5728–5733.

King, W. J., and G. L. Greene. 1984. Monoclonal antibodies localize oestrogen receptor in the nuclei of target cells. *Nature* (London) 307:745–747.

Lee, S. H. 1984. Validity of a histochemical estrogen receptor assay. *Journal of Histochemistry and Cytochemistry* 32:305–310.

McCarty, K. S., D. S. Reintgen, H. F. Seigler, and K. S. McCarty. 1981. Cytochemistry of sex steroid receptors: a critique. *Breast Cancer Research and Treatment* 1:315–325.

McClellan, M. C., N. B. West, D. E. Tacha, G. L. Greene, and R. M. Brenner. 1984. Immunocytochemical localization of estrogen receptors in the macaque reproductive tract with monoclonal antiestrophilins. *Endocrinology* 114:2002–2014.

Notides, A. C., D. E. Hamilton, and H. E. Auer. 1975. A kinetic analysis of the estrogen receptor transformation. *Journal of Biological Chemistry* 250:3945–3950.

Pertschuk, L. P., E. H. Tobin, A. C. Carter, K. B. Eisenberg, V. C. Leo, E. Gaetjens, and
N. D. Bloom. 1982. Immunohistologic and histochemical methods for detection of
steroid binding in breast cancer: a reappraisal. *Breast Cancer Research and Treatment* 1:297–314.
Puca, G. A., E. Nola, A. M. Molinari, N. Medici, D. DeLucia, and V. Sica. 1983. Biochemistry and biology of estrogen receptor: identification of cytoskeletal binding
sites for receptor in a membrane model. In *Steroids and endometrial cancer. Progress in cancer research and therapy,* vol. 25, ed. V. M. Jasonni, I. Nenci, and C.
Flamigni, 1–10. New York: Raven Press.
Sheridan, P. J., J. M. Buchanan, and V. C. Anselmo. 1979. Equilibrium: the intracellular
distribution of steroid receptors. *Nature* (London) 282:579–582.
Sherman, M. R. 1984. Structure of mammalian steroid receptors: evolving concepts and
methodological developments. *Annual Review of Physiology* 46:83–105.
Stumpf, W. E., and M. Sar. 1976. Autoradiographic localization of estrogen, androgen,
progestin, and glucocorticosteroid in 'target tissues' and 'nontarget tissues'. In *Receptors and mechanism of action of steroid hormones, Part 1,* ed J. R. Pasqualini,
41–84. New York: Marcel Dekker.

22

Monoclonal Antibodies
Raised Against Chick Oviduct
Progesterone Receptor:
Cross Reaction with
Human Antigen

DEAN P. EDWARDS, NANCY L. WEIGEL,
WILLIAM T. SCHRADER, SARAH PELEG,
BERT W. O'MALLEY, AND W. L. MCGUIRE

I. INTRODUCTION 396
II. RESULTS 397
   A. PRODUCTION AND CHARACTERIZATION OF MONOCLONAL
      ANTIBODIES TO CHICK PROGESTERONE RECEPTOR B SUBUNIT 397
   B. COMPARISON OF RECEPTOR B PROTEIN AND NON-HORMONE-
      BINDING ANTIGENIC PROTEIN 402
   C. CROSS REACTION WITH ANTIGEN IN HUMAN BREAST CANCER 404
III. DISCUSSION 408
IV. CONCLUSION 411
   REFERENCES 412

I. Introduction

P ROGESTERONE receptor (PgR) is well known to be an important clinical marker of endocrine responsiveness and disease prognosis in breast cancer (Edwards et al. 1979; Bertuzzi et al. 1980; Osborne et al. 1980; Pichon et al. 1980; Saez et al. 1980; Clark et al. 1983) and is now measured routinely in breast cancer patients. PgR is a key regulatory protein in breast cancer cells, since it is known to be modulated by estrogens and antiestrogens (Horwitz et al. 1978) and is also the presumed mediator of the biological actions of progestins (Mockus and Horwitz 1983). The progesterone receptor, therefore, is important not only as a clinical marker but also from the standpoint of basic research as an important protein in our understanding of the fundamental molecular mechanisms of hormone action in breast cancer.

Because of its low abundance in the cell and instability after extraction from tissues, PgR has proven difficult to purify and fully characterize. Receptor studies have had to rely for the most part on the somewhat limited information obtained from radioligand measurement of hormone binding site activities in crude tissue extracts. Development of specific receptor antibodies capable of direct detection of the receptor protein independent of its hormone-binding activity (i.e., by interaction with receptor epitopes outside the hormone binding site) would be an important technological advancement for both clinical and biochemical studies of PgR.

Clinically, an immunological method of PgR detection would offer several advantages over current PgR assays, both for practical reasons (i.e., to eliminate the use of radioisotopes and sucrose density gradients) and because of the limited information obtained from biochemical radioligand assays. As an example, receptor antibodies will allow development of an immunohistochemical procedure for localization of PgR in individual cells not possible by biochemical assays and thus provide information on the cellular heterogeneity of PgR expression in a given tumor. Such data are likely to add to the power of PgR as a predictor of patient prognosis and response to endocrine therapies.

Receptor antibodies will also be important in basic molecular studies as probes to critically examine structural and functional properties of the receptor molecule not presently accessible by conventional hormone-binding methods of receptor analysis. With receptor antibodies, for example, it will be possible to purify receptor by antibody affinity chromatography and map structural and functional domains of the receptor molecule. Antibodies will also allow us to study receptor biosynthesis, isolate receptor mRNA, and ultimately clone the receptor gene and begin to study hormonal regulation of the receptor at the level of gene transcription.

Our approach in producing antibodies reactive with human breast cancer PgR was to immunize animals with highly purified preparations of the more readily available chick oviduct PgR and examine antibodies produced for their cross reaction with human receptor. We chose to produce monoclonal antibodies (MABs) by the method of Köhler and Milstein (1975) rather than produce heteroantisera. The monoclonal antibody technology has the advantage of providing an unlimited supply of antibody produced by hybridoma cells in culture and does not require homogeneous antigen for immunization, since monospecific antibodies can be cloned and selected in the screening procedure. We anticipated being able to isolate cross reactive MABs because of recent evidence of structural similarity between avian and human PgR. By photoaffinity labeling with the synthetic ligand, [³H]R5020, Lessey et al. (1983) found that PgR isolated from T47D human breast cancer cells was composed of two dissimilar hormone-binding polypeptides, analogous and similar in size to the A and B subunits of the avian PgR. Moreover, Renoir et al. (1982) produced polyclonal serum antibodies against purified chick oviduct PgR which showed cross reaction with PgR from human breast cancer, suggesting that there are at least some common determinants between avian and mammalian receptors.

This study describes an overview of our work producing MABs against chick oviduct PgR and an examination of cross reaction with antigen in human breast cancer. An unexpected finding of our study was the presence of what appears to be non-hormone-binding forms, or subunits of receptor, whose presence complicates both our concept of receptor structure and the problem of producing receptor antibodies.

II. *Results*

A. Production and Characterization of Monoclonal Antibodies to Chick Progesterone Receptor B Subunit

The chick PgR is composed of two dissimilar hormone-binding polypeptides, termed A and B, with molecular weights of 79,000 and

108,000, respectively. The receptor is believed to be a dimer composed of A and B subunits, each with different apparent functional properties, since the dissociated A protein binds preferentially to naked DNA, whereas the B protein binds to chromatin but only weakly to DNA (Schrader et al. 1981). In our studies, we used as immunogen only the 108,000 molecular weight receptor B protein. Receptor B protein was purified from hen oviducts as described by Weigel et al. (1981) and material used for immunization was approximately 50% pure as judged by photoaffinity labeling and SDS-gel electrophoresis. Animals used were male Lewis rats and cell fusions were performed with the nonsecreting NS-1 mouse myeloma. All of our hybridomas, therefore, are cross species, rat × mouse hybrids. Details of the fusion and hybridoma procedures are presented elsewhere and will not be given here (Edwards et al. 1984). Hybridomas were screened for antireceptor antibodies in two stages. The initial screening was by a solid phase immunoradiometric assay (IRMA) using a homogeneous preparation of the receptor B protein as the coating antigen bound to the wells of 96-well microtiter plates. Secondary screening was by Western blot analysis. For IRMAs, antigen-coated plates were blocked with a bovine serum albumin (BSA) solution and then incubated with hybridoma culture supernatant followed by plate washing and a secondary incubation with an [125I]-labeled second antibody (goat antirat IgG). Positives were taken as binding of secondary [125I]-labeled antibody, at least 10-fold above background. A two-dimensional gel analysis of the purified receptor B protein preparation used for screening IRMAs is shown in Figure 22.1. For this analysis, the purified receptor was first photoaffinity-labeled with [3H]R5020 (Birnbaumer et al. 1983b) and then resolved by isoelectric focusing in the first dimension followed by SDS-gel electrophoresis in the second dimension (O'Farrell 1975). The second dimension SDS gel was stained with Coomassie blue (Fig. 22.1, left panel) and then dried and fluorographed (right panel). A series of Coomassie-stained spots are visible at 108,000 molecular weight (left panel) and each stained spot contains R5020 binding sites (right panel), thus illustrating the apparent homogeneity of this receptor preparation. Because we had used homogeneous coating antigen, positive reactions by IRMA were considered likely to be MABs against receptor and were screened further by Western blot analysis to determine their monospecificity and define the antigen structure. Western blots were performed as described by Towbin et al. (1979). Preparations containing receptor were electrophoresed on 7.5% SDS-polyacrylamide gels (Laemmli 1970) and the resolved proteins electro-

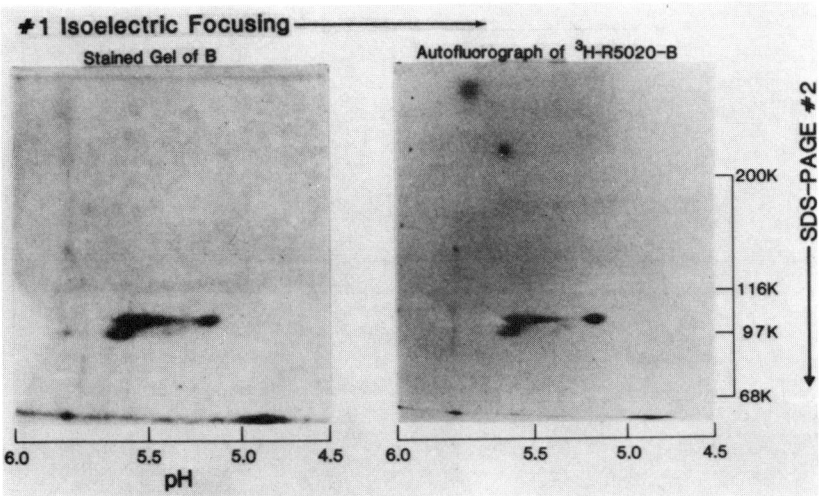

Figure 22.1. Two-dimensional gel analysis of receptor B protein of hen oviduct. The receptor B protein was purified as previously described (Weigel et al. 1981) and photoaffinity labeled with [³H]R5020. Left panel: 10 μg of purified B protein stained with Coomassie blue. Right panel: autofluorography of gel from left panel. (Reprinted with permission from Edwards et al. 1984. Copyright 1984, American Chemical Society.)

phoretically transferred to nitrocellulose filter paper. After unreacted sites were blocked with BSA, the nitrocellulose paper was incubated with MAB followed by a wash step and autoradiography to reveal immunoreactive bands. Figure 22.2 shows the reaction of two of these MABs (9G10 and 3E8) by Western blot using partially purified oviduct receptor B protein as the antigen (panel A = 9G10, panel B = 3E8). Both antibodies react with a 108,000 molecular weight band (right panels), which corresponds with the predominant 108 K protein visualized on Coomassie-stained gels (left panels). This 108,000 molecular weight band has been previously identified as the receptor B protein by photoaffinity labeling with [³H]R5020 (Birnbaumer et al. 1983b). Some smaller molecular weight bands were also reactive but these are degradation fragments of the receptor B protein, which increase with time in storage. Both MABs, therefore, appear to react with the same 108 K protein, but the sensitivity of 3E8 is approximately 20-fold less than that of 9G10. Western blots with homogeneous preparations of the receptor B protein (as judged by silver-stained SDS gels) also give immunoreactivity with a single 108,000 molecular weight protein band (Edwards et al. 1984).

To challenge the sensitivity and monospecificity of our antibodies, fur-

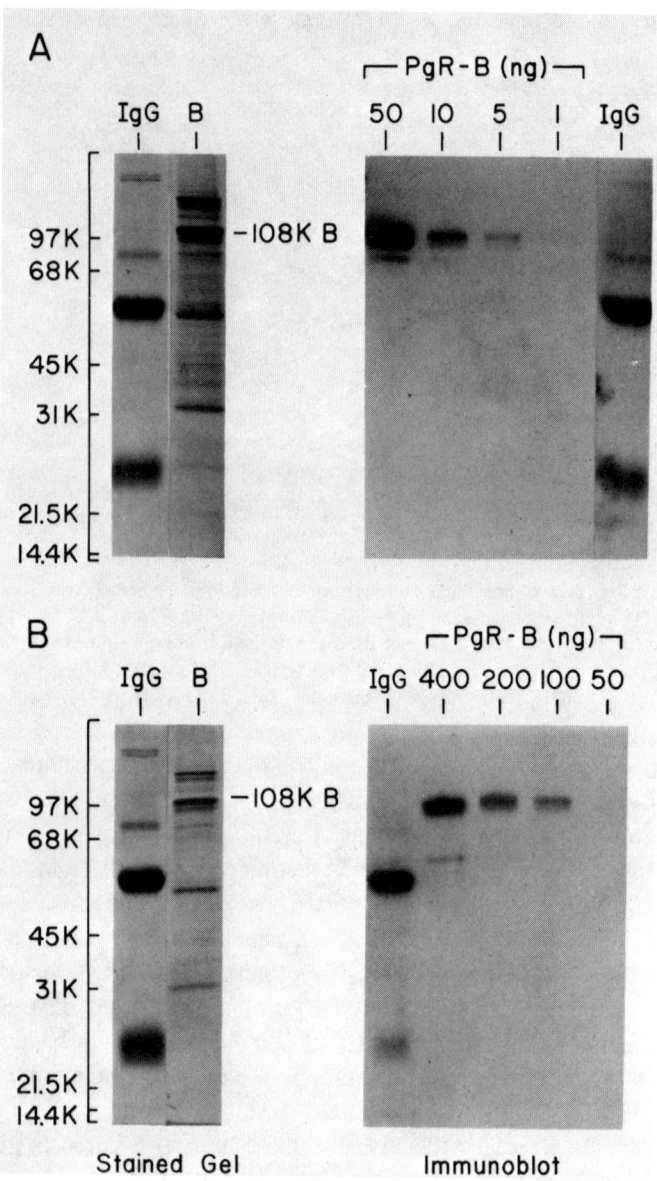

Figure 22.2. Western blot analysis of partially purified hen oviduct receptor B protein. Decreasing amounts of receptor B protein were electrophoresed on SDS-polyacrylamide gels, transferred electrophoretically to nitrocellulose sheets, and the nitrocellulose incubated with MAB followed by ^{125}I-labeled second antibody (rabbit antirat IgG). Coomassie-stained gels of receptor B protein and IgG molecular weight markers are shown in left panels; Western blot autoradiographs in right panels. (A) Reaction with antibody 9G10; (B) with antibody 3E8. (Reprinted with permission from Edwards et al. 1984. Copyright 1984, American Chemical Society.)

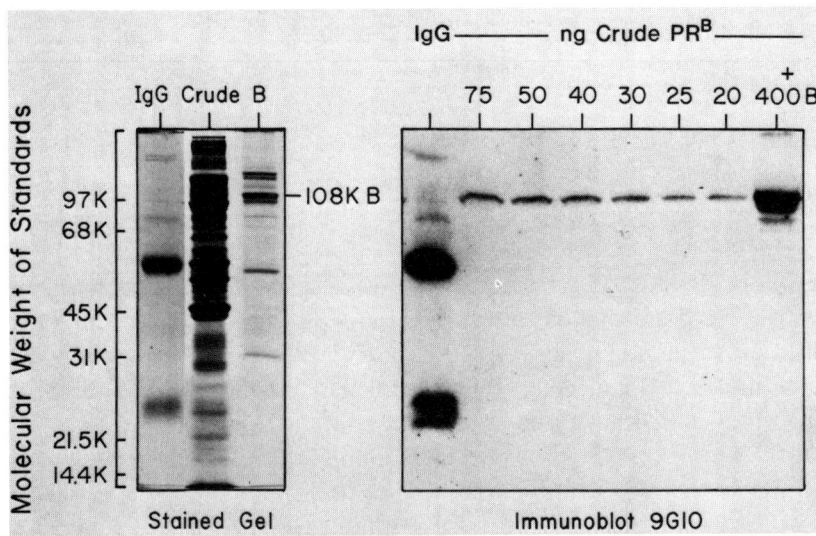

Figure 22.3. Western blot analysis of crude chick oviduct PgR with monoclonal 9G10. Chick oviduct cytosol was fractionated on DEAE to separate receptor A protein and was then immunoblotted as described in Figure 22.2. Coomassie-stained gels of the crude DEAE fraction, a partially purified receptor B protein (B), and IgG molecular weight markers are shown in left panel; right panel is the Western blot autoradiograph with decreasing amounts of the crude receptor B protein fraction. (Reprinted with permission from Edwards et al. 1984. Copyright 1984, American Chemical Society.)

ther Western blot analysis was performed using crude cytosol extracts from chick oviduct. Results with one of the antibodies, 9G10, are shown in Figure 22.3. To illustrate the complexity of proteins in this crude antigen mixture, a Coomassie-stained gel of the crude fraction and, for reference, a partially purified preparation of receptor B protein are also shown. This antibody on Western blot reacted in the various crude receptor preparations analyzed (containing decreasing amounts of antigen) with a single band corresponding with the Coomassie-stained 108 K receptor B protein in partially purified receptor preparations. No cross reaction of antibody was seen with contaminating bands. Three other MABs tested by Western blot similarly reacted with a single 108,000 molecular weight band in crude cytosol receptor preparations, although each with different levels of sensitivity (not shown).

On the basis of the above screening criteria, we have isolated four MABs reactive with the receptor B protein of chick oviduct. The identification code, antibody subtype, and parent myeloma for each antibody are

Table 22.1. Rat monoclonal antibodies produced against chick PgR B protein

Identification code	Antibody class	Subclass	Myeloma
9G10	IgG	2a	NS-1
3E8	IgG	2b	NS-1
413	IgG	?	NS-1
176	IgM	—	NS-1

given in Table 22.1. As a further test of their specificity, cross reactions with purified preparations of the receptor A protein have also been examined by Western blot analysis. None of the MABs, however, cross reacts with the 79,000 molecular weight receptor A protein. Thus by this test, the MABs produced appear to be specific for the receptor B protein.

B. COMPARISON OF RECEPTOR B PROTEIN AND NON-HORMONE-BINDING ANTIGENIC PROTEIN

Despite the apparent specificity of these antibodies for chick receptor B protein, some unexpected results were obtained, which we will summarize instead of presenting data. We have been unable to demonstrate antibody recognition of the native receptor-hormone complex, either by double antibody immunoabsorption techniques or by shifts of receptor on sucrose density gradients. In examining possibilities to explain this we first ruled out that antibodies might be directed toward the hormone binding site of receptor, in which case hormone could subsequently block antibody recognition of receptor. We next considered the possibility that epitopes for these MABs might be hidden in the native receptor such that antibody recognition would require unfolding or denaturation of the receptor molecule. This was suspected because MABs were screened with partially denatured antigen bound to plastic microtiter dishes. This turned out not to be the case, however, since we were unable to observe antibody recognition of receptor photoaffinity labeled with [^{3}H]R 5020 (which will retain its ligand even under denaturing conditions), under various denaturing conditions in solution which do allow immunoprecipitation of the 108,000 molecular weight antigenic protein. Finally, we found that the mass of antigenic material is in large excess over the mass of receptor determined from the number of hormone binding sites per cell. These unexpected findings are consistent with the existence of non-hormone-binding subunits or forms of receptor which are antigenically distinct (at least with these MABs) from hormone-binding receptor subunits. This is supported by the fact that antibodies detect on Western blots a protein (M_r = 108,000) which comigrates with the receptor B subunit. Furthermore, by resolution on two-dimensional electrophoresis, photoaffinity-labeled PgR and antigen appear also to migrate coincidently, yet antigenic protein does not bind hormone.

To begin to resolve the nature of the difference(s) between antigenic 108 K protein and receptor B protein, it was found that the two activities (i.e., immunological and hormone binding) could be separated by ion-exchange chromatographies and the separated proteins were examined by proteolytic enzyme digestion studies and peptide mapping. After separation of receptor A and B subunits on DNA-cellulose and partial purification of the hormone-binding receptor B protein, antigenic activity and hormone-binding activities can be separated by ion-exchange chromatography on DEAE-cellulose (Peleg et al. 1985). Coomassie-stained SDS gels of these separated activities and corresponding Western blot analysis using the 9G10 antibody are shown in Figure 22.4. The separated activities migrate together at 108,000 molecular weight and no detectable antigenic activity was found in the separated hormone-binding fraction. The reverse was also true; no hormone-binding activity was detected in the separated antigen fraction. These findings suggest that the two activities are associated with separate molecules.

To compare proteolytic peptide maps of these separated molecules, the hormone-binding receptor B protein was partially purified, separated from antigenic protein by ion-exchange chromatography, and resolved on SDS-polyacrylamide gels. The 108 K receptor B protein band (which now has no detectable antigenic material) was excised from the gel and digested with increasing amounts of *Staphylococcus aureus* V8 protease as described by Cleveland et al. (1977). Proteolytic peptides were examined by silver staining of SDS gels. The separated 108 K antigenic protein was processed and digested similarly with *Staphylococcus aureus* V8 protease. Results of the Cleveland proteolytic digestion study are shown in Figure 22.5. At all three levels of enzyme digestion, very similar peptide patterns were generated for both hormone-binding receptor B protein and the 108 K antigenic protein. The close similarity in proteolytic digestion patterns strongly suggests that the two activities are associated with either the same or closely related proteins. The precise nature of the difference(s) between antigen and hormone binding is not known as yet. Their similarity in pro-

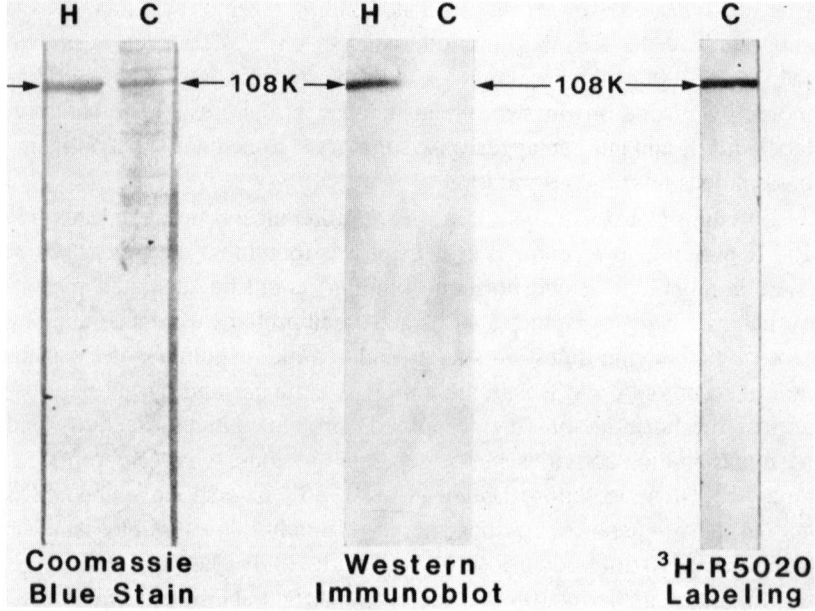

Figure 22.4. Western blot analysis of chick receptor B protein and hen antigenic protein after their partial purification and separation by DEAE chromatography. The [³H]R5020 receptor B complexes from chick oviduct and the 108 K antigenic protein were partially purified and separated as described by Peleg et al. (1985). Left lanes: Coomassie blue staining of the separated antigenic protein (lane 1) and receptor B protein (lane 2). Middle lanes: Western blot autoradiograph of antigenic protein (lane 3) and receptor B protein (lane 4) after reaction with the 9G10 antibody as described in Figure 22.2. Right lane (lane 5): fluorograph of receptor B protein of lane 2 after photoaffinity labeling with [³H]R5020. (From Peleg et al. 1985.)

teolytic peptide maps suggests that receptor and antigenic protein differ by some posttranslational chemical modification, which could account for their different biological activities.

C. Cross Reaction with Antigen in Human Breast Cancer

All four MABs raised against chick receptor B protein were examined for cross reaction with mammalian antigen by Western blot analysis. Results with the 9G10 antibody are shown in Figure 22.6. Cross reaction was observed with a single band in crude cytosol preparations of MCF-7 human breast cancer cells, rabbit uterus, and human uterus. In this particular experiment, the chick oviduct receptor B protein used for comparison

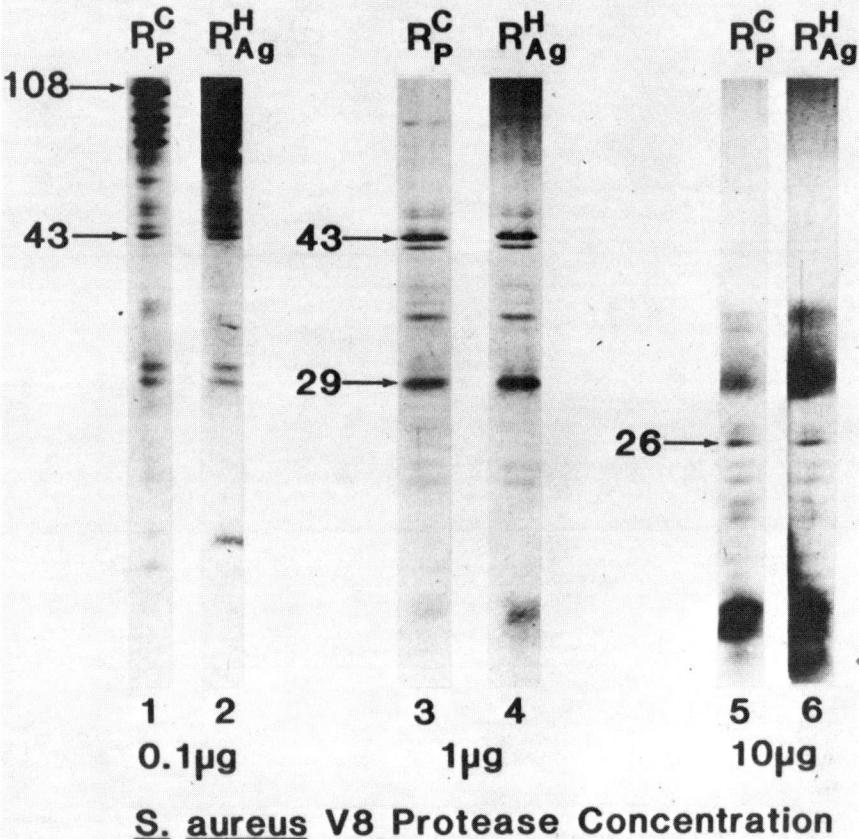

Figure 22.5. Comparison of chick receptor B protein with antigenic protein by Cleveland partial proteolytic peptide mapping. Antigenic protein (R^HAg—even-numbered lanes) and chick receptor B protein (R^cp—odd-numbered lanes) were isolated as single bands on SDS-polyacrylamide gels after their separation and partial purification by DEAE chromatography. Isolated gel bands were digested with the different concentrations of *Staphylococcus aureus* V8 protease indicated and the resulting proteolytic peptides were detected by silver staining as described by Cleveland et al. (1977). (From Peleg et al. 1985.)

was partially degraded, which accounts for the lower molecular bands observed. We have also observed cross reactions with a 108,000 molecular weight antigen in mouse and rat uterus (not shown), so it appears that 9G10 cross reacts with a wide variety of mammalian species. By Western blot, cross reaction with a 108 K antigenic protein in MCF-7 cytosol was also observed for two other MABs, 413 and 3E8 (Fig. 22.7). The fourth antibody, 176, does not, however, detect 108 K antigenic protein but

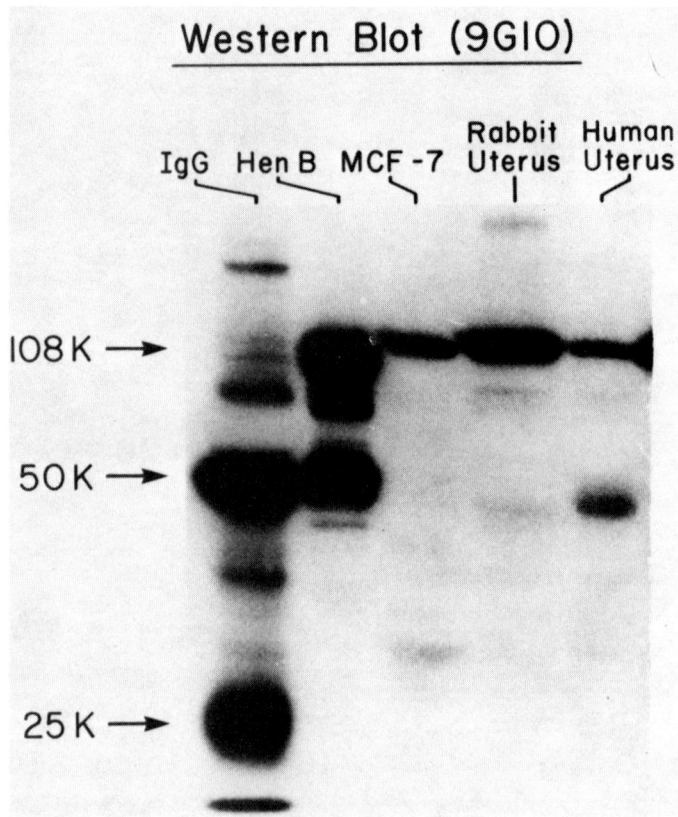

Figure 22.6. Cross reaction of MAB 9G10 with mammalian antigen. Western blot assays as described in Figure 22.2 were performed with crude cytosols of MCF-7 human breast cancer cells, human uterus, and rabbit uterus. Partially purified receptor B protein from chick oviduct (lane 2) was used as a control for comparison and [125I]IgG as a molecular weight standard (lane 1).

reacts weakly in MCF-7 with a band of higher molecular weight. We do not know as yet whether lack of 176 MAB reactivity with the 108 K antigenic protein in MCF-7 is a problem of antibody sensitivity in crude samples or if the reaction observed with higher molecular weight antigen is specific.

As was observed in chick oviduct studies, MABs do not recognize native receptor-hormone complexes in human breast cancer, nor do they interact with photoaffinity-labeled PgR under various conditions of protein denaturation. As with chick antigen, the mass of 108 K antigenic protein

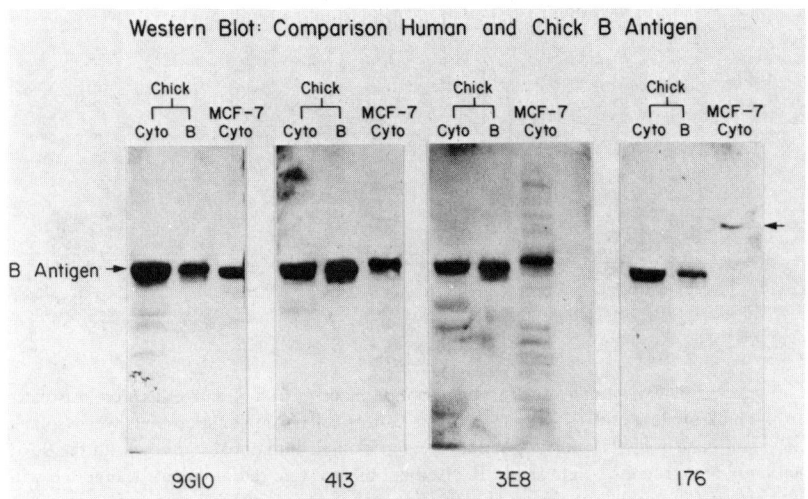

Figure 22.7. Western blot comparison of MAB reactivities with chick and human antigen. Each panel represents Western blot autoradiographs using different MABs (9G10, 413, 3E8, and 176) with crude cytosols of chick oviduct and human MCF-7 cells (cyto) and a partially purified chick receptor B protein (B).

in human breast cancer is in excess of receptor-hormone binding sites per cell.

Since it is known that PgR levels in MCF-7 (Horwitz et al. 1978) are regulated by estrogen, hormone induction of antigenic protein in MCF-7 was examined by semiquantitative Western blot assay. We found the 108 K antigen concentrations in the cell could be stimulated by estradiol but the magnitude of the response varied considerably. Basal levels of antigen were found to vary considerably in estrogen-withdrawn cells, which accounts for the variable inductions observed. This has been a problem as well in this cell line with other known estrogenic responses.

To further characterize human antigen, the 108 K antigenic protein from T47D human breast cancer cells was isolated by immunoaffinity chromatography using MAB 9G10 and protein-A-Sepharose followed by SDS electrophoresis in polyacrylamide. The antigen from chick oviduct cytosols was similarly purified and both purified protein bands were excised from polyacrylamide gels and subjected to proteolytic digestion for comparison of their peptide maps. Digestion with *Staphylococcus aureus* V8 protease by the method of Cleveland (1977), as well as tryptic digestion of iodinated gel bands and analysis by two-dimensional thin-layer electrophoresis (Birnbaumer et al. 1983a), produced similar proteolytic

Tryptic Peptide Maps

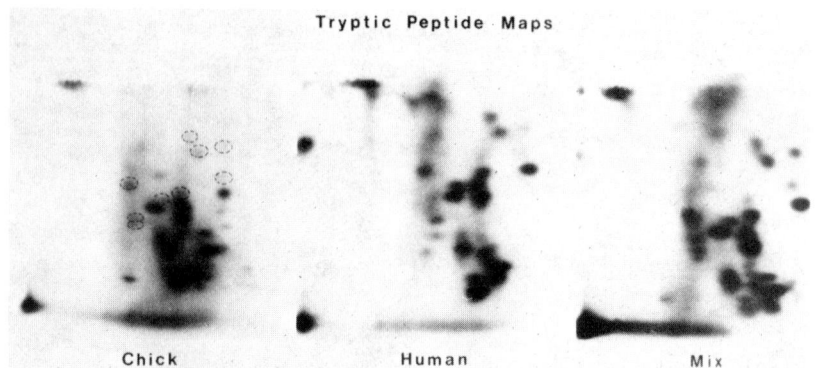

Chick   Human   Mix

Figure 22.8. Two-dimensional tryptic peptide maps of 108 K antigenic protein isolated from chick oviduct and T47D human breast cancer cells. Antigenic proteins were isolated as single bands on SDS-polyacrylamide gels after their immunoabsorption with the 9G10 antibody and protein-A-Sepharose. Excised gel pieces were radio-iodinated, digested with trypsin, and the proteolytic peptide products were resolved in the first dimension by thin-layer electrophoresis followed by thin-layer chromatography in the second dimension (Birnbaumer et al. 1983a). Left panel, chick antigen; middle panel, human antigen; right panel, mix—human plus chick antigen.

peptide patterns for human and chick antigen (Fig. 22.8). Thus, the 108 K antigen in chick and human breast cancer appears to be the same protein and highly conserved.

III. Discussion

The purified chick receptor B protein used as an immunogen and for screening of MABs was assumed to be homogeneous based on two-dimensional gel analysis, which gave superimposable spots of stained protein and [³H]R5020 affinity-labeled binding sites (Fig. 22.1). The present antibody work, however, clearly shows microheterogeneity in this purified receptor preparation and indicates that it contains a mixture of hormone-binding polypeptides and what we define here as 108 K antigenic protein or B antigen. Since we screened for MABs by an IRMA procedure, using this purified material as coating antigen, it appears we have isolated MABs reactive only with the B antigen in this mixture.

The relationship between B antigen and receptor hormone–binding polypeptides is not yet known. In the chick oviduct, the two proteins do share striking structural similarities. They are of the same size and charge by SDS electrophoresis and isoelectric focusing in polyacrylamide, they give similar Cleveland partial proteolytic digestion patterns and tryptic peptide maps. The two molecular entities differ, however, in that B antigen and hormone-binding polypeptides can be resolved on ion-exchange chromatography (which is due largely to an aggregation phenomenon rather than to true charge differences), antigenic sites are in excess of the number of hormone binding sites in the cell, and the B antigen cannot bind hormone *in vitro*.

The structural similarities suggest two possible relationships between B antigen and hormone-binding polypeptide. First, B antigen may be a non-hormone-binding form of the receptor that differs from the hormone-binding polypeptide, not in amino acid sequence but by some posttranslational chemical modification. Posttranslational modification could account for differences in hormone-binding activity as well as in antigenic determinants. A newly synthesized, immature receptor protein (inactive or non-hormone-binding) could be interconvertible to a mature hormone-binding receptor as a result of specific posttranslational events. Phosphorylation would seem a likely possibility, since phosphorylation-dephosphorylation has been shown to be involved *in vitro*, in the interconversion of inactive (non-hormone-binding) to active (hormone-binding) forms of mouse uterus estrogen receptor (Auricchio et al. 1982) as well as glucocorticoid receptors of rat liver (Hausley et al. 1982). Moreover, the purified progesterone receptor B protein used in these studies has previously been shown to be phosphorylated *in vitro* with cyclic AMP-dependent protein kinase (Weigel et al. 1981).

Antibody detection of putative non-hormone-binding forms of steroid receptors has been reported in at least two other systems. Westphal et al. (1984), using MABs to glucocorticoid receptor, reported detection of inactive or non-hormone-binding glucocorticoid receptors in S49.1 lymphoma cells. In variant r− cells (lacking in glucocorticoid receptor binding sites) these same receptor MABs also detect antigenic protein, which on Western blot is indistinguishable from biologically active glucocorticoid receptor of wild-type cells. Thus, r− cells are not lacking in expression of receptor protein but appear rather to contain defective, biologically inactive receptor (which is likely to be the result of conservative changes in receptor structure). In studies related to our own, MABs have now been produced independently against highly purified preparations of chick oviduct progesterone receptor A subunit. Analogous with receptor B protein studies, these MABs also detect protein that is distinct from the hormone-binding A subunit species but shares structural properties with hormone-binding polypeptides (McHale et al. 1984; O'Connor et al. 1984). Thus, non-hormone-binding forms of progesterone receptor may exist for both receptor subunits in the chick oviduct. Whether existence of non-hormone-binding forms of receptors is a phenomenon common to all steroid hormone receptors remains to be seen. Other MABs produced against steroid receptors (estrogen, glucocorticoid, and progesterone receptors) do not detect excess antigenic protein unable to bind hormone. Antibodies in these other studies, however, were screened for their reactivity against hormone-binding activity. The screening, therefore, may have excluded antibodies produced against receptor protein unable to bind hormone (Greene et al. 1980; Logeat et al. 1983; Okret et al. 1984).

There is a second possibility to explain the relationship between B antigen and hormone-binding polypeptide. The two activities may be associated with different proteins, which are products of two separate but closely related genes. If this is true, then an important question that must be considered is whether the B antigen could be a non-hormone-binding subunit of a larger molecular complex (with as yet unknown functions important for the biological action of receptor), or whether antigen is only similar in structure to receptor B protein but has no molecular association or functional relationship with receptor.

In an analogous system, the acetylcholine receptor is known to be a molecular complex (pentamer) composed of four different kinds of subunits, only one of which binds ligand. The other subunits have separate functional properties. Each subunit is synthesized separately by separate genes, but all have extensive homologous amino acid sequences, suggesting that each subunit arose through duplications of a single ancestral gene (Lindstrom 1984). Whether steroid receptor molecules are composed of similar subunit arrangements is not known as yet. There are suggestive data consistent with this concept of receptor structure. Joab et al. (1984), for example, produced a MAB to a 90 kilodalton component of highly purified progesterone receptor from chick oviduct. This 90 K protein is unable to bind hormone but appears to be associated with the 8S receptor molecule, and not with 4S monomers. Similarly, R. J. B. King (King and Coffer, Chapter 21 in this volume) produced a MAB to a non-hormone-binding polypeptide in target tissues which appears to be associated with the activated estrogen receptor. Unlike our studies, these receptor-associated proteins differ in molecular weight from the receptor hormone-binding polypeptides.

To ultimately resolve the issue of the relationship between B antigen and receptor B protein will require isolation and purification of the proteins associated with each activity and comparison of their complete amino acid sequences. As a first step towards this goal, the cDNA coding for the chick B antigen has been cloned in bacteria and partial base sequence has been obtained (Zarucki-Schultz et al. 1984).

Of the four MABs produced against chick progesterone receptor, three appear to cross react with antigen in mammalian tissues, including human breast cancer. Based on its size on SDS electrophoresis and proteolytic peptide mapping studies, the antigen in human and chick tissues appears to be the same protein. As with studies in the chicken, the human antigenic protein is also unable to bind hormone *in vitro*. Because of difficulties in isolation and purification of the receptor hormone-binding polypeptide from human tissues, we have not as yet been able to determine whether the structural and sequence similarities observed between chick antigen and hormone-binding polypeptide will also hold for human antigen and receptor.

Whether the B antigen in human breast cancer is clinically relevant is yet to be determined. We are currently evaluating, by immunohistochemistry, whether the 108 K antigenic protein in human breast tumors is associated with the progesterone receptor detected by conventional radioligand assay. If the B antigen were to represent a non-hormone-binding form or subunit of the receptor molecule, it could well be an important clinical marker of endocrine responsiveness in breast cancer.

IV. *Conclusion*

Our immunological studies with MABs produced against highly purified chick oviduct progesterone receptor may lead to important new information with regard to receptor structure and function. Detection of antigenic protein structurally similar to receptor but unable to bind hormone is consistent with the existence of either non-hormone-binding forms of receptor, non-hormone-binding subunits of a larger molecular complex, or a closely related protein of unknown function. Further studies will be required to determine which of these possibilities is correct.

Acknowledgments

This work was supported by American Cancer Society Grant BC-391A and Public Health Service Grant HD-7857.

References

Auricchio, F., A. Migliaccio, G. Castoria, S. Lastoria, and A. Rotondi. 1982. Evidence that *in vivo* estradiol receptor translocated into nuclei is dephosphorylated and released into cytoplasm. *Biochemical and Biophysical Research Communications* 106:149–157.

Bertuzzi, A., P. Vezzoni, and E. Ronchi. 1980. Prognostic importance of progesterone receptors alone or in combination with estrogen receptors in node-negative breast carcinoma. *Proceedings of the American Association for Cancer Research and the American Society for Clinical Oncology* 22:447.

Birnbaumer, M., W. T. Schrader, and B. W. O'Malley. 1983a. Assessment of structural similarities in chick oviduct progesterone receptor subunits by partial proteolysis of photoaffinity-labeled proteins. *Journal of Biological Chemistry* 258:7331–7337.

Birnbaumer, M., W. T. Schrader, and B. W. O'Malley. 1983b. Photoaffinity labeling of the chick progesterone receptor proteins. *Journal of Biological Chemistry* 255:1637–1644.

Clark, G. M., W. L. McGuire, C. A. Hubay, O. H. Pearson, and J. S. Marshall. 1983. Progesterone receptors as a prognostic factor in Stage II breast cancer. *New England Journal of Medicine* 309:1343–1347.

Cleveland, D. W., S. G. Fischer, M. W. Kirschner, and U. K. Laemmli. 1977. Peptide mapping by limited proteolysis in dodecyl sulfate and analysis by gel electrophoresis. *Journal of Biological Chemistry* 252:1102–1106.

Edwards, D. P., G. C. Chamness, and W. L. McGuire. 1979. Estrogen and progesterone receptor proteins in breast cancer. *Biochimica et Biophysica Acta* 560:457–486.

Edwards, D. P., N. L. Weigel, W. T. Schrader, B. W. O'Malley, and W. L. McGuire. 1984. Structural analysis of chicken oviduct progesterase receptor using monoclonal antibodies to the subunit B protein. *Biochemistry* 23:4427–4435.

Greene, G. L., C. Nolan, J. P. Engler, and E. V. Jensen. 1980. Monoclonal antibodies to human estrogen receptor. *Proceedings of the National Academy of Sciences* 77:5115–5119.

Horwitz, K. B., and W. L. McGuire. 1978. Estrogen control of progesterone receptor in human breast cancer. *Journal of Biological Chemistry* 253:2223–2228.

Horwitz, K. B., Y. Koseki, and W. L. McGuire. 1978. Estrogen control of progesterone receptor in human breast cancer: role of estradiol and antiestrogen. *Endocrinology* 103:1742–1751.

Housley, P. R., M. K. Dahmer, and W. B. Pratt. 1982. Inactivation of glucocorticoid binding capacity by protein phosphatases in the presence of molybdate and complete reactivation by dithiothreitol. *Journal of Biological Chemistry* 257:8615–8618.

Joab, I., C. Radanyi, M. Renoir, T. Buchou, M.-G. Catelli, N. Binart, J. Mester, and E.-E. Baulieu. 1984. Common non-hormone binding component in non-transformed chick oviduct receptors of four steroid hormones. *Nature* (London) 308:850–853.

Köhler, G., and C. Milstein. 1975. Continuous cultures of fused cells secreting antibody of predefined specificity. *Nature* (London) 256:495–497.

Laemmli, U. K. 1970. Cleavage of structural proteins during the assembly of the head bacteriophage T4. *Nature* (London) 227:680–685.

Lessey, B. A., P. S. Alexander, and K. B. Horwitz. 1983. The subunit structure of human breast cancer progesterone receptors characterized by chromatography and photo-affinity labeling. *Endocrinology* 112:1267–1274.

Lindstrom, J. 1984. Nicotinic acetylcholine receptors: use of monoclonal antibodies to study synthesis, structure, function, and autoimmune response. In *Monoclonal and anti-idiotypic antibodies: probes for receptor structure and function,* ed. J. C. Venter and L. C. Harrison, 21–57. New York: Alan R. Liss.

Logeat, F., M. T. VuHai, A. Fournier, P. Legrain, G. Buttin, E. Milgrom. 1983. Monoclonal antibodies to rabbit progesterone receptor: cross reaction with mammalian progesterone receptors. *Proceedings of the National Academy of Sciences* 80:6456–6459.

McHale, A. P., W. T. Schrader, and B. W. O'Malley. 1984. Monoclonal antibodies to chick progesterone receptor subunit. *Proceedings of the Seventh International Congress of Endocrinology,* Quebec. Abstract 1598.

Mockus, M. B., and K. B. Horwitz. 1983. Progesterone receptors in human breast cancer. *Journal of Biological Chemistry* 258:4778–4783.

O'Connor, L., A. P. McHale, W. T. Schrader, and B. W. O'Malley. 1984. Isolation of isoforms of the A-subunit of the progesterone receptor. *Proceedings of the Seventh International Congress of Endocrinology,* Quebec. Abstract 1875.

O'Farrell, P. H. 1975. High resolution two-dimensional electrophoresis of proteins. *Journal of Biological Chemistry* 250:4007–4021.

Okret, S., A.-C. Wikstrom, O. Wrange, B. Andersson, and J.-A. Gustafsson. 1984. Monoclonal antibodies against rat liver glucocorticoid receptor. *Proceedings of the National Academy of Sciences* 81:1609–1613.

Osborne, C. K., M. G. Yochmowitz, W. A. Knight, and W. L. McGuire. 1980. The value of estrogen and progesterone receptors in the treatment of breast cancer. *Cancer Research* 46:2884–2888.

Peleg, S., W. T. Schrader, D. P. Edwards, W. L. McGuire, and B. W. O'Malley. 1985. Immunologic detection of a protein homologous to chicken progesterone receptor B-subunit. *Journal of Biological Chemistry* 260:8492–8501.

Pichon, M. F., C. Pallud, M. Brunet, and E. Milgrom. 1980. Relationship of presence of progesterone receptors to prognosis in early breast cancer. *Cancer Research* 40:3357–3359.

Renoir, J. M., C. Radanyi, C.-R. Yang, and E.-E. Baulieu. 1982. Antibodies against progesterone receptor from chick oviduct. *European Journal of Biochemistry* 127:81–86.

Saez, S., C. Chouvet, M. Mayer, and F. Cheix. 1980. Estradiol and progesterone receptor as prognostic factors in human primary breast cancer. *Proceedings of the American Association for Cancer Research and the American Society of Clinical Oncology* 21:139.

Schrader, W. T., M. E. Birnbaumer, M. R. Hughes, N. L. Weigel, W. W. Grady, and B. W. O'Malley. 1981. Studies on the structure and function of chicken progesterone receptor. *Recent Progress in Hormone Research* 37:583–633.

Towbin, H., T. Staehelin, and J. Garclam. 1979. Electrophoretic transfer of proteins from polyacrylamide gels to nitrocellulose sheets. *Proceedings of the National Academy of Sciences* 76:4350–4354.

Weigel, N. L., J. S. Tash, A. R. Means, W. T. Schrader, and B. W. O'Malley. 1981. Phosphorylation of hen progesterone receptors by cAMP dependent protein kinase. *Biochemical and Biophysical Research Communications* 102:513–519.

Westphal, H. M., K. Mugele, M. Beato, and U. Gehring. 1984. Immunochemical localization of wild type and variant glucocorticoid receptors by monoclonal antibodies.
EMBO Journal 3:1493–1498.

Zarucki-Schulz, T., M. S. Kulomaa, D. R. Headon, N. L. Weigel, M. Baez, D. P. Edwards, W. L. McGuire, W. T. Schrader, and B. W. O'Malley. 1984. Molecular cloning of a cDNA for the chick progesterone receptor B antigen. *Proceedings of the
National Academy of Sciences* 81:6358–6362.

VII

Advanced and
Adjuvant Breast
Cancer Therapy

23

Endocrine Treatment of Advanced Breast Cancer

Baha'Uddin M. Arafah
and Olof H. Pearson

I. Introduction   418
II. Hormone-Ablative Therapy   419
III. Hormone-Additive Therapy   420
IV. Antiestrogen Therapy   421
V. Sequential Endocrine Treatment   423
VI. Discussion   425
References   427

417

I. Introduction

Hormone dependency of some human breast cancer has been known for many years. The first established usefulness of hormone manipulation in the management of advanced breast cancer was reported by Beatson in 1896. In that report, Beatson observed a remission in a premenopausal woman with advanced breast carcinoma following surgical oophorectomy. At the present time, oophorectomy continues to be the main therapeutic modality in premenopausal women with advanced, hormone-responsive breast cancer. Since the pioneering observation of Beatson, hormonal manipulation has been one of the main forms of treatment for advanced breast cancer, and it is well recognized that in an unselected series of patients with advanced breast cancer, objective tumor regression can be induced in 35–40% of patients with endocrine treatments. A number of different modalities of hormone manipulation have been used over the years, including hormone ablation (oophorectomy, hypophysectomy, adrenalectomy), or hormone addition in pharmacological doses (estrogens, progestins, androgens, glucocorticoids), and more recently antihormone therapy such as antiestrogen (tamoxifen). Over the past decade, two major advances have occurred that have had a great impact on the endocrine management of human breast cancer. The first was the discovery of the presence of hormone receptors in some human breast cancer cells (Jensen et al. 1971). Estrogen (ER) and progesterone (PgR) are the two main hormone receptors measured in primary human breast tumors. Their measurement in the cancer tissue has improved our ability to identify and select patients likely to benefit from endocrine therapy. Thus, in patients with ER-positive tumors, a response to hormonal manipulation is seen in 50–65% of the patients; the presence of both hormone receptors (ER and PgR) in tumors will further improve the chance for response to endocrine therapy to roughly 75%. In contrast, responses to hormonal therapies are only rarely seen in patients with ER-negative tumors and thus chemotherapy is the initial treatment of choice for these patients. The introduction of specific antiestrogen in the treatment of these patients provided another major advance in this field.

In this chapter, we review the use of hormone therapy in women with advanced breast cancer, with a major emphasis on the role of antiestrogens in the management of this disease. We also present data on the long-term follow up of 113 patients treated with the antiestrogen tamoxifen, who received sequential forms of endocrine treatments or cytotoxic chemotherapy.

II. *Hormone-Ablative Therapy*

Following the experience of Beatson, oophorectomy continued to be the major hormone-ablative procedure in the treatment of premenopausal women with breast cancer, the rationale for this therapeutic procedure being to eliminate the major source of estrogen in premenopausal women with breast cancer (Pearson et al. 1953).

After cortisone became available, adrenalectomy and hypophysectomy were introduced as effective ablative procedures in the treatment of breast cancer in women. The importance of the adrenal glands as the major source of estrogens in castrated or postmenopausal women was the reason for using adrenalectomy in these patients. Following surgical adrenalectomy, objective remission can be seen in 30–40% of unselected patients. Because of the significant morbidity associated with this surgical procedure, which would limit its use to selected patients, medical alternatives were developed (Santen et al. 1978). The use of enzyme inhibitors of estrogen secretion was one such medical alternative. Aminoglutethimide, an inhibitor of adrenal steroidogenesis as well as an aromatase inhibitor (Santen et al. 1978), is the only such drug available for clinical use in the United States. Medical adrenalectomy in the form of aminoglutethimide-hydrocortisone combination therapy has proven to be an effective treatment for women with advanced breast cancer and its success is comparable to that of surgical adrenalectomy (Santen et al. 1981).

Hypophysectomy for the treatment of advanced breast cancer was introduced in the early 1950s (Pearson and Ray 1960), and with the refinement in the techniques of hypophysectomy, the mortality and morbidity associated with this procedure decreased significantly (Pearson et al. 1978). Objective remissions are seen in 40% of unselected patients following hypophysectomy. It was postulated that hypophysectomy would eliminate the pituitary hormones or delete a "pituitary factor" which might be involved in the growth of human breast cancer. This hypothesis was primarily based on clinical observations that patients commonly respond to surgical hypophysectomy following antiestrogen therapy (Manni et al.

1979, 1981). Fifty-seven percent of patients who initially responded to tamoxifen, and subsequently relapsed, had an objective remission following hypophysectomy (Manni et al. 1981). Furthermore, 27% of patients who had initially failed tamoxifen therapy obtained an objective remission to subsequent hypophysectomy (Manni et al. 1981). The responses to hypophysectomy in these patients suggested that a "pituitary factor" in addition to estrogen is probably involved in the growth of some human breast cancer. However, recent studies obtained on patients treated with aminoglutethimide-hydrocortisone sequentially after tamoxifen challenged this hypothesis (Murray and Pitt 1981; Santen et al. 1982). The response rate to the medical adrenalectomy regimen following tamoxifen is almost identical to that seen with hypophysectomy (Murray and Pitt 1981; Santen et al. 1982). The response seen after surgical hypophysectomy may be secondary to the decrease in estrogen levels rather than the elimination of the "pituitary factor." With the removal of the pituitary gland, the production of the adrenal androgens will diminish and subsequently, because of the decreased substrate for aromatization, estrogen production will decrease. Thus, one mechanism to explain the benefit from hypophysectomy is the drop in estrogen levels following removal of the pituitary gland. However, before this question can be settled, evaluation should be made of the benefit from hypophysectomy after treatment with tamoxifen followed by aminoglutethimide.

III. *Hormone-Additive Therapy*

Hormone-additive therapy represents one of the major forms of treatment for women with advanced breast cancer. The hormones used are estrogens, progestins, androgens, and corticosteroids. Numerous reports in the literature indicate the usefulness of these agents for treating women with advanced breast cancer; estrogens or progestins in pharmacological doses can induce remissions in 30–40% of patients (Kennedy 1970). On the other hand, androgens are reported to induce remissions in 20–30% of the patients (Kennedy 1970).

One of the major limiting factors in the use of additive hormone therapy has been the significance of side effects associated with the use of these hormones in pharmacological doses. Nausea, vomiting, anorexia, fluid retention, and vaginal bleeding are common side effects of estrogen therapy; vaginal bleeding and weight gain are common side effects of progestins. Hirsutism and virilization are commonly associated with andro-gens, and Cushing's syndrome may develop after chronic use of high-dose corticosteroids. The mechanism by which additive hormone therapy influences breast cancer growth is not established.

IV. Antiestrogen Therapy

Nonsteroidal antiestrogens, shown to have potent antitumor activity and to be relatively free of side effects, represent a major advance in the management of breast cancer. Among this class of compounds, tamoxifen has been the most widely used drug. The efficacy of tamoxifen in women with advanced breast cancer has been documented in numerous reports (Cole et al. 1971; Furr et al. 1979; Manni et al. 1979). In a summary of 20 different clinical trials, Furr concluded that 31.7% of the patients obtained partial or complete objective remission and 20% had stabilization of disease (Furr et al. 1979). This was remarkably similar to the conventional ablative or additive hormone therapy with fewer associated side effects. As in the case of other endocrine therapy, objective remissions to tamoxifen were obtained more frequently in patients with ER-positive tumors (Manni et al. 1979, 1981). In our own experience, 63% of patients with ER-positive tumors obtained an objective response to antiestrogen therapy.

After the antitumor effectiveness of tamoxifen was established, several investigators compared the usefulness of this drug to other conventional endocrine treatments. In a randomized clinical trial comparing tamoxifen to estrogen-additive therapy, Ingle et al. (1981) found similar response rates to both agents, yet the side effects associated with tamoxifen were significantly fewer. Similar findings were also reported by Beex (1981). Several randomized clinical trials compared tamoxifen therapy to progestational agents in women with advanced breast cancer. Even though the dose of the progestational agent varied among the studies, the response rates to tamoxifen in all these studies were similar to those seen with progestins (Mattsson 1980). In a randomized study (Westerberg 1980) comparing the effectiveness of tamoxifen and androgens (fluoxymesterone), a higher response rate was found in the tamoxifen-treated group (30% vs 19%).

Aminoglutethimide-hydrocortisone combination therapy has recently been introduced as a means of inducing a medical adrenalectomy in patients with breast cancer. The efficacy of this newly introduced modality was compared in randomized clinical trials to tamoxifen (Lipton et al. 1982). Again, the response rate to tamoxifen was similar to the medical adrenalectomy regimen (Lipton et al. 1982).

These randomized clinical trials have demonstrated that antiestrogen therapy is at least as effective as endocrine-additive therapy and also as effective as aminoglutethimide-hydrocortisone combination in the treatment of women with breast cancer. However, in all these studies, fewer side effects were reported with antiestrogen therapy. It is because of its efficacy and relative lack of side effects that tamoxifen is considered the endocrine treatment of choice in postmenopausal women with advanced breast cancer.

Previous reports have demonstrated the efficacy of the antiestrogen tamoxifen in premenopausal women with breast cancer despite the persistence of regular menses in these patients (Manni and Pearson 1980; Pritchard 1980). In these women treated with tamoxifen, significant elevation in serum estradiol levels was demonstrated (Manni and Pearson 1980). Thus, it is conceivable that the resulting high serum estrogen levels may influence the antiestrogenic effect of tamoxifen. Because of that, it is felt that castration should be considered the hormonal treatment of choice in premenopausal women with advanced breast cancer. Although tamoxifen has been shown to be effective in such women, its use in these patients should be limited to detailed and well-defined research protocols.

It is well known that patients who relapse while receiving one hormone therapy may later respond to another one given subsequently. It is also known that human breast cancer cells are heterogeneous with respect to hormone sensitivity. In combining more than one form of endocrine treatment, therefore, one would expect at least the additive effects of the drugs, but in practice, less than additive effects are seen in combining endocrine treatments. Several randomized clinical trials compared the efficacy of tamoxifen alone to that seen with tamoxifen in combination with different endocrine therapy, such as estrogens (Mouridsen et al. 1980), progestins (Mouridsen et al. 1979), aminoglutethimide (Smith et al. 1982), androgens (Tormey et al. 1983), and corticosteroids (Stewart et al. 1982). The consensus in all these studies is that there is very little overall advantage to combining antiestrogen treatments with other hormonal therapy, since no significant increase in the number or duration of remissions was obtained with combination treatment.

The use of endocrine treatments sequentially rather than in combination appears to offer better results. In fact, this is the approach we advocate in the management of hormone-responsive breast cancer. With this approach, some patients received considerable benefits, resulting in a significantly prolonged period of survival. We will review here our data on 113 patients who were treated with tamoxifen and subsequently with other available forms of treatment.

V. Sequential Endocrine Treatment

The clinical data on 113 selected patients with advanced breast cancer treated with tamoxifen have been previously reported (Manni et al. 1979, 1981) and will be updated here. In this series, 50% of patients obtained objective tumor regression lasting 4–96+ months (mean 23+; median 16 months), with two patients still in remission (Table 23.1). Survival was significantly prolonged in patients who responded to tamoxifen therapy (Table 23.1, Fig. 23.1). It is quite interesting to note that the mean survival from the onset of metastasis in patients who responded to tamoxifen was 67 months, as compared to a mean of 30 months noted in patients who failed tamoxifen therapy (Fig. 23.1). We were particularly interested in evaluating the response to subsequent endocrine treatments in these patients following either a relapse or failure of antiestrogen therapy. In that respect, 44 of this series of patients initially treated with tamoxifen underwent surgical hypophysectomy, and of these, 38 patients were evaluable. Objective remissions (Table 23.2) were seen in 16 patients (42%) and arrest of disease was seen in an additional two patients (5%). The duration of response to hypophysectomy averaged 15 months. Patients who relapsed after a tamoxifen-induced remission benefitted more often

Table 23.1. Result of tamoxifen therapy in 113 patients

	Patients		Duration (months)		Survival[a] (months)		Number still alive
	No.	%	Mean	Median	Mean	Median	
Remissions	56	50	23+[b]	16	49+[c]	44	6
Arrest of disease	8	7	23	19	41	33	0
Failure	49	43	—	—	17	11	0

[a]From the onset of treatment.
[b]Two patients still in remission at 84 and 96 months.
[c]$p < 0.005$ as compared to "failure."

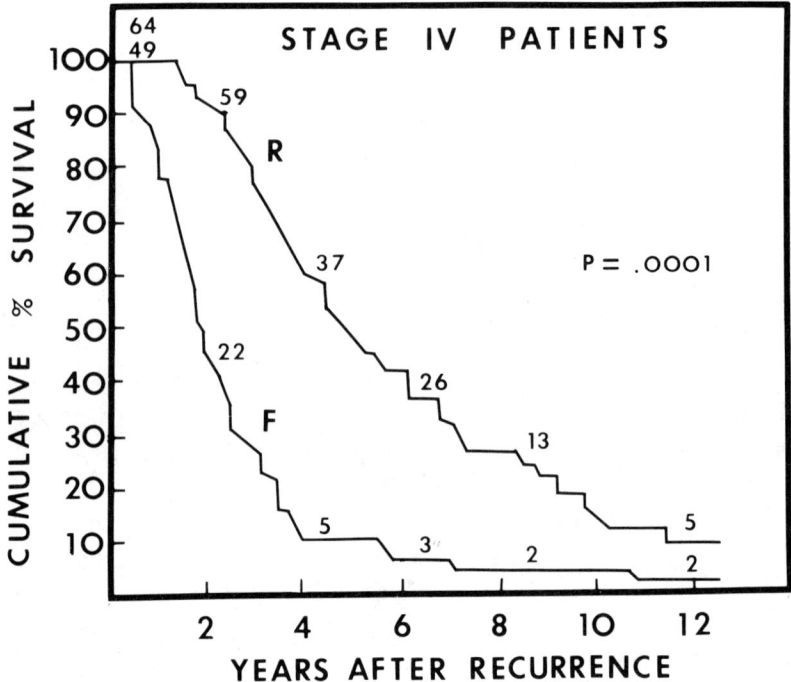

Figure 23.1. Life-table plots of survival from the onset of metastasis in patients who responded (R) (remission and arrest of disease) and those who failed (F) to benefit from tamoxifen therapy.

from hypophysectomy than those who initially failed tamoxifen ($p <$ 0.05).

Similarly, androgen therapy (fluoxymesterone, 20 mg daily) was used in a total of 28 evaluable patients (Table 23.3) in this series. Significant palliation was seen in 15 patients (54%), lasting for a mean of 10.4 months (Table 23.3). We saw responses in patients who benefitted as well as in those who did not benefit from tamoxifen. Of interest is the fact that objective remissions were seen in three of 10 patients who previously underwent hypophysectomy. In this series of 113 patients, too few were treated with progestins or estrogen after tamoxifen to allow proper evaluation of these agents. None of the patients received corticosteroids after tamoxifen therapy.

Chemotherapy was administered to these patients after we thought that maximum benefit from hormonal therapy had been achieved. The chemo-

Table 23.2. The response to hypophysectomy after tamoxifen therapy

Prior response to tamoxifen	Number of patients	Remission		Duration (months)	
		No.	%	Mean	Median
Remission	21	14[a]	67	15	16
Arrest of disease	4	1	25	20	—
Failure	13	3	23	11	—
Total/Average	38	18[a]	47	15	16

[a]Includes two patients who had arrest of disease.

Table 23.3. The response to androgen therapy (fluoxymesterone) in 28 patients

Response to tamoxifen	Number of patients	Remission		Duration (months)		Failure
		No.	%	Mean	Median	
Remissions	22	11[a]	50	10.8	10	11
Arrest of disease	1	1	100	12.0	—	—
Failure	5	3	60	8.3	8	2
Total/Average	28	15[a]	54	10.4	10	13

[a]Includes two patients who had arrest of disease.

therapeutic regimen used included a five-drug combination and has been described in detail previously (Arafah et al. 1984). The response to five-drug chemotherapy was evaluable in 38 patients in this series. A total of 23 patients (60%) had objective remission (18 patients) or arrest of disease lasting for an average of 15 months (median 10 months). The response rate was similar in both tamoxifen responders and failures. Adriamycin was subsequently used in some of these patients as a single agent. With this treatment, nine of 25 patients (36%) obtained objective remission and two additional patients (8%) had arrest of disease lasting for a mean of 6 months.

VI. *Discussion*

Endocrine treatments provide significant palliation for women with advanced hormone-responsive breast cancer. Following relapse or recurrence after mastectomy, our first choice of treatment is hormonal manipulation unless the tumor is known to be ER-negative or the patient has advanced liver metastasis, in which case chemotherapy would be indicated. Measurement of hormone receptors in the primary tumors (ER, PgR) has improved our ability to select patients likely to benefit from endocrine treatments. Recent studies indicate that the presence of ER and PgR in the tumor provides important additional information on the prognosis of patients with stage I and stage II breast cancer (Crowe et al. 1982; Clark et al. 1983).

Antiestrogen therapy has proven to be as effective as, if not better than, conventional endocrine treatments. The lack of significant side effects with this treatment modality is a great additional advantage. Thus treatment with antiestrogens is considered the initial hormonal therapy of choice in postmenopausal women with advanced breast cancer.

In our approach to treating patients with hormone-responsive breast cancer we have utilized the available modalities sequentially, rather than in combination. This approach has provided significant benefit to some patients and has also provided valuable information on the endocrine factors regulating the growth of human mammary cancer. The significant benefit obtained with antiestrogens even in patients who had prior hypophysectomy (Manni et al. 1979) indicates that estrogens are the predominant hormones involved in the growth of human breast cancer cells. However, significant benefit can be obtained with the use of other hormonal treatments after failure of or a relapse from an antiestrogen-induced remission. This suggests that other hormones as well may be implicated in the growth of human mammary carcinoma, a hypothesis that should particularly be considered in explaining the response to androgen therapy in women previously treated with tamoxifen and/or hypophysectomy. We have been intrigued for several years by the response to hypophysectomy following antiestrogen therapy. Initially we thought that elimination of a "pituitary factor" could explain the response to hypophysectomy after antiestrogen therapy. The exact mechanism by which hypophysectomy induces a remission in women with breast cancer is not clearly established, but reduction in the level of circulating estrogen levels following hypophysectomy is undoubtedly a major mechanism. In postmenopausal women with breast cancer previously treated with tamoxifen, the inhibition of estrogen synthesis with aminoglutethimide can result in significant palliation in some patients (Murray and Pitt 1981; Santen et al. 1981, 1982). In fact, current data indicate that the responses to aminoglutethimide treatment after tamoxifen therapy are quite similar to those seen with hypophysectomy after tamoxifen therapy (Murray and Pitt 1981; Santen et al. 1982). We now use aminoglutethimide and hydrocortisone rather than hypophysectomy as the next sequential treatment after tamoxifen. Hypophysectomy is used in patients who are unable to tolerate aminoglutethimide therapy (10–15% of patients).

Several reports in the literature describe the usefulness of other endocrine treatments (aminoglutethimide, progestins) used sequentially after tamoxifen (Murray and Pitt 1981; Ross et al. 1982; Santen et al. 1982). Our data and those reported in the literature indicate that sequential endocrine therapy is highly beneficial for patients with hormone-responsive breast cancer. At the present time our approach is to initiate treatment with tamoxifen, because of its effectiveness and lack of significant side effects. In premenopausal women, oophorectomy would be the initial choice of therapy; we favor aminoglutethimide as a second sequential form of treatment, particularly in patients who responded previously to tamoxifen. Either progestins or androgens can then be used sequentially in these patients.

After maximum benefit is felt to have been obtained with endocrine treatments, we utilized the five-drug combination chemotherapy in these patients. This form of treatment has been effective in patients with hormone-responsive as well as those with hormone-resistant tumors. Obviously the side effects seen with chemotherapy are more significant than those seen with any of the endocrine treatments.

Patients with hormone-responsive tumors represent a favorable group in general. With the use of sequential endocrine treatments and chemotherapy, significant benefit and prolongation of life could be achieved.

References

Arafah, B. M., J. S. Marshall, and O. H. Pearson. 1984. Combination chemotherapy in the treatment of women with advanced breast cancer. In *Fluoropyrimidines in cancer therapy,* ed. K. Kimura et al., *Proceedings of the International Symposium on Fluoropyrimidines,* Nagoya, Japan, November 3–5, 1983. Amsterdam: Elsevier.

Beatson, G. T. 1896. On the treatment of inoperable cases of carcinoma of the mamma: suggestions for a new method with illustrative cases. *Lancet* 2:104–107.

Beex, L., G. Pieters, A. Smals, A. Koenders, T. Benraad, and P. Kloppenborg. 1981. Tamoxifen versus ethinyl estradiol in the treatment of postmenopausal women with advanced breast cancer. *Cancer Treatment Reports* 65:179–185.

Clark, G. M., W. L. McGuire, C. A. Hubay, O. H. Pearson, and J. S. Marshall. 1983. Progesterone receptors as a prognostic indicator for stage II breast cancer. *New England Journal of Medicine* 309:1343–1347.

Cole, M. P., C. T. A. Jones, and I. D. H. Todd. 1971. A new antiestrogenic agent in late breast cancer. *British Journal of Cancer* 25:270–275.

Crowe, J. P., C. A. Hubay, O. H. Pearson, J. S. Marshall, J. Rosenblatt, E. G. Mansour, R. E. Hermann, J. C. Jones, W. J. Flynn, W. L. McGuire, and Other Participating Investigators (Cleveland). 1982. Estrogen receptor status as a prognostic indicator for stage I breast cancer patients. *Breast Cancer Research and Treatment* 2:171–176.

Furr, B. J., J. S. Patterson, D. N. Richardson, S. R. Slater, and A. E. Wakeling. 1979. Tamoxifen. In *Pharmacological and biochemical properties of drug substances,* vol. 2, ed. M. E. Goldberg, 355–399. Washington, D.C.: American Pharmaceutical Association.

Ingle, J. N., D. L. Ahmann, S. J. Green, J. H. Edmonson, H. F. Bisel, L. K. Kvols, W. C. Nichols, E. T. Creagan, R. G. Hahn, J. Rubin, and S. Frytack. 1981. Randomized clinical trial of diethylstilbestrol versus tamoxifen in postmenopausal women with advanced breast cancer. *New England Journal of Medicine* 304:16–21.

Jensen, E. V., G. E. Block, S. Smith, K. Kyser, and E. R. DeSombre. 1971. Estrogen receptors and breast cancer response to adrenalectomy. In *Prediction of response in cancer therapy,* ed. T. C. Hall, 55–70. National Cancer Institute Monograph 34. Bethesda, Md.

Kennedy, B. J. 1970. Hormone therapy in cancer. *Geriatrics* 25:106–112.

Lipton, A., H. A. Harvey, R. J. Santen, A. Boucher, D. White, A. Bernath, R. Dixon, G. Richards, and A. Shafik. 1982. Randomized trial of aminoglutethimide versus tamoxifen in metastatic breast cancer. *Cancer Research* Suppl. 42:3434–3436.

Manni, A., and O. H. Pearson. 1980. Antiestrogen-induced remissions in premenopausal women with stage IV breast cancer: effects on ovarian function. *Cancer Treatment Reports* 64:779–785.

Manni, A., J. E. Trujillo, J. S. Marshall, J. Brodkey, and O. H. Pearson. 1979. Antihormone treatment of stage IV breast cancer. *Cancer* 43:444–450.

Manni, A., J. E. Trujillo, and O. H. Pearson. 1980. Sequential use of endocrine treatment and chemotherapy in metastatic breast cancer: effects on survival. *Cancer Treatment Reports* 64:111–116.

Manni, A., O. H. Pearson, J. S. Marshall, and B. M. Arafah. 1981. Sequential endocrine therapy and chemotherapy in metastatic breast cancer: effects on survival. *Breast Cancer Research and Treatment* 1:97–103.

Mattsson, W. 1980. A phase III trial of treatment with tamoxifen versus treatment with high-dose medroxyprogesterone acetate in advanced postmenopausal breast cancer. In *Role of medroxyprogesterone in endocrine-related tumors. Progress in cancer research and therapy,* vol. 15, ed. S. Iacobelli, and A. DiMarco, 65–71. New York: Raven Press.

Mouridsen, H. T., K. Ellemann, W. Mattsson, T. Palshof, J. L. Daehnfeldt, and C. Rose. 1979. Therapeutic effect of tamoxifen versus tamoxifen combined with medroxyprogesterone acetate in advanced breast cancer in postmenopausal women. *Cancer Treatment Reports* 63:171–175.

Mouridsen, H. T., M. Salimtschik, P. Dombernowsky, K. Gelshoj, T. Palshof, M. Rorth, J. L. Daehnfeldt, and C. Rose. 1980. Therapeutic effect of tamoxifen versus combined tamoxifen and diethylstilbestrol in advanced breast cancer in postmenopausal women. In *Breast cancer: experimental and clinical aspects,* ed. H. T. Mouridsen and T. Palshof, 107–110. Oxford: Pergamon Press.

Murray, R. M. L., and P. Pitt. 1981. Medical adrenalectomy in patients with advanced breast cancer resistant to anti-oestrogen treatment. *Breast Cancer Research and Treatment* 1:91–95.

Pearson, O. H., and B. S. Ray. 1960. Hypophysectomy in the treatment of metastatic mammary cancer. *American Journal of Surgery* 99:544.

Pearson, O. H., C. D. West, and N. Treves. 1953. The role of ovarian function in the growth of mammary carcinoma in man. *Journal of Clinical Investigation* 32:594.

Pearson, O. H., J. S. Brodkey, and A. Manni. 1978. Hypophysectomy for stage IV breast cancer. *Surgical Clinics of North America* 58:809–817.

Pritchard, K. I., D. B. Thomson, R. E. Myers, D. J. A. Sutherland, B. G. Mobbs, and J. W. Meakin. 1980. Tamoxifen therapy in premenopausal patients with metastatic breast cancer. *Cancer Treatment Reports* 64:779–785.

Ross, M. B., A. U. Buzdar, and G. R. Blumenschein. 1982. Treatment of advanced breast cancer with megestrol acetate after therapy with tamoxifen. *Cancer* 49:413–417.

Santen, R. J., S. J. Santner, B. Davis, J. Veldhuis, E. Samojlik, and E. Ruby. 1978. Aminoglutethimide inhibits extraglandular estrogen production in postmenopausal women with breast cancer. *Journal of Clinical Endocrinology and Metabolism* 47:1257–1265.

Santen, R. J., T. J. Worgul, E. Samojlik, A. Interrante, A. E. Boucher, A. Lipton, H. A. Harvey, D. S. White, E. Smart, C. Cox, and S. A. Wells. 1981. A randomized trial comparing surgical adrenalectomy with aminoglutethimide plus hydrocortisone in women with advanced breast cancer. *New England Journal of Medicine* 305:545–551.

Santen, R. J., E. Badder, and S. Lerman. 1982. Pharmacologic suppression of estrogens with aminoglutethimide as treatment of advanced breast carcinoma: mechanistic, hormonal and clinical studies. *Breast Cancer Research and Treatment* 2:375–383.

Smith, I. E., A. L. Harris, and M. Morgan. 1982. Tamoxifen versus aminoglutethimide versus combined tamoxifen and aminoglutethimide in the treatment of advanced breast carcinoma. *Cancer Research Suppl.* 42:3430–3433.

Stewart, J. F., R. D. Rubens, R. J. B. King, M. J. Minton, R. Steiner, D. Tong, P. J. Winter, R. K. Knight, and J. L. Hayward. 1982. Contribution of prednisolone to the primary endocrine treatment of advanced breast cancer. *European Journal of Cancer and Clinical Oncology* 18:1307–1314.

Tormey, D. C., M. E. Lippman, and B. K. Edwards. 1983. Evaluation of tamoxifen doses with and without fluoxymesterone in advanced breast cancer. *Annals of Internal Medicine* 98:139–144.

Westerberg, H. 1980. Tamoxifen and fluoxymesterone in advanced breast cancer: a controlled clinical trial. *Cancer Treatment Reports* 64:17–121.

24

Combined Chemohormonotherapy Approaches for Breast Cancer

D. C. Tormey

I. Introduction   432
II. Selected Combination Systemic Therapy Concepts in Advanced Disease   432
III. Additive Chemohormonotherapy   435
IV. Ablative Hormone Therapy plus Chemotherapy   440
V. Advanced-Disease Versus Postoperative Adjuvant Therapy   441
VI. Comment   443
References   445

431

I. *Introduction*

T HIS chapter provides a brief overview of the development of combined chemohormonotherapy regimens for the treatment of patients with breast cancer. Some of the general principles involved in the development of these regimens are illustrated. Specific conceptual differences between the use of systemic therapy for the palliation of advanced disease and its place in the cure of early postoperative disease are discussed. These principles are illustrated using the results from representative clinical trials.

II. *Selected Combination Systemic Therapy Concepts in Advanced Disease*

The first report of combined chemohormonal therapy for metastatic breast cancer was that of Watson and Turner (1959) using thioTEPA and testosterone. Greenspan's subsequent reports were the first to develop the concept of combination chemotherapy (Greenspan et al. 1963; Greenspan 1966). He utilized combinations of thioTEPA and methotrexate in conjunction with testosterone. However, it was the report of Cooper (1969) that spurred the modern development of combination chemotherapy approaches. He reported a high response rate using cyclophosphamide, methotrexate, 5-fluorouracil, vincristine, and prednisone.

During the early 1970s response rates appeared to reach a maximum when three or four myelosuppressive drugs were present in the regimens (Fig. 24.1). It was also evident that the addition of the very active drug adriamycin to the regimens provided for higher response rates but the plateau using three or four drugs was still evident (Tormey and Neifeld 1977; Aisner et al. 1981). The reason for the response rate plateau, it was thought, was that host toxicity necessitated the reduction of the dose of each drug with each cytotoxic addition. Since chemotherapeutic agents tend to have steep dose-response curves, it appeared that a balance between cell kill and host toxicity was occurring at the level of three or four cytotoxic drugs.

Most studies of chemotherapy regimens, and especially the earlier ones, focused only upon response rate as a measure of cell kill and there-

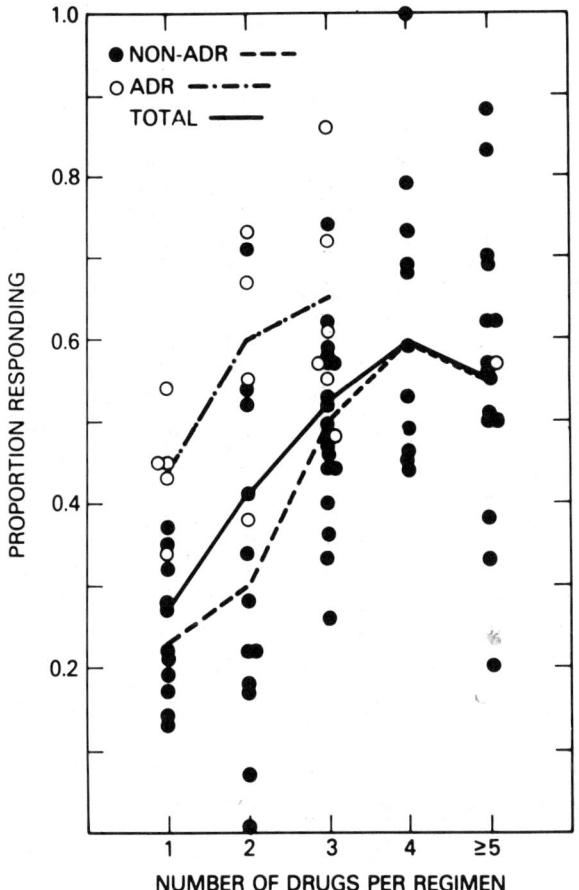

Figure 24.1. The relationship between the number of drugs in chemotherapy treatment regimens and the response rate. ADR refers to adriamycin-containing regimens. Non-ADR refers to regimens not containing adriamycin. (From Tormey and Neifeld [1977] with the permission of the publishers.)

fore of relative treatment effect. The validity of this interpretation was supported by the observation that response durations, i.e., the time from response to treatment to the time of treatment failure, were usually longer in populations treated first with combinations (Canellos et al. 1976; Hoogstraten et al. 1976; Smalley et al. 1976; Mouridsen et al. 1977; Nemoto et al. 1978; Chlebowski et al. 1979). Although the higher response rates and improved response durations with the combinations tended to extend to survival, the advantage was not always statistically significant (Hoogstraten et al. 1976; Nemoto et al. 1978; Chlebowski et al. 1979). A review of the data also suggested that the response durations tended to level off at three or four drugs in the combinations (Tormey and Neifeld 1977). These observations suggested that the combinations achieved their higher cell kill across a broader population of cells than did single agents, i.e., more people responded because of cytotoxicity upon differing resistant cell populations. However, response-duration data are frequently difficult to interpret because of differences in definitions, patient populations, and patient follow-up procedures. Similarly, survival data are difficult to interpret because of dissimilar secondary treatments used in the patients. For these reasons a more uniform population-derived endpoint was developed. This was the "time to treatment failure" endpoint, i.e., the time from initiation of therapy to the time of treatment failure. This endpoint, when applied to the entire treated population, provided greater statistical power to isolate relative cell kill capabilities of the treatments. Thus, two regimens associated with very little difference in response rates could have significantly different times to treatment failure, which could be due to differing net cell kills (Tormey et al. 1983).

Throughout the development of combination regimens, attempts have been made to combine drugs with known activity against the disease. For example, the positive impact of substituting the more active drug, adriamycin, for methotrexate was shown in multiple studies (Smalley et al. 1977; Bull et al. 1978; Aisner et al. 1981; Tormey et al. 1984b). Investigators also attempted to incorporate the principle of using drugs with slightly differing patterns of toxicity. Unfortunately, the majority of active drugs were myelosuppressive even though their relative patterns were slightly different. Occasionally the combinations resulted in unexpected new toxicity patterns. For example, the nonmyelosuppressive drug vincristine, when combined with myelosuppressive drugs, led to an increased myelosuppression (Ahmann et al. 1975). Finally, selected regimens were developed to provide combinations with more widely differing partition coefficients. This was considered important in order to provide combinations of drugs with both lipid- and water-soluble properties to facilitate distribution of multiple drugs into the tumor cells. Adriamycin and dibromodulcitol are more lipid soluble than methotrexate or cyclophosphamide, respectively. Their substitution into appropriate chemotherapy regimens provided for a greater spread of partition coefficients than was observed in the original regimens. Specific examples of this approach include the substitution of adriamycin for methotrexate in the cyclophosphamide, methotrexate, 5-fluorouracil (CMF) regimen (Bull et al. 1978) and of dibromodulcitol for cyclophosphamide in the cyclophosphamide, adriamycin, vincristine regimen (Tormey et al. 1979).

When it became apparent that the three or four drug chemotherapy regimens were not benefitting from the addition of more cytotoxic drugs, investigators began to search for nonmyelosuppressive drugs and for ways to deliver myelosuppressive drugs in a nonmyelosuppressive manner. An example of this latter approach has been the development of continuous intravenous 5-fluorouracil therapy. Unlike bolus 5-fluorouracil injections, myelosuppression with continuous intravenous infusions is seldom dose-limiting. Prior to this more recent approach, multiple investigators combined chemotherapy with hormonal therapies because of their nonmyelosuppressive character. The remainder of this chapter will examine the results and implications of using combined chemohormonotherapy approaches.

III. *Additive Chemohormonotherapy*

It is important to recognize that most of the advanced-disease combined chemohormonotherapy trials were initiated in the mid-1970s when information about the hormone receptor status of the patients was not usually known. Prednisone was used in many of the early combinations. Although it is one of the least active classes of hormone therapies (Stoll 1972), its use was related to the principle that corticosteroids would not increase the toxicity and might provide additional cell kill. Subsequently other hormonal agents were added to the combination regimens.

The first additive hormonal drug to be formally investigated in metastatic disease was prednisone. The Eastern Cooperative Oncology Group (ECOG) compared cyclophosphamide, methotrexate, and 5-fluorouracil (CMF) against CMF + prednisone (CMFP). The addition of the steroid led to a modest response rate improvement (57% vs 63%) and a significant improvement in time to treatment failure (Fig. 24.2) and in survival (Tormey et al. 1982b). The ECOG trials demonstrated that the addition of prednisone resulted in the administration of higher doses of CMF (Fig. 24.3) (Tormey et al. 1983). Previous animal and human experiments provided evidence that the use of corticosteroids causes higher blood counts through peripheral margination of the white blood cells (Daughaday et al. 1948; Hills et al. 1948; Boggs et al. 1964, 1965). Since leukopenia tends to be dose-limiting, it was hypothesized that the reason for the superiority

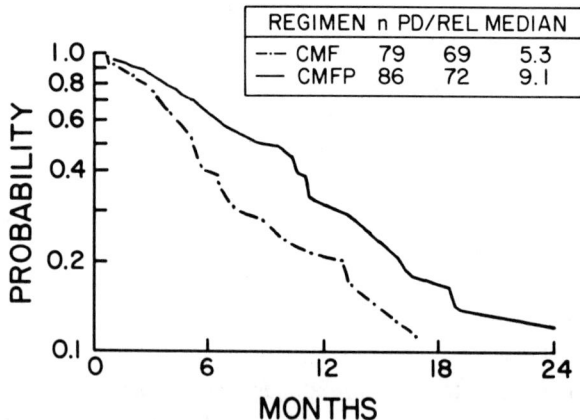

REGIMEN	n	PD/REL	MEDIAN
--- CMF	79	69	5.3
— CMFP	86	72	9.1

Figure 24.2. The impact of adding prednisone (P) to a cyclophosphamide, methotrexate, 5-fluorouracil (CMF) regimen upon time to treatment failure. (Modified from Tormey et al. 1982b.)

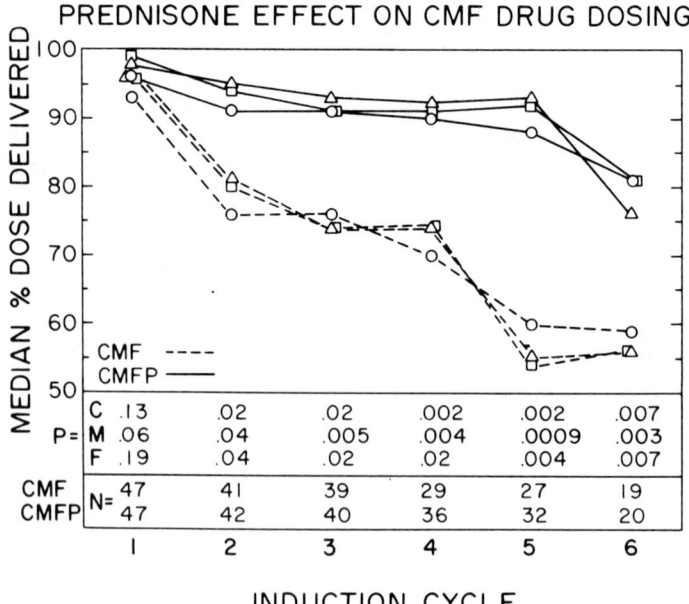

Figure 24.3. The doses of cyclophosphamide (C), methotrexate (M), and 5-fluorouracil (F) delivered with and without the addition of prednisone to a CMF regimen in each of the first six cycles of therapy. ○ = cyclophosphamide (C); □ = methotrexate (M); △ = 5-fluorouracil (F). (Modified from Tormey et al. 1983.)

of CMFP over CMF was related to prednisone's ability to maintain the peripheral blood counts, which in turn led to fewer decreases in CMF dosing. The treatment regimens used in the ECOG studies involved 28-day cycles incorporating 14 days of CMF therapy with 14-day breaks between therapy. Prednisone was given on days 1–14 of each cycle with the CMF. The above interpretation of the drug's effect was supported by observing that there was little or no difference in day 1 blood counts with or without prednisone (Tormey et al. 1982b, 1983). A more recent analysis has provided further evidence by showing that day 8 peripheral white blood counts are significantly higher with prednisone included in the regimen (Table 24.1).

Simultaneously the ECOG prospectively evaluated CMF in advanced disease with and without the addition of continuous therapy with the androgen fluoxymesterone. The patients were randomized after having obtained a response following 6 months of induction therapy. The addition of the androgen led to maintenance of higher day 1 blood counts, greater CMF drug delivery, a longer time to treatment failure, and a suggestion of longer survival (Tormey et al. 1981). This observation was taken as evidence that providing bone marrow support leading to higher blood counts would enable delivery of higher CMF drug doses, resulting in a higher tumor cell kill and resultant greater therapeutic effect.

The alternate explanation, that there was an additional cytotoxic effect from prednisone and fluoxymesterone, was considered but could not be

Table 24.1. Median day 1 and day 8 white blood counts in patients treated with cyclophosphamide, methotrexate, and 5-fluorouracil (CMF) alone or in combination with prednisone (CMFP)[a]

| | Day 1 | | Day 8 | |
Cycle	CMF	CMFP	CMF	CMFP
1	6.10	7.00*	4.05	8.60**
2	4.80	5.10	4.10	8.80**
3	4.70	5.40	4.35	9.50**
4	4.40	5.50	4.00	7.90**
5	4.25	5.15*	4.10	8.50**
6	5.10	4.50	4.00	8.10**

[a]The data are from 99 randomly selected patients from the Eastern Cooperative Oncology Group trials reported by Tormey et al. (1982b, 1983). The statistical analyses for this table were provided by P. Rosenbaum, M.S., at the Wisconsin Clinical Cancer Center. Cyclophosphamide and prednisone were delivered orally days 1–14, and methotrexate and 5-fluorouracil intravenously days 1 and 8 of each 28-day cycle.
$*p < 0.05$; $**p = 0.0001$ (Mann-Whitney tests).

shown to be operating within the context of these trials. Future trials may be designed to investigate how much of the therapeutic enhancement associated with these steroid classes is related to blood count support enabling higher CMF drug delivery versus a direct antitumor effect of the steroids.

There are no large randomized trials of chemotherapy with or without progestins in patients not previously treated with chemotherapy. Since progestins have some of the characteristics of both corticosteroids and androgens, it would be expected that their effects in a combination may be similar. The advanced-disease trials that have been reported are conflicting with respect to any therapeutic benefit from adding progestational agents to chemotherapy (Brunner et al. 1977; Rubens et al. 1978; Pellegrini et al. 1982).

The advanced-disease trials testing the addition of estrogens and antiestrogens to chemotherapy were based upon their nonoverlapping toxicities and potential to kill or prevent growth of the hormone-responsive cell population. The addition of diethylstilbestrol to chemotherapy regimens has not been associated with significant increases in response rates, response durations, or survival in postmenopausal women (Firat and Olshin 1968; Brunner et al. 1977; Holzer et al. 1979; Kiang and Kennedy 1981). The impact upon overall time to treatment failure in these trials was not reported.

The antiestrogen tamoxifen was first added to chemotherapy using a dibromodulcitol and adriamycin regimen in patients who had failed prior chemotherapy for metastatic disease (Tormey et al. 1982a). The resulting combination yielded a higher response rate (55% vs 36%) and time to treatment failure (170 vs 110 days). A recent update (Tormey 1985) has also shown a significant survival advantage (271 vs 416 days). Subsequently, in patients not previously treated for metastatic disease, the addition of tamoxifen to a variety of chemotherapy regimens has been associated with an improved time to treatment failure where evaluated (Cocconi et al. 1983), and with higher response rates either overall or in selected patient subsets (Mouridsen et al. 1980; Cavalli et al. 1983; Cocconi et al. 1983), although the latter has not always been observed (Link et al. 1981; Kardinal et al. 1983).

Several investigators have explored the use of tamoxifen with estrogen reversal to provide for a cell synchronization or recruitment prior to applying chemotherapy. This approach is based upon cell culture work showing that it is possible to manipulate and synchronize hormone-sensitive cell

INDUCTION REGIMEN

DAY OF CYCLE

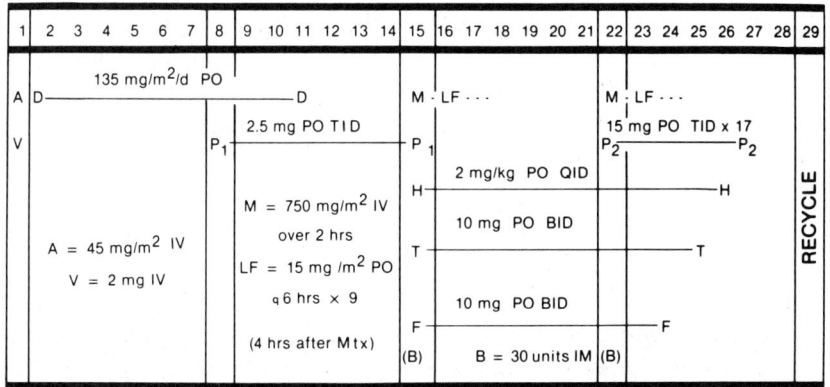

Figure 24.4. The 28-day schema for drug administration of an intensive therapy regimen at the Wisconsin Clinical Cancer Center. A = adriamycin; V = vincristine; D = dibromodulcitol; P = prednisone; M = methotrexate; LF = leukovorin factor; H = hexamethylmelamine; T = tamoxifen; F = fluoxymesterone; B = bleomycin only in first three cycles of patients 1–17. (From Tormey et al. 1985.)

populations (Green et al. 1981; Aitken and Lippman 1982). Both promising (Allegra et al. 1982; Lippman et al. 1984) and negative (Eisenhauer et al. 1984) clinical results with this approach have been reported.

A recent alternate approach conceptually takes advantage of differential normal and tumor cell synchronization approaches with hormone and chemotherapy pulses (Tormey et al. 1985). The regimen, shown in Figure 24.4, was administered over 28 days for six consecutive cycles or to disease stabilization over three consecutive cycles, whichever was longer. The overall response rate in 26 advanced-disease patients was 92%, with a complete remission rate of 77% (Tormey 1985). The parent dibromodulcitol, adriamycin, vincristine, tamoxifen, and fluoxymesterone regimen had an overall response rate of 58% and a complete remission rate of only 19% (Loprinzi et al. 1984). The time to treatment failure with the regimen in Figure 24.4 was also comparably longer, supporting the concept that a higher cell kill was achieved. As with many combination studies, it is not clear what the specific contributions of the hormones were in this trial. However, because of the high complete response rate, a modification of this regimen is now under test in the Eastern Cooperative Oncology Group.

Thus, response rate and time to treatment failure indices suggest that a cell kill advantage is achieved by adding hormone therapies to cytotoxic regimens. It is not clear in all cases what the reason is for the benefit of adding exogenous hormones to chemotherapy. In some cases there may be an additional cytotoxic or cytostatic effect, whereas in other cases there may also be an element of bone marrow and peripheral blood count support resulting in delivery of greater chemotherapy doses.

IV. *Ablative Hormone Therapy plus Chemotherapy*

The major randomized advanced-disease trials using ablative therapy in combination with chemotherapy have been in premenopausal women using bilateral oophorectomy (Brunner et al. 1977; Falkson et al. 1979; Ahmann et al. 1982; Rossof et al. 1982). Each of these studies has shown an increase in the response rate and an associated increased time to treatment failure using the two approaches together as compared to oophorectomy alone; however, there has not been an improvement in survival in any of the larger randomized studies. It is unclear why these initial indicators of cell kill have not translated into a survival advantage. It is possible that the rescue 50% response rate with chemotherapy after oophorectomy failure may have been sufficient to ablate any potential differences (Falkson et al. 1979). This would suggest that there is little overlap between chemotherapy- and oophorectomy-sensitive cell populations in these patients. A critical trial in this regard is a current ECOG metastatic disease study testing chemotherapy with or without a bilateral oophorectomy. This study is currently showing that a cyclophosphamide, adriamycin, 5-fluorouracil (CAF) regimen is not significantly different from the same drugs plus a bilateral oophorectomy in both estrogen receptor–positive (ER +) and ER-unknown patients, and the results in ER + patients are similar to the same chemotherapy alone in estrogen receptor–negative (ER −) patients (Falkson et al. 1984). If continued follow-up substantiates these results, it may indicate that the amenorrhea induced by chemotherapy is equivalent in its cell kill capability to adding a surgical castration to the chemotherapy. An analysis of the results in the CAF-alone-treated patients by the presence or absence of drug-induced amenorrhea would be helpful for the interpretation of the relative benefits of the chemotherapy and oophorectomy. Such an analysis in the postoperative adjuvant setting has suggested that those patients developing a CMF-induced amenorrhea have a better therapeutic effect than those whose menses continue (Tormey 1984).

Thus, the current evidence would suggest that a bilateral oophorectomy does not add to the effects of chemotherapy because of the chemical castration provided by chemotherapy alone, whereas chemotherapy added to oophorectomy may enhance the initial cell kill because of effects on an oophorectomy-insensitive population.

There are as yet insufficient randomized trial data available with surgical adrenalectomy or hypophysectomy approaches with and without chemotherapy. The recent advent of medical ablative approaches, as well as peripheral aromatase inhibitors, has provided the impetus to develop such studies. It might be predicted that the results and interpretations from such trials will be similar to those with surgical castration.

V. Advanced-Disease Versus Postoperative Adjuvant Therapy

Although the recent introduction of intensive systemic therapy programs (Tormey et al. 1985), autologous bone marrow transplantation (Knight et al. 1984), and hyperthermia (Robins 1984) may lead to cures in metastatic disease, the regimens in common use today are clearly palliative. In contrast, the intent in postoperative adjuvant therapy is clearly curative. In advanced disease, although there is seldom benefit to combining chemotherapy and hormonal therapy with respect to survival, there does appear to be a benefit in selected patients in order to achieve the higher cell kill associated with the combined approach. The identification of this higher cell kill leads to a different approach in the postoperative setting. Instead of attempting to *manipulate* differing resistant and sensitive cell population ratios, the approach is to kill or control *all* such populations. To this end, it is theoretically desirable to maximize the cell kill by combining chemotherapy and hormonotherapy. Similarly, it is desirable to control or kill both the hormone-sensitive and insensitive populations of the residual tumor. Irrespective of the ER or progesterone (PgR) analysis of the total tumors, it is generally accepted that the majority of tumors are heterogeneous. Thus, in the adjuvant setting there would appear to be a role for combined chemohormonotherapy in almost all cases. Multiple adjuvant trials have been developed since 1976 to assess the effects of CMF-based chemotherapy with and without hormone therapy in stratified ER + and

ER − patient cohorts. The added hormone therapy to date has been tamoxifen or a bilateral oophorectomy. Other drugs and approaches are only now coming under study. It is still too early to make definitive statements about the results within the initial adjuvant trials. The suggestion at present is that there is an advantage to CMF chemotherapy with hormonal therapy in the earlier relapsing ER − cohorts, whereas the later relapsing ER + cohorts require further follow-up before "early data" become available (Ludwig 1984; Tormey 1984; Tormey et al. 1984a). The suggested benefit in ER − patients is consonant with the concepts of disease heterogeneity with respect to hormone sensitivity.

The advanced-disease and adjuvant settings are also considered to differ with respect to the heterogeneity of their treatment-resistant cell populations. This concept is based upon the presumed lower tumor burden and number of previous doubling times present at the time of primary surgery as opposed to the time of documentation of metastatic disease—a concept still awaiting proof. In advanced disease the control of one population of cells leads to the emergence or overgrowth of a resistant population that is frequently sensitive to a different treatment approach. In this clinical setting it appears that hormone sensitivity as measured by a positive ER or PgR assay only implies that the majority population of tumor cells are hormone sensitive. However, lack of responsiveness to one hormone but not another, as well as the observation that development of resistance to one hormone is frequently associated with sensitivity to a different hormone, underscores our lack of knowledge concerning the *in vivo* effects of hormonal therapy and the clinical meaning of hormonal sensitivity as measured by a positive ER or PgR assay. Extrapolations from these observations in advanced disease to the adjuvant setting have not yet been made but could provide a rationale for combined or sequential hormonal therapy additions to chemotherapy.

Finally, the observation that hormonal therapy provides a G_1 block, at least in hormone-sensitive cells (Green et al. 1981; Goldenberg and Froese 1982; Brandes and Hermonat 1983), provides a rationale to continue the hormonal therapy indefinitely past the cessation of chemotherapy in adjuvant patients. It is unlikely that cells held in G_1 during chemotherapy will be killed by the chemotherapy, which generally requires a replicating population. It is tempting to suggest that the induction of a hormonal block removes hormone-sensitive cells from the replicating pool, thereby enabling transfer of more hormone-insensitive cells from the nonreplicating to the replicating pool, thus enabling a greater chemotherapy effect. However, one then has to consider whether to stimulate the remaining hormone-sensitive cells into cycle prior to a chemotherapy cycle, or administer the hormone therapy for a long enough period of time to induce cell death, if not definitely. On the basis of these considerations, as well as experiments in the DMBA-induced rat mammary tumor system (Jordan et al. 1979), we initiated adjuvant treatment with chemotherapy alone or with tamoxifen in 1976 (Tormey and Jordan 1984). The group receiving tamoxifen either stopped the drug at the completion of chemotherapy or continued it indefinitely. This pilot study demonstrated that tamoxifen, N-desmethyltamoxifen, and metabolite Y levels remained constant for at least 5 years. A recent clinical update of this study continues to show no demonstrable side effects from the tamoxifen continuation after stopping chemotherapy, and the disease-free survival and survival to 8 years continue to be favorable for the patients who have continued tamoxifen (Figs. 24.5, 24.6). The curves in the group in which tamoxifen was terminated are slowly approaching the chemotherapy-only group. Of interest is that no relapses have occurred after 5 years in the patients continuing tamoxifen. This is similar to a trial comparing radiation castration to radiation castration plus 5 years of prednisone (Meakin et al. 1983). The relative specific relapse rate beyond 5 years appeared to remain further reduced in the group that received prednisone. Whether this means cell death is induced by 5 years, thereby allowing drug discontinuation, must await further follow-up and studies. The approach of using tamoxifen for 1 vs 5 years has been under test in the Eastern Cooperative Oncology Group since 1982. The results from this national trial will be critical with respect to these concepts.

VI. *Comment*

Although the results of combined chemohormonotherapy in advanced disease have not been uniformly as positive as originally hoped, there are several positive attributes. The trials do show that combining hormone therapy with chemotherapy generally results in improved response rates and/or times to treatment failure. These indices suggest that a higher cell kill is achieved with the addition of hormonotherapies to chemotherapy

TIME TO RELAPSE WITH SYSTEMIC THERAPY +/-LONG-TERM TAMOXIFEN

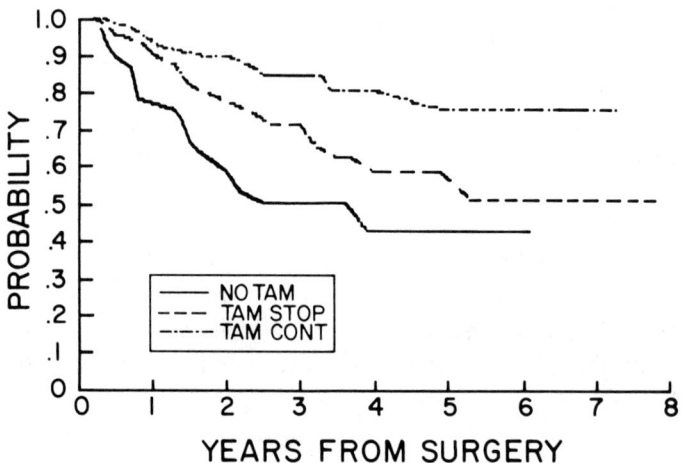

Figure 24.5. The disease-free survival life-table plots for node-positive postoperative adjuvant patients treated with chemotherapy alone (NO TAM), chemotherapy and tamoxifen (TAM STOP), and chemotherapy and tamoxifen followed by continued tamoxifen (TAM CONT). The chemotherapy duration was a median of 14 months. (See Tormey and Jordan 1984 for details.)

SURVIVAL WITH SYSTEMIC THERAPY +/- LONG-TERM TAMOXIFEN

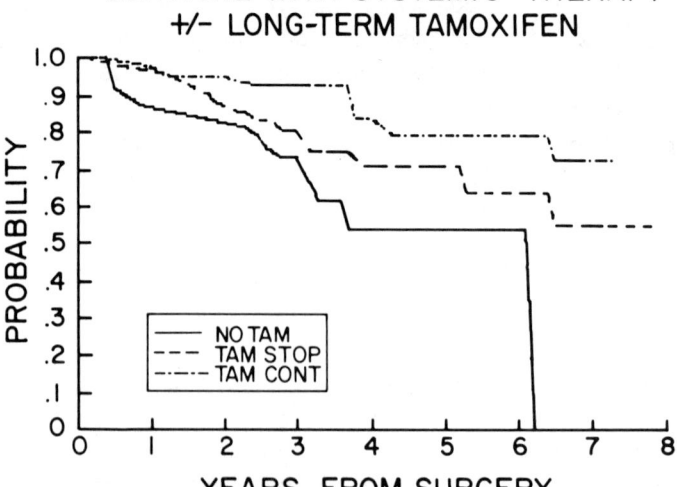

Figure 24.6. The survival life-table plots for node-positive postoperative adjuvant patients treated with chemotherapy alone (NO TAM), chemotherapy and tamoxifen (TAM STOP), and chemotherapy and tamoxifen followed by continued tamoxifen (TAM CONT). The chemotherapy duration was a median of 14 months. (See Tormey and Jordan 1984 for details.)

regimens. There are also suggestions that the two approaches are additive, i.e., are primarily affecting different cell populations. It is also of interest that in the adjuvant therapy situation the early results suggest improvement in predominantly hormone-insensitive patient populations. Assuming that the cell populations present in postoperative adjuvant patients are heterogeneous with respect to hormone-sensitive cells, the cell kill results in metastatic disease would suggest that the probability of cure would be enhanced postoperatively by using combined chemohormonotherapy. Additional clinical and laboratory data suggest that the hormone therapy used in the adjuvant setting should continue for at least 5 years. Adjuvant trials testing these concepts are currently maturing.

Acknowledgments

Supported in part by NIH grants P30-CA-14520, P01-CA-20432, and U10-CA-21076.

References

Ahmann, D. L., H. F. Bisel, R. G. Hahn, R. T. Eagan, J. H. Edmonson, J. L. Steinfeld, D. C. Tormey, and W. F. Taylor. 1975. An analysis of a multiple-drug program in the treatment of patients with advanced breast cancer utilizing 5-fluorouracil, cyclophosphamide, and prednisone with or without vincristine. *Cancer* 36:1925–1935.

Ahmann, D. L., S. J. Green, H. F. Bisel, J. N. Ingle, R. G. Hahn, R. A. Lee, and J. H. Edmonson. 1982. An evaluation of early or delayed adjuvant chemotherapy in premenopausal patients with advanced breast cancer undergoing oophorectomy: a later analysis. *American Journal of Clinical Oncology* (CCT) 5:355–358.

Aisner, J., V. Weinberg, M. Perloff, R. Weiss, P. Raich, M. Perry, and P. H. Wiernik, for CALGB. 1981. Chemoimmunotherapy for advanced breast cancer: a randomized comparison of 6 combinations (CMF, CAF vs CAFVP) and with or without MER immunotherapy. A CALGB study. *Proceedings of the American Society of Clinical Oncology* 22:443. Abstract C-433.

Aitken, S. C., and M. E. Lippman. 1982. Hormonal regulation of net DNA synthesis in MCF-7 human breast cancer cells in tissue culture. *Cancer Research* 42:1727–1735.

Allegra, J. C., T. M. Woodcock, S. P. Richman, K. I. Bland, and J. L. Wittliff. 1982. A phase II trial of tamoxifen, premarin, methotrexate and 5-fluorouracil in metastatic breast cancer. *Breast Cancer Research and Treatment* 2:93–100.

Boggs, D. R., J. W. Athens, G. E. Cartwright, and M. M. Wintrobe. 1964. The effect of adrenal glucocorticosteroids upon the cellular composition of inflammatory exudates. *American Journal of Pathology* 44:763–773.

Boggs, D. R., J. W. Athens, G. E. Cartwright, and M. M. Wintrobe. 1965. Leukokinetic studies. IX. Experimental evaluation of a model of granulopoiesis. *Journal of Clinical Investigation* 44:643–656.

Brandes, L. J., and M. W. Hermonat. 1983. Receptor status and subsequent sensitivity of subclones of MCF-7 human breast cancer cells surviving exposure to diethylstilbestrol. *Cancer Research* 43:2831–2835.

Brunner, K. W., R. W. Sonntag, P. Alberto, H. J. Senn, G. Martz, P. Obrecht, and P. Maurice. 1977. Combined chemo- and hormonal-therapy in advanced breast cancer. *Cancer* 39:2923–2933.

Bull, J. M., D. C. Tormey, S-H. Li, P. P. Carbone, G. Falkson, J. Blom, E. Perlin, and R. Simon. 1978. A randomized comparative trial of adriamycin versus methotrexate in combination drug therapy. *Cancer* 41:1649–1657.

Canellos, G. P., S. J. Pocock, S. G. Taylor, III, M. E. Sears, D. J. Klaasen, and P. R. Band. 1976. Combination chemotherapy for metastatic breast carcinoma: prospective comparison of multiple drug therapy with L-phenylalanine mustard. *Cancer* 38:1882–1886.

Cavalli, F., M. Beer, G. Martz, W. F. Jungi, P. Alberto, J. P. Obrecht, B. Mermillod, and K. W. Brunner. 1983. Concurrent or sequential use of cytotoxic chemotherapy and hormone treatment in advanced breast cancer: report of the Swiss Group for Clinical Cancer Research. *British Medical Journal* 286:5–8.

Chlebowski, R. T., L. E. Irwin, R. P. Pugh, L. Sadoff, R. Hestorff, J. M. Wiener, and J. R. Bateman. 1979. Survival of patients with metastatic breast cancer treated with either combination or sequential chemotherapy. *Cancer Research* 39:4503–4506.

Cocconi, G., V. DeLisi, C. Boni, P. Mori, P. Malacarne, D. Amadori, and E. Giovanelli. 1983. Chemotherapy versus combination of chemotherapy and endocrine therapy in advanced breast cancer: a prospective randomized study. *Cancer* 51:581–588.

Cooper, R. G. 1969. Combination chemotherapy in hormone resistant breast cancer. *Proceedings of the American Association for Cancer Research* 10:15.

Daughaday, W. H., R. H. Williams, and G. A. Daland. 1948. The effect of endocrinopathies on the blood. *Blood* 3:1342–1366.

Eisenhauer, E. A., D. M. Bowmann, K. I. Pritchard, A. H. G. Paterson, J. Ragaz, P. H. S. Geggie, and I. Maxwell. 1984. Tamoxifen and conjugated estrogens (Premarin) followed by sequenced methotrexate and 5-FU in refractory advanced breast cancer. *Cancer Treatment Reports* 68:1421–1422.

Falkson, G., H. C. Falkson, O. Glidewell, V. Weinberg, L. Leone, and J. G. Holland. 1979. Improved remission rates and remission duration in young women with metastatic breast cancer following combined oophorectomy and chemotherapy: a study by Cancer and Leukemia Group B. *Cancer* 43:2215–2222.

Falkson, G., R. Gelman, and D. C. Tormey. 1984. Personal communication: preliminary results from EST 2177 comparing CAF to CAF + oophorectomy.

Firat, D., and S. Olshin. 1968. Treatment of metastatic carcinoma of the female breast with combination of hormones and other chemotherapy. *Cancer Chemotherapy Reports* (Part 1) 52:743–750.

Goldenberg, G. J., and E. K. Froese. 1982. Drug and hormone sensitivity of estrogen receptor-positive and -negative human breast cancer cells in vitro. *Cancer Research* 42:5147–5151.

Green, M. D., A. M. Whybourne, I. W. Taylor, and R. L. Sutherland. 1981. Effects of antioestrogens on the growth and cell cycle kinetics of cultured human mammary carcinoma cells. In *Non-steroidal antioestrogens: molecular pharmacology and antitumour activity,* ed. R. L. Sutherland and V. C. Jordan, 397–412. Sydney: Academic Press.

Greenspan, E. M. 1966. Combination cytotoxic chemotherapy in advanced disseminated breast carcinoma. *Journal of Mt. Sinai Hospital, New York* 33:1–27.

Greenspan, E. M., M. Fieber, G. Lesnick, and S. Edelman. 1963. Response of advanced breast carcinoma to the combination of the antimetabolite, methotrexate, and the alkylating agent, Thio-TEPA. *Journal of Mt. Sinai Hospital, New York* 30:246–267.

Hills, A. G., P. H. Forsham, and C. A. Finch. 1948. Changes in circulating leukocytes induced by administration of pituitary adrenocorticotrophic hormone (ACTH) in man. *Blood* 3:755–768.

Holzer, D., H. A. Harvey, and A. Lipton. 1979. Comparison of DES vs DES + chlorambucil in women with first recurrence of breast cancer. *Journal of Surgical Oncology* 12:1–9.

Hoogstraten, B., S. L. George, B. Samal, S. E. Rivkin, J. J. Costanzi, J. D. Bonnet, T. Thigpen, and H. Braine. 1976. Combination chemotherapy and adriamycin in patients with advanced breast cancer: a Southwest Oncology Group study. *Cancer* 38:13–20.

Jordan, V. C., C. J. Dix, and K. E. Allen. 1979. The effectiveness of long-term tamoxifen treatment in a laboratory model for adjuvant hormone therapy of breast cancer. In *Adjuvant therapy of cancer II,* ed. S. E. Jones and S. E. Salmon, 19–26. New York: Grune and Stratton.

Kardinal, C. G., M. C. Perry, V. Weinberg, W. Wood, S. Ginsberg, and R. N. Raju, for the Cancer and Leukemia Group B. 1983. Chemoendocrine therapy vs chemotherapy alone for advanced breast cancer in postmenopausal women: preliminary report of a randomized study. *Breast Cancer Research and Treatment* 3:365–372.

Kiang, D. T., and B. J. Kennedy. 1981. Chemoendocrine therapy of advanced breast cancer. *Breast Cancer Research and Treatment* 1:105–109.

Knight, W. A., III, C. P. Page, J. G. Kuhn, G. M. Clark, and T. F. Newcomb. 1984. High-dose *L*-Pam with autologous bone marrow infusion for advanced, steroid hormone receptor negative, breast cancer. *Breast Cancer Research and Treatment* 4:336.

Link, H., H. Rückle, H. D. Waller, and K. Wilms. 1981. Kombinierte Chemoantiöstrogentherapie beim metastasierten Mammakarzinom: eine randomisierte Vergleichsstudie zwischen AVC and AVC plus Tamoxifen. *Deutsche Medizinische Wochenschrift* 106:1260–1262.

Lippman, M. E., J. Cassidy, M. Wesley, and R. C. Young. 1984. A randomized attempt to increase the efficacy of cytotoxic chemotherapy in metastatic breast cancer by hormonal synchronization. *Journal of Clinical Oncology* 2:28–36.

Loprinzi, C. L., D. C. Tormey, G. Falkson, A. Chang, and T. Read. 1984. Prospective evaluation of dibromodulcitol, doxorubicin, vincristine, tamoxifen and fluoxymesterone therapy and carcinoembryonic antigen levels in metastatic breast cancer. *Clinical Research* 32:766A.

Ludwig Breast Cancer Study Group. 1984. Adjuvant therapy for postmenopausal women with operable breast cancer. Part I. A randomized trial of chemoendocrine versus endocrine therapy versus mastectomy alone. In *Adjuvant therapy of cancer IV,* ed. S. E. Jones and S. E. Salmon, 379–391. New York: Grune and Stratton.

Meakin, J. W., W. E. C. Allt, F. A. Beale, R. S. Bush, R. M. Clark, P. J. Fitzpatrick, N. V. Hawkins, R. D. T. Jenkin, J. F. Pringle, J. G. Reid, W. D. Rider, J. L. Hayward, and R. D. Bulbrook. 1983. Ovarian radiation and prednisone following surgery and radiotherapy for carcinoma of the breast. *Breast Cancer Research and Treatment* 3 Suppl. 1:45–48.

Mouridsen, H. T., T. Palshof, M. Brahm, and I. Rahbek. 1977. Evaluation of single-drug versus multiple-drug chemotherapy in the treatment of advanced breast cancer. *Cancer Treatment Reports* 61:47–50.

Mouridsen, H. T., T. Palshof, E. Engelsman, and R. Sylvester. 1980. CMF versus CMF plus tamoxifen in advanced breast cancer in postmenopausal women. An EORTC trial. In *Breast cancer: experimental and clinical aspects,* ed. H. T. Mouridsen and T. Palshof, 119–123. Oxford: Pergamon Press.

Nemoto, T., D. Rosner, R. Diaz, T. Dao, R. Sponzo, T. Cunningham, J. Horton, and R. Simon. 1978. Combination chemotherapy for metastatic breast cancer: comparison of multiple drug therapy with 5-fluorouracil, cytoxan and prednisone with adriamycin or adrenalectomy. *Cancer* 41:2073–2077.

Pellegrini, A., G. Robustelli Della Cuna, B. Massidda, B. Bernardo, V. Mascia, and L. Pavesi. 1982. Medroxyprogesterone acetate plus chemotherapy versus chemotherapy alone: 3 randomized clinical trials. In *Proceedings of the International Symposium on Medroxyprogesterone Acetate,* ed. F. Cavalli, W. L. McGuire, F. Pannuti, A. Pellegrini, and G. Robustelli Della Cuna, 265–275. Amsterdam: Elsevier.

Robins, H. I. 1984. Role of whole-body hyperthermia in the treatment of neoplastic disease: its current status and future prospects. *Cancer Research* 44 (Suppl.):4878–4883.

Rossof, A. H., R. Gelman, and R. H. Creech. 1982. Randomized evaluation of combination chemotherapy vs observation alone following response or stabilization after oophorectomy for metastatic breast cancer in premenopausal women. *American Journal of Clinical Oncology* (CCT) 5:253–259.

Rubens, R. D., R. H. J. Begent, R. K. Knight, S. A. Sexton, and J. L. Hayward. 1978. Combined cytotoxic and progestogen therapy for advanced breast cancer. *Cancer* 42:1680–1686.

Smalley, R. V., S. Murphy, C. M. Huguley, Jr., and A. A. Bartolucci. 1976. Combination versus sequential five-drug chemotherapy in metastatic carcinoma of the breast. *Cancer Research* 36:3911–3916.

Smalley, R. V., J. Carpenter, A. Bartolucci, C. Vogel, and S. Krauss. 1977. A comparison of cyclophosphamide, adriamycin, 5-fluorouracil (CAF) and cyclophosphamide, methotrexate, 5-fluorouracil, vincristine, prednisone (CMFVP) in patients with metastatic breast cancer—a Southeastern Cancer Study Group report. *Cancer* 40: 625–632.

Stoll, B. A. 1972. Androgen, corticosteroid and progestin therapy. In *Endocrine therapy in malignant disease,* ed. B. A. Stoll, 165–191. London: W. B. Saunders.

Tormey, D. C. 1984. Adjuvant systemic therapy in postoperative node positive patients with breast carcinoma: the CALGB trial and the ECOG premenopausal trial. *Recent Results in Cancer Research* 96:155–165.

Tormey, D. C. 1985. Updated analysis.

Tormey, D. C., and V. C. Jordan. 1984. Long-term tamoxifen adjuvant therapy in node-positive breast cancer: a metabolic and pilot clinical study. *Breast Cancer Research and Treatment* 4:297–302.

Tormey, D. C., and J. P. Neifeld. 1977. Chemotherapeutic approaches to disseminated disease. In *Breast cancer management early and late,* ed. B. A. Stoll, 117–131. London: Heinemann.

Tormey, D. C., G. Falkson, R. M. Simon, J. Blom, J. M. Bull, M. E. Lippman, S-H. Li, J. Cassidy, and H. C. Falkson. 1979. A randomized comparison of two sequentially administered combination regimens to a single regimen in metastatic breast cancer. *Cancer Clinical Trials* 2:247–256.

Tormey, D. C., R. Gelman, P. R. Band, M. Sears, M. Bauer, J. C. Arseneau, and G. Falkson. 1981. A prospective evaluation of chemohormonal therapy remission maintenance in advanced breast cancer. *Breast Cancer Research and Treatment* 1:111–119.

Tormey, D. C., G. Falkson, J. Crowley, H. C. Falkson, J. Voelkel, and T. E. Davis. 1982a. Dibromodulcitol and adriamycin ± tamoxifen in advanced breast cancer. *American Journal of Clinical Oncology* (CCT) 5:33–39.

Tormey, D. C., R. Gelman, P. R. Band, M. Sears, S. N. Rosenthal, W. DeWys, C. Perlia, and M. S. Rice. 1982b. Comparison of induction chemotherapies for metastatic breast cancer: an Eastern Cooperative Oncology Group trial. *Cancer* 50:1235–1244.

Tormey, D. C., R. Gelman, and G. Falkson. 1983. Prospective evaluation of rotating chemotherapy in advanced breast cancer: an Eastern Cooperative Oncology Group trial. *American Journal of Clinical Oncology* (CCT) 6:1–18.

Tormey, D. C., S. G. Taylor, IV, R. Gray, and J. E. Olson. 1984a. Postmenopausal node-positive comparison of observation with CMFP and CMFP + tamoxifen adjuvant therapy: an Eastern Cooperative Oncology Group trial. In *Adjuvant chemotherapy of breast cancer. Recent results in cancer research,* vol. 96, ed. H. J. Senn, 110–116. Berlin: Springer-Verlag.

Tormey, D. C., V. E. Weinberg, L. A. Leone, O. J. Glidewell, M. Perloff, B. J. Kennedy, E. Cortes, R. T. Silver, R. B. Weiss, J. Aisner, and J. F. Holland. 1984b. A comparison of intermittent vs. continuous and of adriamycin vs. methotrexate 5-drug chemotherapy for advanced breast cancer: a Cancer and Leukemia Group B study. *American Journal of Clinical Oncology* (CCT) 7:231–239.

Tormey, D. C., J. C. Kline, M. Palta, T. E. Davis, R. R. Love, and P. P. Carbone. 1985. Short term high density systemic therapy for metastatic breast cancer. *Breast Cancer Research and Treatment* 5:177–188.

Watson, G. W., and R. L. Turner. 1959. Breast cancer, a new approach to therapy. *British Medical Journal* 1:1315–1321.

25

Antihormone Therapy as an Adjuvant to Mastectomy

NOLVADEX ADJUVANT TRIAL ORGANIZATION

PAPER PRESENTED BY

DIANA BRINKLEY

MEMBERS OF THE STEERING COMMITTEE
M. BAUM (CHAIRMAN), D. M. BRINKLEY,
J. A. DOSSETT, K. MCPHERSON, J. S. PATTERSON,
R. D. RUBENS, F. G. SMIDDY, B. A. STOLL,
A. WILSON, D. RICHARDS, AND S. H. ELLIS

I.   INTRODUCTION   452
II. THE NOLVADEX TRIAL ORGANIZATION   453
III. IMPLICATIONS OF THE STUDY   455
     REFERENCES   456

I. *Introduction*

MASTECTOMY fails to cure breast cancer because the disease has a propensity to spread to distant sites of the body and in a high proportion of patients secondary disease will develop and will sooner or later result in death.

Many types of surgery and radiotherapy are successful in achieving loco-regional control of breast cancer but as yet there is no certain treatment which will eradicate distant metastatic disease. Long-term follow-up studies show that even in so-called "early disease" 70% of patients will die of breast cancer (Brinkley and Haybittle 1984).

It has been known for many years that changes in hormone balance can affect the growth of breast cancer (Beatson 1896). Removal of hormone-producing endocrine glands or administration of hormones has been shown to influence the growth of primary and metastatic breast cancer. More recently, the antiestrogen tamoxifen has been shown to be an active agent in the treatment of advanced breast disease.

If treatment for early breast cancer is to become more successful, a means of eradicating micrometastatic disease must be developed. It is a logical step to bring in the agents known to be effective in advanced disease and to use them at the time of the primary loco-regional treatment, when metastases are subclinical.

Many clinical trials of adjuvant chemotherapy have been and are being conducted and the results are still being evaluated. There seems no doubt that cytotoxic drugs used in conjunction with primary treatment will delay recurrence of disease, and may improve patient survival, although many years must elapse before there can be certainty of "cure."

Clinical trials have also been carried out to establish the place of adjuvant endocrine therapy (Meakin 1980) and more recently to establish the place of antihormone therapy, particularly with tamoxifen.

The preliminary results of a number of studies have already been reported using tamoxifen as an adjuvant to primary treatment, either as a single agent or in association with chemotherapy. Of particular interest are the studies reported from Manchester by Riberio (Riberio and Palmer 1983), from Stockholm by Wallgren and Glas (1983), and a review by Mouridsen and Palshof (1983).

II. *The Nolvadex Adjuvant Trial Organization*

In the United Kingdom in 1977 a controlled trial was started to investigate the use of tamoxifen as a single adjuvant agent in the management of early breast cancer. Over the following 3½ years, 1285 patients were recruited from 37 centers. The primary treatment comprised a total mastectomy with either axillary node clearance or axillary node sampling. The eligible patients were either premenopausal with one or more histologically proven ipsilateral axillary lymph nodes or postmenopausal women aged 75 years or less with or without nodal involvement. Standard regional postoperative radiotherapy was restricted to those patients with involved axillary lymph nodes where the sampling operation alone had been used.

Patients were randomized to receive either tamoxifen 10 mg twice a day or no further treatment, the duration of trial medication being 2 years or until relapse if this occurred earlier. (The dose and duration of tamoxifen was selected empirically.) Treatment was started within 8 weeks of mastectomy and the two groups were followed up identically. The treatment used on relapse was not specified in the protocol and was left to the discretion of the participating clinicians, who were informed of the estrogen receptor status of the primary tumor, if known, at the time of relapse. Randomization between the two treatment arms was carried out centrally, checks were made to exclude prerandomization bias, compliance studies were carried out on 5% of the patients, and the events which were recorded during follow-up were the subject of medical audit.

Estrogen receptor levels were measured on 46% of the patients. The assays were conducted at seven different laboratories, all using modifications of the dextran-coated charcoal method. Exceptional care was taken to ensure as far as possible that this study was fair and unbiased.

Of the entire group, 151 patients were found to be ineligible at entry; thus 1129 patients were available for comparison, 562 treated with tamoxifen and 567 controls.

Analysis was on the basis of "intention to treat." Two separate endpoints were analyzed: the first endpoint ("an event") was the first recurrence of breast cancer including contralateral disease, or death without confirmed recurrence. The second endpoint was death alone. The log rank test was used to assess the treatment effect on both events and deaths, and the Kaplan-Meier method was used to construct life tables.

Analysis of events at a median follow-up time of 45 months revealed that 152 had occurred in the tamoxifen-treated group and 220 in the con-

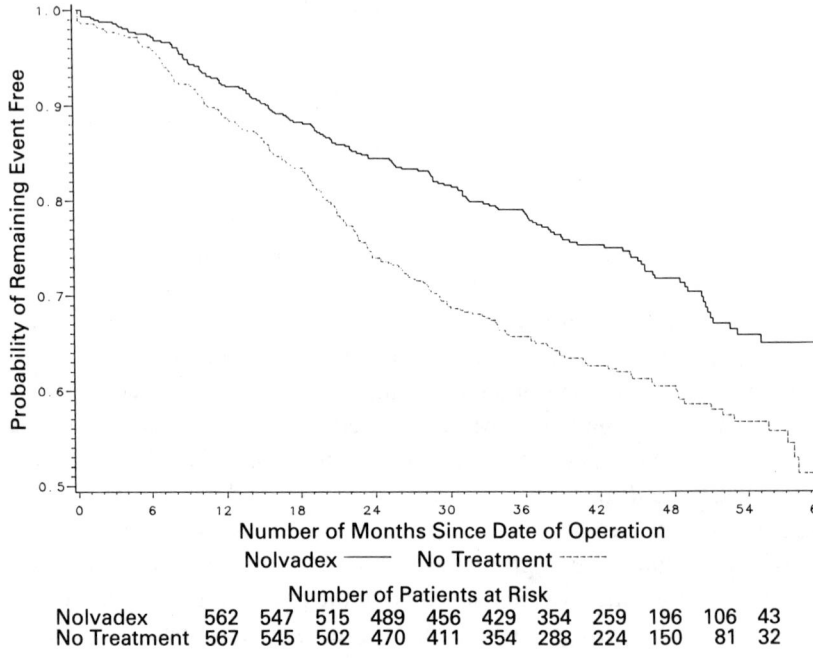

Figure 25.1. Life table for Nolvadex, showing the probability of remaining event free.

trol group. These figures showed a significant reduction in treatment failure in the tamoxifen-treated group—41% fewer events. These results are
shown in Figure 25.1 as a life table (p = 0.0001, log rank analysis).

The effect seemed to be apparent in all groups, whether premenopausal
node negative or postmenopausal node negative or positive.

Both loco-regional and distant recurrence was reduced in the treatment
groups.

Analysis of survival is shown on a life table in Figure 25.2. There were
45 fewer deaths in the tamoxifen-treated group. This reduction was statistically significant (p = 0.0019), and again, the beneficial effect of prophylactic or adjuvant tamoxifen was seen in all the subgroups.

Estrogen receptor measurements were available on 524 patients.

At a cutoff point of 5 fmol/mg cytosol protein, estrogen receptor status
was of prognostic significance in relation to survival but did not appear to
predict the effect of treatment on survival. At 30 fmol/mg cytosol protein,
the prognostic significance of estrogen receptor status was further enhanced but again the receptor status did not predict the treatment effect.

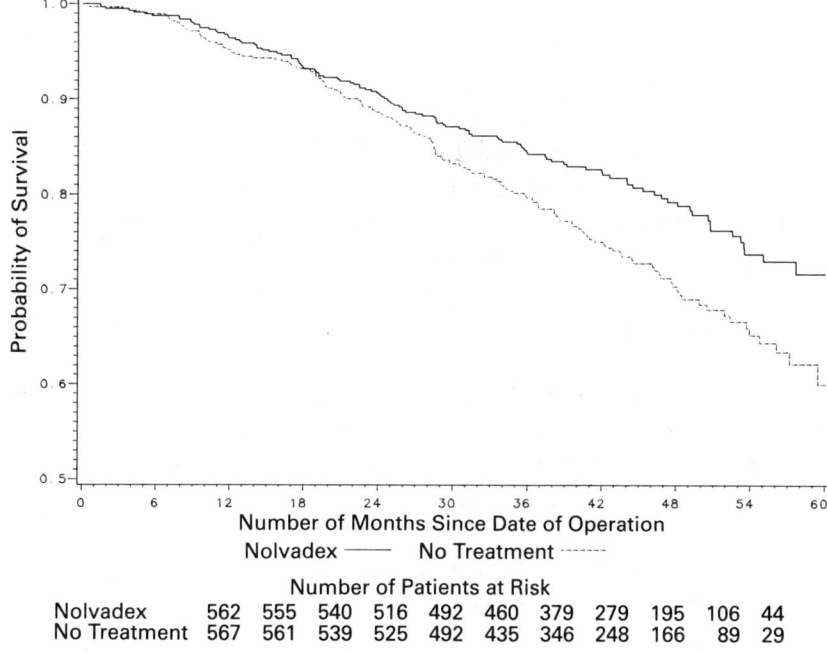

Figure 25.2. Life table for Nolvadex, showing the probability of survival.

The treatment was well tolerated with few side effects and the compliance studies showed excellent results.

III. *Implications of the Study*

The results of this study, which has become known as the NATO Trial (Baum et al. 1983) (Nolvadex Adjuvant Trial Organization), are important because they demonstrate that at a maximum follow-up time of 6 years, adjuvant tamoxifen prolongs the disease-free interval and significantly increases survival, with 34% fewer deaths observed in the treatment group than in the control group. Comparable results are reported by Riberio and Palmer (1983) and Wallgren and Glas (1983). Much can be learned from a careful study of the results of this controlled trial, and further questions become apparent.

Care must be taken in interpreting the results, as the follow-up time is still short, and the pattern of improved survival may change as time passes. Continued follow-up is essential to determine if an accelerated mortality occurs following the completion of prophylactic tamoxifen and if the postrecurrence survival time of the controls is similar to that of the treated group.

The results should be assessed in parallel with other studies and if the apparent benefits of tamoxifen are confirmed, further work will be needed to determine what dose is optimal and for how long the preparation should be taken—2 years, 5 years, indefinitely.

It is interesting that in the hands of the NATO investigation, estrogen receptors give a guide to prognosis but not to treatment response. This unexpected result has been observed in other trials.

With the development of adjuvant treatments, the detection of micro-metastases is becoming increasingly important and at the same time it will be of immense value to know whether or not a particular tumor would be sensitive to hormones and/or chemotherapy. The method of action of tamoxifen in breast cancer is still the subject of intense investigation. It seems likely that only a part of its effect is due to hormonal component and another effect may be in an alternative biological pathway (Patterson et al. 1982).

There seems little doubt that adjuvant tamoxifen used as a single agent prolongs the disease-free interval and increases the survival time in patients with breast cancer. The beneficial effects are not associated with any short-term or long-term toxicity. Because it infers benefit and is nontoxic, trials are being conducted to evaluate the effect of chemotherapy given with tamoxifen. Interpretation of the results of such trials becomes difficult, as there is as yet no clear understanding of the mechanism of action of chemotherapy in this situation and adding tamoxifen adds further uncertainties. The role of adjuvant tamoxifen in relation to adjuvant chemotherapy needs more clinical and laboratory research so that the advantages offered by this nontoxic drug can be used to maximum effect in the treatment of early breast cancer.

References

Baum, M., D. M. Brinkley, J. A. Dossett, K. McPherson, J. S. Patterson, R. D. Rubens, F. G. Smiddy, B. A. Stoll, A. Wilson, J. C. Lea, D. Richards, and S. H. Ellis. 1983. Controlled trial of tamoxifen as adjuvant agent in management of early breast cancer. *Lancet* 1:257–261.

Beatson, G. T. 1896. On the treatment of inoperable cases of carcinoma of the mamma: suggestions for a new method of treatment with illustrative cases. *Lancet* 1:104.

Brinkley, D., and J. L. Haybittle. 1984. Long-term survival of women with breast cancer. *Lancet* 1:1118.

Meakin, J. W. 1980. Ovarian irradiation and prednisone therapy following surgery for carcinoma of the breast. *European Journal of Cancer* Suppl. 1:179–181.

Mourisden, H. T., and T. Palshof. 1983. Adjuvant systemic therapy in breast cancer, a review. *European Journal of Cancer and Clinical Oncology* 19:1755–1770.

Patterson, J., B. Furr, A. Wakeling, and L. Battersby. 1982. The biology and physiology of Nolvadex (tamoxifen) in the treatment of breast cancer. *Breast Cancer Research and Treatment* 2:263–374.

Riberio, G., and M. K. Palmer. 1983. Adjuvant tamoxifen for operable carcinoma of the breast: report of clinical trial by the Christie Hospital and Holt Radium Institute. *British Medical Journal* 286:827–830.

Wallgren, A., and U. Glas. 1983. Adjuvant tamoxifen in operable breast cancer in Stockholm. *Thirteenth International Congress of Chemotherapy,* Vienna.

26

The Ludwig Breast Cancer Studies: Adjuvant Therapy for Early Breast Cancer

Franco Cavalli, Aron Goldhirsch, and Richard Gelber,

for the

Ludwig Breast Cancer Study Group

I.	Introduction	460
II.	LBCS I	460
III.	LBCS II	463
IV.	LBCS III	464
V.	Combined LBCS III and IV	465
VI.	LBCS V	466
	Ludwig Breast Cancer Study Group	467
	References	469

I. *Introduction*

Postoperative adjuvant treatment in operable breast cancer can significantly reduce the rate of disease relapse and the early mortality of breast cancer (Bonadonna et al. 1977; Fisher et al. 1977; Nissen-Meyer 1978; Howat et al. 1981; Senn et al. 1981). Multidrug regimens were apparently superior to a single-agent therapy (Howat et al. 1981; Joint BCTCS/WHO/UICC 1984). Adjuvant endocrine therapy delayed recurrence and prolonged the survival of premenopausal patients who underwent oophorectomy and received additional low-dose continuous prednisone (Meakin et al. 1979). Adjuvant endocrine therapy with tamoxifen was effective in reducing relapse rate and mortality rate in postmenopausal patients (Baum et al. 1983; NATO 1983).

In 1978 the Ludwig Breast Cancer Study Group initiated four complementary randomized controlled clinical trials to evaluate adjuvant therapy in both premenopausal and postmenopausal patients with operable breast cancer and axillary lymph node involvement. By August 1981, 1713 patients had been entered into the studies. All of the follow-up data on 1601 patients (93.5%) have been analyzed.

The studies were concerned with adjuvant treatment with chemotherapy, chemo- and endocrine therapy, or endocrine therapy alone in operable breast cancer after at least total mastectomy with axillary clearance. Post-surgery treatment was started after wound healing.

II. *LBCS I*

This trial concerned the impact of adding low-dose continuous prednisone (p) 7.5 mg daily to the adjuvant cyclophosphamide, methotrexate, and 5-fluorouracil (CMF) chemotherapy regimen in premenopausal women with 1–3 positive axillary lymph nodes. In this trial, 491 patients were evaluable (97% of the 505 patients who were randomly allocated to the two treatment arms). Of these, 241 received CMF and 250 CMF + prednisone (CMFp). Patient characteristics are described in Table 26.1.

The patients in the CMFp-treated group received significantly higher doses of CMF than did those who did not receive prednisone ($p = 0.001$

SCHEMA

	S U R G E R Y		R A N D O M	
LBCS I		Pre- & perimenopausal 1–3 N+		CMF CMFp
LBCS II	S U R G E R Y	Pre- & perimenopausal 4 or more N+	R A N D O M	CMFp Oophorectomy + CMFp
LBCS III	S U R G E R Y	Postmenopausal All N+, 65 years or less	R A N D O M	Observation CMFp + TAM p + TAM
LBCS IV	S U R G E R Y	Postmenopausal All N+, 66 years up to 80 years	R A N D O M	Observation p + TAM

C: Cyclophosphamide	100 mg/m^2 p.o., days 1–14 of each cycle	
M: Methotrexate	40 mg/m^2 i.v., days 1 & 8 of each cycle	
F: 5-Fluorouracil	600 mg/m^2 i.v., days 1 & 8 of each cycle	
p: Prednisone	7.5 mg/day p.o. (5 mg A.M., 2.5 mg P.M.)	
TAM: Tamoxifen	20 mg p.o. daily	
	CMF for 12 28-day cycles	
	p + TAM for 12 monthly cycles	

log rank analysis). On average 72% of the full CMF dose in cycles 1 to 6 was received by CMF-treated patients as compared with 83% for CMFp-treated patients. The toxic effects of the chemotherapy regimen were reported and graded for each cycle given. Fifty-two percent of the treatment cycles for the CMF group were modified because of hematological toxicity, whereas this toxicity was recorded as the reason for dose modification of only 31% of the CMFp cycles ($p < 0.0001$). However, at 48 months median follow-up, no improvement in disease-free survival (DFS) or overall survival was observed (Table 26.2).

Table 26.1. LBCS I: patient entry and characteristics

		Treatment	
	Total	CMF	CMFp
Randomized number of patients	505	250	255
Number of evaluable patients[a]	491	241	250
(% of total)	(97)	(96)	(98)
Age (%)			
≤ 39 years	24	24	24
≥ 40 years	76	76	76
Nodes (%)			
1 N+	45	43	47
2–3 N+	55	57	53
Tumor size (%)			
≤ 2 cm	48	49	47
> 2 cm	52	51	53
Hormone receptor status[b] (%)			
ER+ ≥ 10	28	27	28
ER− 0–9	24	24	24
ER unknown	48	49	48
PgR+ ≥ 10	24	23	24
PgR− 0–9	26	27	26
PgR unknown	50	50	50

[a]Reasons nonevaluable: noncompliant institutions (n = 5), tumor stage more than T_{3A} (n = 2), randomization to the wrong study on the basis of menopausal status or number of positive nodes (n = 4), previous other malignancy (n = 1), inadequate renal function (n = 1), and previous treatment for cancer (n = 1).
[b]In fmol/mg cytosol protein. ER = estrogen receptor; PgR = progesterone receptor.

Table 26.2. LBCS I: four-year results at a median follow-up time of 48 months

	Total (%)	CMF (%)	CMFp (%)	p-Value
Disease-free survival	75	77	73	0.35
Overall survival	86	86	86	0.75

Induced amenorrhea was associated with a longer DFS for younger patients, patients who received lower CMF doses, and patients with estrogen receptor–positive tumors. It is suggested that the chemotherapy regimen, with or without prednisone, may also influence tumor growth by suppression of ovarian endocrine function.

III. LBCS II

This trial studied the effect of chemotherapy with cyclophosphamide, methotrexate, 5-fluorouracil, and prednisone, with or without oophorectomy, in high-risk premenopausal patients with four or more axillary lymph nodes involved. In this trial, 327 (92%) of 356 randomized patients were evaluated. Patient characteristics are described in Table 26.3. At 48 months of median follow-up no statistically significant differences between regimens in terms of DFS or overall survival were demonstrated

Table 26.3. LBCS II: patient entry and characteristics

		Treatment	
	Total	CMFp	Oophorectomy + CMFp
Randomized number of patients	356	179	177
Number of evaluable patients[a]	327	161	166
(% of total)	(92)	(90)	(94)
Age (%)			
≤ 39 years	27	30	25
≥ 40 years	73	70	75
Nodes (%)			
4–6 N+	48	49	46
7–10 N+	24	20	29
> 10 N+	28	31	25
Hormone receptor status[b] (%)			
ER+ ≥ 10	33	28	37
ER− 0–9	28	26	31
ER unknown	39	46	32
PgR+ ≥ 10	26	26	26
PgR− 0–9	30	23	36
PgR unknown	44	51	38
ER+/PgR+	20	21	20
ER−/PgR−	21	18	24
Pathological grade[c] (%)			
1	17	14	19
2	49	50	48
3	32	31	32

[a]Reasons nonevaluable: noncompliant institutions (n = 9), patient refused treatment and follow-up (n = 3), tumor stage > T_{3A} (n = 4), randomization to the wrong study based upon menopausal status or number of positive nodes (n = 11), previous other malignancy (n = 1), low blood cell counts (n = 1).
[b]In fmol/mg cytosol protein. ER = estrogen receptor; PgR = progesterone receptor.
[c]Available for 98% of cases (8 unknown: 5 CMFp, 3 oophorectomy + CMFp).

Table 26.4. LBCS II: four-year results at a median follow-up time of 48 months

	Total (%)	CMFp (%)	Oophorectomy + CMFp (%)	p-Value
Disease-free survival	53	51	54	0.33
Overall survival	70	70	71	0.67

(Table 26.4); this was true even for patients with steroid hormone receptor–containing tumors. A high incidence of amenorrhea (89%) due to ovarian function suppression was observed for the group receiving CMFp alone. Supplementation of the adjuvant therapy regimen by surgical oophorectomy might have been rendered superfluous by this effect of cytotoxic treatment.

IV. LBCS III

This trial involved combined chemo-endocrine therapy as adjuvant treatment in postmenopausal patients with operable breast cancer and axillary nodal metastasis. In this trial, 463 (92%) of the 503 randomized patients were analyzed. The 3-year results have been extensively reported (LBCSG 1984). Patient characteristics are described in Table 26.5.

At a median follow-up of 48 months, 57/154 (37%) patients treated with CMFp + tamoxifen (TAM) failed, as did 77/153 (50%) patients who were treated with prednisone + tamoxifen (p + TAM), and 106/156 (68%) patients who did not have adjuvant treatment after mastectomy and axillary clearance. DFS was significantly longer in the patients with

Table 26.5. LBCS III: clinical details of patients

	CMFp + TAM	p + TAM	Control
Number randomized	171	164	168
Number (%) evaluable	154 (90)	153 (93)	156 (93)
Median (range) age in years	60	59	59
	(46–65)	(45–65)	(40–65)
Nodal status (%)			
N+ 1–3	58	54	55
N+ 4 or more	42	46	45
Estrogen receptor status (%)			
Positive	38	29	34
Negative	12	20	21
Unknown	50	51	45

CMFp + TAM than in patients with p + TAM or control. There were no significant differences in overall survival among the randomized groups at this point. The retrospective analysis of treatment effects in subpopulations with known steroid hormone receptor status in the primaries revealed that the DFS of the CMFp + TAM–treated and of the p + TAM–treated patients were similar for those whose tumors were estrogen receptor–positive. In patients with estrogen receptor–negative tumors, the DFS of those treated with CMFp + TAM was longer than that of patients treated with p + TAM or with mastectomy alone; the DFS of the latter two were similar.

V. Combined LBCS III and IV

The combined LBCS III and IV evaluated adjuvant endocrine therapy in postmenopausal patients treated with prednisone and tamoxifen, or with surgery alone. The data analyses on the 629 evaluable patients treated in LBCS III and IV have also been extensively reported elsewhere (LBCSG 1984). Patient entry and characteristics are described in Table 26.6. DFS was significantly longer in women who received p + TAM than in the control patients in both studies. At a median follow-up time of 48 months, 152/320 (47%) patients who received p + TAM as adjuvant treatment failed, whereas 195/309 (63%) control patients relapsed. At this point there were no significant differences in overall survival between the randomized groups. The analysis of treatment effect within subpopulations with a known hormone receptor content in the primary revealed that the

Table 26.6. LBCS III and IV: clinical details of patients

	p + TAM	Control
Number randomized	346	335
Number (%) evaluable	320 (92)	309 (92)
Median (range) age in years	66	65
	(45–80)	(40–80)
Nodal status (%)		
N+ 1–3	58	58
N+ 4 or more	42	42
Estrogen receptor status (%)		
Positive	32	32
Negative	16	16
Unknown	52	52

effect of p + TAM as adjuvant treatment was restricted to patients who had higher concentrations of estrogen receptors in their primaries. The patients with low estrogen receptor content (< 10 fmol/mg cytosol) did not benefit in terms of DFS from the endocrine adjuvant treatment.

These findings from the LBCS I, II, III, and IV are regarded as preliminary and should be substantiated by further follow-up.

VI. LBCS V

This trial, of perioperative and conventionally timed chemotherapy in operable breast cancer, has been designed to pose a biologically important question, namely, whether the timing of the start of adjuvant therapy is important in terms of averting relapses and reducing the number of deaths due to breast cancer. Two-thirds of the patients are randomized to receive perioperative chemotherapy and one-third to receive no perioperative

SCHEMA OF TRIAL V

		Therapy Assigned	
		Node-negative	Node-positive
R	Perioperative therapy[a]	None	None
A			
N			
D	Perioperative therapy[a]	None	Conventionally timed therapy[b]
O			
M	No treatment	None	Conventionally timed therapy[b]
OPERATION			

[a]*Perioperative therapy* (begun within 36 hours after mastectomy)

Cyclophosphamide	400 mg/m² i.v.	⎱
Methotrexate	40 mg/m² i.v.	⎰ days 1 & 8
5-Fluorouracil	600 mg/m² i.v.	
Leucovorin®	15 mg i.v. 24 hours after day 1 and	
	15 mg p.o. 24 hours after day 8	

[b]*Conventionally timed adjuvant therapy* (begun 25–32 days after mastectomy)

Cyclophosphamide	100 mg/m² p.o., days 1–14	
Methotrexate	40 mg/m² i.v., days 1 & 8	Every
5-Fluorouracil	600 mg/m² i.v., days 1 & 8	28 days,
Prednisone	7.5 mg p.o., daily	for six
For postmenopausal patients:		cycles
Tamoxifen also	20 mg p.o., daily	

chemotherapy, with subsequent treatment assigned according to nodal status. Node-negative patients receive no further treatment, and node-positive patients receive the treatment to which they were randomized: one-third of the latter will have been allocated to receive no treatment after the perioperative therapy, one-third of those who received no perioperative treatment will receive conventionally timed therapy for 6 months, and one-third of those who received perioperative therapy will also receive conventionally timed chemotherapy.

The objectives of the trial are to assess the value of a combination of perioperative chemotherapy and conventionally timed chemotherapy as compared with perioperative therapy alone and conventionally timed therapy alone in node-positive patients, and to assess the value of perioperative chemotherapy in patients with proven breast cancer who are classified as node-negative postsurgically.

From November 1981 until December 1985, when accrual was terminated, 2628 patients had entered the trial. In November 1982 the perioperative treatment was altered because of unpredictable and severe toxic effects of the perioperatively administered intravenous CMF regimen (LBCSG 1983). These changes were the addition of Leucovorin to the treatment, better hydration of the patients after mastectomy, and a more accurate control of the patients, including more stringent dose modification criteria. Patients older than 65 years were also excluded from entry into the trial. There has been no life-threatening toxicity due to treatment since these modifications have been in effect. The treatment results will be evaluated after all patients are off treatment.

The two generations of the Ludwig Breast Cancer Studies could provide important information about the treatment of patients with early breast cancer. Long-term follow-up, however, is needed for meaningful and definitive conclusions.

Ludwig Breast Cancer Study Group

Ludwig Institute for Cancer Research, Bern Branch, Inselspital, Bern, Switzerland
A. Goldhirsch (*Study Coordinator*), J. Stjernsward, D. Zava, V. C. Jordan;
W. Hartmann, B. Davis (*Study Pathologists*), A. Zimmermann, A. H. Baggenstoss,
M. Castiglione, C. Wiedmer
Harvard School of Public Health and Dana-Farber Cancer Institute, Boston, Mass.,
U.S.A.
R. Gelber (*Study Statistician*), K. Stanley, M. Zelen
Frontier Science & Technology Research Foundation, Buffalo, N.Y., U.S.A.
M. Isley, L. Szymoniak

Groote Schuur Hospital, Cape Town, South Africa
P. Helman, A. Hacking, A. Gudgeon, A. Tiltman, E. Dowdle
University of Essen, Cancer Research Center, Essen, West Germany
C. G. Schmidt, R. Zchaber, F. Schüning, K. Höffken, L. D. Leder, H. Ludwig, R. Callies
West Swedish Breast Cancer Study Group, Goteborg, Sweden
C.-M. Rudenstam, J. Säve-Söderbergh, E. Cahlin, C. Johnsen, J. Mattsson, H. Salander, J. O. Svensson, S. Nilsson, J. Fornander, L. Mattsson, C.-G. Bäckström, S. Bergegardh, S. Dahlin, N. Fahl, Y. Hessman, S. Holmberg, O. Ruusvik, L.-G. Niklasson, U. Ljungqvist, C. Andersson, L. Ivarsson, J. Mark, G. Ostberg, I. Dahl
The Institute of Oncology, Ljubljana, Yugoslavia
J. Lindtner, J. Novak, M. Naglas, J. Cervek, A. Vodnik, E. Majdic, P. Mavec, R. Golouh, J. Lamovec, S. Sebek, M. Sencar, B. Stabuc
The Royal Free Hospital, London, Great Britain
S. Parbhoo, K. Hobbs, E. Boessen, D. Skeggs, B. Stoll, F. Sennanyake, G. Scott, K. Griffiths
Madrid Breast Cancer Group, Madrid, Spain
H. Cortés Funes, F. Martinez Tello, F. Cruz Caro, P. L. Madrigal Alonso, I. Requena, J. Lizon, C. Cerquella, P. Espana, M. A. Figueras, M. L. Marcos, M. L. Coba, B. de Quiros, A. Lecona, M. Hall
Anti-Cancer Council of Victoria, Melbourne, Australia
I. Russell, M. A. Schwarz, R. Bennett, W. I. Burns, G. Brodie, J. Colebatch, J. Collins, J. Forbes, J. Funder, E. Guli, P. Jeal, P. Kitchen, R. Reed, L. Sisely, R. Snyder, A. Shaw
SAKK (Swiss Group for Clinical Cancer Research)
Bern, Inselspital
K. Brunner, H. Cottier, R. Joss, G. Locher, M. Walther, E. Dreher, U. Herrmann, P. Herrmann
St. Gallen, Kantonsspital
W. F. Jungi, A. Mutzner, U. Schmid, H. J. Senn
Bellinzona, Ospedale San Giovanni
F. Cavalli, P. Luscieti, G. Losa, L. Passega, H. Neuenschwander
Zürich, Kantonsspital
G. Martz, J. R. Rüttner, H. Sulsen, M. Makek
Neuchatel, Hôpital des Cadolles
P. Siegenthaler, R. P. Baumann
Basel, Kantonsspital
J. P. Obrecht, F. Harder, A. Almendral, J. Torhorst, U. Eppenberger
Ludwig Institute for Cancer Research, and Royal Prince Alfred Hospital, Sydney, Australia
M. Tattersall, R. Fox, R. Wood, D. Hedley, D. Glenn, F. Niesche, R. West, S. Renwick, D. Green, J. Donovan, P. Duval, T. Jelihovsky, A. Ng, A. Coates
Wellington Hospital, Wellington, New Zealand
J. S. Simpson, E. C. Watson, C. T. Collins, A. J. Gray, J. W. Logan, J. J. Landreth, W. Brander, P. Cairney, L. Hollaway, I. M. Holdaway, C. Unsworth

References

Baum, M., D. M. Brinkley, J. A. Dossett, K. McPherson, J. S. Patterson, R. D. Rubens, F. G. Smiddy, B. A. Stoll, A. Wilson, J. C. Lea, D. Richards, and S. H. Ellis. 1983. Improved survival among patients treated with adjuvant tamoxifen after mastectomy for early breast cancer. *Lancet* 2:450.

Bonadonna, G., A. Rossi, T. Valagussa, A. Banfi, and U. Veronesi. 1977. The CMF program for operable breast cancer with positive axillary nodes. *Cancer* 39:2904–2915.

Fisher, B., A. Glass, C. Redmond, E. Fisher, B. Barton, E. Such, P. Carbone, S. Economou, R. Foster, R. Frelick, H. Lerner, M. Levitt, R. Margolese, J. MacFarlane, D. Plotkin, H. Shibata, H. Volkand, and other cooperating investigators. 1977. L-phenylalanine mustard (L-PAM) in the management of primary breast cancer. *Cancer* 39:2883–2903.

Howat, J. M. T., R. Hughes, and P. Durning. 1981. A controlled clinical trial of adjuvant chemotherapy in operable cancer of the breast. In *Adjuvant therapy of cancer III*, ed. S. E. Salmon and S. E. Jones, 371–376. New York: Grune and Stratton.

Joint BCTCS/WHO/UICC. 1984. Overview of mortality results in randomized trials in early breast cancer. *Lancet* 2:1205.

Ludwig Breast Cancer Study Group (LBCSG). 1983. Toxic effects of early adjuvant chemotherapy for breast cancer. *Lancet* 2:542–544.

Ludwig Breast Cancer Study Group (LBSCG). 1984. Randomized trial of chemo-endocrine therapy, endocrine therapy, and mastectomy alone in postmenopausal patients with operable breast cancer and axillary node metastasis. *Lancet* 1:1256–1260.

Meakin, J. W., W. E. C. Allt, F. A. Beale, T. C. Brown, R. S. Bush, R. M. Clark, P. J. Fitzpatrick, N. V. Hawkins, R. D. Jenkin, J. F. Pringle, J. G. Reid, W. D. Rider, J. L. Hayward, and R. D. Bulbrook. 1979. Ovarian irradiation and prednisone following surgery and radiotherapy for carcinoma of the breast. *Canadian Medical Association Journal* 120:1221–1231.

Nissen-Meyer, R., K. Kjellgren, K. Malmio, B. Mansson, and T. Norin. 1978. Surgical adjuvant chemotherapy: results with one short course with cyclophosphamide after mastectomy for breast cancer. *Cancer* 41:2088–2098.

Nolvadex Adjuvant Trial Organization (NATO). 1983. Controlled trial of tamoxifen as adjuvant agent in management of early breast cancer. *Lancet* 1:257–261.

Senn, H. J., W. F. Jungi, and R. Amgwerd. 1981. Chemoimmunotherapy with LMF plus BCG in node-negative and node-positive breast cancer. In *Adjuvant therapy of cancer, III*, ed. S. E. Salmon and S. E. Jones, 385–390. New York: Grune and Stratton.

27

Adjuvant Tamoxifen and Chemotherapy in Stage II Breast Cancer: Interim Findings from NSABP Protocol B-09

NORMAN WOLMARK AND BERNARD FISHER

I. INTRODUCTION 472
II. METHODS 472
III. RESULTS 473
   A. DISEASE-FREE SURVIVAL AND SURVIVAL REGARDLESS OF TUMOR
      RECEPTOR STATUS 473
   B. DISEASE-FREE SURVIVAL RELATIVE TO QUANTITATIVE ER STATUS 474
IV. DISCUSSION 478
V. SUMMARY 481
   REFERENCES 482

I. *Introduction*

In 1977 the National Surgical Adjuvant Breast and Bowel Project (NSABP) initiated a randomized prospective clinical trial (protocol B-09) in order to address the propriety of adding tamoxifen to chemotherapy in women with primary operable breast cancer and histologically positive axillary nodes. Between January 1977 and May 1980, 1891 patients were randomized to receive adjuvant chemotherapy consisting of L-phenyl-alanine mustard (L-PAM) and 5-fluorouracil (5-FU) with and without tamoxifen. This effort represented a component part of a continuum of protocols in which the efficacy of adjuvant therapy was addressed in stage II breast cancer. The selection of the chemotherapeutic agents employed as well as the decision not to utilize tamoxifen without chemotherapy was directly based on the results of the three previous NSABP chemotherapy trials reviewed elsewhere in this volume. These latter studies indicated that adjuvant chemotherapy with L-PAM-containing combinations resulted in the prolongation of disease-free survival and survival in specific patient subsets. The comparison of L-PAM with a placebo disclosed a benefit in patients ≤ 49 years of age, particularly those with 1–3 positive nodes; the addition of 5-fluorouracil to L-PAM (PF) resulted in a transient increment in disease-free survival for patients ≥ 50 years of age with ≥ 4 positive nodes. The initiation of protocol B-09 was therefore conducted on a background that had demonstrated that PF could alter the natural history of breast cancer. Accordingly, the PF combination provided a logical base-line upon which the effect of tamoxifen could be assessed. The data analyzed at 2 and 3 years have indicated that the consequences of adding tamoxifen to PF were dependent on patient age as well as on hormone receptor status (Fisher et al. 1981, 1983). The data presented in this review are derived from a mean time on study of 50 months.

II. *Methods*

The details of the protocol design, patient characteristics, therapeutic regimens, and statistical analyses employed have been presented in earlier NSABP publications. Women with one or more histologically positive axillary nodes who had a mastectomy and axillary node dissection were eligible for this study (protocol B-09) provided they fulfilled specific criteria identical to those used in previous NSABP trials of adjuvant therapy (Fisher et al. 1975). Patients were stratified according to age ($\leq$ 49 years and $\geq$ 50 years) and number of positive nodes (1–3 and $\geq$ 4 nodes). Tumor estrogen receptor (ER) values were a prerequisite for entry on study shortly after its inception; the requirement for a progesterone receptor (PgR) value was added following the first year of patient accrual.

There were 1891 patients randomized to either PF or PFT (with tamoxifen) between January 1, 1977, and May 16, 1980; 1862 (98.5%) were eligible for the study. The mean time on study for patients is 50 months (range of 33–73 months).

Tumor specimens were assayed for both ER and PgR utilizing the sucrose density gradient, dextran-coated charcoal titration with Scatchard analysis, or dextran-coated charcoal with a single saturating dose; all receptor values are reported in fmol/mg of cytosol protein.

L-PAM was administered at a dose of 4 mg/m^2 for the first 5 days of each cycle; 5-FU (300 mg/m^2) was given intravenously on each of the same 5 days. Each cycle was repeated every 6 weeks for a total of 17 times (approximately 2 years). The dose of tamoxifen in the PFT treatment group was 10 mg by mouth twice a day for the entire 2 years of therapy. Treatment was commenced within 2–4 weeks following operation. Doses were modified according to the presence and degree of hematological and gastrointestinal toxicity.

The statistical significance of the differences between the life-table distributions by treatment was determined by a summary chi square (log rank) test adjusted for the number of positive nodes (Mantel 1966; Cox 1972; Peto and Peto 1972). All p values given are related to a two-sided test of significance.

III. *Results*

A. DISEASE-FREE SURVIVAL AND SURVIVAL REGARDLESS OF TUMOR RECEPTOR STATUS

The assessment of tamoxifen efficacy in this study was not restricted to patients whose tumors contained estrogen and progesterone receptor. In fact, since the initial aims of this study specifically did not include any restrictions on tumor receptor status, it became mandatory to first analyze

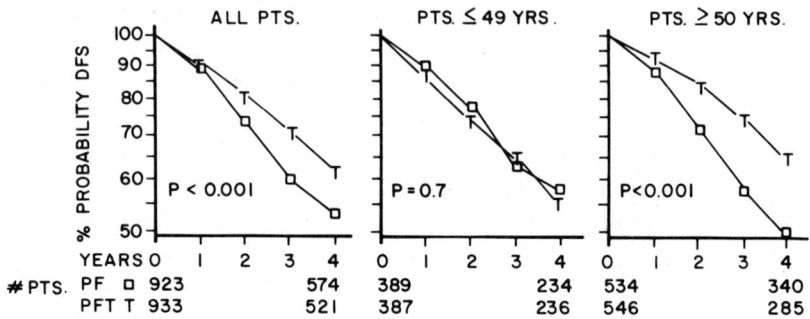

Figure 27.1. Disease-free survival according to age without regard for tumor estrogen receptor status.

the data according to traditional patient subsets without regard for tumor receptor content.

Examination of disease-free survival for all patients irrespective of age and the number of positive nodes disclosed a significant prolongation when tamoxifen was added to PF ($p = 0.0001$, Fig. 27.1). Further analysis according to age demonstrated a disparate response, in that patients ≥ 50 years of age benefitted from tamoxifen ($p < 0.001$), whereas women ≤ 49 years of age appeared to be resistant. Subdivision of the ≥ 50-year cohort according to the number of positive nodes indicated that the largest increment in disease-free survival occurred in the ≥ 4 positive nodes subset ($p < 0.0001$, Fig. 27.2). Thus, the benefit attributed to tamoxifen for all patients without regard for receptor status was derived exclusively from the contribution of women ≥ 50 years, particularly if they had ≥ 4 positive nodes. The disease-free survival benefit noted in women ≥ 50 years with ≥ 4 positive nodes has been translated into a significant prolongation in actual survivorship (Fig. 27.3, $p = 0.03$).

B. DISEASE-FREE SURVIVAL RELATIVE TO QUANTITATIVE ER STATUS

Examination of disease-free survival according to quantitative tumor estrogen receptor content indicated that no benefit for tamoxifen was observed in patients whose tumor estrogen receptors were < 10 fmol (data not shown).

The results were then evaluated according to quantitative tumor estrogen receptor content irrespective of age and nodal status. There appeared to be a relationship between the degree of estrogen receptor positivity and

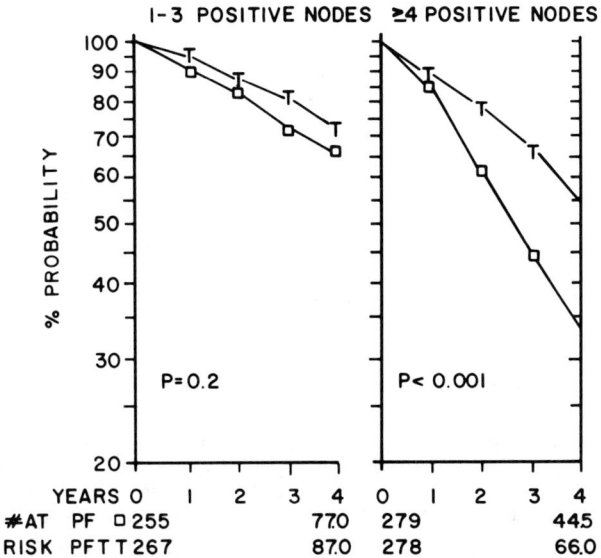

Figure 27.2. Disease-free survival regardless of receptor status according to the number of positive nodes in women ≥ 50 years of age.

the benefit attributable to the addition of tamoxifen to chemotherapy (Fig. 27.4); highly significant differences in disease-free survival were demonstrable for tumor estrogen receptor levels ≥ 10 fmol. Had the analysis been stopped at this juncture, it would have been possible to erroneously conclude that the addition of tamoxifen to PF resulted in a prolongation in disease-free survival for all positive-node patients with tumor estrogen

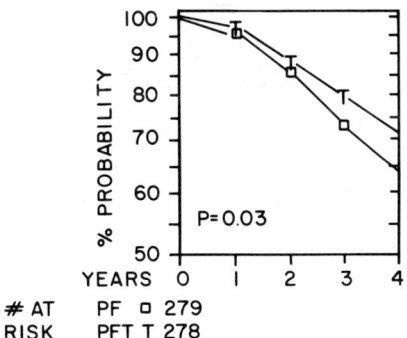

Figure 27.3. Survival regardless of receptor status in women ≥ 50 years of age with ≥ 4 positive nodes.

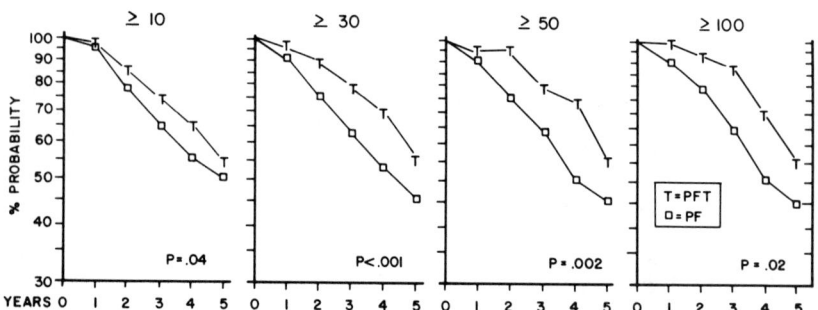

Figure 27.4. Disease-free survival according to quantitative tumor estrogen receptor content—all patients.

receptors ≥ 10 fmol regardless of age. As a consequence of the results obtained from the previous NSABP studies, it is apparent that the presentation of data for "all" patients obscures the heterogeneous response to chemotherapy. When the tamoxifen data were analyzed according to patient age and quantitative ER, once again, a marked heterogeneous response to the addition of tamoxifen was encountered. Women ≤ 49 years

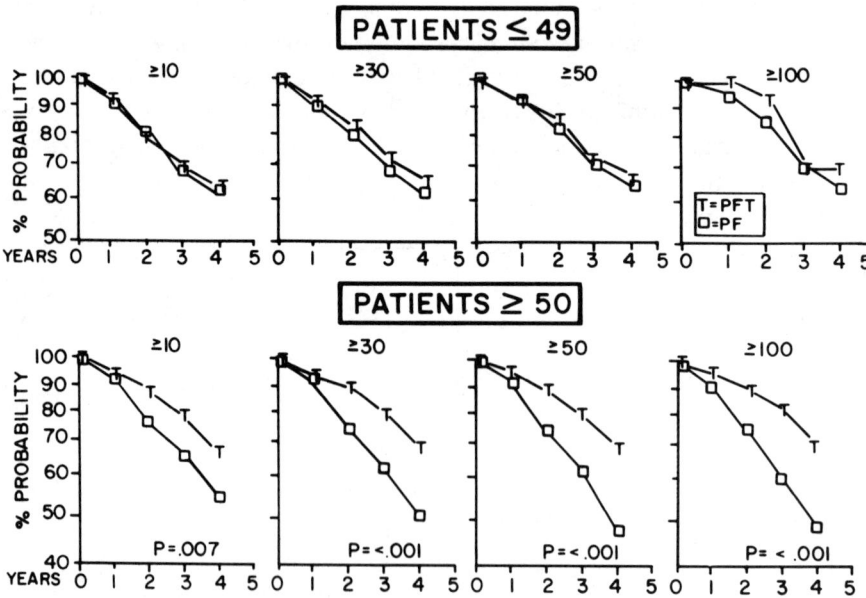

Figure 27.5. Disease-free survival according to age and quantitative tumor estrogen receptor content.

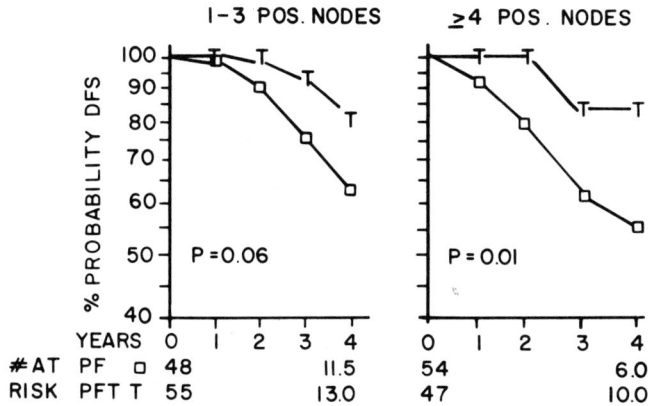

Figure 27.6. Disease-free survival in women ≥ 50 years of age with tumor estrogen receptor ≥ 50 fmol according to the number of positive nodes.

of age failed to benefit from the addition of tamoxifen even if the tumor ER content was ≥ 100 fmol/mg (Fig. 27.5). It became evident that the prolongation in disease-free survival noted for all receptor-positive patients was derived exclusively from women ≥ 50 years of age where highly significant differences were apparent; these differences have not as yet been translated into a survival advantage. Further examination of the cohort of patients ≥ 50 years according to the number of positive nodes indicated that the tamoxifen benefit was present in both the 1–3 and ≥ 4 positive node subsets but was more impressive in the latter group (Fig. 27.6).

The subset characterized by women ≥ 50 with ≥ 4 positive nodes provided an opportunity to assess the effect of tamoxifen according to location of treatment failure (Fig. 27.7). There was a significant diminution in both local and distant treatment failure as a result of the addition of tamoxifen. Since the incidence of regional disease was small with PF alone, it is not surprising that an improvement could not be detected with the addition of tamoxifen.

When the same analyses were carried out using progesterone receptor levels instead of estrogen receptor, similar results were obtained (data not shown).

This study was also instructive in underscoring the potential dangers of the injudicious application of adjuvant therapy. In contrast to the benefit achieved by tamoxifen, there was also observed an unanticipated negative influence. It was previously pointed out that women ≤ 49 years of age

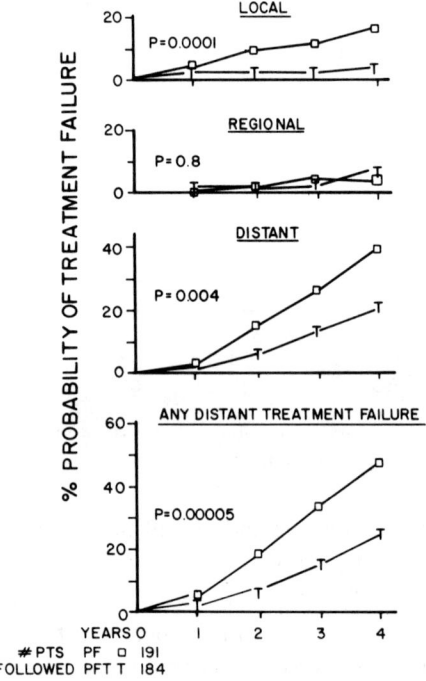

Figure 27.7. Effect of tamoxifen according to site of first treatment failure in patients ≥ 50 years of age and tumor estrogen receptor ≥ 50 fmol.

failed to benefit from the addition of tamoxifen to PF chemotherapy regardless of receptor level. If tamoxifen was administered to patients ≤ 49 years whose tumor progesterone receptors were < 10 fmol, not only did these patients not benefit from tamoxifen but there was a significant decrease in disease-free survival and survival when compared to similar patients receiving only PF (Fig. 27.8). This negative effect did not reduce disease-free survival and survival to levels below those documented in patients not treated with *any* adjuvant therapy, but the addition of tamoxifen to this group appeared to attenuate the beneficial response observed with chemotherapy.

IV. Discussion

These results indicate that the addition of tamoxifen to PF can prolong disease-free survival over and above that noted with PF alone. The re-

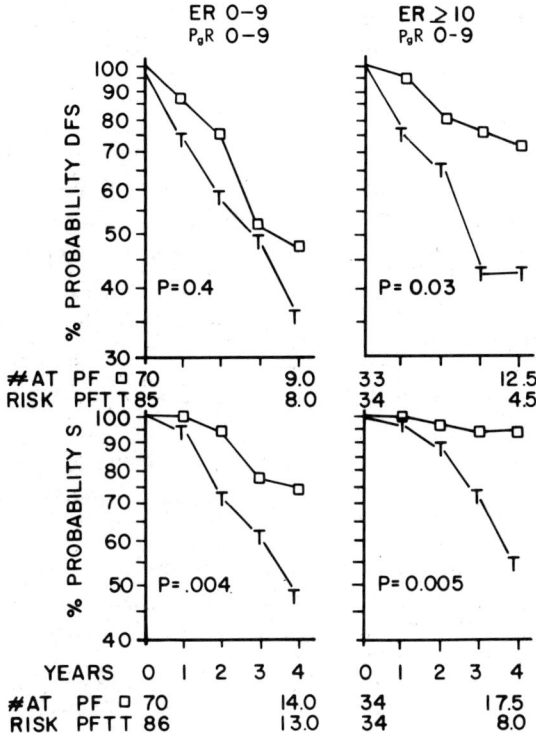

Figure 27.8. Disease-free survival and overall survival in women ≤ 49 years of age according to tumor estrogen and progesterone receptor status.

sponse to tamoxifen was not uniform and the benefit observed when all patients were evaluated was contributed exclusively by women ≥ 50 years of age and was associated with tumor ER and PgR content. In this latter group (≥ 50 years), as the tumor quantitative ER level increased there appeared to be a corresponding decrease in the incidence of treatment failure. This was true in both the 1–3 and ≥ 4 positive node categories. When the data were examined without regard for tumor receptor status, the disease-free survival advantage attributable to tamoxifen in women ≥ 50 years of age with ≥ 4 positive nodes was translated into an actual survival benefit.

The failure of women ≤ 49 years of age to respond to the addition of tamoxifen to chemotherapy is noteworthy. When tamoxifen was added to chemotherapy in patients ≤ 49 years with tumor PgR < 10 fmol, not only was no benefit observed but a significant decrease in disease-free survival and survival was apparent. This negative effect underscores the dangers of abstracting the seemingly attractive features of various protocols solely on the basis of intuitive perception and synthesizing a regimen that has not been adequately tested.

Despite the negative effects of tamoxifen in younger patients with negative receptors, it is essential that the beneficial response be placed into perspective. The data at 3 (Fisher et al. 1983) and at 4 years continue to corroborate the 2-year results initially published in 1981 (Fisher et al. 1981). The prolongation in disease-free survival, albeit limited to women ≥ 50 years of age, is still amongst the most impressive positive effects thus far documented in the NSABP adjuvant therapy experience. The data underscore the heterogeneous response to PFT, recapitulating previous observations with adjuvant chemotherapy alone. This phenomenon may be unique to the PFT combination, or it may be an intrinsic biological property of stage II breast cancer; further investigation is needed to determine this point.

In order to place the effect of tamoxifen into perspective, it may be of some value to review the NSABP cumulative observations with the first generation of adjuvant therapy trials (Table 27.1). If one selects PF as being illustrative of responsiveness to chemotherapy, it is evident that those women ≤ 49 years of age demonstrate the greatest sensitivity to adjuvant chemotherapy. Of this group, patients with 1–3 positive nodes are most responsive. In contrast there was a small benefit noted in women ≥ 50 years of age, which was derived exclusively from patients with ≥ 4 positive nodes. The addition of tamoxifen to PF failed to improve on the prolongation in disease-free survival noted in the group most sensitive to chemotherapy, namely, patients ≤ 49 years. On the contrary, those women that were relatively resistant to PF, women ≥ 50 years, sustained the greatest benefit from the addition of tamoxifen.

Table 27.1. NSABP cumulative PF experience

	PF	PFT
≤ 49 years	+ + +	−
1–3 nodes	+ + +	−
≥ 4 nodes	−	−
≥ 50 years	+	+ + +
1–3 nodes	−	+ +
≥ 4 nodes	+	+ + +

The data give rise to a number of questions that address the activity of tamoxifen. The adverse effects of tamoxifen in young patients with receptor-poor tumors and the lack of an effect in young patients with positive receptors may be a result of tamoxifen-induced alteration in metabolism of PF. Thus in younger patients PFT may have had no effect because the advantage of chemotherapy observed in this group was nullified. If this theory is relevant, then it would be of interest to determine whether tamoxifen administration alone or tamoxifen sequenced with chemotherapy would have resulted in a benefit. The beneficial effect of tamoxifen in older patients also leads to further questions. If the addition of tamoxifen to a chemotherapeutic regimen of limited efficacy in women ≥ 50 years of age resulted in a substantial benefit, could this benefit have been achieved with tamoxifen alone? Because the chemotherapy effect was of limited magnitude in this group, any putative interference with chemotherapy metabolism by tamoxifen would not be enough to defeat the overall tamoxifen advantage observed. The propriety of administering tamoxifen alone or tamoxifen together with chemotherapy is a theme being explored in the current generation of NSABP protocols. A major study now underway, NSABP protocol B-14, is limited to node-negative receptor-positive patients and randomizes women to tamoxifen or placebo; it has thus far accrued over 900 patients. The results will no doubt contribute to the elucidation of the role of tamoxifen as a single agent.

V. *Summary*

Data are presented from a prospective clinical trial in which 1891 patients with histologically confirmed stage II breast cancer were randomized to receive adjuvant therapy consisting of L-phenylalanine mustard (L-PAM) and 5-fluorouracil (5-FU) with and without tamoxifen (T). The findings indicate that the benefit previously noted for the addition of tamoxifen at 2 and 3 years mean follow-up time is still apparent at 4 years. Although the tamoxifen-containing regimen prolongs disease-free survival and overall survival, this effect is not uniform and is dependent upon patient age and tumor receptor content. Only those patients ≥ 50 years of age demonstrated a benefit from the addition of tamoxifen to chemotherapy. The benefit was influenced by the degree of quantitative tumor receptor content. Patients ≤ 49 years of age failed to demonstrate a prolongation in disease-free survival with tamoxifen, even when the tumor estrogen receptor content was > 100 fmol. Not only was there no benefit attributable to tamoxifen in patients ≤ 49 years, if the tumor progesterone receptors were < 10 fmol there was a signification diminution in disease-free survival and overall survival. The results continue to indicate that the response to PFT therapy is heterogeneous, in that only specific patient subsets demonstrate a salutary effect. Whether this phenomenon of heterogeneity is unique to the PFT combination or is an intrinsic biological property of stage II breast cancer remains to be ascertained.

Acknowledgments

Supported by Public Health Service grants from the National Cancer Institute (NCI U10-CA-12027 and NCI U10-CA-34211) and by a grant from the American Cancer Society (ACS-RC-13).

References

Cox, D. R. 1972. Regression models and life-tables. *Journal of the Royal Statistical Society* (B) 34:187–220.

Fisher, B., P. Carbone, S. G. Economou, R. Frelick, A. Glass, H. Lerner, C. Redmond, M. Zelen, P. Band, D. L. Katrych, N. Wolmark, E. R. Fisher, and other cooperating investigators. 1975. L-phenylalanine mustard (L-PAM) in the management of primary breast cancer: a report of early findings. *New England Journal of Medicine* 292:117–122.

Fisher, B., C. Redmond, A. Brown, N. Wolmark, J. Wittliff, E. R. Fisher, D. Plotkin, S. Sachs, J. Wolter, R. Frelick, R. Desser, N. LiCalzi, P. Geggie, T. Campbell, E. G. Elias, D. Prager, P. Koontz, H. Volk, N. Dimitrov, B. Gardner, H. Lerner, H. Shibata, and other NSABP investigators. 1981. Treatment of primary breast cancer with chemotherapy and tamoxifen. *New England Journal of Medicine* 305:1–6.

Fisher, B., C. Redmond, A. Brown, D. L. Wickerham, N. Wolmark, J. Allegra, G. Escher, M. Lippman, E. Savlov, J. Wittliff, and E. R. Fisher, with the contributions of D. Plotkin, D. Bowman, J. Wolter, R. Bornstein, R. Desser, R. Frelick, and other NSABP investigators. 1983. Influence of tumor estrogen and progesterone receptor levels on the response to tamoxifen and chemotherapy in primary breast cancer. *Journal of Clinical Oncology* 1:227–241.

Mantel, N. 1966. Evaluation of survival data and two new rank order statistics arising in its consideration. *Cancer Chemotherapy Reports* 50:163–170.

Peto, R., and J. Peto, 1972. Asymptomatically efficient rank invariant test procedures. *Journal of the Royal Statistical Society* (A) 135:185–206.

28

Breast Cancer 1984: Role of Tamoxifen

PAUL P. CARBONE

I.	INTRODUCTION	484
II.	MINIMAL SURGERY	485
III.	ADJUVANT THERAPY	485
IV.	IMPACT OF THERAPY IN METASTATIC DISEASE	488
V.	TAMOXIFEN AND HORMONAL THERAPY	490
VI.	FUTURE ISSUES WITH TAMOXIFEN	491
VII.	TAMOXIFEN AND PREVENTION OF BREAST CANCER	492
VIII.	HORMONE RECEPTORS AND BREAST CANCER	493
IX.	SUMMARY	494
	REFERENCES	495

483

I. Introduction

B̲REAST cancer is the number 1 cause of deaths from cancer in women between the ages of 35 and 55. In 1984, 40,000 deaths in the United States were attributable to this disease. Over the past 50 years the overall mortality due to breast cancer has not changed dramatically (Silverberg 1984). Because of these gloomy figures, one should ask, "Are there rays of hope indicating we are making progress in our knowledge or therapy of this disease?"

In this chapter I would like to present a clinical perspective of where we are now in the management of breast cancer, stressing the role of Nolvadex (tamoxifen). In this discussion, I would propose that although the advances in knowledge and therapy may not have improved survival, they have resulted in a better quality of life for more women.

Over the past 20 years, in my opinion there have been four major advances in the management of breast cancer (Table 28.1). First, the domination of radical surgery as the most common primary treatment of breast cancer has been supplanted by the acceptance and use of less extensive surgery with resultant improved functional status and increased acceptance by the patient. Second, we have seen the introduction of modern postoperative adjuvant therapy based on the realization that a high probability of recurrence can be predicted and that chemotherapy after surgery may eliminate micrometastases. Third, the antiestrogen tamoxifen has become the first-line endocrine-therapy, supplanting ablative endocrine surgery and additive hormonal therapy for a large segment of metastatic breast cancers. This widespread acceptance of tamoxifen is undoubtedly due to its relative lack of side effects as well as its effectiveness. Fourth, the widespread use of laboratory methodology to measure hormone receptors has not only increased our knowledge of the biology of the disease

Table 28.1. Major clinical advances in past 20 years

Acceptance of minimal surgery
Use of adjuvant therapy
Use of tamoxifen (Nolvadex)
Hormone receptors

but also has enhanced the prognostic and therapeutic implications of the receptor content of the tumor.

II. *Minimal Surgery*

Although the movement away from the radical Halsted mastectomy has markedly decreased the morbidity associated with primary treatment, it has not improved the mortality. The use of segmental mastectomy or tumorectomy with postoperative radiation has become more common. While the minimal surgery results in preservation of normal-looking breasts, the modified mastectomy is still the most common primary operation. At the University of Wisconsin Hospital and Clinics, only 10–15% of women elect minimal surgery. We see less limitation of motion of the shoulder and less arm swelling with the modified mastectomy operation, and the patient also feels more normal and less restricted in her options for clothing and physical activity.

III. *Adjuvant Therapy*

Breast cancer presents primarily as localized disease, clinically restricted to the breast or regional lymph nodes (Vana et al. 1981). However, the impact of nodal status on prognosis, recurrence of breast cancer, and eventual mortality in those women with positive nodes is well known (Fisher et al. 1983). Beginning with the ECOG-NSABP trials with L-PAM (Fisher et al. 1975) and the studies of the National Cancer Institute of Milan (Bonadonna et al. 1976), the use of long-term postoperative chemotherapy has been employed in many countries and studies. The ultimate goal of these adjuvant studies, namely the cure of significantly more patients with breast cancer, has not been clearly achieved, but I believe we have made some progress (Table 28.2). Results of these protocols are presented in other chapters in this volume.

Several important concepts appear to be emerging from these adjuvant studies. First, the use of minimal chemotherapy, i.e., low-dose, single-agent treatment, has little impact on disease-free survival or mortality except in a single subset of patients, namely, premenopausal and with 1–3 positive nodes (Fisher et al. 1977). Second, there are suggestions that the duration of cytotoxic therapy to achieve a benefit need not be extended

Table 28.2. Impact of therapy

Stage	Modality	Survival		Reference
		5 years (%)	10 years (%)	
I	Surgery	82	76	Vana et al. 1981
II	Surgery	48	30	Bonadonna and Valagussa 1985
	Surgery + chemotherapy	58	47	Bonadonna and Valagussa 1985
	Surgery + tamoxifen	65	—	Mouridsen et al. 1984
III	Surgery	25	—	
	Surgery + chemotherapy + x-ray therapy	45	—	Loprinzi et al. 1984

beyond 4–6 months (Tancini et al. 1983). Third, the content of estrogen receptor in the primary tumor may not only be of prognostic value, but is also important in selecting the use of hormonal adjuvant therapy (Clark et al. 1983).

There are still many questions that need to be answered. Most important, the use of tamoxifen in postmenopausal patients clearly may be as effective as adjuvant chemotherapy (Carbone 1977; Fisher et al. 1981; Baum and NATO 1983). Another important finding has been the effectiveness of prednisone plus oophorectomy (Meakin et al. 1983) and prednisone plus tamoxifen as adjuvant therapies (Gelber 1984; Goldhirsch 1984).

Additional issues that need to be addressed in future studies are shown in Table 28.3. In the past we have been inclined to believe that the average tumor burdens in stage I and the 1–3 node-positive stage III group were small. Therefore, we tended to use less aggressive therapy in these patients. Skipper has published an interesting series of data (Figs. 28.1, 28.2) that suggest that although the *average* tumor burden for a stage I patient is less than for stage II or III patients, the actual residual burden in a patient destined to fail is actually not much different in the various stages (Skipper 1982). This fact suggests that to develop strategies that assume lesser tumor burdens for stage I patients may be misleading. Instead we

Table 28.3. Primary disease: future problems

Selecting out cures
Determining optimal therapy
Defining duration of therapy

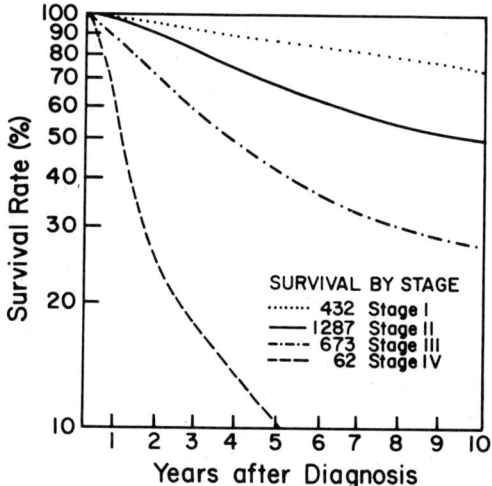

Figure 28.1. Survival of breast cancer patients according to stage, including cures.

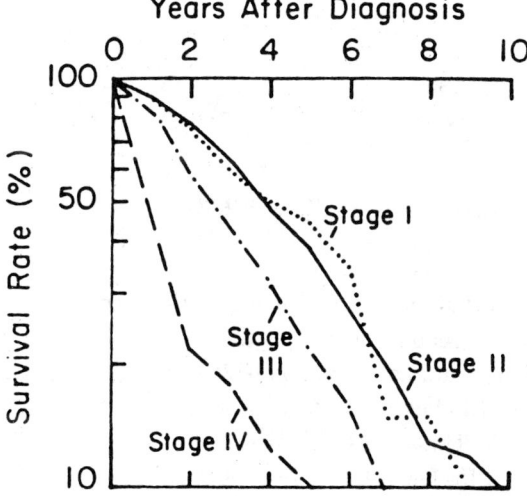

Figure 28.2. Survival of breast cancer patients by stage, excluding 10-year survivors.

need to devise specific methods to estimate tumor burden in individual patients (Carbone 1977). Based on our current concepts it is also obvious that the optimal adjuvant chemotherapy still needs to be defined. Again, in my opinion, we are probably underutilizing, in most adjuvant therapies, the most effective agent against breast cancer, namely adriamycin.

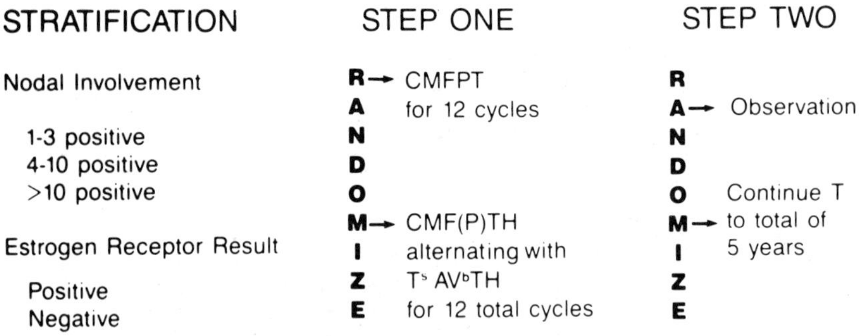

STRATIFICATION
STEP ONE
STEP TWO
Nodal Involvement
1-3 positive
4-10 positive
>10 positive
Estrogen Receptor Result
Positive
Negative
RANDOMIZE
CMFPT for 12 cycles
CMF(P)TH alternating with T^{s} $AV^{b}TH$ for 12 total cycles
RANDOMIZE
Observation
Continue T to total of 5 years

Figure 28.3. Schema showing treatment in ECOG study 5181 for premenopausal women.

STRATIFICATION
Nodal Involvement
1-3 positive
4-10 positive
>10 positive
Estrogen Receptor Result
Positive
Negative
RANDOMIZE
CMFPT × 12 cycles + continuous TAM to a total of 5 years
CMFPT for 12 cycles + Observation
CMFPT × 4 cycles + Observation

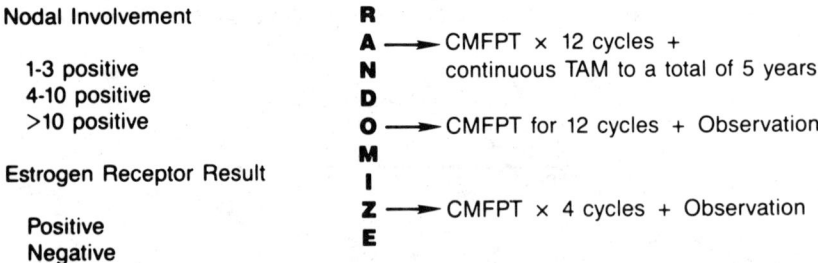

Figure 28.4. Schema showing treatment in ECOG study 4181 for postmenopausal women.

Another important clinical challenge is to determine the optimal duration of treatment. Much has been said about the duration of chemotherapy, but until recently little attention has been paid to the length of treatment with tamoxifen. Studies by Jordan in the laboratory (Jordan et al. 1980) and Tormey at the University of Wisconsin Hospital and Clinics in Madison (Tormey and Jordan 1984) have suggested rather strongly that tamoxifen should be continued almost indefinitely. This is being done in two current ECOG studies (5181 and 4181) (Figs. 28.3, 28.4) (Carbone and Tormey 1984).

IV. *Impact of Therapy in Metastatic Disease*

The therapies that are currently being used in patients with metastatic breast cancer are shown in Table 28.4. The options are surprisingly simple

Table 28.4. Metastatic disease: current therapies, 1984

	Estrogen receptor–positive	Estrogen receptor–negative
Premenopausal	Oophorectomy + chemotherapy (?) Chemotherapy	Chemotherapy
Postmenopausal	Tamoxifen Chemotherapy + tamoxifen (?)	Chemotherapy

Table 28.5. Metastatic disease: impact of therapy, 1984

Modality	Number of patients	Percent response	Percent complete response	Time to treatment failure (median months)	Survival (median months)	Reference
Chemotherapy	1617	47	15	8.5	16.3	Bonadonna and Valagussa 1983
Tamoxifen	461	42	—	5–13	—	Furr and Jordan 1984
Chemohormono-therapy	26	92	77	13	22	Tormey et al. 1985

Table 28.6. Metastatic disease: future problems

Increase disease control to maximize duration of control:
Hormones
Modest chemotherapy
Increase disease control by maximal therapy:
High-intensity
Rotating combinations
X-ray therapy to disease sites
Retreatment
Better definition of hormone refractoriness

when looked at in generic terms such as chemotherapy (CT) or hormonal therapy. If we examine the impact of therapy in terms of responses and complete responses (CR), we see good response rates, and even dramatic effects using intensive combinations (Table 28.5). However, when measured in terms of time to treatment failure or survival, we see relatively modest effects. The future challenges that need to be met in the treatment of metastatic breast cancer are shown in Table 28.6.

The first question that a clinician or clinical investigator must consider is whether the objective in treating breast cancer patients is to control the disease and maximize *quality of life* or to aim for maximal therapy with a hope of *achieving long-term cure*. Obviously, in the usual clinical practice situation the former usually prevails as the objective. In the research setting with good, well-designed protocols, one can aim to increase the CR rate and the overall survival. This would involve a variety of strategies shown in Table 28.6.

Finally, more research needs to be done to define hormonal refractoriness. An important clinical fact is that response to one hormonal maneuver after failure of the hormonal therapy will predict for a second hormonal therapy. The mechanism of resistance to the first hormone is unlikely to be due to loss of all hormonal receptors. We do not understand why the tumor recurs after hormonal therapy and how a second response occurs from either stopping the hormonal therapy or changing to another. There are challenging biological questions.

V. *Tamoxifen and Hormonal Therapy*

Since the nineteenth century the use of ovarian ablation has been known to cause remissions in breast cancer in premenopausal women. The development of other hormonal therapies has occurred over the past 30 years. However, the introduction of tamoxifen into clinical practice in the late 1970s has been a remarkable success story. Its ability to cause regressions in metastatic breast cancer has clearly been shown to be equivalent to all other forms of hormone manipulation (Table 28.7) (Legha et al. 1978). Not only is the response rate equivalent, but the morbidity and toxicity are significantly less than with most other available endocrine therapies.

The mechanisms of action of the hormones in causing cell death and

Table 28.7. Metastatic breast disease: hormonal therapy

Therapy	Number of patients	Percent response
Oophorectomy	550	29
Adrenalectomy	690	28
Hypophysectomy	340	33
Androgens	423	18
Estrogens	243	36
Tamoxifen	370	36

From Legha et al. 1978.

Table 28.8. Tamoxifen combinations with hormones

Tamoxifen alone				In combination		
Number of patients	Number of responses	Percent response	Agent	Number of patients	Number of responses	Percent response
61	25	41	Diethylstilbesterol	53	21	40
94	18	19	Fluoxymesterone	100	39	39
68	29	42	Progestins	78	18	23
240	80	33	Aminoglutethimide	180	55	31

From Furr and Jordan 1984.

stasis are not known. A logical clinical maneuver would be to combine diverse hormone therapies to improve response rates. This has not been shown to have any clinical advantage (Table 28.8) (Furr and Jordan 1984). The fact that second responses occur after tamoxifen failures is clear, yet the simultaneous administration of these agents is not associated with improved responses. More recently, an interesting strategy is being proposed by Iacobelli and colleagues, namely, that tamoxifen causes an increase in progesterone receptors (Iacobelli et al. 1984). This increase would suggest that progestins should be more effective if used in some sequential fashion after tamoxifen. This approach needs a rigid controlled comparison of tamoxifen, progestin alone, and the combination given sequentially.

VI. *Future Issues with Tamoxifen*

The clinical use of tamoxifen as a primary hormone therapy as well as adjuvant treatment has increased enormously. Several clinical issues need to be resolved regarding its use and its potential utility in other clinical situations (Table 28.9). First, tamoxifen has agonal estrogen effects. Abnormal uterine bleeding and vaginal cornification are known to occur with

Table 28.9. Clinical issues: tamoxifen

Impact on uterus:
Bleeding
? Cancer
Vaginal cornification
Premenopausal women
Prevention

patients on tamoxifen. These effects suggest that estrogenic action may still be possible despite the apparent primary antiestrogen effect on the breast cancer cells. I have seen at least one endometrial carcinoma occur in a patient while on long-term tamoxifen for 4 years. This case may be completely coincidental. Other cases of endometrial cancer occurring while on tamoxifen have been suggested in personal communication from other researchers. Whether this association will turn out to be a serious problem needs to be considered as more patients are being treated with tamoxifen for long periods of time.

Second, tamoxifen in premenopausal patients causes a marked increase in plasma estrogens, presumably through inhibition of the estrogen receptor in the pituitary and subsequent increased driving of the ovaries through increased follicle-stimulating hormone (FSH) levels (Rose and Davis 1980). Some women who are premenopausal continue to menstruate while on tamoxifen despite having a clinical response in their breast cancer. There are no clear data, although the ovaries of these women on tamoxifen are said to be cystic (Pritchard et al. 1980). Finally, tamoxifen may have exciting possibilities as a chemopreventive agent in breast cancer.

VII. *Tamoxifen and Prevention of Breast Cancer*

Jordan and colleagues have shown that tamoxifen, when given long term, may inhibit the development of breast tumors in rats given DMBA (Jordan et al. 1980). With the idea of preventing breast cancer, the Eastern Cooperative Oncology Group has proposed controlled clinical studies in women with two clinical situations. The incidence of developing breast cancer in the contralateral breast after the primary tumor is resected is about 0.8% per year ($8/10^5$ women/year). Likewise, there is an increased incidence of primary breast cancer in women who have a strong family history of breast cancer (at least one blood relative with cancer, i.e., mother, sister, aunt). These two clinical situations offer the possibility of the use of tamoxifen to prevent breast cancer.

The basic plan would be to randomly allocate women to tamoxifen or a placebo in two separate protocols, one for women with one breast cancer to prevent the development of a second breast cancer and the other for unaffected women with strong family history and between the ages of 45 and 55. These women would be treated at doses of 20 mg/day for 5 years,

Table 28.10. Tamoxifen and prevention of breast cancer

Proposed clinical study, Eastern Cooperative Oncology Group
First-degree relatives, $4/10^5$
Stage I opposite breast, $8/10^5$
Impact on cancer incidence
Effect on estrogen receptor of tumors
Relationship of tamoxifen blood levels to cancers
Relationship of hormones to cancers
Effect on tumor histology
Effect on breast pathology

with results to show the impact on a variety of parameters shown in Table 28.10. The obvious concerns in such a study would be the possibility of inducing other cancers, the accentuation of osteoporosis, or cardiovascular disease. To date none of these possibilities seems to have been seen in the women treated with tamoxifen. Data on bone effects have been collected but the results are inconclusive (Gotfredsen 1984). The cardiovascular morbidities on tamoxifen seem to occur in patients receiving chemotherapy with prednisone (Lipton et al. 1984). The other concern would be the side effect of tamoxifen, which seems to cause "hot flashes" or menopausal symptoms. If those women who are in the menopause or just prior to the menopause are selected, symptoms could be expected on the placebo group as well. Finally, the use of tamoxifen for this purpose must be done in well-controlled prospective trials, since differences, namely a 50% decrease in cancer risk, will require large numbers of women (8–12,000) followed for 5 years. This might be as few as 60 expected cancers in the control group and an expected 30 or fewer in the treated group. This change would need to be carefully documented and measures taken to check for compliance and continued participation. On the other hand, this reduction in disease incidence could be extremely important if the effective treatment is applied to larger samples of women. Likewise, the incidence of side effects must be documented as well to make sure that we have not created other types of damage than breast cancer.

VIII. *Hormone Receptors and Breast Cancer*

Hormone receptors in the management of patients with breast cancer have been used for the past 10 years for the purpose of selecting therapy, determining prognosis, and studying the biology of the disease. The receptors and their role in breast cancer treatment and research are beyond the scope of my presentation.

IX. Summary

The outcome and improvement in quality of life as manifested by cure for most breast cancers still remain a challenge (Table 28.11). Surgery cures some women of their disease, although radical surgery is associated with physical and/or emotional disabilities. The current trend towards using lesser surgery offers hope to those women who present with relatively small tumors. Effective therapy can be given with preservation of the normal appearance of the breasts. Adjuvant therapy, although it offers much promise, has not resulted in major gains in decreased mortality. The improvement is a 10–25% lessened mortality (Peto 1984), although the questions of what are the best treatments, the optimal duration, and the role of tamoxifen or oophorectomy and prednisone alone relative to chemotherapy remain to be answered (Bonadonna and Valagussa 1983). Tamoxifen alone seems to be an effective adjunctive treatment, although most of the data thus far support an improvement in disease-free period rather than survival.

In the treatment of metastatic disease, hormonal therapy seems still to play a major role in controlling the disease. Tamoxifen has become the standard initial therapy for postmenopausal patients. The use of combination chemotherapy can produce complete responses in 15–20% and partial responses in 30–50%, yet the ability to cure patients with metastatic disease has not been shown (Carbone and Tormey 1985). Attempts to increase the complete response rates with high intensity therapies (Allegra et al. 1982; Tormey et al. 1985) or with sequential hormonal and chemotherapy have been undertaken experimentally in small numbers of patients. The ultimate utility of this approach remains to be seen.

Table 28.11. Summary

Outcome improvement remains challenge
Hormonal therapy continues to play important role
Future strategies:
Intensification of therapy
Duration of therapy
Overcoming resistance
Prevention
Tumor markers

Future strategies in the management of metastatic breast cancer, besides intensification, include studies of the duration of therapies, particularly in the adjuvant situation. The use of shorter courses of chemotherapy (Tancini et al. 1983) and the long-term use of tamoxifen are being tested (Carbone and Tormey 1984). Also, the use of alternating combinations is being tested to overcome or prevent resistance.

The possibility of using tamoxifen as a way to prevent breast cancer in two populations was presented. This approach based on animal data should be tested clinically. The concept of trying to prevent breast cancer, particularly in high-risk groups, is exciting. The clinical problems associated with this approach were described.

As I indicated in 1977 during my Richard and Hinda Rosenthal Lecture (Carbone 1977), one of the major stumbling blocks to early diagnosis and treatment is lack of an effective tumor marker that correlates with cell number. Having this marker, if it were specific for tumor cell numbers, would allow for monitoring of therapy as well as leading to a change of therapy when the marker indicates progression and before clinical failure occurs. Not only would one be able to treat more satisfactorily, but one could avoid therapy in those patients who have no residual disease despite adverse prognostic signs (large tumor size, positive nodes, estrogen receptor–negative tumors). Ultimately, therapy must be specific, nontoxic, effective, and tailored to the individual patient. Until then, one should do high-quality clinical trials to determine what is best and to determine whether there is potential harm done by the new therapies.

Acknowledgments

Supported by Cancer Center Core Grant P30-CA-14520 and ECOG Grant U10-CA-21115. I must offer my gratitude and appreciation to Professor V. C. Jordan for all the effort he put into organizing this meeting. I also want to thank the many donors who provided support so that this meeting could take place, especially Stuart Pharmaceuticals and ICIplc (Pharmaceuticals Division) England.

References

Allegra, J., T. M. Woodcock, S. P. Richman, K. I. Bland, and J. L. Wittliff. 1982. A phase II trial of tamoxifen, premarin, methotrexate, and fluorouracil in metastatic breast cancer. *Breast Cancer Research and Treatment* 2:93–99.

Baum, M., and the Nolvadex Adjuvant Trial Organization (NATO). 1983. Controlled trial of tamoxifen as adjuvant therapy in management of early breast cancer. *Lancet* 1:257–261.

Bonadonna, G., and P. Valagussa. 1983. Chemotherapy of breast cancer: current views and results. *International Journal of Radiation Oncology Biology Physics* 9:279–297.

Bonadonna, G., and P. Valagussa. 1985. Adjuvant systemic therapy for resectable breast cancer. *Journal of Clinical Oncology* 3:259–275.

Bonadonna, G., E. Brusamolino, P. Valagussa, A. Rossi, L. Brugnatelli, C. Brambilla, M. De Lena, G. Tancini, E. Bajetta, R. Musumeci, and U. Veronesi. 1976. Combination chemotherapy as an adjuvant treatment in operable breast cancer. *New England Journal of Medicine* 294:405–410.

Carbone, P. P. 1977. Tumor biology and clinical trials: the Richard and Hinda Rosenthal Foundation award lecture. *Cancer Research* 37:4239–4245.

Carbone, P. P., D. C. Tormey, for the Eastern Cooperative Oncology Group. 1984. Personal Communication.

Carbone, P. P., and D. C. Tormey. 1985. Clinical chemotherapy trials in advanced breast cancer. In *Clinical trials in cancer medicine,* ed. U. Veronesi and G. Bonadonna, 343–361. San Diego, Calif.: Academic Press.

Clark, G. M., W. L. McGuire, C. A. Hubay, O. H. Pearson, and J. S. Marshall. 1983. Progesterone receptors as a prognostic factor in stage II breast cancer. *New England Journal of Medicine* 309:1343–1347.

Fisher, B., P. Carbone, S. G. Economou, R. Frelick, A. Glass, H. Lerner, C. Redmond, M. Zelen, P. Band, D. L. Katrych, N. Wolmark, and E. R. Fisher. 1975. L-Phenylalanine mustard (L-PAM) in the management of primary breast cancer: a report of early findings. *New England Journal of Medicine* 292:117–122.

Fisher, B., A. Glass, C. Redmond, E. R. Fisher, B. Barton, E. Such, P. P. Carbone, S. Economou, R. Foster, R. Frelick, H. Lerner, M. Levitt, R. Margolese, R. MacFarlane, D. Plotkin, H. Shibata, and H. Volk. 1977. L-Phenylalanine mustard (L-PAM) in the management of primary breast cancer: an update of earlier findings and a comparison with those utilizing L-PAM plus 5-fluorouracil (5-FU). *Cancer* 39:2883–2903.

Fisher, B., C. Redmond, A. Brown, N. Wolmark, J. Wittliff, E. R. Fisher, D. Plotkin, D. Bowman, S. Sachs, J. Wolter, R. Frelick, R. Desser, N. Licalzi, P. Geggie, T. Campbell, E. G. Elias, D. Prager, P. Koontz, H. Volk, N. Dimitrov, B. Gardner, H. Lerner, and H. Shibata. 1981. Treatment of primary breast cancer with chemotherapy and tamoxifen. *New England Journal of Medicine* 305:1–6.

Fisher, B., M. Bauer, D. L. Wickerham, C. K. Redmond, E. R. Fisher, A. B. Cruz, R. Foster, B. Gardner, H. Lerner, R. Margolese, R. Poisson, H. Shibata, and H. Volk, 1983. Relation of number of positive axillary nodes to the prognosis of patients with primary breast cancer: an NSABP update. *Cancer* 52:1551–1557.

Furr, B. J. A., and V. C. Jordan. 1984. The pharmacology and clinical use of tamoxifen. *Pharmacology and Therapeutics* 25:127–205.

Gelber, R. D. 1984. Ludwig Breast Cancer Trials LBCS III: chemo and endocrine adjuvant therapy in post menopausal patients. In *Adjuvant chemotherapy of breast cancer. Recent results in cancer research,* vol. 96, ed. H. J. Senn, 102–109. Berlin: Springer-Verlag.

Goldhirsch, A. 1984. Ludwig Breast Cancer Trials LBCS III and IV: adjuvant endocrine treatment in post menopausal patients. In *Adjuvant chemotherapy of breast cancer. Recent results in cancer research,* vol. 96, ed. H. J. Senn, 204–209. Berlin: Springer-Verlag.

Gotfredsen, A., C. Christiansen, and T. Palshof. 1984. The effect of tamoxifen on bone mineral content in premenopausal women with breast cancer. *Cancer* 53:853–857.

Iacobelli, S., M. Forcucci-Zulli, G. Scambia, F. De Cicco, and N. Gentiloni. 1984. Effect of tamoxifen on estrogen and progesterone receptors in human breast cancer. *Proceedings of the Second International Symposium on Anti-Hormones in Breast Cancer,* 21–24 October, Berlin (in press).

Jordan, V. C., K. E. Naylor, C. J. Dix, and G. Prestwich. 1980. Anti-oestrogen action in experimental breast cancer. In *Endocrine treatment of breast cancer: a new approach. Recent results in cancer research,* vol. 71, ed. B. Henningsen, F. Linder, and C. Steichele, 30–44. Berlin: Springer-Verlag.

Legha, S. S., H. L. Davis, and F. M. Muggia. 1978. Hormonal therapy of breast cancer: new approaches and concepts. *Annals of Internal Medicine* 88:69–77.

Lipton, A., H. A. Harvey, and R. W. Hamilton. 1984. Venous thrombosis as a side effect of tamoxifen treatment. *Cancer Treatment Reports* 68:887–889.

Loprinzi, C. L., P. P. Carbone, D. C. Tormey, P. R. Rosenbaum, W. Caldwell, J. C. Kline, R. A. Steeves, and G. Ramirez. 1984. Aggressive combined modality therapy for advanced local-regional breast cancer. *Journal of Clinical Oncology* 2:157–163.

Meakin, J. W., W. E. C. Allt, F. A. Beale, T. C. Brown, R. S. Bush, R. M. Clark, P. J. Fitzpatrick, N. V. Hawkins, R. D. T. Jenkin, J. F. Pringle, W. D. Rider, J. L. Hayward, and R. D. Bulbrook. 1983. Ovarian irradiation and prednisone following surgery and radiation for carcinoma of the breast. *Breast Cancer Research and Treatment* 3:45–48.

Mouridsen, H. T., C. Rose, H. Brincker, S. M. Thorpe, F. Rank, K. Fischerman, and K. W. Anderson. 1984. Adjuvant systemic therapy in high risk breast cancer: the Danish Breast Cancer Cooperative Group's trials of cyclophosphamide or CMF in premenopausal and tamoxifen in postmenopausal patients. In *Adjuvant chemotherapy of breast cancer. Recent results in cancer research,* vol. 96, ed. H. J. Senn, 117–128. Berlin: Springer-Verlag.

Peto, R. 1984. Personal communication.

Pritchard, K. I., D. B. Thomson, R. E. Myers, D. J. A. Sutherland, B. G. Mobbs, and J. W. Meakin. 1980. Tamoxifen therapy in premenopausal patients with metastatic breast cancer. *Cancer Treatment Reports* 64:787–796.

Rose, D. P., and T. E. Davis. 1980. Effects of adjuvant chemohormonal therapy on the ovarian and adrenal function of breast cancer patients. *Cancer Research* 40:4043–4047.

Silverberg, E. 1984. Cancer statistics, 1984. *CA* 34:7–34.

Skipper, H. 1982. Human Cancers: shapes and slopes of remission and survival curves and variables that affect them. Part III. Breast cancer. Booklet 17. Birmingham, Ala.: Southern Research Institute.

Tancini, G., G. Bonadonna, P. Valagussa, S. Marchini, and U. Veronesi. 1983. Adjuvant CMF in breast cancer: comparative 5-year results of 12 versus 6 cycles. *Journal of Clinical Oncology* 1:2–10.

Tormey, D. C., and V. C. Jordan. 1984. Long term tamoxifen adjuvant therapy in node positive breast cancer: a metabolic and pilot clinical study. *Breast Cancer Research and Treatment* 4:297–302.

Tormey, D. C., J. C. Kline, M. Palta, T. E. Davis, R. R. Love, and P. P. Carbone. 1985. Short term high density systemic therapy for metastatic breast cancer. *Breast Cancer Research and Treatment* 5:177–188.

Vana, J., R. Bedwani, C. Mettlin, and G. P. Murphy. 1981. Trends in the diagnosis and management of breast cancer in the U.S. from the surveys of the American College of Surgeons. *Cancer* 48:1043–1052.

VIII

Summary

29

Laboratory and Clinical Research
on the Hormone Dependence
of Breast Cancer:
Current Studies and
Future Prospects

V. Craig Jordan, N. F. Fritz,
Marco M. Gottardis, D. M. Mirecki,
P. M. Ravdin, and Wade V. Welshons

I.	Introduction	502
II.	Growth Factors	503
III.	Monoclonal Antibodies	505
IV.	Clinical Endocrinology	508
	A. Chemotherapy	509
	B. Tamoxifen	509
	C. Chemotherapy and Tamoxifen	511
V.	Failure of Tamoxifen Therapy	512
	References	519

I. Introduction

Tʜᴇ aim of this book has been to present in a single volume a broad overview of the evolution of steroid hormone action, the development of specific antihormonal therapies, and the current strategies for the treatment of breast cancer. The value of the book is increased for research students and for academicians because the contributions offered are written by many of the investigators who conducted the original studies. In this chapter, we will focus upon some of the topics not covered in detail and propose areas of research which may be of interest in the future.

In 1966, Dr. Steven Carter discovered the unique ability of cytochalasins (Fig. 29.1) to enucleate mouse L cells (Carter 1967). This discovery provided a powerful new tool to study the subcellular localization of proteins. The use of the technique to establish that DNA polymerase α is a nuclear (Herrick et al. 1976) rather than a cytosolic enzyme raised the possibility that the technology could be used to study estrogen receptors in cell lines. The successful application of the technique to identify estrogen receptors in the nuclear compartment of GH_3 rat pituitary cells (Wel-

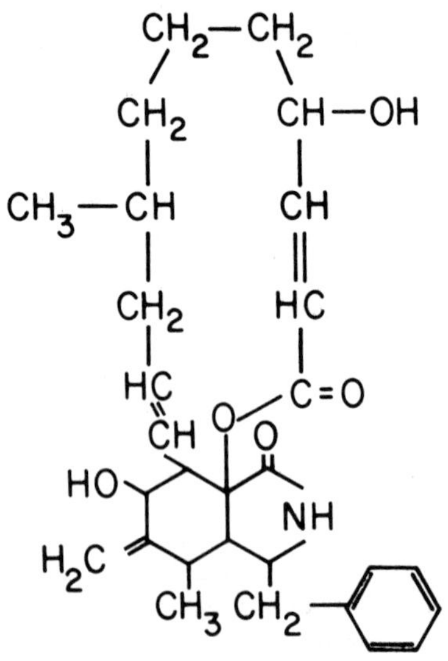

Figure 29.1. The structure of cytochalasin B.

502

Table 29.1. Receptor levels in human breast cancer cell lines[a]

Cell line	ER	PgR	GR	EGF-R$_c$	EGF-R$_m$
MDA-MB-231	5	11	248	560	256
T47D	46	1600	8	70	26
MCF-7	206	177	909	40	20

ER = estrogen receptor; PgR = progesterone receptor; GR = glucocorticoid receptor; EGF-R$_c$ = epidermal growth factor receptor on intact cells; EGF-R$_m$ = epidermal growth factor receptor on plasma membrane preparations.
[a]All values are expressed as fmol/mg protein.

shons et al. 1984) and the proposition that the unoccupied estrogen receptor may be a nuclear protein (Sheridan et al. 1979; King and Greene 1984; Welshons et al. 1984; Jordan et al. 1985b) raise important questions about the subcellular localization of progesterone and glucocorticoid receptors. The numerous breast cancer cell lines with different steroid hormone receptor profiles (Table 29.1) provide an exciting opportunity to consolidate (or refute) the generality of the hypothesis that all steroid receptors are nuclear proteins. The availability of techniques to enucleate cells by centrifugation following incubation with cytochalasin B provides a possible experimental approach.

It is interesting to point out that while Steven Carter was conducting a search for novel anticancer agents in fermentation broths at the laboratories of Imperial Chemical Industries (Pharmaceuticals Division), across the corridor Arthur Walpole was screening synthetic compounds as potential contraceptive agents. Steven Carter discovered the properties of the cytochalasins and Arthur Walpole discovered tamoxifen—two compounds that continue to play important roles in laboratory and clinical investigations.

II. Growth Factors

In Chapter 13, Dr. Lippman and coworkers proposed that estrogen causes the secretion of growth factor in breast cancer cells. The concept that autocrine growth factors may play an important role in breast cancer has been investigated by examining cell lines and breast tumors for the presence of receptors for epidermal growth factor (EGF-R) (Fitzpatrick et al. 1984a; Perez et al. 1984; Sainsbury et al. 1985) and by workers who have investigated the effects of epidermal growth factor (EGF) on cell growth in culture (Imai et al. 1982; Osborne et al. 1982; Fitzpatrick et al. 1984b).

EGF, like other peptide hormones, saturates specific receptors at very low concentrations. The concentration dependence of EGF binding to breast cancer cell lines has been reported by several authors who all found major binding sites with K_ds between 0.2 and 4.0 nM but who have disagreed on whether there were one or more different affinity binding sites on some cell lines. Using ^{125}I EGF concentrations between 0.4 and 40.0 nM, we have found the major binding sites' K_d on MDA-MB-231 breast cancer cells to be 1.8 nM, T47D cells 0.5 nM, and on MCF-7 cells to be 0.7 nM. Fitzpatrick et al. (1984b) found K_d values of 0.2 nM for MDA-MB-231, 4.0 nM for T47D, and the MCF-7 binding curve to be complex, suggesting more than one site but with a half-maximal binding concentration of 1–2 nM.

Human breast tumor specimens have been examined for EGF-R and in these studies there was a significant association between high EGF-R values and low estrogen receptor values. This relationship is illustrated in Figure 29.2 from samples received by the steroid receptor laboratory at the Wisconsin Clinical Cancer Center. Tumors with high levels of estrogen receptor have low levels of EGF-R and the converse is true. This association has been noted in cell lines in culture, with lines with high EGF-R levels having low estrogen receptor values. We have measured the EGF-R levels in three breast cancer cell lines in culture (Table 29.1). Similar EGF-R levels have been observed by Fitzpatrick et al. (1984b), who reported EGF-R levels of 220 fmol/mg for MDA-MB-231, 85 fmol/mg for T47D, and site densitites per cell of approximately one-quarter of T47D values for MCF-7.

The reported EGF-R levels measured in breast tumor specimens have usually been lower than those measured on breast cell lines in culture. Fitzpatrick et al. (1984a) reported an average EGF-R level of only 8 fmol/mg protein in breast cancer tumor membrane preparations but when EGF-R was measured by binding to intact cells in tissue culture even the T47D cell line had EGF-R 80 fmol/mg total protein.

We have found that the methods used to prepare tumor specimen membrane fractions seem to cause losses in measurable EGF-R. MDA-MB-231 cells were grown in culture and EGF-R was measured by direct binding to intact cells and also to a membrane preparation of these cells prepared and assayed by the technique used on breast biopsy specimens. The EGF-R value as measured on intact cells was 401 fmol/mg total protein, whereas the membrane preparation was only 256 fmol/mg. Similar losses were noted during the homogenization of MCF-7 and T47D cells

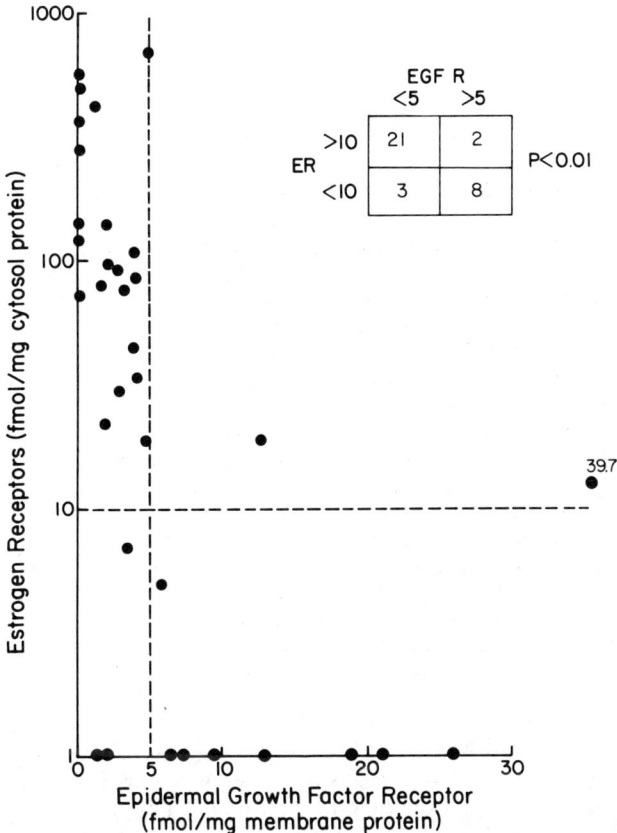

Figure 29.2. The relationship between estrogen receptor (ER) levels in human breast tumor cytosols and the epidermal growth factor receptor (EGF-R) levels in the membrane fraction.

(Table 29.1). Nevertheless, the very low dose levels of EGF-R noted in breast tumors is still rather perplexing, but it may be a reflection of the adaptive changes that must occur to produce a breast cancer cell line.

Clinical assays to measure EGF-R on breast tumor may, however, provide additional useful information about the hormone dependence or perhaps the metastatic potential of a tumor.

III. *Monoclonal Antibodies*

The development of monoclonal antibodies to the human estrogen receptor has proved to be a significant advance in our ability to measure estro-

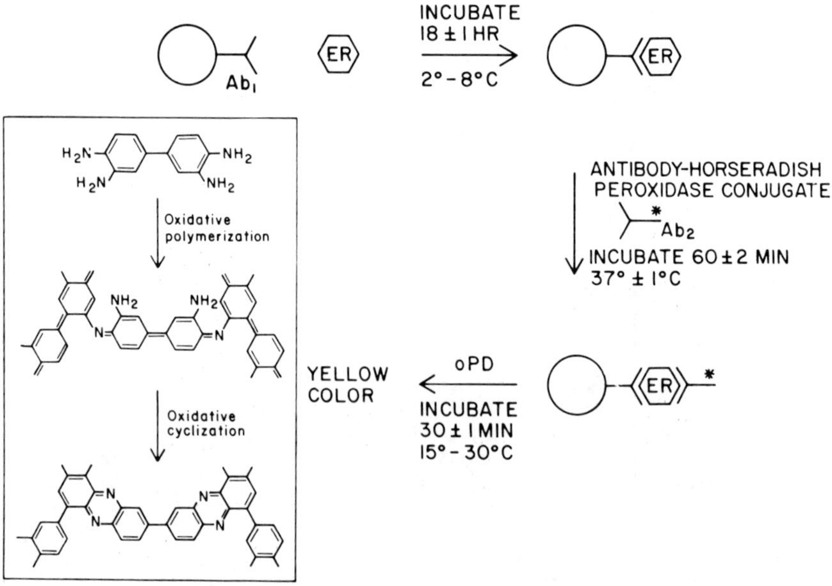

Figure 29.3. A schematic diagram to illustrate the technique employed in the estrogen receptor enzyme-linked immunoassay (ER-EIA). The color reaction developed by the monoclonal antibody linked to the peroxidase enzyme system is shown as an insert.

gen receptors (Greene et al. 1980). The technique for the detection of estrogen receptors in frozen sections of tumors (ER-ICA) has been described in Chapters 17 and 20; however, the technology cannot, as yet, be used to quantitate the receptor level. Another technique, the estrogen receptor enzyme-linked immunoassay (ER-EIA), is available to quantify estrogen receptors in cytosols. The methodology is illustrated in Figure 29.3 and depends upon quantification by a simple colorimetric assay using a preprogrammed Quantum spectrophotometer (Abbott Laboratories). The technique provides distinct advantages for laboratories where liquid scintillation counting facilities are limited and the use of radioactivity is restricted.

The ER-EIA assay system has been evaluated in a number of laboratories against several types of steroid-binding assays (Mirecki and Jordan 1985; Jordan et al. 1986). We have compared the assay of unoccupied estrogen receptors in breast tumor cytosols by commercially available steroid-binding kits from New England Nuclear with results obtained using the ER-EIA (Fig. 29.4). This and previous studies show a slight tendency of the ER-EIA to overestimate estrogen receptors, compared with steroid-

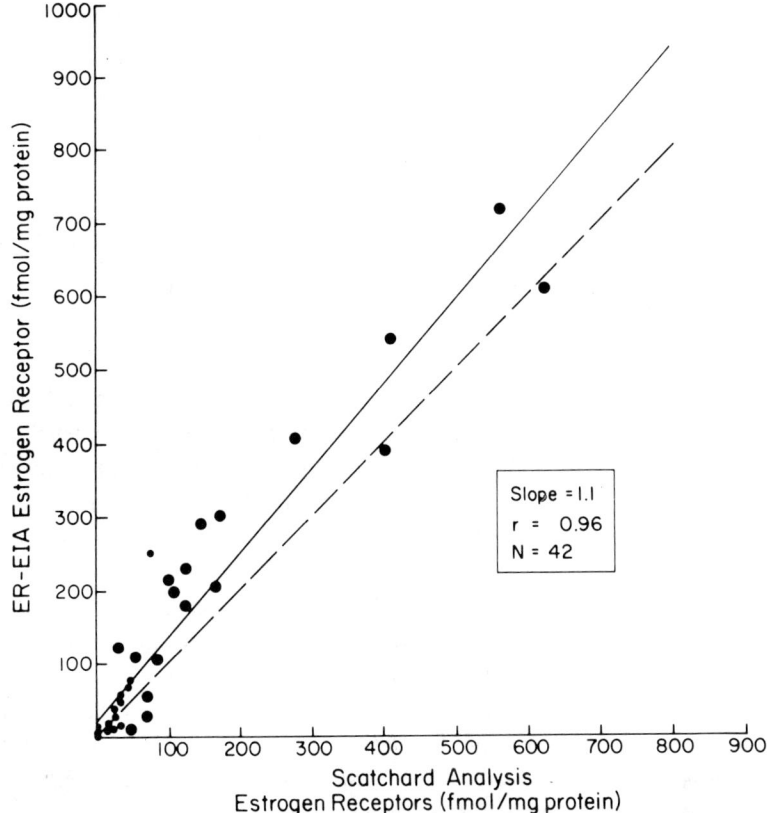

Figure 29.4. The relationship between the level of cytosolic estrogen receptors from human breast tumors measured by commercially available saturation assays (Scatchard analysis) and ER-EIA. The dashed line is the ideal slope of 1 (45°); the solid line is the experimentally determined slope.

binding assays. This situation may result from an estimate of filled and unfilled sites by ER-EIA or an ability of the monoclonal antibodies to detect receptor fragments that do not bind radiolabeled ligand. Alternatively, the result may reflect differences between two steroid-binding assays: (1) the assay to calibrate the standards used in the ER-EIA, and (2) the steroid-binding assay used by a particular laboratory. It is well known that there is considerable variation among clinical steroid receptor laboratories when they assay prepared standards (Jordan et al. 1983).

A particular advantage of the ER-EIA methodology is its ability to quantitate estrogen receptors whether they are occupied or unoccupied.

Table 29.2. The effect of buffer containing 0.4 M KCl or estradiol on the ability of the ER-EIA to measure human breast tumor estrogen receptor[a]

	A	B	C
No additions	37 ± 1	60 ± 2	440 ± 65
+ 10 nM estradiol	42 ± 4	69 ± 5	430 ± 20
+ 0.4 M KCl	41 ± 5	66 ± 5	460 ± 20
+ 0.4 M KCl and 10 nM estradiol	39 ± 1	62 ± 2	470 ± 15

[a]Results are represented as fmol/ml for the different standards (A–C). Values represent mean ± SE of three determinations.

This is illustrated in Table 29.2. This property permits a determination of tumor estrogen receptor status in the presence of high circulating levels of estrogen. Filled estrogen receptors can be extracted with 0.4 M KCl buffer from the nuclear compartment of breast cancer cells so that total estrogen receptor levels can be estimated. The 0.4 M KCl buffer does not interfere with the ER-EIA (Table 29.2).

We are currently evaluating the ability of the assay to determine the hormone receptor status of human breast cancer cell lines grown in athymic mice with estrogen pellets. Two results are shown in Figure 29.5. Panel A shows tumors grown in athymic mice which are progesterone receptor positive but would not be classified as estrogen receptor positive if a non-KCl buffer was used. If 0.4 M KCl homogenization buffer is used, the occupied receptors are extracted and the ER-EIA measures high levels of estrogen receptor. If the implanted estrogen pellet is permited to become exhausted, then the non-KCl buffer can extract more estrogen receptor. However, buffer that contains KCl again extracts the full complement of receptors from the tumor tissue.

The monoclonal antibody technology should, after thorough laboratory evaluation in models similar to the ones described above, be very useful to monitor the level of breast tumor receptors during estrogen or antiestrogen therapy.

IV. Clinical Endocrinology

The preceding chapters have described and reviewed the genesis and evolution of endocrine therapy and chemotherapy for the treatment of breast cancer. However, for completeness, the impact of the therapies upon the ovarian hypothalmo-pituitary axis must be considered, to demonstrate the ablative effects of chemotherapy on the endocrine system.

A. CHEMOTHERAPY

Treatment of premenopausal patients with combination chemotherapy is associated with menstrual irregularities and amenorrhea. Earlier studies analyzed the incidence of amenorrhea and the response to adjuvant chemotherapy but no positive correlation was noted (Bonadonna et al. 1977). Analysis of steroid hormones and gonadotrophins also showed few alterations (Sherman et al. 1979b). Be that as it may, chemotherapy has been shown to have a powerful effect on ovarian steroidogenesis (Koyama et al. 1977; Rose and Davis 1977; Samaan et al. 1978). Young women (less than 35 years of age) have amenorrhea during chemotherapy but there is often a recovery of regular menstrual cycles (Dnistrian et al. 1983). In contrast, older women have a premature menopause with a decrease in circulating steroids and a rise in gonadotrophins. This is illustrated in Figure 29.6. Under these conditions, it is perhaps not surprising that amenorrhea does not correlate with disease-free interval during adjuvant therapy, as circulating estrogen is still detectable and adrenal steroids have the potential to be converted to estrone in peripheral sites. A therapeutic strategy (long-term tamoxifen) to limit the effectiveness of the estrogen may be indicated (Tormey and Jordan 1984).

B. TAMOXIFEN

Tamoxifen produces many different effects upon the endocrinology of pre- and postmenopausal patients (Fig. 29.7). In premenopausal patients tamoxifen causes a reduction in the midcycle peak of circulating prolactin (Groom and Griffiths 1976). This can be ascribed to the antiestrogenic actions of the drug. In contrast, there is a rise in circulating level of estrogens (Groom and Griffiths 1976; Sherman et al. 1979a). This action of the drug in premenopausal patients, may, in fact, become limiting to the therapy for breast cancer because the increase in estrogens may reverse the blockade by tamoxifen in the breast tumor cells and stimulate regrowth. However, a successful response to tamoxifen followed by failure may be followed by a subsequent response to oophorectomy.

Tamoxifen has no effect on circulating estrogens in postmenopausal women but produces an interesting spectrum of effects in the pituitary gland. Luteinizing hormone (LH) and follicle-stimulating hormone (FSH)

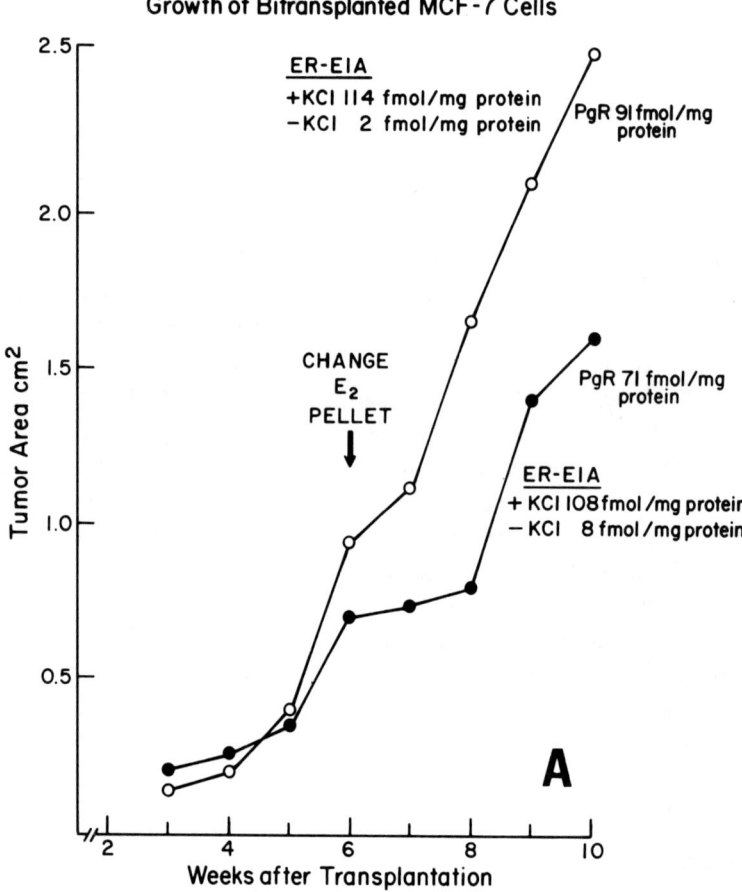

Figure 29.5. The growth of MCF-7 breast cancer cells into solid tumors in athymic mice. In panel A, the estrogen pellet (1.7 mg 8-week release) was exchanged at week 6 and assays performed at week 10. In panel B, the pellet was allowed to become exhausted before assays were performed. The progesterone receptor (PgR) levels were determined by six-point Scatchard analysis using buffer without KCl. The ER-EIA was used to determine estrogen receptors in cytosols prepared using KCl or non-KCl (0.4 M) buffer.

are partially decreased in postmenopausal patients as an expression of partial estrogenicity (Golder et al. 1976; McFadyen et al. 1979). Other weak estrogenic actions have been noted in the vaginal cytology and the composition of serum proteins. Paradoxically, the level of antithrombin III is not consistently depressed and tamoxifen is not sufficiently estrogenic

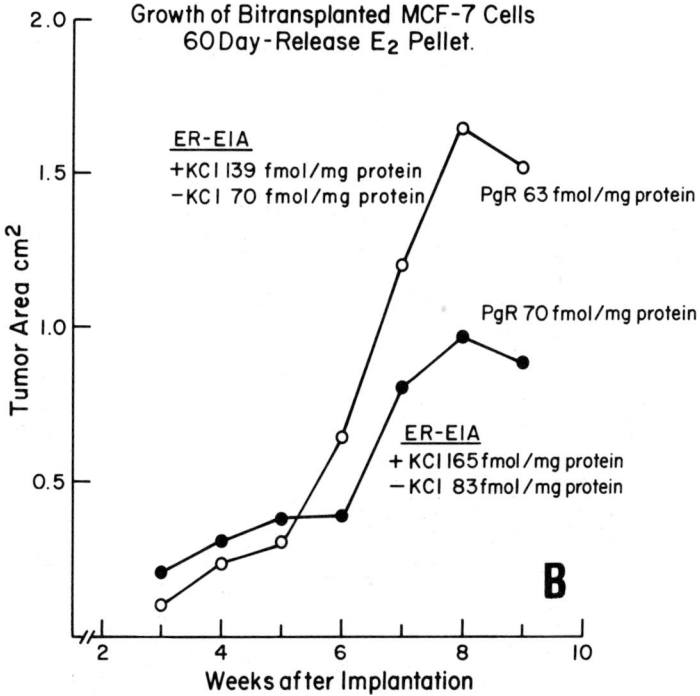

to increase circulating levels of prolactin (unpublished observations). Indeed, tamoxifen decreases prolactin levels in some patients (Helgason et al. 1982).

C. CHEMOTHERAPY AND TAMOXIFEN

The therapeutic interaction of chemotherapy and tamoxifen in premenopausal patients results in an initial increase in circulating estrogens before the destruction of ovarian tissue by the chemotherapy. This is illustrated in Figure 29.8. The reduction in circulating estrogens results in a rise in both LH and FSH (Rose and Davis 1980); however, this is prevented from attaining the level that is observed in postmenopausal women by the partial agonistic actions of tamoxifen. Gonadotrophin levels remain constant for as long as tamoxifen treatment is continued (Fig. 29.9). Indeed, determination of LH or FSH could be used as a marker of patient compliance during long-term tamoxifen therapy. The clinical pharmacology of tamoxifen has recently been reviewed (Furr and Jordan 1984).

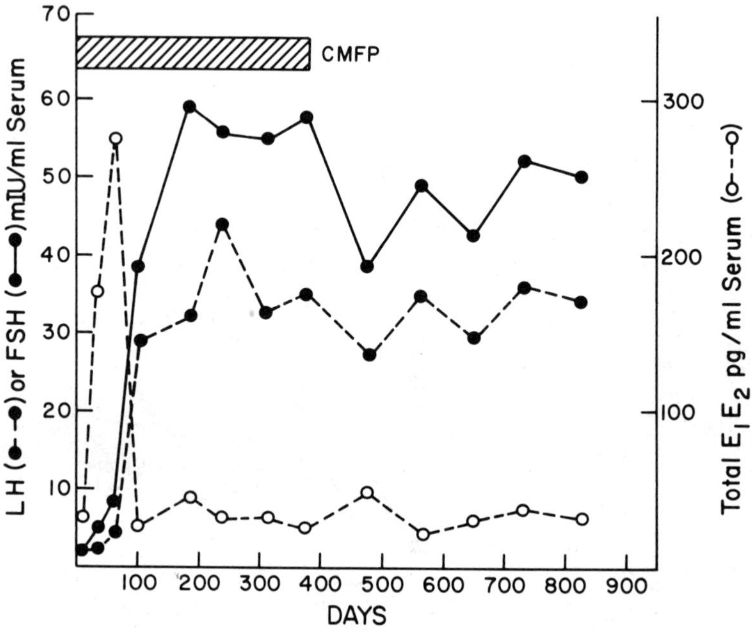

Figure 29.6. The effect of cycles of CMFP adjuvant chemotherapy on the estrogen (E_1 and E_2) luteinizing (LH) or follicle-stimulating hormone (FSH) in a premenopausal woman with node-positive breast cancer.

V. *Failure of Tamoxifen Therapy*

We have listed several possibilities to explain the inability of tamoxifen to prevent the growth of breast cancer (Table 29.3). Clearly, noncompliance is of primary concern during prolonged therapy with tamoxifen. Under these circumstances, there may be a temptation, after years of therapy, to avoid taking the drug or at least miss days or weeks of drug administration. The resulting rise and fall in the drug levels may, in fact, be a disadvantage, as low concentrations of tamoxifen can stimulate tumor cell division (Darbre et al. 1984; Reddel and Sutherland 1984). In the case of

Table 29.3. Potential mechanisms for the therapeutic failure of tamoxifen

Noncompliance
Inadequate dosage
Dietary changes
Drug resistance

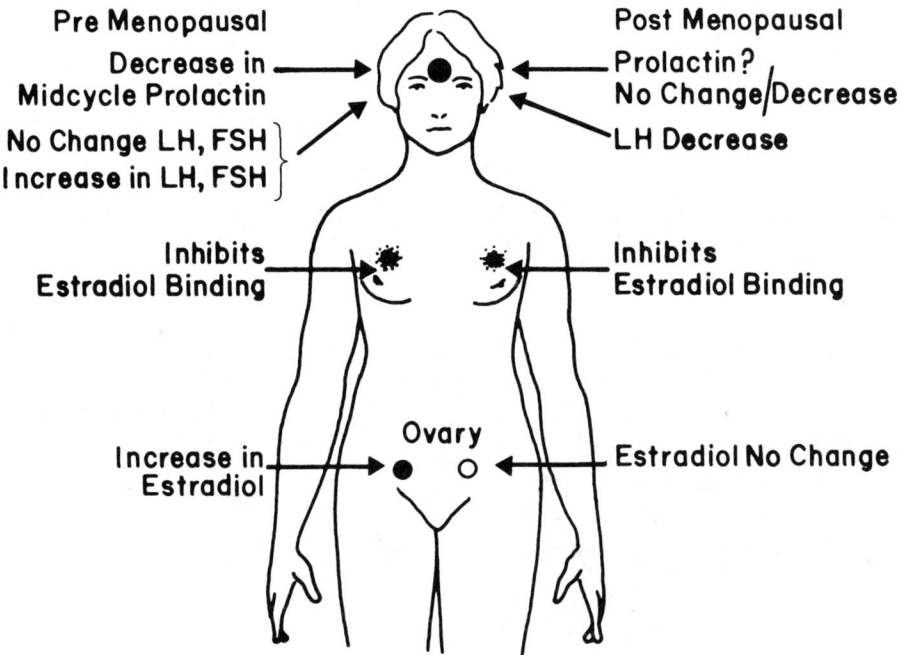

Pre Menopausal
Decrease in Midcycle Prolactin
No Change LH, FSH
Increase in LH, FSH

Post Menopausal
Prolactin?
No Change/Decrease
LH Decrease

Inhibits Estradiol Binding

Inhibits Estradiol Binding

Increase in Estradiol

Ovary

Estradiol No Change

Figure 29.7. The endocrine effects of tamoxifen in pre- and postmenopausal women.

the noncompliant patient described in Figure 29.9, serum levels of tamoxifen and metabolites fell as the level of gonadotrophins rose. These events occurred several months prior to an estrogen receptor–positive recurrence. The concerns raised by this patient argue in favor of routine monitoring of drug levels, especially during clinical trials that aim to evaluate the efficacy of the drug.

The possibility that fluctuating blood levels of tamoxifen may stimulate tumor growth can be avoided by using higher daily doses of tamoxifen. In the United States, 10 mg tamoxifen twice a day is recommended, whereas in other countries 20 mg twice a day or 30 mg daily is used. Since tamoxifen has such a prolonged biological half-life, the higher steady state levels achieved with larger dosages may ultimately be an advantage to the patient. The issue of inadequate dosage becomes more important during long-term therapy, when bioavailability is critical.

Successful therapy with tamoxifen over a period of several years may be associated with changes in the dietary habits of the patients. Weight increases may be very important, because tamoxifen is extremely lipo-

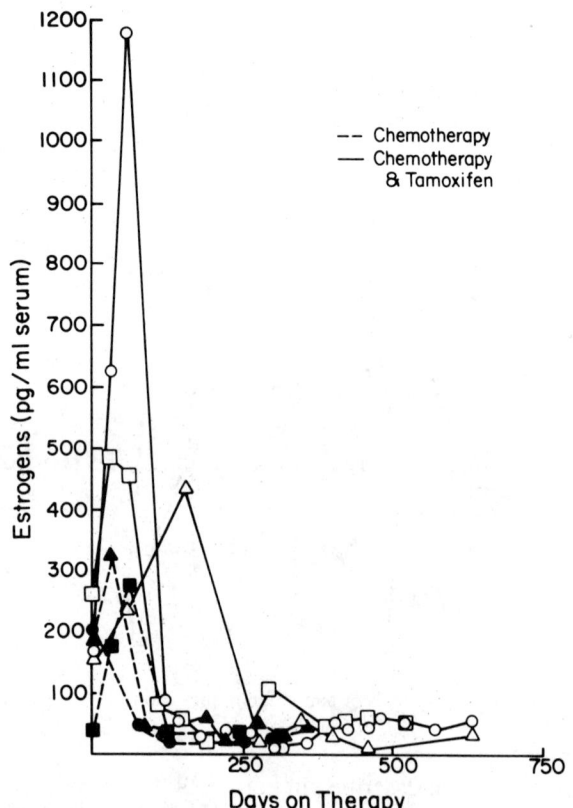

Figure 29.8. The effect of adjuvant chemotherapy (CMFP) or chemotherapy plus tamoxifen on the circulating serum estrogen (E_1 and E_2) levels in premenopausal women with node-positive breast cancer.

philic and may depot in the body fat, thereby reducing bioavailability to the tumor.

Should a patient change her diet to become a vegetarian, then there will be an increase in estrogenic compounds (phytoestrogens) which can compete with tamoxifen and metabolites at the tumor. Furthermore, the recent finding that enterolactone (Fig. 29.10) (Setchell et al. 1980; Stitch et al. 1980), a product of intestinal bacteria (Setchell et al. 1981), is a very weak estrogen (Jordan et al. 1985a) suggests that it can contribute to the total level of potential estrogens in the patient. Indeed, the broad range of potential estrogens in the diet that might activate a hormone-dependent tumor (Adlercreutz et al. 1982) argues against the long-term usefulness of

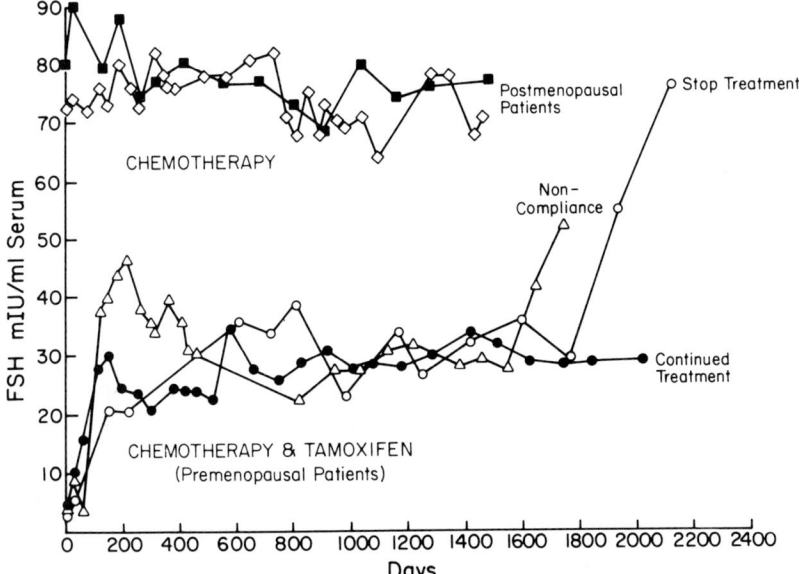

Figure 29.9. The effect of chemotherapy (CMFP) in postmenopausal patients or chemotherapy (CMFP) plus tamoxifen in premenopausal patients on serum follicle-stimulating hormone (FSH) levels. Chemotherapy was administered for up to 2 years ($\approx$ 700 days) and in premenopausal patients tamoxifen (10 mg twice a day) was continued alone.

aromatase inhibitors which specifically prevent the conversion of androstenedione to estrone.

Thus far we have considered the reasons for the failure of tamoxifen that can be avoided by careful monitoring of the patient. However, the development of drug resistance to tamoxifen may be more difficult to avoid using the current range of therapeutic tools (Table 29.4).

One important potential mechanism for the resistance of a patient to tamoxifen therapy is the metabolic conversion of the parent drug to estro-

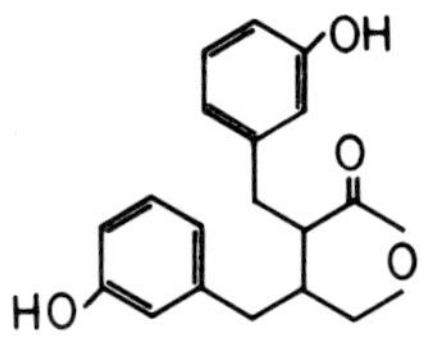

Figure 29.10. Structure of the bacterial product, enterolactone.

Table 29.4. Drug resistance to tamoxifen

Metabolic tolerance
Partial agonist action of tamoxifen
Change in hormonal sensitivity of cells
Selective growth of hormone-independent cells

---

genic metabolites that might stimulate, rather than prevent, tumor growth. On one hand, there are no reports to lend weight to this mechanism of drug resistance, but on the other hand there are no reports of the careful monitoring of patient sera and their target tissues. Clearly, this is required in the future.

The possibility that metabolic resistance occurs would be supported if the species differences observed with tamoxifen were found to be the result of differential metabolism; i.e., tamoxifen is converted into potent estrogens in the mouse to account for the estrogenic actions. However, no unique estrogenic metabolites have been found in the mouse (Lyman and Jordan 1985). A line of evidence that argues against the metabolic conversion of tamoxifen to estrogens in the mouse is that tamoxifen does not support the growth of MCF-7 cells transplanted into athymic mice, although uterine size increases. These results argue in favor of the target (or species) site specificity to tamoxifen. Thus, the mouse uterus is stimulated to grow by the ligands that are sequestered within uterine cells, whereas the transplanted human tumor is prevented from translating the signal from the ligand receptor complex into growth (Gottardis et al. 1985; Osborne et al. 1985).

The intrinsic estrogenicity of tamoxifen in some tissues and test systems (Jordan 1984) may eventually be self-defeating over many years of administration. This concept has recently been illustrated *in vitro* by Sonnenschein and coworkers (1985). It is proposed that serum contains a target tissue–specific inhibitory factor called estrocolyone. Estradiol binds preferentially to estrocolyone, which dissociates from the target cell membrane to permit cell replication. The antiestrogen tamoxifen partially binds to estrocolyone to produce a small increase in cell division. However, it is interesting to observe that the known estrogens, metabolite E and ICI 47,699 (*cis* isomer of tamoxifen), cause maximal cell division and the antiestrogens (4-hydroxytamoxifen, N-desmethyltamoxifen, and metabolite Y) do not. Since all of the biological activities noted are consistent with their estrogen receptor binding activities these data could therefore be interpreted as an effect modulated through the estrogen receptor to control inhibitory factors which bind to the cell membrane and modify growth factor action. Nevertheless, Sonnenschein's hypothesis might be useful to aid the development of nonestrogenic estrogen antagonists. The current interest in the weakly estrogenic antiestrogens, LY 117018 and LY 156758 (keoxifine), has demonstrated their poor performance as antitumor agents *in vivo* (Clemens et al. 1983; Wakeling and Valacaccia 1983; Gottardis and Jordan 1984). It is possible that an evaluation of the estrogenicity in a mouse uterine assay is of no relevance in developing effective antitumor agents for human disease. Further studies should consider alternate mechanisms for the regulation of neoplastic cell division.

A change in the hormonal sensitivity of the tumor may result in the failure of tamoxifen therapy. Most of the research has focused upon estrogen-stimulated growth, but the conversion from hormone dependence to hormone independence is probably the most critical of transition points for our ability to control tumor replication. If estrogens do induce growth factors (see Chapter 13) which ultimately control cell replication, then antiestrogens may prevent this estrogen-stimulated response. In Section II we pointed out that hormone-independent cells have a higher concentration of epidermal growth factor receptors; however, the mechanism for the continued production of the receptors is unknown. It is possible that other hormonal factors regulate growth factor receptors. These pathways may be targets for future drug development.

The fact that patients who initially respond to tamoxifen therapy and then fail may subsequently respond to other hormonal modalities argues either in favor of the poor bioavailability of tamoxifen or a change in hormone dependency. Approximately 50% of patients who eventually fail tamoxifen therapy respond to aminoglutethimide (Stuart-Harris and Smith 1984). Aminoglutethimide is primarily believed to be an inhibitor of aromatase enzyme systems but the drug also prevents the production of pregnenolone from cholesterol (Fig. 29.11). This in turn reduces the production of progesterone (Salhanick 1982). The overall effect of reduced progesterone has never been considered, although there are reports from studies conducted with carcinogen-induced rat mammary carcinoma models that progesterone is able to facilitate the induction of tumors (Cantarow et al. 1948; Huggins and Yang 1962; Jabara 1967). Clearly, antiprogestins should be systematically tested to determine their role as potential anticancer agents (Baulieu 1984). The primary problem is that the agent of current interest, RU 38486 (Fig. 29.12), has significant antiglucocorticoid activity (Moguilewsky and Philibert 1984). This is not surprising because

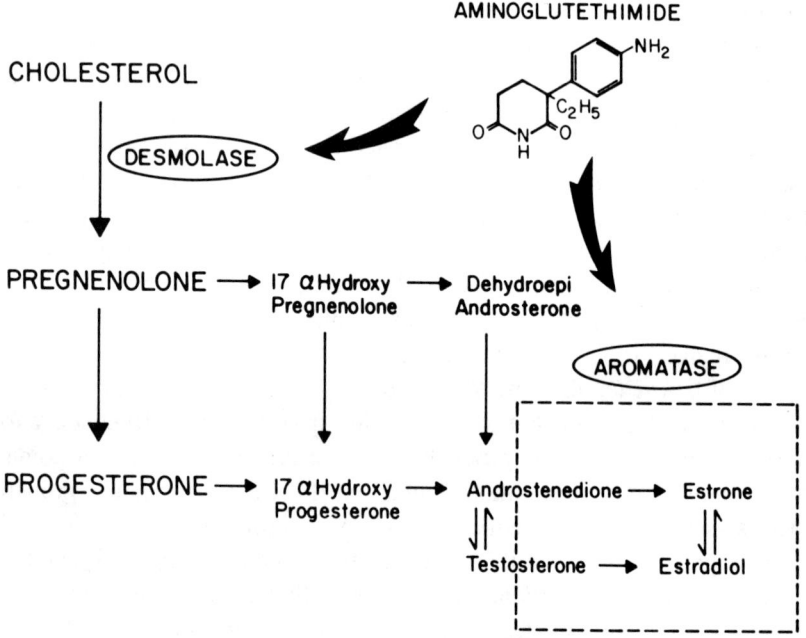

Figure 29.11. Mode of action of aminoglutethimide on steroid biosynthesis.

of the similarity of fit of progestins, androgens, and glucocorticoids for the receptor. As with the antiandrogens (cyproterone acetate) that have progestational activity, the problem has been resolved with nonsteroidal agents (flutamide and R 23908). A similar effort to develop a nonsteroidal antiprogestin would aid progress to determine the subcellular role of progestins in breast cancer cell growth.

Tamoxifen resistance can be studied at the subcellular level by the development of tamoxifen-resistant strains of breast cancer cells (Nawata

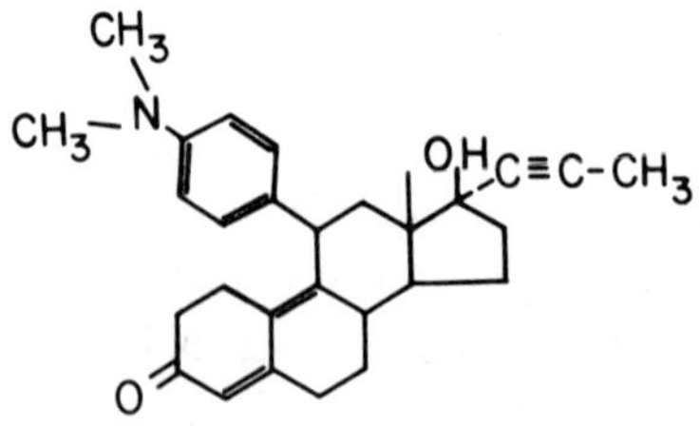

Figure 29.12. Structure of the antiprogestin RU 38486.

et al. 1981a,b). Hormone receptors appear to remain intact in tamoxifen-resistant strains, although secretion of some glycoproteins (52 K) that are associated with estrogen stimulation is now induced by antiestrogen (Westley et al. 1984). Strategies that confound these changes must be a primary goal for future studies.

Acknowledgments

These studies were supported by grants P30-CA-14520, P01-CA-20432 and CA-32713.

References

Adlercreutz, H., T. Fotsis, R. Heikkinen, J. T. Dwyer, M. Woods, B. R. Goldin, and S. L. Gorbach. 1982. Excretion of the lignans, enterolactone and enterodiol, and of equol by omnivorous and vegetarian postmenopausal women and in women with breast cancer. *Lancet* 2:1295–1299.

Baulieu, E. E. 1984. Pharmacology of steroid receptors: from molecular and cellular studies to efficient antihormonal drugs. *Biochemical Pharmacology* 33:905–912.

Bonadonna, G., A. Rossi, P. Valagussa, A. Bangi, and U. Veronesi. 1977. The CMF program for operable breast cancer with positive axillary nodes. *Cancer* 39:2904–2915.

Cantarow, A., J. Stasney, and K. E. Paschkis. 1948. The influence of sex hormones on mammary tumors induced by 2-acetaminofluorene. *Cancer Research* 8:412–417.

Carter, S. B. 1967. Effects of cytochalasins on mammalian cells. *Nature* (London) 213:261–264.

Clemens, J. A., D. R. Bennett, L. J. Black, and C. D. Jones. 1983. Effect of a new antiestrogen, keoxifene (LY 156758), on growth of carcinogen-induced mammary tumors and on LH and prolactin levels. *Life Sciences* 32:2869–2875.

Darbre, P. D., S. Curtis, and R. J. B. King. 1984. Effects of estradiol and tamoxifen on human breast cancer cells in serum-free culture. *Cancer Research* 44:2790–2793.

Dnistrian, A. M., M. K. Schwartz, A. A. Fracchia, R. J. Kaufman, T. B. Hakes, and V. E. Currie. 1983. Endocrine consequences of CMF adjuvant therapy in premenopausal and postmenopausal breast cancer patients. *Cancer* 51:803–807.

Fitzpatrick, S. L., J. Brightwell, J. L. Wittliff, G. H. Barrows, and G. S. Schultz. 1984a. Epidermal growth factor binding by breast tumor biopsies and relationship to estrogen and progestin receptor levels. *Cancer Research* 44:3448–3453.

Fitzpatrick, S. L., M. P. Lachance, and G. S. Schultz. 1984b. Characterization of epidermal growth factor receptor and action on human breast cells in culture. *Cancer Research* 44:3442–3447.

Furr, B. J. A., and V. C. Jordan. 1984. The pharmacology and clinical uses of tamoxifen. *Pharmacology and Therapeutics* 25:127–205.

Golder, M. P., M. E. A. Phillips, D. R. Fahmy, P. E. Preece, V. Jones, J. M. Henk, and K. Griffiths. 1976. Plasma hormones in patients with advanced breast cancer treated with tamoxifen. *European Journal of Cancer* 12:719–723.

Gottardis, M. M., and V. C. Jordan. 1984. A comparative study of antiestrogens,

LY 156758 and tamoxifen, on N-nitrosomethylurea-induced rat mammary carcinomas: a potential model for adjuvant therapy. *Journal of Steroid Biochemistry* 20:1031.

Gottardis, M. M., S. P. Robinson, and V. C. Jordan. 1985. Control of estrogen-responsive human breast cancer cell lines in athymic mice by long-term tamoxifen therapy. *Breast Cancer Research and Treatment* 6:173.

Greene, G. L., F. W. Fitch, and E. V. Jensen. 1980. Monoclonal antibodies to estrophilin: probes for the study of estrogen receptors. *Proceedings of the National Academy of Sciences* 77:157–161.

Groom, G. V., and K. Griffiths. 1976. Effect of the antioestrogen, tamoxifen, on plasma levels of luteinizing hormone follicle-stimulating hormone, prolactin, oestradiol and progesterone in normal premenopausal women. *Journal of Endocrinology* 70:421–428.

Helgason, S., N. Wilking, K. Carlström, M.-G. Domber, and B. von Schoultz. 1982. A comparative study of the estrogenic effects of tamoxifen and 17β-estradiol in postmenopausal women. *Journal of Clinical Endocrinology and Metabolism* 54:404–408.

Herrick, G., B. B. Spears, and G. Veomett. 1976. Intracellular localization of mouse DNA polymerase α. *Proceedings of the National Academy of Sciences* 72:1136–1139.

Huggins, C., and N. C. Yang. 1962. Induction and extinction of mammary cancer. *Science* 137:257–262.

Imai, Y., C. K. Leung, H. G. Friesen, and R. P. Shiu. 1982. Epidermal growth factor receptors and effect of epidermal growth factor on the growth of human breast cancer cells in long-term culture. *Cancer Research* 42:4394–4398.

Jabara, A. G. 1967. Effect of progesterone of 9,12-dimethyl-1,2 benzanthracene-induced mammary tumors in Sprague-Dawley rats. *British Journal of Cancer* 21:418–429.

Jordan, V. C. 1984. Biochemical pharmacology of antiestrogen action. *Pharmacological Reviews* 36:245–276.

Jordan, V. C., D. T. Zava, U. Eppenburger, A. Kiser, S. Sebek, E. Dowdle, Z. Krosnowski, R. C. Bennett, J. Funder, I. M. Holdaway, and J. L. Wittliff. 1983. Reliability of steroid hormone receptor assays: an international study. *European Journal of Cancer and Clinical Oncology* 19:357–363.

Jordan, V. C., S. Mital, B. Gosden, R. Koch, and M. E. Lieberman. 1985a. Structure-activity relationship of estrogens. *Environmental Health Perspectives* 61:97–110.

Jordan, V. C., A. C. Tate, S. D. Lyman, B. Gosden, M. Wolf, R. R. Bain, and W. V. Welshons. 1985b. Rat uterine growth and induction of progesterone receptor without estrogen receptor translocation. *Endocrinology* 116:1845–1857.

Jordan, V. C., H. I. Jacobson, and E. J. Keenan. 1986. Determination of estrogen receptor in breast cancer using monoclonal antibody technology: results of a multi-center study in the United States. *Cancer Research* (in press).

King, W. J., and G. L. Greene. 1984. Monoclonal antibodies localize oestrogen receptor in the nuclei of target cells. *Nature* (London) 307:745–747.

Koyama, H., T. Wada, Y. Wishezawa, T. Iwanaga, Y. Aoki, T. Terasawa, G. Kosaki, T. Yamamoto, and A. Wada. 1977. Cyclophosphamide-induced ovarian failure and its therapeutic significance in patients with breast cancer. *Cancer* 39:1403–1409.

Lyman, S. D., and V. C. Jordan. 1985. Metabolism of tamoxifen and its uterotrophic activity. *Biochemical Pharmacology* 34:2787–2794.

McFadyen, I. J., G. Raab, A. P. M. Forrest, A. O. Langlands, H. J. Stewart, M. M. Roberts, T. Hamilton, M. P. Golder, G. V. Groom, and K. Griffiths. 1979. The effect of tamoxifen and stilboestrol on plasma hormone levels in postmenopausal women with advanced breast cancer. *Clinical Oncology* 5:251–256.

Mirecki, D. M., and V. C. Jordan. 1985. Steroid receptors and human breast cancer. *Laboratory Medicine* 16:287–294.

Moguilewsky, M., and D. Philibert. 1984. RU 38486: potent antiglucocorticoid activity correlated with strong binding to the cytosolic glucocorticoid receptor followed by an impaired activation. *Journal of Steroid Biochemistry* 20:271–276.

Nawata, H., D. Bronzert, and M. E. Lippman. 1981a. Isolation and characterization of a tamoxifen-resistant cell line derived from MCF-7 human breast cancer cells. *Journal of Biological Chemistry* 256:5016–5021.

Nawata, H., M. T. Chang, D. Bronzert, and M. E. Lippman. 1981b. Estradiol-independent growth of a subline of MCF-7 human breast cancer cells in culture. *Journal of Biological Chemistry* 256:6895–6902.

Osborne, C. K., B. Hamilton, G. Titus, and R. B. Livingston. 1982. Receptor binding and processing of epidermal growth factor by human breast cancer cells. *Journal of Clinical Endocrinology and Metabolism* 55:86–93.

Osborne, C. K., K. Hobbs, and G. M. Clark. 1985. Effect of estrogens and antiestrogens on growth of human breast cancer cells in athymic nude mice. *Cancer Research* 45:584–590.

Perez, R., M. Pascual, A. Macias, and A. Lage. 1984. Epidermal growth factor receptors in human breast cancer. *Breast Cancer Research and Treatment* 4:189–193.

Reddel, R. R., and R. L. Sutherland. 1984. Tamoxifen stimulation of human breast cancer cell proliferation *in vitro:* a possible model for tamoxifen tumor flare. *European Journal of Cancer and Clinical Oncology* 20:1419–1424.

Rose, D. P., and T. E. Davis. 1977. Ovarian function in patients receiving adjuvant chemotherapy for breast cancer. *Lancet* 1:1174–1176.

Rose, D. P., and T. E. Davis. 1980. Effect of adjuvant chemohormonal therapy on the ovarian and adrenal function of breast cancer patients. *Cancer Research* 40:4043–4047.

Sainsbury, J. R., G. V. Sherbet, J. R. Farndon, and A. L. Harris. 1985. Epidermal growth factor receptors and oestrogen receptors in human breast cancer. *Lancet* 1:364–366.

Salhanick, H. A. 1982. Basic studies on aminoglutethimide. *Cancer Research* 42:3315s–3321s.

Samaan, N. A., D. N. deAsis, A. U. Buzdar, and G. R. Blumenschein. 1978. Pituitary-ovarian function in breast cancer patients on adjuvant chemoimmunotherapy. *Cancer* 41:2084–2087.

Setchell, K. D. R., A. M. Lawson, F. L. Mitchell, H. Adlercreutz, D. N. Kirk, and M. Axelson. 1980. Lignans in man and in animal species. *Nature* (London) 287:740–742.

Setchell, K. D. R., A. M. Lawson, S. P. Boppiello, R. Harkness, H. Gordon, and D. M. L. Morgan. 1981. Lignan formation in man-microbial involvement and possible roles in relation to cancer. *Lancet* 2:4–7.

Sheridan, P. J., V. C. Alselmo, J. M. Buchanan, and P. M. Martin. 1979. Equilibrium: the intracellular distribution of steroid receptors. *Nature* (London) 282:579–582.

Sherman, B. M., F. K. Chapler, K. Crickard, and D. Wycoff. 1979a. Endocrine consequences of continuous antiestrogen therapy with tamoxifen in premenopausal women. *Journal of Clinical Investigation* 64:398–404.

Sherman, B. M., R. B. Wallace, and P. R. Jochimsen. 1979b. Hormonal regulation of the menstrual cycle in women with breast cancer: effect of adjuvant chemotherapy. *Clinical Endocrinology* 10:287–296.

Sonnenschein, C., J. T. Papendorp, and A. M. Soto. 1985. Estrogenic effect of tamoxifen and its derivatives on the proliferation of MCF-7 human breast tumor cells. *Life Sciences* 37:387–394.

Stitch, S. R., J. K. Toumba, M. B. Groen, C. W. Funke, J. Leemhius, J. Vink, and G. F. Woods. 1980. Excretion, isolation and structure of a new phenolic constituent of female urine. *Nature* (London) 287:738–740.

Stuart-Harris, R. C., and I. E. Smith. 1984. Aminoglutethimide in the treatment of advanced breast cancer. *Cancer Treatment Reviews* 11:189–204.

Tormey, D. C., and V. C. Jordan. 1984. Long-term adjuvant therapy in node positive breast cancer—a metabolic and pilot clinical study. *Breast Cancer Research and Treatment* 4:297–302.

Wakeling, A. F., and B. Valacaccia. 1983. Antioestrogenic and antitumour activities of a series of non-steroidal antioestrogens. *Journal of Endocrinology* 99:455–464.

Welshons, W. V., M. E. Lieberman, and J. Gorski. 1984. Nuclear localisation of unoccupied oestrogen receptors. *Nature* (London) 307:747–749.

Westley, B., F. E. B. May, A. M. C. Brown, A. Krust, P. Chambon, M. E. Lippman, and H. Rochefort. 1984. Effects of antiestrogens on the estrogen regulated pS2 RNA, 52 kDa and 160 kDa proteins in MCF-7 cells and two tamoxifen resistant sublines. *Journal of Biological Chemistry* 259:10030–10035.

Index

2AAF. *See* 2-Acetylaminofluorene
2-Acetylaminofluorene (2AAF), structure
    of, 285
2-Acetylaminofluorene (2AAF)-induced
    mammary cancer, 284–285
Acetylcholine receptor, 410
Adjuvant therapy, 441–445, 451–456,
    459–467, 471–488, 494
Adrenalectomy, 304, 311, 343, 418–422,
    441, 490
Adriamycin therapy, 425, 432–435, 438–
    440, 487
AEBS. *See* Antiestrogen binding site
Affinity chromatography, for isolation of
    estrogen receptor, 360–361
Amenorrhea, induced, 462, 509
Aminoglutethimide-hydrocortisone therapy,
    421–422, 427
Aminoglutethimide therapy, 222–228,
    419–420, 426–427, 491, 518
Androgen, aromatization to estrogen, 223
Androgen therapy, 420–422, 424–426,
    490
Anethole, 21–22
Animal models, of breast cancer, 283–294
Anol, 22
Antibodies. *See* Monoclonal antibodies;
    Polyclonal antibodies
Antiestrogen. *See also* specific compounds
    activation of, 136
    activity of
        in vitro, 157–164
        in vivo, 154–157
    agonistic action of, 116–119, 165, 174
    antagonistic action of, 116–119, 165,
        174–175
    antitumor activity of, in carcinogen-
        induced mammary cancer, 287–289
    binding to estrogen receptor, 74–77,
        127–145, 175–177, 184–185
    in chicken, 171–186

Antiestrogen (*continued*)
    covalent labeling of estrogen receptor
        with, 80–81
    effect of
        on cell cycle, 265–278
        on cell proliferation, 129–130
        on estrogen-regulated mRNA (pS2),
            251–259
        on estrogen-regulated proteins, 249–
            261
        on progesterone receptor production,
            151–165
    in liver, 174–182
    metabolism of, 74–79, 173, 191–215
    mode of action of, 289–293
    pharmacokinetics of, 173
    potency of, 165
    radiolabeled, 73–87
        as estrogen receptor probes, 74–83
        synthesis of, 74
    regulation of secreted 52 K protein by,
        250–254
    site of action of, 290
    structure-activity relationships of, 19–
        37, 157, 159–164, 273–276
Antiestrogen binding site (AEBS), 275.
        See also Triphenylethylene binding
        site
    antiestrogen action and, 115–125
    in antiestrogen-resistant cells, 259
    binding properties of, 97–99
    binding specificity of
        competition studies of, 99–101
        tissue differences in, 101
    in breast cancer cells, 127–145
    cytosolic, 178–179
    detergent-solubilized, 104–108
    endogenous ligand for, 101–103, 119–
        120, 123–125, 180–182
    enzyme susceptibility of, 104–105
    function of, 109–111

Antiestrogen binding site (*continued*)
  hormonal control of, 97
  ligand specificity of, 179–180
  in liver, 177–180, 186
  molecular properties of, 104–108
  molecular weight of, 106
  nuclear, 177–178
  in oviduct, 185–186
  properties of, 93–111
  subcellular distribution of, 94–98, 131–
    133, 178–179
  tissue distribution of, 94–98, 130–131
Antiestrogen binding site inhibitory activ-
    ity, 180–182
Antiestrogen-receptor complex, physico-
    chemical analysis of, 136–139
Antiestrogen-resistant cells, 255–259
Antiestrogen therapy, 128, 421–423, 426
  with chemotherapy, 438
  with other hormonal therapy, 422
Antiprogestin, 517–518
Antitumor activity
  of antiestrogens, 287–289
  of 4-hydroxyandrostenedione, 226–228
  of tamoxifen, 226–228
Arachidonic acid, 14–15
Aromatase enzyme system, 517–518
  inhibition by 4-hydroxyandrostenedione,
    221–233
    in vitro, 223–226
    in vivo, 223–226
Aryl hydrocarbon hydroxylase, 201
Athymic mouse, transplantation of breast
    tumor to, 292–294, 508–511
Autocrine control of cell proliferation,
    255–261

Belleau's macromolecular perturbation
    theory, 34–35
Benzocaine, 101
Biochanin A, 25
Bisphenol, 27, 33–35, 196
  effect on progesterone receptor produc-
    tion, 159–160, 162
  potency of, 165
  structure of, 153
Bleomycin therapy, 439

BPEA. *See* t-Butylphenoxyethyl diethy-
    lamine
Brain
  antiestrogen binding sites in, 130–131
  progesterone receptor in, 156–157
Breast cancer. *See also* Mammary tumor
  advanced, 347–348, 417–427
  age at occurrence of, 330
  animal models of, 283–294
  antiestrogen binding sites in, 97–98
  carcinogen-induced, 283–284
  clinical trials in, 325–338, 341–351,
    417–427, 431–445, 451–456, 459–
    467, 471–482
  cytosol inhibitor in, 63–65, 69
  disease-free interval, 336–337
  early, 344–346, 459–467
  epidermal growth factor receptor in,
    503–505
  estrogen receptor in, 308–312, 325–338,
    342–346, 366–367, 418, 473–478
  growth factors in, 237–245, 503–505
  heterogeneity of, 387–391
  hormone dependency of, 304–305
    changes in, 517
  metastatic, 347–348, 488–490, 494–495
  mitotic index of, 329–330, 336–337
  natural history of, 326–338
  p29 in, 380–391
  postmenopausal, 304, 309–310, 315,
    336, 338, 419, 422, 426
  premenopausal, 304, 309, 315, 418–
    419, 422, 427, 440, 490
  prevention of, 492–493, 495
  progesterone receptor in, 311, 341–351,
    396, 404–408, 411, 418, 477, 491
  prognosis for, 330–332, 344
  prognostic index for, 328–333
  rapidly progressive, 325–338
  recurrence of, 318–319, 328–333, 344–
    346
    site of, 335–336, 477–478
    survival after, 333–338
    tumor growth rate and, 336–338
  stage I, 486–487
  stage II, 471–482, 486–487
  stage III, 486–487
  stage IV, 487
  survival of, 330–338, 344–346, 473–
    478

Breast cancer (*continued*)
  therapy for. *See* Adjuvant therapy;
    Chemotherapy; Endocrine therapy;
    specific drug therapies; specific op-
    erations
  thymidine-labeling index of, 329–330
  tissue fixation, 313
  transplantation to athymic mice, 292–
    294
Breast cancer cells. *See also* specific cell
    lines
  antiestrogen binding sites in, 127–145
  antiestrogen-resistant, 255–259
  asynchronous, effects of antiestrogens
    on, 266–268
  effect of antiestrogens on, 129–130,
    249–261, 271–273
  estrogen receptor in, 137
  turnover of, 140–144
  growth in athymic mice, 292–294, 508–
    511
  proliferation of, 129–130
  synchronous, effect of antiestrogens on,
    269–271
Breast tumor
  antiestrogen binding sites in, 97–98
  receptor-positive, imaging agents for,
    83–84
BT-20 cells
  antiestrogen binding sites in, 98
  cell cycle effects of tamoxifen in, 272–
    274
BT-474 cells
  antiestrogen binding sites in, 98
  cell cycle effects of tamoxifen in, 272–
    274
t-Butylphenoxyethyl diethylamine (BPEA),
    144
  binding to antiestrogen binding site, 135
  binding to estrogen receptor, 135

CAF regimen, 440
Calmodulin, 110
Cancer. *See* specific organ cancers
Carcinogen-induced breast cancer, 283–
    284
Cell cycle, 442–443
  effect of antiestrogens on, 265–278
Cell proliferation, 69–71, 116–119, 129–
    130, 238–239, 250

Cell proliferation (*continued*)
  autocrine control of, 255–261
  effect of antiestrogens on, 265–278
  stimulation by tamoxifen, 276–278
Chemohormonotherapy, 431–445, 489
Chemotherapy, 387, 418, 424–427, 471–
    482, 489, 494–495
  combination, 432–445
  endocrine effects of, 509, 512
  with hormone-ablative therapy, 440–441
  postoperative, 485
  tamoxifen therapy and, 511, 514–515
  time to treatment failure, 434
Chicken
  antiestrogen action in, 171–186
  estrogen action in, 172–173
  tamoxifen metabolism in, 197
Chlorotrianisene, metabolism of, 212–213
5-Cholestene-3β-ol-7-one, 100, 102
Δ4-Cholestene-3-one, 180
Cholesterol, metabolism of, 122, 124–125,
    517–518
Chromatin, 172, 184–185, 308, 358–359,
    369–370
CI 628, 28–29
  binding to antiestrogen binding site,
    134–135, 185
  binding to estrogen receptor, 7, 134–
    135, 184
  effect of
    on breast cancer tissue, 305–306
    on DMBA-induced mammary cancer,
      289
    on liver, 174
    on progesterone receptor production,
      154, 157, 159
  metabolism of, 75–76, 136, 208–211,
    214
  radiolabeled, 74–75
  structure of, 29, 153, 288
CI 628M, 75–76, 134–139, 165, 209, 211
CI 680, binding to estrogen receptor, 184
Clomid. *See* Clomiphene
Clomiphene, 28, 30
  binding to antiestrogen binding site, 99–
    101, 109–110, 275
  binding to estrogen receptor, 275
  cell cycle effects of, 275
  effect on progesterone receptor produc-
    tion, 154
  inhibition of nuclear type II sites, 56

CMF regimen, 434–442, 460–462, 467
CMFP regimen, 435–437, 488, 512–515
CMFp regimen, 460–465
Compound 10222
  binding to estrogen receptor, 275
  cell cycle effects of, 275
Compound 13, 102
Compound 14, 102
Compound 145680, 102
Compound 47108, 102
Compound 6866
  binding to estrogen receptor, 275
  cell cycle effects of, 275
Compound 9599, 99–101
  binding to estrogen receptor, 275
  cell cycle effects of, 275
Conalbumin, 182–183
Conditioned medium, growth factors in,
  237–245
Corticosteroid therapy, 420–422
Coumestans, 24
Coumestrol, 24, 26
Cyclophosphamide therapy, 432, 434–442,
  460–467, 488, 512–515
Cytochalasin B, 45–47, 502–503
  structure of, 503
Cytochrome P_{450}, 109, 201–202, 222–223
Cytoplast
  estrogen receptor in, 48–52
  preparation of, 45–47
Cytosol, uterine, effect on estrogen binding
  to nuclear type II sites, 58–61
Cytosol inhibitor
  in liver, 65, 68, 70
  in malignant tissue, 63–65
  physiological function of, 69
  uterine
    chromatography of, 61–62
    detection and measurement of, 56–60
    purification and characterization of,
      64–67
Cytosol inhibitor binding protein, 71
Cytosol type II site, 70–71

D5 antigen, 379–383. *See also* p29
DDT, 27
DES. *See* Diethylstilbestrol
N-Desethylenclomiphene, 208, 210
Desmethyl chlorotrianisene, 212–213

Desmethylnafoxidine, 85–86
N-Desmethyltamoxifen, 99–101,110, 136,
  177, 193–207, 213, 443, 516
Dexamethasone, 56, 69, 183
Dextran sulfate, 11
Diadzein, 25–26
Dianethole, 22
Dianol, 21–22
Diaphragm, cytosol inhibitor in, 70
Dibromodulcitol therapy, 434, 438–439
N-Didesmethyltamoxifen. *See* Tamoxifen:
  metabolite Z
Diet, estrogens in, 514–515
Diethylstilbestrol (DES), 22–23, 363, 438,
  491
  structure of, 153
Diethylstilbestrol (DES) diproprionate, 23
Dihydrofolate reductase, 239
Dihydroxyhexahydrochrysene, 22
3,4-Dihydroxytamoxifen. *See* Tamoxifen:
  metabolite D
7,12-Dimethylbenz[a]anthracene (DMBA),
  structure of, 285
7,12-Dimethylbenz[a]anthracene (DMBA)-
  induced mammary cancer, 285–286,
  492
  effect of antiestrogens on, 287–291
  estradiol uptake by, 306
α,α-Di-(p-ethoxyphenyl)βphenylbromo-
  ethylene, 23
DMBA. *See* 7,12-Dimethylbenz[a]-
  anthracene
DNA
  interaction with estrogen receptor, 12–13
  synthesis of, 118
    estrogen-induced, 69, 239
Dog, tamoxifen metabolism in, 197
Drug metabolism, interactions in, 201–202

Eastern Cooperative Oncology Group
  breast cancer prevention study by, 492–
    493
  breast cancer therapy studies by, 435–
    440, 488
EGF. *See* Epidermal growth factor
Egg white protein, 172
ELISA. *See* Enzyme-linked immunosor-
  bent assay
Enclomiphene, 34

Enclomiphene (*continued*)
activity of, 201
binding to antiestrogen binding site, 99–101
binding to estrogen receptor, 184
effect on progesterone receptor production, 154, 156–157
effect on prolactin synthesis, 32
metabolism of, 207–210, 214
structure of, 33
Enclomiphene N-oxide, 208, 210
Endocrine therapy, 205, 308–312, 326, 333–337, 342–343, 347–350, 387, 417–427. *See also* Chemohormonotherapy; specific operations
adjuvant, 459–467
combination, 422
sequential, 423–427
tamoxifen therapy and, 490–491
Endometrium
cancer of, 493
p29 in, 382
Endoplasmic reticulum, antiestrogen binding sites in, 95–111, 133–134
Enterolactone, 514–515
structure of, 515
Enucleation procedure, 45–47, 502–503
Enzyme immunoassay of estrogen receptor (ER-EIA), 366, 506–508
Enzyme-linked immunosorbent assay (ELISA) of p29, 383
Epidermal growth factor (EGF), 503–504
Epidermal growth factor (EGF) receptor, 503–505, 517
Equol, 26
ER-EIA. *See* Enzyme immunoassay of estrogen receptor
ER-ICA. *See* Immunocytochemical assay of estrogen receptor
Esophagus, antiestrogen binding sites in, 97, 130–131
Estradiol (17β-Estradiol), 25. *See also* Estrogen
binding assay, 381–382
binding in uterine nuclear fractions, 56–71
binding to estrogen receptor, 177, 184
concentration by target tissues, 5
displacement from estrogen receptor, 8–12

Estradiol (*continued*)
effect on progesterone receptor production, 159–162, 164
metabolism of, 23–24, 173
priming effect of, 153–154
structure of, 153
uptake by target tissue, 205–207
uterine growth and, 116–119
16α-Estradiol
effect on progesterone receptor production, 159–160
structure of, 153
Estradiol receptor. *See* Estrogen receptor
Estriol
effect on progesterone receptor production, 159–160
structure of, 153
Estrocolyone, 516
Estrogen. *See also* Estradiol
in breast cancer, 237–245
in chicken, 172–173
fluorescent, 85–87
formation from androgen, 223
gamma-emitting, 83–84
interactions with target cells, 305–308
normal versus neoplastic, 305–312
interaction with progesterone receptor, 151–165
multiple binding sites for, 55–71
photofluorogenic, 85–87
regulation of growth factors by, 237–245
regulation of nucleic acid synthesis by, 239
structure-activity relationships of, 19–37
synthesis of, ovarian, 291
Estrogen-fluorophore conjugate, 85–86
Estrogen-noncompetable binding site. *See* Antiestrogen binding site
Estrogen receptor, 503
activation of, 6–7, 14–15, 184, 255, 308
antibodies to, 312–320, 357–370
monoclonal, 363–370, 378, 505–508
polyclonal, 362–363, 377–378
specificity of, 377–378
antiestrogen binding to, 74–77, 127–145, 175–177, 184–185
antigenic determinants in, 366–367
assay of, 312–320, 327–328, 505–508
antibody-based, 312–314
in breast cancer, 366–367
immunocytochemical, 313–320

Estrogen receptor (*continued*)
    with monoclonal antibodies, 365–370
    steroid-binding, 313–320
    binding to chromatin, 369–370
    in breast cancer, 308–312, 325–338,
        342–346, 418, 473–478
    clinical studies involving, 303–320
    complexes with estrogens versus anties-
        trogens, 77–80
    conformational changes in, 8–12
    covalently labeled, 80–81
    in cytoplasts, 48–52
    cytosol, 44–45, 59–60, 155, 172, 307–
        308, 368–369, 376
    cytosol type II, 70–71
    displacement of estradiol from, 8–12
    in DMBA-induced mammary cancer,
        290
    DNA-binding domain of, 366–367
    effect of estradiol on, 117
    effect of nafoxidine on, 117
    functional domains of, 365–370
    gene for, 370
    half-life of, 143
    historical aspects of, 4–7
    interaction with DNA, 12–13
    interaction with histones, 11–13
    intracellular distribution of, 45–52, 359
    isolation of, 10–12
    in liver, 186
    mammalian, 360–362
    molecular properties of, 361–362
    in myometrium, 375–392
    in normal tissue, 307–308
    nuclear, 43–52, 155, 175–177, 183–186,
        358–359, 368–369, 376
    nuclear retention time of, 155, 158–159
    in nucleoplasts, 48–52
    in oviduct, 186
    probes for, 73–87
        in single cells, 85–87
    processing of, 156, 158, 376
    properties of, 6–7
    purification of, 360–362, 365–366, 377
    relationship to p29, 383–391
    4S form of, 77, 139, 308, 361
    5S form of, 77, 308, 361
    5.5S form of, 137–140
    8S form of, 376–378
    steroid-binding domain of, 366–367
    structure of, 10–11, 14–15, 361–362

Estrogen receptor (*continued*)
    subcellular distribution of, 132–133, 502
    as transducer, 13–15
    turnover in breast cancer cells, 140–144
    type II site. *See* Nuclear type II site
    type I site, 56
    unoccupied, 43–52
Estrogen-receptor complex
    affinity-labeled, characterization of,
        139–140
    physicochemical analysis of, 136–139
Estrogen-regulated proteins, 249–261
Estrogen synthetase. *See* Aromatase en-
        zyme system
Estrogen therapy, 420–422, 490
Estrone, metabolism of, 23–24
17α Ethinyl estradiol, 23–25
7-Ethoxycoumarin-O-deethylase, 201
Ethylmorphone-N-demethylase, 201
Euchromatin, 370

Fallopian tube, p29 in, 382, 386
Fatty acids, 14–15
Fixation techniques, 313
Flavones, 24
Fluorescent estrogens, 85–87
16α-Fluoroestradiol, 84
5-Fluorouracil therapy, 432–442, 460–
        467, 471–482, 488, 512–515
Fluoxymesterone therapy, 424–425, 437,
        439, 491
Flutamide, 518
Follicle-stimulating hormone (FSH), 492,
        509, 511–513, 515
Formononetin, 25–26
FSH. *See* Follicle-stimulating hormone

Gamma-emitting estrogens, 83–84
Gene, for estrogen receptor, 370
Genistein, 24–26
GH₃ cells, estrogen receptor in, 45–52
Glucocorticoid receptor, 409, 502–503
Glucocorticoids, with tamoxifen, 183–184
Gonadotrophin release, 291
G₀ phase, 267–269, 273
G₁ phase, 267–271, 273, 275, 277, 442
Growth factors, 517
    in breast cancer, 237–245, 503–505
    estrogen-induced, 237–245
    insulin-like, 241–242

Growth factors (*continued*)
  in vivo tests of, 243–244
  transforming, 241–243

H 1285, 134–135
Hamster, progesterone receptor in, 154–155
HBL-100 cells
  antiestrogen binding sites in, 98
  cell cycle effects of tamoxifen in, 272–274
Heparin, 8–9, 11
Heterochromatin, 370
Hexamethylmelamine therapy, 439
Hexestrol, 305
Histones, interaction with estrogen receptor, 11–13
Hormone-ablative therapy, 418–422
  with chemotherapy, 440–441
Hormone therapy. *See* Endocrine therapy
Hs0578T cells
  antiestrogen binding sites in, 98
  cell cycle effects of tamoxifen in, 272–274
Hs578t cells
  insulin-like growth factor in, 241–242
  monoclonal antibodies to secreted proteins, 245
Human, tamoxifen metabolism in, 198–201
4-Hydroxyandrostenedione
  androgenic activity of, 228
  antitumor activity of, 226–228
  inhibition of aromatase enzyme system, 221–233
  toxicity of, 228, 232
4-Hydroxyandrostenedione therapy, 229–233
4-Hydroxyenclomiphene, 207–208
17β-Hydroxysteroid dehydrogenase, 226
Hydroxystilbene, 20–21
4-Hydroxytamoxifen, 34, 75–77, 84, 199, 201, 213, 516
  agonistic action of, 182
  analytical measurement of, 204–207
  binding of
    to antiestrogen binding site, 99–101, 110, 134–135, 178
    to antiestrogen receptor, 137–139
    to estrogen receptor, 134–135, 175–177, 184–185, 202, 363

4-Hydroxytamoxifen (*continued*)
  biological properties of, 202
  effect of
    on cytochrome P_{450}, 202
    on DMBA-induced mammary cancer, 289
    on liver, 175–177
    on progesterone receptor production, 156, 159–161, 163–164
    on prolactin secretion, 291
    on secreted 52 K protein, 251–254
  formation of, 193–200, 204
  isomerization of, 81–83
  metabolism of, 173
  potency of, 165
  in prolactin synthesis assay, 30–31, 35
  radiolabeled, 74–75
  structure of, 29, 153, 288
Hyperplasia, cellular, 69–71, 116–119
Hypertrophy, cellular, 69–71, 116–119
Hypophysectomy, 304, 311, 418–420, 423–427, 441, 490

ICI 46,474. *See* Tamoxifen
ICI 47,699, 34, 516
  binding to antiestrogen binding site, 109
  binding to estrogen receptor, 184
  effect on progesterone receptor production, 162
  effect on prolactin synthesis, 32
  structure of, 33, 153
ICI 77,949. *See also* Tamoxifen: metabolite E
  effect on progesterone receptor production, 157, 159, 162
  potency of, 165
  structure of, 153
Imaging agent, for breast tumor, 83–84
2-Iminothiolane, 139–140
Immunocytochemical assay of estrogen receptor (ER-ICA), 313–314, 359, 368–369, 506
  clinical applications of, 313–320
Immunohistochemical assay
  of estrogen receptor, 313
  of p29, 382, 386–391
Immunoradiometric assay (IRMA)
  of estrogen receptor, 366–367
  of p29, 381–386, 390–391
  of progesterone receptor B protein, 398–399

Inhibitor, cytosol. *See* Cytosol inhibitor
Insulin-like growth factor I, 241–242
Intestine, antiestrogen binding sites in, 97
IRMA. *See* Immunoradiometric assay
Isoflavones, 24–25

Keoxifene, 29–30, 517
    effect on carcinogen-induced mammary
        cancer, 289
    structure of, 288
Kepone, 27
7-Ketocholesterol, 180
Ketohydroxy estrin, 20–21
1-Keto-1,2,3,4, tetrahydrophenanthrene,
    20–21
Kidney
    antiestrogen binding sites in, 97, 130–
        131
    concentration of estradiol by, 5

LDL. *See* Low density lipoproteins
Leukovorin therapy, 439, 466–467
LH. *See* Luteinizing hormone
Lignocaine, 101
Liver
    antiestrogen binding site inhibitory activ-
        ity in, 180
    antiestrogen binding sites in, 97–98,
        101–103, 110, 130–134, 177–180,
        186
    antiestrogens in, 174–182
    chick, 172, 174–182
    concentration of estradiol by, 5
    cytosol inhibitor in, 65, 68, 70
    estrogen receptor in, 186
    tamoxifen metabolism in, 195, 197–198
    triphenylethylene binding sites in, 119–
        124
LN 1643, 207–209, 212
LN 2839, 209, 212
Low density lipoproteins (LDL), 180
    triphenylethylene binding sites and,
        120–124
Ludwig Breast Cancer Study, 459–467
    Trial I, 460–462
    Trial II, 463–464
    Trial III, 464–466
    Trial IV, 465–466
    Trial V, 466–467

Lung, antiestrogen binding sites in, 97,
    130–131
Luteinizing hormone (LH), 509, 511–513
LY 117018, 30, 100, 517
    binding to antiestrogen binding site, 102,
        134–135
    binding to estrogen receptor, 134–135,
        275
    cell cycle effects of, 275
    effect on progesterone receptor produc-
        tion, 156, 159–161, 163
    structure of, 153
LY 156758. *See* Keoxifene

MAB. *See* Monoclonal antibodies
Macromolecular perturbation theory, Bel-
    leau's, 34–35
Malignant tissue, cytosol inhibitor in, 63–
    65
Mammary gland, cytosol inhibitor in, 63–
    65, 68–69
Mammary tumor. *See also* Breast cancer
    cytosol inhibitor in, 63–65, 68–69
    progesterone receptor in, 156
Mastectomy, 464, 465, 485
    antihormone therapy adjuvant to, 451–
        456
MCF-7 cells
    antiestrogen binding sites in, 98, 101–
        105, 131–133, 136
    cell cycle effects of antiestrogens in,
        265–278
    defined medium for, 241
    effect of antiestrogens on, 129–130
    epidermal growth factor receptor in,
        503–505
    estrogen receptor in, 81, 133, 137–144,
        343, 365–370, 503
        purification of, 361
    estrogen-regulated mRNA in, 251–256
    glucocorticoid receptor in, 503
    growth in athymic mice, 292–294, 510–
        511
    growth pattern of, 240
    insulin-like growth factor in, 241–242
    monoclonal antibodies to secreted pro-
        teins, 244–245
    p29 in, 380, 382
    progesterone receptor in, 157–159, 404–
        407, 503, 510

MCF-7 cells (*continued*)
  secreted 52 K protein of, 250–254
  synchronization of, 240
  tamoxifen metabolism in, 198
  tamoxifen-resistant, 109
  transforming growth factors in, 242–243
MDA-MB-134 cells
  antiestrogen binding sites in, 98
  cell cycle effects of tamoxifen in, 272–274
MDA-MB-231 cells
  antiestrogen binding sites in, 98, 131–132
  cell cycle effects of tamoxifen in, 272–274
  effect of antiestrogens on, 129–130
  epidermal growth factor receptor in, 503–505
  estrogen receptor in, 503
  glucocorticoid receptor in, 503
  insulin-like growth factor in, 241–242
  monoclonal antibodies to secreted proteins, 245
  progesterone receptor in, 503
MDA-MB-330 cells
  antiestrogen binding sites in, 98
  cell cycle effects of tamoxifen in, 272–274
MDA-MB-361 cells
  antiestrogen binding sites in, 98
  cell cycle effects of tamoxifen in, 272–274
Medroxyprogesterone acetate therapy, 348
Menstrual cycle, effect of chemotherapy on, 509, 512
MER 25, 28, 154
  structure of, 153
Messenger RNA (mRNA), estrogen-regulated
  effect of antiestrogens on, 251–260
  synthesis of, 239
Mestranol, 23–25
Metastasis, of breast cancer, 335–336, 347–348, 488–490, 494–495
Methotrexate therapy, 432, 434–442, 460–467, 488, 512–515
Methoxychlor, 27–28
3-Methylcholanthrene, structure of, 285
3-Methylcholanthrene-induced mammary cancer, 285

Microsomes, antiestrogen binding sites in, 95–111, 133–134, 179
Mitogen, autocrine, 255–261
Mitotic index, of breast cancer specimen, 329–330
Monkey, tamoxifen metabolism in, 197
Monoclonal antibodies (MAB)
  to estrogen receptor, 312–314, 363–370, 378, 505–508
  to progesterone receptor, 383, 395–411
    A subunit, 410
    B subunit, 397–411
  to proteins secreted by breast cancer cells, 244–245
Monohydroxytamoxifen. *See* 4-Hydroxytamoxifen
Monophenol, 27
Mouse
  athymic, 508–511
    transplantation of breast tumor to, 292–294
  tamoxifen metabolism in, 195
MRL 41. *See* Clomiphene
mRNA. *See* Messenger RNA
Muscle, antiestrogen binding sites in, 103, 130–131
Myometrium
  estradiol receptor in, 374–392
  p29 in, 382

NADPH-cytochrome c reductase, 222
Nafoxidine, 28–30
  binding to antiestrogen binding site, 177–178
  binding to estrogen receptor, 7, 184
  effect
    on breast cancer tissue, 305–306
    on DMBA-induced mammary cancer, 289
    on estrogen receptor, 117
    on liver, 174
    on progesterone receptor production, 154, 156, 158
  inhibition of nuclear type II sites, 56
  structure of, 29, 153, 288
National Surgical Adjuvant Breast and Bowel Project (NSABP)
  protocol B-09, 471–482
  protocol B-14, 281

5-Nitro-2-furaldehyde-induced mammary
cancer, 286
5-Nitro-2-furaldehyde semicarbazone,
structure of, 285
Nitromiphene. *See* CI 628
N-Nitrosobutylurea, structure of, 285
N-Nitrosobutylurea-induced mammary can-
cer, 286
N-Nitrosomethylurea (NMU), structure of,
285
N-Nitrosomethylurea (NMU)-induced
mammary cancer, 287, 289
NMU. *See* N-Nitrosomethylurea
Nolvadex. *See* Tamoxifen
Nolvadex Adjuvant Trial Organization
Study, 453–456
Nottingham-Tenovus breast cancer study,
326–338
NSABP. *See* National Surgical Adjuvant
Breast and Bowel Project
Nuclear type II site, 56
inhibitor of, 56–71. *See also* Cytosol in-
hibitor
Nucleic acids, synthesis of, regulation by
growth factors, 239
Nucleoplast
estrogen receptor in, 48–52
preparation of, 45–47
Nucleus
estrogen binding sites in, 56–71
estrogen receptor in. *See* Estrogen recep-
tor: nuclear

Oophorectomy, 304, 311, 418–419, 427,
440–441, 460–464, 486, 489–490,
494, 509
Ovalbumin, 182–183
Ovary, antiestrogen binding sites in, 97,
130–131
Oviduct
antiestrogen binding sites in, 185–186
chick, 172–173, 182–186, 395–411
estrogen receptor in, 186
progesterone receptor in, 395–411
tamoxifen metabolism in, 198
12-Oxo-9(11)-dehydroestradiol, 85–86
Oxonitromiphene, 211

p29, 379–383
in breast tumor, 383–391

p29 (*continued*)
immunoassay of, 382–386
immunohistochemical studies of, 382,
386–391
tissue distribution of, 382, 386
L-PAM. *See* L-Phenylalanine mustard
Perphenazine, 291
Pesticides, 27–28
PF regimen, 471–482
PFT regimen, 471–472
L-Phenylalanine mustard (L-PAM) therapy,
471–482
Photofluorogenic estrogen, 85–87
Phytoestrogens, 23–27, 514
Pituitary factors, 285–287, 419–420, 426,
492
Polyclonal antibodies
to estrogen receptor, 362–363, 377–378
to progesterone receptor, 362, 397
Polysaccharide, sulfated, 8–9, 11
Postoperative adjuvant therapy, 441–445
Prednisone therapy, 432, 435–439, 443,
460–466, 486, 488, 493–494, 512–
515
Procaine, 101
Progesterone, 56, 69
metabolism of, 517–518
with tamoxifen, 183–184
Progesterone receptor, 151–165, 250, 260,
312, 503
antibodies to
monoclonal, 383, 395–411
polyclonal, 362, 397
in antiestrogen-resistant cells, 257–259
assay of, 348–351, 395–411
sequential, 349–351
simultaneous, 349
A subunit of, 410
in breast cancer, 311, 341–351, 396,
404–408, 411, 418, 477, 491
B subunit of
in breast cancer, 404–408
compared to non-hormone-binding antigenic protein, 402–411
monoclonal antibodies to, 397–411
effect of tamoxifen on, 250, 257–259
human, 395–411
induction of, 153–154
loss of, 350–351
non-hormone-binding subunit of, 402–
408

Progesterone receptor (*continued*)
  oviduct, 395–411
  phosphorylated, 409
  posttranslational modification of, 409
  regulation by antiestrogens, 154–165
  structure of, 397–398
  subcellular distribution of, 502
Progestin receptor. *See* Progesterone receptor
Progestin therapy, 420–422, 438, 491
Prolactin, 509, 513
  gene for, 13
  secretion of, effect of antiestrogens on, 291
  synthesis of, 25–26
Prolactin synthesis assay, for estrogens and antiestrogens, 30–31
Propranolol, 101–102
Proteins
  estrogen-regulated, 249–261
  secreted. *See* Secreted 52 K protein; Secreted 160 K protein
  secreted by breast cancer cells, 237–245

R 23908, 518
R27 cells, 254–259
R5020, 397, 399, 402
Rabbit, progesterone receptor in, 154–155
Rat
  progesterone receptor in, 156
  tamoxifen metabolism in, 196
Receptors. *See* specific receptors
5-α-Reductase, 226
RNA polymerase, 117, 254
RTx6 cells, 254–259
RU 38486, 517–518
  structure of, 518

*p*SAP. *See p*-Secondary amyl phenol
p-Secondary amyl phenol (*p*SAP), 8–9
Secreted 52 K protein, 250, 255–260
  in antiestrogen-resistant cells, 257–259
  regulation by antiestrogens, 250–254
Secreted 160 K protein, 260
  in antiestrogen-resistant cells, 257–259
Serum
  antiestrogen binding site inhibitory activity in, 180–182
  antiestrogen binding sites in, 186
  antiestrogen metabolism in, 214

Serum (*continued*)
  triphenylethylene binding sites in, 120–124
SKF-525A, 101–102, 109, 201–202
Somatomedin C. *See* Insulin-like growth factor I
S phase, 269, 273, 275, 277
Spleen
  antiestrogen binding sites in, 97, 130–131
  cytosol inhibitor in, 70
Steroid biosynthesis, effect of aminoglutethimide on, 518
Stomach, antiestrogen binding sites in, 97
Suicide inhibitor, 224
Surgery, 484–486, 494
  minimal, 494

T47D cells
  antiestrogen binding sites in, 98, 131–132
  in athymic mice, 294
  cell cycle effects of tamoxifen in, 272–274, 277
  effect of antiestrogens on, 129–130
  epidermal growth factor receptor in, 503–505
  estrogen receptor in, 503
  glucocorticoid receptor in, 503
  progesterone receptor in, 154, 397, 503
TABS. *See* Triphenylethylene binding site
TACE. *See* Trianisylchloroethylene
Tamoxifen, 28–31, 94
  agonistic action of, 182–183, 491–492
  antagonistic action of, 182–183
  antitumor effects of, 226–228
  binding to antiestrogen binding site, 98–111, 134–135, 178, 185, 275
  binding to estrogen receptor, 7, 134–135, 175–177, 184, 275
  conjugates of, 196–197
  cytotoxicity of, 269–270, 273
  effect of
    on breast cancer cells, 129–131
    on cell cycle, 265–268, 275–278
    on DMBA-induced mammary cancer, 287–290
    on estrogen-regulated mRNA, 257–259
    on estrogen synthesis, 291
    on gonadotrophin release, 291

Tamoxifen (*continued*)
on liver, 174–177
on MCF-7 cells in athymic mice, 293–294
on metabolism of other drugs, 201–202
on NMU-induced mammary cancer, 289
on progesterone receptor production, 156–161, 163, 250, 257–259
on prolactin synthesis, 32, 291
on proteins secreted by breast cancer cells, 257–259
on secreted 52 K protein, 251–254
fluorescent phenanthrene derivatives of, 204–207
with glucocorticoids, 183–184
half-life of, 200
metabolism of, 75–77, 110, 136, 173, 193–195, 213–215, 515–516
analytical measurement of metabolites, 204–207
by animals *in vivo*, 195–197
biological properties of metabolites, 202–204
in humans, 198–201
in vitro, 197–198
metabolite A, 194
metabolite B. *See* 4-Hydroxytamoxifen
metabolite C, 197
metabolite D, 193, 197, 203, 213
metabolite E, 102, 193–194, 197, 203, 206, 214, 516
metabolite F, 198
metabolite X. *See* N-Desmethyl-tamoxifen
metabolite Y, 193, 195, 200, 203, 206, 213, 443, 516
metabolite Z, 193, 195, 200–201, 203, 213
potency of, 165
with progesterone, 183–184
radiolabeled, 74–75
structure of, 29, 33, 153, 288
Tamoxifen aziridine, 80–81, 140–142, 144
radiolabeled, 74–75
Tamoxifen N-oxide, 193, 195, 197, 204
Tamoxifen-resistant cells, 255–259
Tamoxifen therapy, 195, 198–201, 288, 319, 421–423, 439, 464–466, 483–495

Tamoxifen therapy (*continued*)
adjuvant, 443–444, 453–456, 471–482
androgen therapy and, 424–425
chemotherapy and, 424–425, 438, 511, 514–515
chronic administration, 199–201
development of drug-resistant cells during, 259–260
duration of, 488
endocrine effects of, 509–513
with estrogen reversal, 438–439
failure of, 512–519
hormonal therapy and, 490–491
with hypophysectomy, 423–425
patient age and, 471–482
in prevention of breast cancer, 492–493
resistance to, 515–519
side effects of, 478–481, 493
single dose, 198–199
Testosterone therapy, 222–223, 432
Tetracaine, 8–11, 15, 101–102
2-Tetrahydronaphthol (THN), 8–9
ThioTEPA therapy, 432
THN. *See* 2-Tetrahydronaphthol
Thymidine kinase, 239
Thymidine-labeling index, of breast cancer, 329–330
Transforming growth factor, 241–243
Trianisylchloroethylene (TACE), 23
effect on progesterone receptor production, 154
structure of, 153
Tricin, 24–25
Trioxifene, 29–30
effect on NMU-induced mammary cancer, 289
effect on progesterone receptor production, 156
structure of, 288
Triphenylchloroethylene, 23
Triphenylethylene, 23, 28
Triphenylethylene binding site (TABS), 119–120
endogenous ligand for, 123–125
low density lipoproteins and, 120–124
Tumorectomy, 484
Two-step model of receptor action, 44

U 11,100. *See* Nafoxidine
U 23,469
binding to antiestrogen binding site, 102

U 23,469 (*continued*)
binding to estrogen receptor, 184
effect on progesterone receptor production, 159
metabolism of, 75–79, 136, 208–209, 211–212, 214
radiolabeled, 74–75
structure of, 153
U 23,469M, 75–76, 165, 209, 212
Uterine cell culture, progesterone receptor, in 159–164
Uterus
abnormal bleeding from, 491–492
antiestrogen binding sites in, 97–98, 102, 130–131
concentration of estradiol by, 5
cytosol inhibitor in, 56–71
estrogen binding sites in, 56–71
estrogen receptor in, 307–308, 369
priming of, 153–154
progesterone receptor in, 404–407
tamoxifen metabolism in, 195–196
triphenylethylene binding sites in, 119–122

Vagina
concentration of estradiol by, 5
cornification of, 23, 491–492

Very low density lipoproteins (VLDL), 172, 174
Vincristine therapy, 432, 434–435, 439
Vitellogenin, 174–175
VLDL. *See* Very low density lipoproteins

Western blot analysis, of progesterone receptor B protein, 398–401

ZR-75 cells
estrogen receptor in, 137
p29 in, 382
ZR-75-1 cells
antiestrogen binding sites in, 98
cell cycle effects of tamoxifen in, 272–274
monoclonal antibodies to secreted proteins, 244–245
progesterone receptor in, 158
Zuclomiphene, 34
binding to antiestrogen binding site, 109
binding to estrogen receptor, 184
effect on progesterone receptor production, 154
effect on prolactin synthesis, 32
structure of, 33

DESIGNED BY HERBERT JOHNSON
COMPOSED BY GRAPHIC COMPOSITION, INC., ATHENS, GEORGIA
MANUFACTURED BY FAIRFIELD GRAPHICS, FAIRFIELD, PENNSYLVANIA
TEXT AND DISPLAY LINES ARE SET IN TIMES ROMAN

Library of Congress Cataloging-in-Publication Data
Estrogen/antiestrogen action and breast cancer.
Proceedings of a satellite symposium entitled
"Estrogen and antiestrogen action: basic and clinical
aspects" held at the Wisconsin Clinical Cancer Center,
Madison, in June 1984 in conjunction with the 7th
International Congress of Endocrinology and sponsored
by Imperial Chemical Industries and others.
Includes bibliographies and index.
1. Breast—Cancer—Chemotherapy—Congresses.
2. Breast—Cancer—Endocrine aspects—Congresses.
3. Estrogen—Therapeutic use—Congresses.   4. Estrogen—
Antagonists—Therapeutic use—Congresses.   5. Estrogen
—Receptors—Congresses. I. Jordan, V. Craig (Virgil
Craig)   II. International Congress of Endocrinology
(7th:1984:Québec, Québec)   III. Imperial Chemical
Industries, ltd. [DNLM: 1. Breast Neoplasms—drug
therapy—congresses.   2. Estrogen Antagonists—
therapeutic use—congresses.   3. Estrogens—
therapeutic use—congresses.   WP 870 E79 1984]
RC280.B8E7   1986   616.99'449061   85-40763
ISBN 0-299-10480-X